ATI NURSEN...

Medical–Surgical *E. Cunha*
Core Content At-A-Glance

Includes "Study and Memory Aids"

Edited by:
Sally Lambert Lagerquist, RN, MS

Authors:
Christine Hooper, RN, EdD

Robyn M. Nelson, RN, DNSc

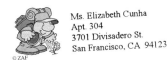

E. Cunha

ATI NurseNotes
Medical–Surgical
Core Content At-A-Glance

Edited by:
Sally Lambert Lagerquist, RN, MS

Former Instructor in Undergraduate and Graduate Programs
and Continuing Education in Nursing
University of California, San Francisco, School of Nursing
President, Review for Nurses, Inc., and RN Tapes Company
San Francisco, California

Contributing Authors:
Christine Hooper, RN, EdD

Associate Professor
San Jose State University
San Jose, California

Robyn M. Nelson, RN, DNSc

Dean, College of Health and Human Services
Touro University, Nevada

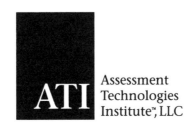

Assessment
Technologies
Institute™, LLC

Acquisitions Editor: Bob Cole
Assistant Editor: Bonnie Bergstrom
Project Editor: Sally Volkoff
Production Manager: Don Walde
Programmer: Trevor Gunter
Art Director: Hara Allison
Graphic Design-Illustrators: Allen Croswhite and Eric Osterback
Design Production: Cheryl Appel
Indexer: Laura Steen

Library of Congress Cataloging-in-Publications Data

NurseNotes: Medical–Surgical/Hooper, Christine; Nelson, Robyn M.; edited by Sally Lambert Lagerquist.
p.cm.
Includes bibliographical references and index.
ISBN 0-9760063-1-6
1. Medical–Surgical Nursing—Outlines, syllabi, etc. 2. Medical–Surgical Nursing—Examinations, questions, etc. I. Hooper, Christine. II. Lagerquist, Sally L. III. Title.
[DNLM: 1. Medical–Surgical Nursing—examination questions. 2. Medical–Surgical Nursing—outlines. WY 18.2 C718n 1997]
RT52.N45 2006
610.73'076–dc20
DNLM/DLC
for Library of Congress   96-20788
                                                                 CIP

Care has been taken to confirm the accuracy of the information presented and to describe generally accepted practices. However, the authors, editors, and publisher are not responsible for errors or omissions or for any consequences from application of the information in this book and make no warranty, express or implied, with respect to the contents of the publication.

The authors, editor and publisher have exerted every effort to ensure that drug selection and dosage set forth in this text are in accordance with current recommendations and practice at the time of publication. However, in view of ongoing research, changes in government regulations, and the constant flow of information relating to drug therapy and drug reactions, the reader is urged to check the package insert for each drug for any change in indications and dosage and for added warnings and precautions. This is particularly important when the recommended agent is a new or infrequently employed drug.

Some drugs and medical devices presented in this publication have Food and Drug Administration (FDA) clearance for limited use in restricted research settings. It is the responsibility of the health care provider to ascertain the FDA status of each drug or device planned for use in their clinical practice.

Last digit indicates print number   9   8   7   6   5   4   3   2   1

Dedications

For everything there is a *season*, a *time*, a *purpose* . . .

To my husband, Tom
I wish this "year of the 7 books" to become an everlasting *season* of celebrating health and joyfulness, and reaping the benefits of all that overload that we shared side-by-side.

Your gentle, nurturing ways,
    Your quiet strength
        Your remarkable humor
            provided all the love and support
                I've needed these 40 years together.
                    L'chaim!

It is our *time* . . .

    To reap what we have "planted"
    To laugh contagiously
    To dance spontaneously
    To follow our dreams of "if only we had time..."
    To reflect joyously on all that we have accomplished in 40 years!

May our *purpose* be to discover all the best that life's about.
    With your gift of enthusiasm and many capabilities,
    We can turn challenges into opportunities (lemons → lemonade).
As we start our "trips" to somewhere new,
    I look with hope and pride in you.

To our daughter, Elana
    I am grateful for your sensitivity, all the special things you've done for our family, and all the "firsts" that we've shared (e.g. parenthood).
    You've been someone on whom I know I can depend, someone kind who will help anyway that you can.
    We are grateful to you and Dan for our first very special granddaughter, Kaya. She brings such joy to our life with her own brand of humor and incredible verbal and conceptual abilities.

To our son, Kalen
    May you always continue...to see life as an adventure...to have time to reminisce...to savor new experiences...to bring joy into our lives as your family.
    We continue with our hearts full of pride in your professional and personal accomplishments. Your multi–task abilities are amazing!

                                                                    Sally

This book is dedicated to all who aspire to become nurses; may you continue to grow as professionals in knowledge, compassion and caring. I hope this book makes your journey a little better.

And, to my husband and son, who put up with a lot—I couldn't grow as a professional without you.

Christine Hooper

To borrow from a very powerful phrase..."it takes a village to raise a child"—thus it takes a family to produce a book. Thank you to my husband Dean for enduring yet one more publishing project; to my mother Patty for providing the copy machine; to my daughter Kelly for being a sounding board and daughter Tina for exemplifying what patients value in a nurse; and to Sage and Stirling, my precious grandsons, for always loving their "Gammie". A special thank you to those who have chosen nursing...it takes many books to prepare for the NCLEX...thanks for choosing one of the best.

Robyn Nelson

Contributing Author to Previous Edition

Janice Horman Stecchi, RN, EdD
Dean Emerita, College of Health Professions
University of Massachusetts–Lowell
Lowell, Massachusetts

Acknowledgements

A special tribute to Sally Volkoff, who took on the herculean task of being the authors' own special project coordinator in developing this and five other exam prep books for publication—from conception to completion!

Even with all the stops, starts, spurts and changes ("add this," "replace that," "move this," "find that"), she delivered this manuscript with smiles that increased her face value!

A big thank you to Don Walde and Angie Rothrock at ATI and to Hara Alison, Cheryl Appel, Allen Croswhite, Eric Osterback, and Molly Obetz at Element Media Productions for being remarkably accommodating to my need for "perfection," and for being willing to put in that extra effort to make this complex book stand out from all the rest in the field.

Sally L. Lagerquist

Foreword

It is a pleasure to endorse resources for students and faculty that really work!

Faculty now has an important role in assisting the student in condensing and organizing the essential knowledge that can be translated into competent and safe nursing practice. With the exploding amount of knowledge in nursing and health care, students are often frustrated because they need to know so much. They ask questions from faculty like, "what is on the test?" and "what do I need to know?" The *ATI NurseNotes* are an incredibly easy synthesis of critical material that students need to master. Using the *NurseNotes* series along with the major nursing textbooks enhances students' comprehension of complex concepts and their application to clinical practice. The feedback from students themselves has been very positive. They comment that the *NurseNotes* save them time as they learn and review core content because concepts are graphically presented, chapters are short (yet comprehensive), with summaries and test questions at the end of each chapter to identify their problem areas.

The faculty finds that the *NurseNotes* series helps to organize their own presentations of material to students in a way that helps elevate the students' mastery of core content.

John M. Lantz, RN, PhD
Dean and Professor
School of Nursing
University of San Francisco
2130 Fulton Street
San Francisco, CA 94117

Sally Higgins, RN, PhD, FAAN
Professor and Chair of the Department of Family Health
University of San Francisco
2130 Fulton Street
San Francisco, CA 94117

"I am writing to acknowledge the high value of your book: *NurseNotes: Medical-Surgical Nursing.*

I use the book to supplement our textbook in the instruction of adult nursing therapeutics. The book is written in very concise language, very well indexed, and summarizes the most important points, which greatly assists nursing students in their focused study. The greatest value of the book is the effect it has helping students to bridge the transition between memorization of facts and the application of critical elements of nursing therapeutics.

(continued on next page)

I am the faculty of record for the Therapeutics II course at University of San Francisco (taken in the junior I semester). This course is extremely difficult as the course is designed and taught to move students' thinking from knowing THE WHAT, to knowing the SO WHAT(implications), the WHEN (the critical thinking about conditions and context), and the WHY (rationale). Your book is extremely beneficial in this pedagogical task as students apply clinical reasoning to plan, implement, and evaluate therapeutic care for acutely ill adults.

Our student body is very diverse, and therefore for many students in our program, English is a second language. The concise writing style and the effective organization promotes success for ALL our students, but most importantly, those students struggling with the English language and medical terminology report that the *NurseNotes* book is invaluable to them.

I hope your valuable resource will continue to be published as I intend to use it in future semesters."

Dr. Gregory A. DeBourgh,
Associate Professor & Chair,
Department of Adult Health
University of San Francisco
2130 Fulton Street
San Francisco, CA 94117-1080

Preface

There are numerous outstanding, comprehensive medical–surgical textbooks on the market today–some over 2000 pages long! Nursing students preparing for professional nursing practice must understand the "art and science" of nursing—the theory and techniques—that can be covered thoroughly only in a textbook. However, students frequently ask for help to *focus* their studying and preparation before caring for clients in the clinical setting. Review books used to prepare for the nursing licensure examination, particularly *Davis's NCLEX-RN® Success*, have successfully condensed the world of nusing practice in all clinical areas, but several trends in nursing have led to the need to provide students with condensed review material specific to just one clinical area at a time for use as they rotate from one area to another.

What's New In This Edition

Extensive new content has been added in the areas of: **cultural and ethnic** variations in assessment, nutrition, and pain management; the impact of **lifestyle choices** on health; assessment, nursing care, and medication use by the **elderly; infection control** and standard precautions; **alternative and complementary therapies; herbal** medications; and **bioterrorism.** In addition, new disease conditions have been added, including **Raynaud's Phenomenon, Syndrome of Inappropriate Antidiuretic Hormone,** and **Multi-Organ Dysfunction Sydrome.**

    Eleven new tables were added including: *immunization* guidelines for adults and the elderly; comparison of *acute and chronic pain*; assessment and care of *venous and arterial ulcers*, a summary of current guidelines for *isolation precautions* in health facilities; and common *herb/drug interactions*.

Intended Audience

ATI's NurseNotes: Medical–Surgical: Core Content At–A–Glance is particularly useful to students in nursing programs who spend the greatest amount of clinical time in medical–surgical settings, including acute care and long–term care. The book concisely presents selected clinical disorders for each body system within the nursing process framework. A brief overview of the *pathophysiologic* basis for each disorder is followed by *risk factors, objective* and *subjective* physical assessment and findings, NANDA– approved *nursing diagnoses,* current approaches to *nursing care,* and criteria to determine achievement of desired client *outcomes.* Common *pharmacologic* therapies, recommended *diets,* and *diagnostic procedures* are integrated with the dicussion of the clinical disorder. Students no longer have to refer to separate chapters for this information.

    Although the NCLEX® tests knowledge of all clinical areas, a major focus of the exam is physiologic integrity and safe and effective nursing care. A student may feel the need to review only medical–surgical nursing care in preparation for the test. *ATI's*

NurseNotes: Medical–Surgical may also be helpful to nurses facing work transformation or job redesign who must move to a new clinical unit, or prepare for certification exams.

Features

Special added features include end-of-chapter *Study and Memory Aids* ☼, *Summary of Key Points* 🗝, and **questions and answers** covering the steps of the nursing process, categories of human function and client needs/subneeds with fact-packed *rationale*. Also included is a disk containing additional questions with answers and rationale. The questions follow the NCLEX® test plan.

Unique to this book are visual features that include numerous text figures (30), easy-to-read charts (92), shaded boxes for emphasis, and special symbols to highlight phases of the nursing process ⧑, hands-on nursing care ☞, diagnostic tests and procedures ⧓, laboratory data, shaded boxes, and medications ⬤, diets 🍎; *standard precautions* ▲, *hazard/danger* ⚡; *positions*, and *tubes* appear in *italics*. **Health teaching** 📖 sections stand out in bold face.

How to Benefit from this Book

The extensive *appendices* should be very useful in providing even more study and review material under one cover. They include over 300 need-to-know common *acronyms* and *abbreviations*; review of *nutrition* and **pharmacology** (over 300 drugs are reviewed); *indices* to quickly locate 60 *diets*, 105 common **diagnostic studies** and **procedures**, **lab data**, 25 common **tubes**, a checklist of over 100 need-to-know **hands–on nursing treatment/care**, 40 examples of *positioning* of the client, and questions and answers related to the steps of the nursing process as well as 4 client needs and 6 client subneeds, and 8 categories of human function; an index to 28 *mnemonics/memory aids* for various conditions; quick guide to 25 *common clinical signs; home health care* situations; NCLEX–RN® test plan; and health and welfare agencies and resources for client education.

Preparation of care plans and test review will be easier with this clinically focused book. The author and editor of this book have brought together over 60 years of their combined clinical expertise and nursing education experience to assist the nursing student , new graduate, re-entry nurse, or international graduate in achieving theoretical and clinical competence in the care of medical–surgical clients as easily as possible.

Sally Lambert Lagerquist, RN, MS
Editor, *ATI's NurseNotes series*

Christine Hooper, RN, EdD
Robyn M. Nelson, RN, DNSc
Authors of *ATI's NurseNotes: Medical–Surgical*

How to Use the ATI NurseNotes Series

The *ATI NurseNotes* series was written to lower students' stress while increasing mastery of essential subjects (i.e. core content), by presenting concise information in a visual way to enable an at-a-glance approach to increasing understanding and retention.

Students can use this series as a basis for doing care plans (care maps) at the *beginning* of and *throughout* a course, as well as an *end–point* review for the course exam.

Steps To the Most Effective Use of This book By Students

❖ Quickly glance at the *outline* at the start of each chapter to see what topics/conditions will be covered.

❖ Look over the outline format that is used, noting that there is a brief *description*, followed by concisely worded *pathophysiology* paragraph and a list of relevant *risk factors/causes*.

❖ Spend significant time going over: 1) the *assessment* section, especially noting how *subjective data* is differentiated from *objective*; 2) diagnostic tests/procedures and any related lab data. Note that the symbol in the margins ⌇, quickly identifies diagnostic tests.

❖ Briefly glance at the *nursing diagnosis*, which can relate to pathophysiology, with implications for nursing interventions.

❖ Spend the most concentrated time in the section: *nursing plan* (i.e., the general goals)/*implementation* (i.e., specific interventions). Pay special attention to *diets* 🍎, *positioning, hands-on care aspects* ☞, *medications* ⬤, *infection control situations* ▲, and *health teaching* 🎓.

❖ Next, study all the information in table format, the words and phrases that are in **boldface** (very important) and *italic* type as well as boxed content and shaded areas. These visual cues are time-savers for the reader because they serve the same purpose as when students spend time doing their own highlighting and underlining for emphasis. These visual cues allow for faster learning!

❖ Carefully read the **summaries** of key points 🔑 at the end of each chapter to check what you understood and retained as the key points when you read through the chapter. Also, look at the end of each chapter for a synthesis of need-to-remember diets, drugs and diagnostic tests/procedures.

❖ Now take the *test questions* at the end of each chapter. Read the rationale not only for the best answer, but also the rationale for all the other options. Determine your percentage correct; if it was less than 85% correct (this is a higher benchmark than you'd expect to find on the licensure exam), then we suggest that you re-read that chapter.

❖ When you have completed all the chapters in the book for an end-point review, be sure to go through the content-packed **appendices**. The indices there can also lead you to pages where specific content (e.g. diets) and specific questions (e.g. safety and infection control) are located in the book. For example, this means that you can go through the book and do a review of all the diets; then you can go through the book and do a review of all the tubes or positioning etc.

❖ Follow this approach before you use the additional 275 questions on the *CD* in each book as your final "test and assess."

Suggestions for Instructor's Use of the Books in the ATI NurseNotes Series

While these books offer a synthesis of essential content in a condensed format, the instructor can then use lecture time to focus on expansion of content, to illustrate key concepts with clinical scenarios (to use in conjunction with *ATI Nursing Q&A: Critical Thinking Exercises* and the 75 case scenarios).

❖ These books can increase time for the focus of the instructor's lecture to be on a re-emphasis of more complex concepts (e.g. acid-base).

❖ If any clinical experience in the nursing program is reduced in scope, the instructor can select from these books certain chapters for special supplemental coverage to fill in those gaps. In that way, their lectures can be tailored to the particular needs of the nursing program.

❖ Instructors can use these books to point out major nursing care problems, to separate them from secondary ones; and to provide a *hands-on care skills assessment checklist* (see ☞ throughout the chapters), with an opportunity to learn and fill in gaps in the how-to aspects of nursing care.

❖ A focus on sections in these books that cover **assessment** data is another way the instructor can point out patterns, relationships and make appropriate inferences based on assessment data.

❖ The instructor should also call students' attention to the many appendices that provide **multiple ways** that students can use these books for self-assessment in addition to the usual end-of-chapter questions and questions on the *CD*. For example, show students how they can do a focused review of special topics (e.g. use the index in an Appendix to locate throughout the book a review of diets, diagnostic studies/procedures, common tubes, positioning of the client.) They can also review by questions throughout the book which directly relate to the NCLEX-RN® Test Plan (e.g. by client needs/subneeds), by nursing process steps; and by level of complexity of questions (from basic knowledge/comprehension to application and analysis.)

❖ These books can help *new* instructors to zero-in on core content, and can give *experienced* lecturers more time to focus on clinically-based anecdotal illustrations.

Contents

Appendixes

List Of Illustrations

List of Tables

Nursing Assessment of the Adult

Assessment, Analysis, and Nursing Diagnosis of the Adult

Assessment is the process of gathering a comprehensive database about the client's present, past, and potential health problems, as well as a description of the client as a whole in the context of his or her environment. It includes a comprehensive nursing history, a physical examination, and laboratory/x-ray data, and it concludes with the formulation of nursing diagnoses. In the following units, possible nursing diagnoses are listed under each disorder.

Subjective Data

Nursing History

The nursing history obtains data for the planning and implementation of nursing actions.

I. **General information**: reason for admission; duration of present illness; previous hospitalization; history of illnesses; diagnostic procedures prior to admission; allergies—type and severity of reactions; medications taken at home—over-the-counter, prescription, and herbal remedies.

II. **Information relative to growth and development**: age; menarche—age at onset; heavy menses; dysmenorrhea; vaginal discharge; date of last Papanicolaou smear; pregnancies; abortions; miscarriages.

III. **Information relative to psychosocial functions**: feelings (anger, denial, fear, anxiety, guilt, lifestyle changes); language barriers; family support; spiritual needs; history of trauma/rape.

IV. **Information relative to nutrition**: appetite—normal, changes; dietary habits; food preferences or intolerances; difficulty swallowing or chewing; dentures; use of caffeine/alcohol; weight changes; excessive thirst, hunger, sweating; acid reflux or indigestion.

V. **Information relative to fluid and gas transport**: difficulty breathing; shortness of breath; history of cough/smoking; colds; sputum; swelling of extremities; chest pain; palpitations; varicosities; excessive bruising; blood transfusions; excessive bleeding.

VI. **Information relative to protective functions**: skin problems—rash, itch; current treatment; unusual hair loss.

VII. **Information relative to comfort, rest, activity, mobility**: usual activity (ADL); present ability and restrictions; rest and sleep pattern; weakness; joint or muscle stiffness, pain, or swelling; occupation; interests.

VIII. **Information relative to elimination**: bowel habits; changes—constipation, diarrhea; ostomy; emesis; nausea; voiding—retention, frequency, dysuria, incontinence.

IX. **Information relative to sensory/perceptual functions**: pain—verbal report; quality, location; precipitating factors; duration; limitations in vision (glasses), hearing, touch, smell; orientation to person, place, time; confusion; headaches; fainting; dizziness; convulsions.

Objective Data

Physical Assessment

▶ I. **Physical assessment**—requires knowledge of normal findings, organization, and keen senses, i.e., visual, auditory, touch, smell. For abnormal findings, refer to the *Assessment* section of each health problem discussed under the categories of human functioning.

FACTORS AFFECTING VITAL SIGNS

Factor	Infection (Fever)	↑ K+	↓ K+	↑ Blood Sugar (DKA)	↓ Blood Sugar (Insulin Shock)	MI (acute)
Temp.	↑	(ok)	(ok)	↑	↓	↑
Pulse	↑	↓	↑	↑	(ok) (↑)	↑
Resp.	↑	Shallow	Shallow	↑	(ok)	↑
B.P.	(ok)	(ok) (↑)	↓	↓	(ok) (↑)	↑ initially, then ↓

A. **Components**
   1. **Inspection**—uses observations to detect deviations from normal.
   2. **Auscultation**—to perceive and interpret sounds emanating from various organs, particularly heart, lungs, and bowel.
   3. **Palpation**—to assess for discomfort, temperature, pulsations, size, consistency, and texture.
   4. **Percussion**—to elicit vibrations produced by underlying organ structures; used less frequently in nursing practice.
      a. *Flat*—normal percussion sound (quiet, short) over muscle or bone.
      b. *Dull*—normal percussion sound (quiet, thudding) over organs such as liver.
      c. *Resonance*—normal percussion sound (hollow, loud) over emphysematous lungs.
      d. *Tympany*—normal percussion sound over stomach or bowel.

B. **Sequence**
   1. *General appearance*—well or poorly developed or nourished. Color (black, white, jaundiced, pale). Mobility (smooth, steady gait with full ROM of joints). Behavior (facial expression, mood, affect appropriate for situation). In distress (acute or chronic)?
   2. *Vital signs*—(see text table above) *blood pressure* (which arm or both, orthostatic change). *Pulse* (regular or irregular, orthostatic change). *Respirations* (labored or unlabored, wheeze). *Temperature* (axillary, rectal, or oral). Weight. Height.

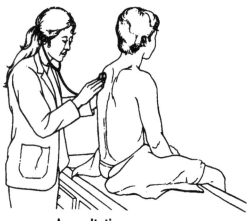

Auscultation

   3. *Skin, hair, and nails*—pigmentation, scars, lesions, bruises, turgor, moisture, texture. Describe or draw rashes.
      a. *Skin color:*
         Red—fever, allergic reaction, CO poisoning.
         Yellow—jaundice
         White (pallor)—excessive blood loss, fright.
         Blue (cyanosis)—hypoxemia, peripheral vasoconstriction.
         Mottled—cardiovascular embarrassment.
      b. *Skin temperature*:
         Hot, dry—excessive body heat (heat stroke).
         Hot, wet—reaction to increased internal or external temperature.
         Cool, dry—exposure to cold.
         Cool, clammy—shock.
      c. *Hair*:
         Color, texture, distribution.
      d. *Nails*:
         Shape, contour, consistency, color
   4. *Nodes*—any cervical, supraclavicular, axillary, epitrochlear, inguinal lymphadenopathy? If so, size of nodes (in cm), consistency (firm, rubbery, tender), mobile or fixed.
   5. *Head*—scalp, skull (configuration), scars, tenderness, bruits, headache, facial symmetry.
   6. *Eyes*:
      a. External eye: conjunctivae, sclerae, lids, cornea, pupils (including reflexes), visual fields, extraocular motions, visual acuity.
      b. Fundus: disk, blood vessels, pigmentation.
   7. *Ears*—shape of pinnae, lumps on or near ear, skin lesions around ear, external canal, tympanic membrane, acuity, air conduction versus bone conduction (**Rinne test**), lateralization (**Weber's test**), discharge.
   8. *Nose*—septum, mucosa, polyps, discharge.
   9. *Mouth and throat*—lips, teeth, tongue (size, papillation), buccal mucosa, palate, tonsils, oropharynx.

10. *Neck*—suppleness, (trachea, larynx, thyroid).
11. *Thorax and lungs*:
    a. **Inspection:** contour, symmetry, expansion.
    b. **Palpation:** expansion, rib tenderness, tactile fremitus; tracheal deviation.
    c. **Percussion:** diaphragmatic excursion, dullness, (possible hemothorax) or hyperresonance (possible pneumo-thorax).
    d. **Auscultation:** crackles, rubs, wheezes, bronchophony, egophony, pectoriloquy.
       (1) Use diaphragm. Normal breath sounds.
           (a) *Vesicular*—heard over alveoli.
           (b) *Bronchovesicular*—heard over major bronchi: posteriorly between scapulae, anteriorly around upper sternum.
              (c) *Bronchial*—heard over trachea and larynx.
       (2) *Crackles*—discontinuous noises heard on auscultation; caused by popping open of air spaces; usually associated with increased fluid in the lungs; formerly called *rales*.
       (3) *Wheezes*—high-pitched, whistling sounds made by air flowing through narrowed airways; formerly called *rhonchi*.
12. *Heart and neck vessels*:
    a. **Inspection:**
       Heart—PMI (point of maximal impulse), chest contour, heaves, or lifts.
       Neck vessels—jugular venous pulse.
    b. **Palpation:**
       Heart—apical impulse, thrills.
       Neck vessels—carotid artery pulses (be sure to palpate each carotid artery separately and avoid the carotid sinus area in upper half of neck).
    c. **Auscultation:**
       Heart—Listen in 4 valve areas: aortic, pulmonic, tricuspid, and mitral. Use *diaphragm* for *higher*-pitched sounds, and *bell* for *lower*-pitched sounds. Listen for S_1 and S_2, extra heart sounds (S_3 and S_4), murmurs, rubs, or clicks.
       Neck vessels—listen for carotid bruit.
13. *Breasts*—symmetry, retraction, lesions, nipples (inverted, everted), masses, tenderness, discharge, skin texture, color changes.
14. *Abdomen*:
    a. **Inspection:** scars (draw these), contour, masses, vein pattern.
    b. **Auscultation:** bowel sounds (normal: every 15–20 sec.), rubs, bruits. Use diaphragm. Auscultate *after* inspection and *before* palpation and percussion. Listen to each quadrant for at least 1 min. If bowel sounds are present, they will be heard in *lower right* quadrant (area of ileocecal valve).
    c. **Percussion:** organomegaly, hepatic dullness.
    d. **Palpation:** tenderness, masses, rigidity, liver, spleen, kidneys.
    e. **Hernia:** femoral, inguinal, ventral.
15. *Genitalia*:
    a. **Men:** penile lesions, scrotum, testes. Circumcised?
    b. **Women:** labia, Bartholin's and Skene's glands, vagina, cervix. Bimanual examination of internal genitalia.
16. *Rectum*—perianal lesions, sphincter tone, tenderness, masses, prostate, stool color, occult blood.
17. *Extremities*—pulses (symmetry, bruits, perfusion). Capillary refill (normal = < 3 sec.). Joints (mobility, deformity); cyanosis; varicosities; muscle mass; edema (o = none observed; +1 = < 2mm depression; +2 = 2-4 mm depression; +3 = 5-8mm depression; +4 = > 8mm)
18. *Back*—contour spine, tenderness. Sacral edema.
19. *Neurologic*:
    a. **Mental status:** alertness, memory, judgment, mood, cognition, behavior.
    b. **Cranial nerves:** (I-XII).
       (1) Olfactory—smell.
       (2) Optic—vision/visual fields.
       (3) Oculomotor—pupil reactions.
       (4) Trochlear—eyeball moves down and laterally.
       (5) Trigeminal—skin, eye, mandibular sensation.
       (6) Abducens—eyeballs move laterally.
       (7) Facial—facial expressions and taste (smile, frown, close eyes, tastes: sweet, salt, sour, bitter).
       (8) Auditory—equilibrium, hearing.
       (9) Glossopharyngeal—swallowing, gag.
       (10) Vagus—speech.
       (11) Accessory—head and shoulders.
       (12) Hypoglossal—tongue movement.
    c. **Motor:** muscle mass, strength, gait, balance, rapid alternating movements.
    d. **Sensory:** touch, pain, vibration. Heat and cold as indicated.
    e. **Reflexes:** DTRs, pathologic or primitive.

◄ II. **General assessment**—provides information on the client as a whole.
    A. *Race, sex, apparent age* in relation to stated age.

TABLE 1.1 ◄ ASSESSMENT: COMMON VARIATIONS AMONG CULTURAL AND ETHNIC GROUPS

Skin, hair, nails	In dark skinned individuals, check for: *pallor* & *cyanosis* on palms of hands, soles of feet, buccal mucosa, conjunctiva. Check for: *jaundice* in sclera of eyes, soft palate, palms of hands. Erythema can be difficult to see—palpate for warmth, swelling, tenderness.
Eyes	Note narrowed palpebral fissures characteristic of persons of Asian descent. Dark irides usually coincide with darker retinas.
Ears	Incidence of otitis media increased in Native American, Alaskan, and Canadian Inuit children. Asians, Native Americans tend to have dry, flaky cerumen. African-American, Caucasians tend to have wet cerumen.
Nose, mouth, throat	Cleft lip and cleft palate more common in Native Americans and Asians. Leukoedema and hyperpigmentation of buccal mucosa more common in African-Americans than Caucasians. Tooth decay and loss of teeth more common in Caucasians than African-Americans. Caucasians have the smallest teeth, followed by African-Americans, Asians, & Native Americans; larger teeth cause some groups to have protruding jaws.
Breasts and sexual development	African-American girls tend to develop secondary sex characteristics earlier than Caucasian girls. Incidence of breast cancer is higher in United States, Britain, and Netherlands; may correlate with high fat diets in those countries.
Thorax and lungs	Size of chest cavity decreases in order: Caucasian, African-American, Asian, Native-American; size of chest cavity affects pulmonary function.
Heart and neck vessels	Risk factors (hypertension, smoking, obesity, hyperlipidemia, diabetes) for heart disease and stroke are increased among African-Americans (see **Chapters 2, 3, &4**).
Musculoskeletal	African-Americans tend to have greater bone density and decreased incidence of osteoporosis than other populations. Most people have 24 vertebrae; some African-American women have 23, while some Inuit and Native Americans have 25.
Genitalia	Most newborn boys in the United States are circumcised. Some religious groups such as Jews and Muslims practice circumcision as part of religious value system. Prostate cancer is more common in North America and northwestern Europe; highest incidence of prostate cancer is among African-Americans.

B. *Nutritional status*—well hydrated and developed or obesity, cachexia—include weight.
  1. Assess for obesity acccording to body mass index (BMI). Formula weight/height^2
     a. BMI 25-29.9 kg/m^2=overweight
     b. BMI 30-39.9 kg/m^2=obese
     c. BMI > 40 kg/m^2=clinically severe obesity (see **Appendix B p. 384** for information about managing **obesity**)
C. *Apparent health status*—general good health or mild, moderate, severe debilitation.
D. *Posture and motor activity*—erect, symmetric, and balanced gait and muscle development or: ataxic, circumducted, scissor, or spastic gait; slumped or bent-over posture; mild, moderate, or hyperactive motor responses.
E. *Behavior*—alert; oriented to person, time, place; hears and comprehends instructions, or tense, anxious, angry; uses abusive language; slightly or largely unresponsive; delusions, hallucinations.
F. *Odors*—noncontributory, or acetone, alcohol, fetid breath, incontinent of urine or feces.

G. *Cultural and ethnic variations.* (See **Table 1.1**)
◄ **III. Health assessment of the older adult**
  A. *Skin*:
    1. Decrease in elasticity → wrinkles and lines, dryness.
    2. Loss of fullness → sagging.
    3. Wasting appearance due to generalized loss of adipose and muscle tissue.
    4. Decrease of adipose tissue on extremities, redistributed to hips and abdomen in middle age.
    5. Bony prominences become visible.
    6. Excessive pigmentation → age spots.
    7. Dry skin and deterioration of nerve fibers and sensory endings → pruritus.
    8. Pallor and blotchiness due to decreased blood flow.
    9. Overgrowth of epidermal tissue leads to lesions (some benign, some premalignant, some malignant).
    10. Decreased skin thickness → decubitus ulcers.

11. Skin breakdown (decubitus ulcers) stages:
    a. *Stage I*—intact, non-blanching erythemic area.
    b. *Stage II*—abrasion, blister or crater.
    c. *Stage III*—full-thickness crater down to, but not penetrating, the fascia.
    d. *Stage IV*—same as III, but penetrating the fascia, involving muscle, bone, tendon, joint.
12. Decreased skin vascularity → altered thermoregulation → ↑ risk for heatstroke.
13. Loss of subcutaneous tissue → decreased insulation → ↑ risk for hypothermia.

B. *Nails*:
1. Dry, brittle.
2. Increased susceptibility to fungal infections.
3. Decreased growth rate.
4. Toenails thick, difficult to cut.

C. *Hair*:
1. Loss of pigment → graying, white.
2. Decreased density of hair follicles → thinning of hair.
3. Baldness due to decreased blood flow to skin and decreased estrogen production.
    a. Hair distribution thin on scalp, axilla, pubic area, upper and lower extremities.
    b. Decreased facial hair in *men*.
4. Increased facial (chin, upper lip) hair in *women* due to decreased estrogen production.

D. *Eyes*:
1. Loss of soluble protein with loss of lens transparency → development of *cataracts*.
2. Decrease in pupil size limits amount of light entering the eye → elderly need more light to see.
3. Decreased pupil reactivity → decrease in rate of light changes to which a person can readily adapt.
4. Diminished night vision due to decreased accommodation to darkness and dim light.
5. Shrunken appearance due to loss of orbital fat.
6. Blink reflex—slowed.
7. Eyelids—loose.
8. Visual acuity—decreased.
9. Peripheral vision—diminished.
10. Visual fields—diminished.
11. Lens accommodation—decreased; requires corrective lenses.
12. *Presbyopia*—lens may lose ability to become convex enough to accommodate to nearby objects; starts at age 40 (*farsightedness*).
13. Color of iris—fades.
14. Conjunctiva—ectropion (lower lid drops away) or entropion (lower lid folds under) may occur.
15. Lacrimal apparatus—decreased tearing causes dryness and burning.
16. Increased intraocular pressure leads to *glaucoma*.
17. *Macular degeneration*—increased incidence of loss of central vision, inability to read fine print, do fine work.

E. *Ears*:
1. Changes in cochlea: decrease in average pitch of sound.
2. Hearing loss: decreased ability to hear high frequencies and consonants.
3. Tympanic membrane: atrophied, thickened, causing hearing loss.
4. *Presbycusis*—progressive loss of hearing in old age.

F. *Mouth*:
1. Dental caries.
2. Poorly fitting dentures.
3. Cancer of the mouth—increased risk.
4. Decrease in taste buds → inability to taste sweet/salty foods.
5. Olfactory bulb atrophies → decreased ability to smell.

G. *Cardiovascular*:
1. Blood pressure increased due to lack of elasticity of vessels →↑ diastolic blood pressure → increased resistance to blood flow; decreased diameter of arteries.
2. Atherosclerotic plaques → thrombosis.
3. Valves become sclerotic, less pliable → reduced filling and emptying.
4. Diastolic murmurs heard at base of heart.
5. Loss of elasticity, decreased contractility → decreased cardiac output.
6. Pumping action of the heart is reduced due to changes in the coronary arteries → pooling of blood in systemic veins and shortness of breath.
7. Dysrhythmias due to disturbance of the autonomic nervous system.
8. Extremities—pedal pulses weaker due to arteriosclerotic changes; colder extremities, mottled color.

H. *Respiratory*:
1. Efficiency reduced with age.
2. Greater residual air in lungs after expiration.
3. Decreased vital capacity.
4. Decreased capacity to cough because of weaker expiratory muscles.
5. Decreased ciliary, activity → stasis of secretions → susceptibility to infections.
6. Dyspnea on exertion (DOE) due to oxygen debt in the muscles.
7. Reduced chest wall compliance.

I. *Breasts*:
1. Atrophy.
2. Cancer risk—increased with age.

J. *Gastrointestinal*:
   1. *Pernicious anemia* due to lack of intrinsic factor.
   2. Gastric motility—decreased.
   3. Esophageal peristalsis—decreased.
   4. *Hiatal hernia*—increased incidence.
   5. Digestive enzymes—gradual decrease of ptyalin (which converts starch), pepsin and trypsin (which digest protein), lipase (fat-splitting enzyme).
   6. Absorption—decreased.
   7. Constipation due to improper diet.

K. *Endocrine*:
   1. Basal metabolism rate lowered → decreased temperature.
   2. Cold intolerance.
   3. *Women*; decreased ovarian function → increased gonadotropins.
   4. Decreased renal sensitivity to ADH → unable to concentrate urine as effectively as younger persons.
   5. Decreased clearance of blood glucose after meals → elevated postprandial blood glucose.
   6. Risk of diabetes mellitus increased with age.

L. *Urinary*:
   1. Renal function—impaired due to poor perfusion.
   2. Filtration—impaired due to reduction in number of functioning nephrons.
   3. Urgency and frequency: *men*—often due to prostatic hypertrophy; *women*—due to perineal muscle weakness.
   4. Nocturia—both men and women.
   5. Urinary tract infection—increased incidence.
   6. Incontinence—especially with dementia.
      a. *Stress*: leakage with cough, sneeze.
      b. *Overflow*: difficulty starting stream; dribbling; feeling of fullness after voiding; weak stream; small amount.
      c. *Functional*: manual or mobility impairment; meds (sedatives, hypnotics, diuretics, anticholinergics, CNS depressants) pain; depression, delirium, dementia.

M. *Musculoskeletal*:
   1. Muscle mass—decreased.
   2. Bony prominences—increased.
   3. Demineralization of bone.
   4. Shortening of trunk due to narrowing of intervertebral space.
   5. Posture—normal; some kyphosis.
   6. Range of motion—limited.
   7. *Osteoarthritis*—related to extensive physical activities and joint use.
   8. Gait—altered.
   9. *Osteoporosis* related to menopause, immobilization, elevated levels of cortisone.
   10. Calcium, phosphorus, and vitamin D levels decreased.

N. *Neurologic*:
   1. Voluntary, automatic reflexes—slowed.
   2. Sleep pattern—shorter periods of sleep.
   3. Mental acuity—decreased ability to respond to multiple stimuli.
   4. Sensory interpretation and movement—changes; reduced tactile sensation → ↑ risk for self-injury.
   5. Pain perception—diminished due to decreased nerve conduction.
   6. Dexterity and agility—lessened.
   7. Reaction time—slowed due to loss of nerve fibers/neurons.
   8. Memory—past more vivid than recent memory.
   9. Depression.
   10. *Alzheimer's* disease.

O. *Sexuality*:
   1. *Women*
      a. Estrogen production—decreased with menopause.
      b. Breasts atrophy.
      c. Vaginal secretions—reduced lubricants.
      d. Sexuality—drive continues; sexual activity declines.
   2. *Men*
      a. Testosterone production—decreased.
      b. Testes—decrease in size; decreased sperm count.
      c. Libido and sexual satisfaction—no changes.

IV. **Routine laboratory studies—see Appendix G for normal ranges.**
   A. *Hematology*:
      1. *Complete blood count*—detects presence of anemia, infection, allergy, and leukemia.
      2. *Prothrombin time*—increase may indicate need for vitamin K therapy.
      3. *Serology* (VDRL)—determines presence of syphilis; false positives may indicate collagen dysfunctions.
   B. *Urinalysis*:
      1. *Physical*—color, appearance, odor, specific gravity.
      2. *Chemical*—pH, protein, glucose, ketones, bilirubin.
      3. *Microscopic*—RBC, WBC, casts, crystals, bacteria.
   C. *Chest x-ray*—detects tuberculosis or other pulmonary dysfunctions, as well as changes in size and/or configuration of heart.
   D. *Electrocardiogram*—detects rhythm and conduction disturbances, presence of myocardial ischemia or necrosis, and ventricular hypertrophy.

TABLE 1.2 ⬭ IMMUNIZATION SCHEDULE FOR ALL ADULTS	
Immunization	**Age Group**
Influenza	**19-49:** yearly for all persons with medical indication. **50 or older:** yearly for all persons.
Pneumococcal pneumonia	**19-64:** once. **65 or older:** once if not vaccinated previously, or 1 re-vaccination if vaccinated in earlier years. *Note:* some health care providers recommend a booster at 6-8 years
Tetanus	**All adults:** 1 booster dose every 10 years.
Hepatitis B	Series is recommended for **all adults** who were not vaccinated as children.
Hepatitis A	Series is recommended for **all adults** who were not vaccinated as children.
Measles, mumps, rubella (MMR)	**19-49:** complete series from childhood **50 or older:** all older adults should have this series completed.
Varicella	**All adults** complete the vaccination if not already done in childhood.

E. *Blood chemistries*—detect deviation in electrolyte balance, presence of tissue damage, and adequacy of glomerular filtration.

〰️ V. **Common diagnostic procedures**

A. **Noninvasive diagnostic procedures**—procedures that provide an indirect assessment of organ size, shape, and/or function; these procedures are considered safe, are easily reproducible, need less complex equipment for recording, and generally do not require the written consent of client and/or guardian.

  1. **General nursing responsibilities:**

     a. Reduce client's anxieties and provide emotional support by:

        (1) Explaining purpose and procedure of test.

        (2) Answering questions regarding safety of the procedure, as indicated.

        (3) Remaining with client during procedure when possible.

     ☞ b. Utilize procedures in the collection of specimens that prevent contamination and facilitate diagnosis—clean-catch urine and sputum specimens after deep breathing and coughing, for example.

〰️ B. **Invasive diagnostic procedures**—procedures that directly record the size, shape, or function of an organ and that are often complex or expensive or that need to be performed by highly trained personnel; these procedures may result in morbidity and occasionally mortality of the client and therefore require the written consent of the client or guardian.

  1. **General nursing responsibilities:**

     ☞ a. *Prior to procedure*: institute measures to provide for client's safety and emotional comfort.

        (1) Have client sign permit for procedure.

        (2) Ascertain and report any client history of allergy or allergic reactions.

        (3) Explain procedure briefly, and accurately advise client of any possible sensations, such as flushing or a warm feeling, when a contrast medium is injected.

        (4) Keep client NPO 6-12 h before procedure if anesthesia is to be used.

        (5) Allow client to verbalize concerns, and note attitude toward procedure.

     ⬭ (6) Administer preprocedure sedative, as ordered.

        (7) If procedure done at bedside:

           (a) Remain with client, offering frequent reassurance.

           (b) Assist with optional positioning of client.

           (c) Observe for indications of complications—shock, pain or dyspnea.

     ☞ b. *Following procedure*: institute measures to prevent complications and promote physical and emotional comfort.

        (1) Observe and record vital signs.

        (2) Check injection, cut-down or biopsy sites for bleeding, infection, tenderness, or thrombosis.

           (a) Report untoward reactions to physician.

           (b) Apply warm compresses to ease discomfort, as ordered.

        (3) If topical anesthetic is used during procedure (e.g., gastroscopy, bronchoscopy), *do not* give food or fluid until gag reflex returns.

(4) Encourage relaxation by allowing client to discuss experience and verbalize feelings.

VI. 🔲 **Immunizations:** See **Table 1.2** Immunization schedule for all adults.

Growth and Development

Young Adulthood (20–30 Years of Age)

I. **Stage of development**—psychosocial stage: *intimacy versus isolation.*

II. **Physical development**
   A. At the *height* of bodily vigor.
   B. *Maximum* level of strength, muscular development, height, and cardiac and respiratory capacity; also, period of peak sexual capacity for men.

III. **Cognitive development**
   A. Close to *peak* of intelligence, memory, and abstract thought.
   B. Maximum ability to solve problems and learn new skills.

IV. **Socialization**
   A. Has a vision of the future and imagines various possibilities for self.
   B. Defines and tests out what can be accomplished.
   C. Seeks out a mentor to emulate as a guiding, though transitional, figure; the mentor is usually a mixture of parent, teacher, and friend who serves as a role model to support and facilitate the developing vision of self.
   D. Grows from a beginning to a fuller understanding of own authority and autonomy.
   E. Transfers an interest into an occupation or profession; crucial work choice may be made after one has knowledge, judgment, and self-understanding, usually at the end of young adulthood; when the choice is deferred beyond these years, valuable time is lost.
   F. Experiments with and chooses a life-style.
   G. Forms mature peer relationships with the opposite sex.
   H. Overcomes guilt and anxiety about the opposite sex and learns to understand the masculine and feminine aspects of self as well as the adult concept of roles.
   I. Learns to take the opposite sex seriously and may choose someone for a long-term relationship.
   J. Accepts the responsibilities and pleasures of parenthood.

Adulthood (31–45 Years of Age)

I. **Stage of development**—psychosocial stage: *generativity versus self-absorption.*

II. **Physical development**
   A. Gradual decline in biologic functioning, although in the late 30s the individual is still near peak.
   B. Period of peak sexual capacity for women occurs during the mid-30s.
   C. Distinct sense of bodily decline occurs around 40 years of age.
   D. *Circulatory* system begins to slow somewhat after 40 years of age.

III. **Cognitive development**
   A. Takes longer to memorize.
   B. Still at peak in abstract thinking and problem solving.
   C. Generates new levels of awareness.
   D. Gives more meaning to complex tasks.

IV. **Socialization**
   A. Achieves a realistic self-identity.
   B. Perceptions are based on reality.
   C. Acts on decisions and assumes responsibility for actions.
   D. Accepts limitations while developing assets.
   E. Delays immediate gratification in favor of future satisfaction.
   F. Evaluates mistakes, determines reasons and causes, and learns new behavior.
   G. Struggles to establish a place in society.
      1. Begins to settle down.
      2. Pursues long-range plans and goals.
      3. Has a stronger need to be responsible.
      4. Invests self as fully as possible in social structure, including work, family, and community.
   H. Seeks advancement by improving and using skills, becoming more creative, and pursuing ambitions.

Middle Life (46–64 Years of Age)

I. **Stage of development**—psychosocial stage: *continuation of generativity versus self-absorption.*

II. **Physical development**
   A. Failing *eyesight*, especially for close vision, may be one of the first symptoms of aging.
   B. Hearing loss is very gradual, especially for low sounds; hearing for *high-pitched* sounds is impaired more readily.
   C. There is a gradual loss of *taste* buds in the 50s and gradual loss of sense of *smell* in the 60s, causing the individual to have a diminished sense of taste.
   D. *Muscle strength* declines because of decreased levels of estrogen and testosterone; it takes more time to accomplish the same physical task.
   E. *Lung* capacity is impaired, which decreases endurance.
   F. The *skin* begins to wrinkle, and hair begins to gray.

TABLE 1.3 IMMUNIZATIONS FOR OLDER ADULTS	
Immunization	**Frequency**
Influenza	Yearly
Pneumococcal pneumonia	Once *Note*: some health care providers recommend a booster at 6-8 years
Tetanus	Booster every 10 years

    G. *Postural changes* take place due to loss of calcium and reduced activity.

III. Cognitive development

    A. *Memory* begins to decline slowly around 50 years of age.

    B. It takes longer to *learn* new tasks, and old tasks take longer to perform.

    C. *Practical judgment* is increased due to experiential background.

    D. May tend to withdraw from mental activity or overcompensate by trying the impossible.

IV. Socialization

    A. The middle years can be very rewarding if previous stages have been fulfilled.

    B. The years of responsibility for raising children are over.

    C. Husbands and wives usually find a closer bond.

    D. There is less financial strain for those with steady employment.

    E. Individuals are usually at the height of their careers; most leaders in their field are in this age group.

    F. Self-realization is achieved.

        1. There is more inner direction.

        2. There is no longer a need to please everyone.

        3. Individual is less likely to compare self with others.

        4. Individual approves of self without being dependent on standards of others.

        5. There is less fear of failure in life because past failures have been met and dealt with.

Early Late Years (65–79 Years of Age)

I. Stage of development—psychosocial stage: *ego integrity and acceptance versus despair and disgust.*

II. Physical development

    A. Continues to decrease in vigor and capacity.

    B. Has more frequent aches, pains, and falls.

    C. Likely to have at least one major illness.

    D. Urinary incontinence may occur.

III. Cognitive development

    A. Mental acuity continues to slow down.

    B. Judgment and problem solving remain intact, but the processes may take longer.

    C. May have problems in remembering *names* and *dates*.

IV. Socialization

    A. Individual is faced with the reality of the experience of physical decline.

    B. Physical and mental changes intensify the feelings of aging and mortality.

    C. Increasing frequency of death and serious illness among friends, relatives, and associates reinforces further the concept of mortality.

    D. Constant reception of medical warnings to follow certain precautions or to run serious risks otherwise adds to general feeling of decline.

    E. Individual is less interested in obtaining the rewards of society and is more interested in utilizing own inner resources.

    F. Individuals feel that they have earned the right to do what is important for self-satisfaction.

    G. Retirement allows time for expression of own creative energies.

    H. Overcomes the splitting of youth and age; gets along well with adolescents.

    I. Learns to deal with the reality that only old age remains.

    J. Provides moral support for grandchildren; more tolerant of grandchildren than was of own children.

    K. Tends to release major authority of family to children while holding self in the role of consultant.

  V. Immunization—See **Table 1.3**, Immunizations for Older Adults.

Late Years (80 Years of Age and Older)

I. Stage of development—psychosocial stage: *continuation of ego integrity and acceptance versus despair and disgust.*

II. Physical development

    A. Additional sensory problems occur, including diminished sensation to *touch and pain*.

    B. Increase in loss of muscle tone occurs, including *sphincter* (urinary and anal) control.

    C. Individual is insecure and unsure about orientation to *space* and sense of *balance*, which may result in falls and injury.

III. Cognitive development

    A. Has better memory for the *past* than the present.

    B. *Repetition* of memories occurs.

C. Individual may use *confabulation* to fill in memory gaps.

D. Forgetfulness may lead to serious *safety* problems, and individual may require constant supervision.

E. Increased arteriosclerosis may lead to mental illness (dementia and other cognitive disorders).

IV. **Socialization**

A. Few significant relationships are maintained; deaths of friends, family, and associates cause isolation.

B. Individual may be preoccupied with immediate bodily needs and personal comforts; the *gastrointestinal tract* frequently becomes the major focus.

C. Individuals see they can provide others with an example of wisdom and courage.

D. Individuals come to terms with themselves.

E. Individuals are concerned with own mortality.

F. Individuals come to terms with the process of dying and prepare for own death.

Lifestyle Factors That Impact Health

I. **Diet**

A. Diet may increase risk for future illness.

1. High fat, high cholesterol may increase risk of *cardiovascular disease* or *obesity*.

2. Excess sodium may increase risk of *hypertension*.

3. Caloric intake in excess of caloric needs, especially of a poorly balanced diet, increases risk of *obesity* which increases risk of *cardiovascular disease, hypertension*, and *diabetes*.

4. High fat may increase risk for *prostate cancer*.

5. High fat and low fiber may increase risk for *colon cancer*.

II. **Exercise**

A. Sedentary lifestyle increases risk for *hypertension, cardiovascular disease, insomnia*, increased *fatigability, stress*, and *tension*.

III. **Occupational hazards**

A. Occupational exposure to chemicals (such as asbestos, vinyl chloride, benzene, chromium, arsenic, and petroleum distillates) increases risk for certain *cancers*.

IV. **Substance abuse**

A. Tobacco

1. Smoking increases risk for *lung cancer* and *emphysema*.

2. Chewing tobacco increases risk of *mouth* and *throat cancers*.

B. Alcohol—short term use: increases risk for *accidents, violence*, and *occupational injuries*. Chronic alcohol use: affects nearly all body systems.

C. Sedative-hypnotics—may cause memory impairment, respiratory depression, increases risk for accidents.

D. Amphetamines—increases risk for *cardiac arrhythmias, myocardial ischemia and infarction, brain cell death*.

E. Use of injectable drugs increases risk of *HIV* and *Hepatitis C*.

V. **Susceptibility to STD, Hepatitis ABCDEG**

A. AIDS: increased risk of infection with unsafe sexual practices, sharing of hypodermic needles.

B. STDs: increased risk of infection with unsafe sexual practices.

C. Hepatitis

1. *Hepatitis A*—transmitted via fecal-oral route: poor sanitation, poor hygiene, contaminated food, infected food handlers.

2. *Hepatitis B*—transmitted via percutaneous exposure to blood and blood products, and sexual contact: contaminated needles and syringes, sexual activity with infected partners, tattoos, body piercing.

3. *Hepatitis C*—transmitted via percutaneous exposure to blood and blood products, and high-risk sexual contact: needles and syringes, sexual activity with infected partners.

4. *Hepatitis D*—transmission routes same as *Hepatitis B*; can cause infection only together with *Hepatitis B*.

5. *Hepatitis E*—transmitted via fecal-oral route, associated with contaminated water supply in developing countries: found in Asia, Africa, and Mexico; not common in US or Canada.

6. *Hepatitis G*—parenterally and sexually transmitted, but is poorly characterized; can be transmitted via transfusion.

VI. **Homelessness**

A. Exposure to hazardous environment, poor nutrition, multiple stressors, little or no consistent health care.

VII. **Sun exposure**—increases risk of skin cancer.

🔑 Summary of Key Points

1. *Avoid* bias, prejudice, or stereotyping during an assessment. For example, a 34-year-old man complaining of chest pain on exertion is not too young to have severe coronary artery disease.

2. Use an organized approach for completing an assessment (e.g., head-to-toe, systems).

3. *Subjective* data are the information given by the client or family member.

4. *Objective* data consist of what the nurse observes, hears on auscultation or percussion, feels during palpation, or smells. These data validate the subjective findings.

5. Assessment always begins with *inspection*.

Questions

1. Which information about a client is an example of subjective data?
   1. Vital signs
   2. Reason for admission
   3. Chest x-ray
   4. Color of urine

2. The first step in performing a physical assessment is:
   1. Inspection
   2. Palpation
   3. Percussion
   4. Auscultation

3. On auscultation of the lungs the nurse hears a popping sound. The correct assessment would most likely be:
   1. Fremitus
   2. Crepitus
   3. Crackles
   4. Wheezes

4. A normal physical assessment finding in the older adult would be:
   1. Increased taste
   2. Thinning of toenails
   3. Increased lung compliance
   4. Decreased elasticity of skin

Answers/Rationale

1. (2) Subjective data includes what the client or family members tell the nurse. The information gathered during the nursing history is subjective data. Objective data are observations made during physical assessment or the results from laboratory/diagnostic tests (1,3,4). **AS, KN/RE, 5, HPM, Health promotion and maintenance**

2. (1) Regardless of the system being assessed, the sequence *always* begins with inspection or observation. The *next* step is usually palpation (2), followed by percussion (3), and finally auscultation (4). The *exception* is the GI system, where auscultation *follows* inspection. **AS, KN/RE, 5, HPM, Health promotion and maintenance**

3. (3) Crackles (*formerly* called rales) are the discontinuous sounds heard on auscultation, produced by the popping open of airways; usually associated with fluid accumulation in the lungs. Fremitus (1) is sound vibration felt with the hand placed on the chest. Crepitus (2) is the crackling sound of air in the subcutaneous tissue when palpation is done. Wheezes (4) are high-pitched sounds produced by air through narrowed airways. **AS, COM, 6, PhI, Physiological adaptation**

4. (4) With aging, the skin loses moisture and elasticity, developing wrinkles and lines. Taste buds (1) decrease, not increase; in particular there is a decrease in the ability to taste salt and sweet. Toenails (2) thicken, *not* thin, as peripheral circulation decreases. Lung compliance (3) decreases with age; consequently, the older adult tends to hypoventilate and is at greater risk for pulmonary problems. **AS, KN/RE, 5, HPM, Health promotion and maintenance**

Key to Codes

Nursing process: AS, assessment; AN, analysis; PL, planning; IMP, implementation; EV, evaluation. (See **Appendix M** for explanation of nursing process steps.)

Cognitive level: RE/KN, recall/knowledge; COM, comprehension; APP, application; ANL, analysis; EVL, evaluation; SYN, synthesis. (See **Appendix M** for explanation.)

Category of human function: 1, protective; 2, sensory-perceptual; 3, comfort, rest, activity, and mobility; 4, nutrition; 5, growth and development; 6, fluid-gas transport; 7, psychosocial-cultural; 8, elimination. (See **Appendix 0** for explanation.)

Client need: SECE, safe, effective care environment; PhI, physiological integrity; PsI, psychosocial integrity; HPM, health promotion and maintenance. (See **Appendix P** for explanation.)

Client subneed: (See **Appendix P** for explanation)

Peripheral Vascular Disorders

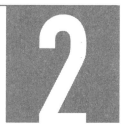

Chapter Outline

- Hypertension
- Arteriosclerosis
- Arteriosclerosis Obliterans
- Raynaud's Phenomenon
- Aneurysms
- Varicose Veins
- Arterial and Venous Ulcers
- Vein Ligation and Stripping
- Thrombophlebitis

- Peripheral Embolism
- Summary of Key Points
- Study and Memory Aids
  — Positioning
  — Diagnostic Study: Venography
  — Diets
  — Drug review
- Questions
- Answers/Rationale

Hypertension

Hypertension in adults is defined as a systolic pressure equal to or greater than 140 mm Hg, *or* a diastolic blood pressure equal to or greater than 90 mm Hg on at least 3 occasions over the course of several weeks (**Table 2.1**).

I. **Pathophysiology:** increased peripheral resistance leading to thickened arteriole walls and left ventricular hypertrophy.

II. **Risk factors/causes:**
   A. *Non-modifiable*
      1. African-Americans (2:1).
      2. Age.
      3. Gender.
      4. Family history.
      5. Socioeconomic status.
   B. *Modifiable*
      1. Obesity.
      2. Smoking.
      3. Elevated serum lipids.
      4. Excessive alcohol use.
      5. Lack of activity.
      6. Stress.
      7. Excessive sodium intake.
      8. Diabetes mellitus.

III. **Classifications:**
   A. *Primary* (essential): occurs in 90% of clients; etiology unknown; systolic pressure is ≥ 140 mm Hg or diastolic pressure is ≥ 90 mm Hg, and other causes of hypertension are absent. *Pre-hypertension* (systolic pressure 120-139 mm Hg) is considered controllable; *malignant* hypertension (diastolic >140-150 mm Hg) is uncontrollable.
   B. *Secondary*: occurs in remaining 10%; usually renal, endocrine, neurogenic, and/or cardiac in origin.

C. *Labile* (prehypertensive): a fluctuating blood pressure; increases during stress, otherwise normal or near normal.
D. See **Table 2.1** for comparison of hypertension and hypotension.

▶ IV. **Assessment**
   A. *Subjective data:*
      1. Light-headedness, tinnitus.
      2. Palpitations.
      3. Fatigue, insomnia.
      4. Forgetfulness, irritability.
      5. Altered vision: white spots, blurring or loss.
      6. Reduced tolerance for activity.
      7. Angina.
      8. Dyspnea.
      9. If BP is very high: headache, dizziness.
   B. *Objective data:*
      1. Epistaxis (nosebleeds).
      2. Elevated blood pressure: systolic > 140 mm Hg, diastolic > 90 mm Hg; narrowed pulse pressure.
      3. Retinal changes; papilledema.
      4. Shortness of breath on slight exertion.
      5. Cardiac, cerebral, and renal changes.

▶ V. **Analysis/nursing diagnosis**
   A. *Altered peripheral tissue perfusion* related to increased peripheral resistance.
   B. *Decreased cardiac output* related to ventricular hypertrophy.
   C. *Risk for injury* related to altered vision.
   D. *Risk for activity intolerance* related to inadequate oxygenation.
   E. *Fatigue* related to poor perfusion.
   F. *Non-compliance* related to life-long need for treatment of hypertension.

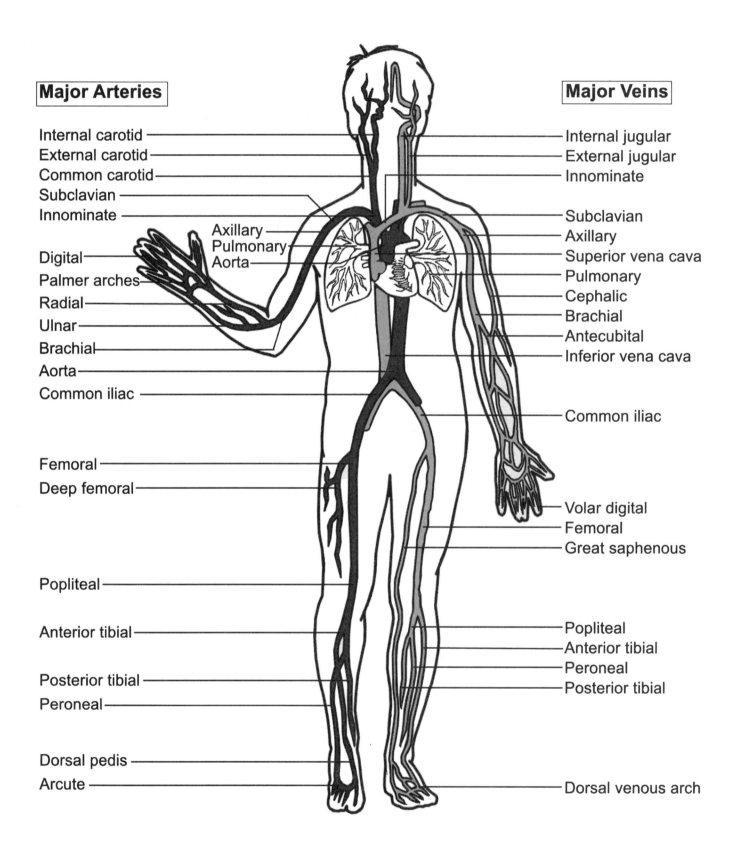

Major Arteries

Internal carotid
External carotid
Common carotid
Subclavian
Innominate

Axillary
Pulmonary
Aorta

Digital
Palmer arches
Radial
Ulnar
Brachial
Aorta
Common iliac

Femoral
Deep femoral

Popliteal

Anterior tibial

Posterior tibial
Peroneal

Dorsal pedis
Arcute

Major Veins

Internal jugular
External jugular
Innominate

Subclavian
Axillary
Superior vena cava
Pulmonary
Cephalic
Brachial
Antecubital
Inferior vena cava

Common iliac

Volar digital
Femoral
Great saphenous

Popliteal
Anterior tibial
Peroneal
Posterior tibial

Dorsal venous arch

Peripheral Vascular System: major arteries and major veins

TABLE 2.1 IMBALANCES IN BLOOD PRESSURE: COMPARATIVE ASSESSMENT OF HYPOTENSION AND HYPERTENSION

	Hypotension	Hypertension
Common causes		
	Angina pectoris	Essential hypertension
	Myocardial infarction	Iron deficiency anemia
	Acute and chronic pericarditis	Pernicious anemia
	Valvular defects	Arteriosclerosis obliterans
	Heart failure	Polycythemia vera
	Loss of fluid volume	
	Vasodilation	
▶ Assessment		
Behavior	Anxiety, apprehension, decreasing mentation, confusion	Nervousness, mood swings, irritability, difficulty with memory, depression, confusion
Neurologic	Essentially noncontributory	Decreased vibratory sensations, increased/decreased reflexes, *Babinski* reflex, changes in coordination
Head/neck	Worried expression	Bruits over carotids, distended neck veins, epistaxis, diplopia, ringing in ears, dull occipital headaches on arising
Skin	Pale, cool, moist	Dry, pale, glossy, flaky, cold; decreased or absent hair
GI	Anorexia, nausea, vomiting, constipation	Anorexia, flatulence, diarrhea, constipation
Respiratory	Dyspnea, orthopnea, paroxysmal nocturnal dyspnea, tachypnea, moist crackles, cough	Dyspnea, orthopnea, moist crackles
Cardiovascular	Tires easily	Decreased exercise tolerance, weakness, palpitations
	Blood pressure—decreased systolic, decreased systolic/diastolic	Blood pressure—increased systolic or diastolic
	Pulse—increased/decreased, weak, thready, irregular, arrhythmias	Decreased or absent pedal pulses
Renal	Orthostatic changes	
	Oliguria	Oliguria, nocturia, proteinuria
Extremities	Dependent edema	Tingling, numbness, or cold hands and feet, dependent edema, ulcers of legs or feet

Source: ©Lagerquist, SL: *Little, Brown's NCLEX-RN® Examination Review*. Boston: Little, Brown, (out of print)

▶ **VI. Nursing care plan/implementation**

  A. Goal: *provide for physical and emotional rest.*

  1. Rest periods before/after eating, visiting hours; *avoid* upsetting situations.

  ▭ 2. Give *tranquilizers, sedatives,* as ordered.

  B. Goal: *provide for special safety needs.*

  ☞ 1. Monitor blood pressure: both arms; *standing, sitting, lying positions.*

  2. Limit/prevent activities that increase pressure (anxiety, anger, frustration, visitors who are upsetting, fatigue).

  3. Assist with ambulation; change position gradually to prevent dizziness and light-headedness (*postural hypotension*).

  ⩗ 4. Monitor for electrolyte imbalance when
  🍎 on *low sodium diet, diuretic therapy;* monitor intake and output to prevent fluid depletion and arrhythmias resulting from potassium loss.

  5. Observe for signs of hemorrhage, shock, and stroke, which may occur after surgery.

  ⌂ C. Goal: **health teaching** (client and family).

  1. Procedures to decrease anxiety; relaxation techniques, stress management.

  2. Importance of taking meds as prescribed for most rapid improvement of condition.

  ▭ 3. Side effects of: *hypotensive* drugs, *diuretics, adrenergic blockers, vasodilators, calcium channel blockers* (faintness, nausea, vomiting, postural hypotension, sexual dysfunction). See **Appendix D** for specific pharmacologic actions.

  4. Weight control to reduce arterial pressure.

  🍎 5. *Restrictions:* stimulants (tea, coffee, tobacco), sodium, calories, fat.

  6. Lifestyle adjustments: daily exercise needed; reduce occupational and environmental stress; importance of rest.

7. Blood pressure measurement: daily, same conditions, position preference of physician.
8. Signs, symptoms, complications of disease (headache, confusion, visual changes, nausea/vomiting, convulsions).
9. Causes of intermittent hypotension: alcohol, hot weather, exercise, febrile illness, hot bath.

◄ **VII. Evaluation/outcome criteria**
   A. Blood pressure within normal range for age (systolic <140 mm Hg, diastolic <90 mm Hg)—stable.
   B. Minimal or no pathophysiologic or therapeutic complications (e.g., visual changes, stroke, drug side effects).
   C. Reduces weight to reasonable level for height, bone structure.
   D. *Takes prescribed medications* regularly, even when symptoms have resolved.
   E. Complies with restrictions: no smoking; restricted sodium, fat.
   F. Exercises regularly—program compatible with personal and health care goals.

Arteriosclerosis

Arteriosclerosis is a loss of elasticity, thickening, and hardening of arterial walls. The common type is atherosclerosis. Arteriosclerosis precedes angina pectoris and myocardial infarction.

I. **Pathophysiology:**
   A. Atherosclerotic plaque, discrete lumpy thickening of arterial wall.
   B. Narrows lumen, can occlude vessel.

II. **Risk factors/causes:**
   A. Increased serum cholesterol (low-density lipids) level.
   B. Hypertension.
   C. Cigarette smoking.
   D. Diabetes mellitus.

(See **Angina pectoris, p. 46**, and **Myocardial infarction, p. 46–48**, for nursing implications.)

Arteriosclerosis Obliterans

Arteriosclerosis obliterans is the most common obstructive disorder of the arterial system (aorta, large and medium-size arteries). It frequently involves the femoral artery.

I. **Pathophysiology**: fatty deposits in intimal, medial layer of arterial walls; plaque formation → narrowed arterial lumens; decreased distensibility → decreased blood flow; ischemic changes in tissues.

II. **Risk factors/causes:**
   A. Age (>50).
   B. Sex (men).
   C. Diabetes mellitus.
   D. Hyperlipidemia—obesity.
   E. Cigarette smoking.
   F. Hypertension.
   G. Polycythemia vera.

◄ **III. Assessment**
   A. *Subjective data:*
      1. Pain:
         a. *Type*—cramplike.
         b. *Location*—foot, calf, thigh, buttocks.
         c. *Duration*—variable, may be relieved by rest.
         d. *Precipitating causes*—exercise (*intermittent claudication*), but occasionally may occur when at rest.
      2. Tingling, numbness in toes, feet.
      3. Persistent coldness of one or both lower extremities.
   B. *Objective data:*
      1. Lower extremities:
         a. Pedal pulses—absent or diminished.
         b. Skin—shiny, glossy, dry, cold, chalky white, decreased/absent hair, ulcers, gangrene.
      2. Lab data: *increased* serum cholesterol, triglycerides, CBC, platelets.
      3. *Angiography*—indicates location, nature of occlusion.

◄ **IV. Analysis/nursing diagnosis**
   A. *Altered tissue perfusion* related to decreased arterial blood flow.
   B. *Risk for activity intolerance* related to pain and sensory changes.
   C. *Pain* related to ischemia.
   D. *Risk for impaired skin integrity* related to poor circulation.
   E. *Risk for injury* related to numbness of extremities.

◄ **V. Nursing care plan/implementation**
   A. Goal: *promote circulation; decrease discomfort.*
      1. *Position*: elevate *head* of bed on blocks (3–6 in.), as gravity aids perfusion to thighs, legs; elevating legs increases pain.
      2. Comfort: keep warm; *avoid* chilling or use of heating pads, which may burn skin; apply bed socks.
      3. Circulation: check pedal pulses, skin color, capillary refill, temperature qid.
      4. Medications:
         a. *Vasodilators.*
         b. *Anticoagulants*—heparin sodium, dicumarol, ASA.
         c. *Antihyperlipidemics*—clofibrate, cholestyramine resin, nicotinic acid.

B. Goal: *prevent infection, injury.*

☞ 1. Skin care: use bed cradle; sheepskin; heel pads; mild soap, dry thoroughly; lotion; to prevent release of thrombus, do **not** massage.

2. Foot care: wear properly fitting shoes, slippers when out of bed; inspect for injury or pressure areas; nail care by podiatrist.

🍎 3. *Diet*: *high* in vitamins B and C to improve cardiovascular functioning and skin integrity; *low* fat

🏠 C. Goal: **health teaching.**

1. Skin care; inspect daily.

2. Activity: balance exercise, rest to increase collateral circulation; walk only until painful.

3. Exercises: walking, Buerger-Allen exercises (gravity alternately fills and empties blood vessels).

4. *Avoid* smoking.

5. Recognizes and reports signs of occlusion (e.g., pain, cramping, numbness in extremities, color changes—white or blue, temperature changes—cool to cold).

🕊 VI. **Evaluation/outcome criteria**

A. Decreased pain.

B. Skin integrity preserved; no loss of limb.

C. Quits smoking.

D. Does exercises to increase collateral circulation.

Raynaud's Phenomenon

Intermittent vasospasm of small cutaneous arteries.

I. **Pathophysiology**: unclear—may occur as an exaggerated response to sympathetic nervous system stimulation, or may be a result of abnormalities in endothelium and endothelium-derived vasoactive substances.

II. **Risk factors/causes:**

A. Women, between 15 and 40 years old.

B. Collagen diseases, (e.g. rheumatoid arthritis, systemic lupus erythematosus).

C. Episodes precipitated by: cold exposure, caffeine, tobacco, emotional upsets

D. Repetitive trauma or pressure to the fingertips, (e.g. pianists, typists).

E. Exposure to heavy metals.

🕊 III. **Assessment**

A. *Subjective data:*

1. Coldness, numbness in affected digits, followed by throbbing ache and tingling.

B. *Objective data:*

1. Color changes in affected digits: initially pallor due to decreased perfusion, followed by cyanosis, then rubor from a hyperemic response as the episode subsides and perfusion is restored.

2. Swelling of the affected digits during the hyperemic phase.

3. Skin of affected digits may become thickened and nails brittle.

🕊 IV. **Analysis/nursing diagnosis**

A. *Ineffective tissue perfusion* related to decreased arterial blood flow.

🕊 V. **Nursing care plan/implementation**

A. Goal: *manage episodes of vasospasm.*

1. Immerse hands in warm (*not hot*) water.

💊 2. For severe cases administer calcium channel blocker medications as ordered: nifedipine (*Procardia*) 30-60 mg sustained release PO q day; diltiazem (*Cardizem*) 30 mg PO qid, increasing to 180-360mg q day.

🏠 B. Goal: **health teaching.**

1. Prevention of recurrent episodes of vasospasm: *avoid* temperature extremes, caffeine and tobacco.

2. Learn coping strategies for stress.

3. Clothing should be loose and warm.

4. Biofeedback is useful for some clients.

🕊 VI. **Evaluation/outcome criteria**

A. Vasospasm episodes are less frequent.

B. Avoidance of controllable risk factors.

Aneurysms

Aneurysms can form in either the thoracic or abdominal aorta and are defined as localized or diffuse dilatations or outpouchings of a vessel wall, usually an artery, that exert pressure on adjacent structures. They primarily occur in men over 60 years of age. Conventional surgical repair involves reconstruction with a synthetic or vascular graft. The newest procedure is an endovascular graft in which a Dacron cylinder is inserted into the aorta via the femoral artery.

I. **Risk factors/causes:**

A. Atherosclerosis.

B. Trauma.

C. Syphilis.

D. Congenital weakness.

E. Local infection, e.g. *salmonella*.

🕊 II. **Assessment**

A. *Subjective data:*

1. Pain:

a. Constant, boring, neuralgic, intermittent—low back, abdominal.

b. Angina—sudden onset may mean rupture or dissection, which are **emergency** conditions.

2. Dyspnea; orthopnea.

3. Dysphagia, hoarseness.

B. *Objective data:*
1. Vital signs:
   a. Radial pulses differ.
   b. Tachycardia.
   c. Hypotension after rupture, leading to shock.
2. Pulsating mass: abdominal, chest wall pulsation; edema of chest wall (*thoracic aneurysm*); periumbilical pulsation (*abdominal aneurysm*); audible bruit over aorta.
3. Cyanosis, mottled below level of aneurysm.
4. Veins: (distended) dilated, superficial—neck, chest, arms.
5. Cough: paroxysmal, brassy.
6. Diaphoresis, pallor, fainting after rupture.
7. Peripheral pulses:
   a. Femoral present.
   b. Pedal weak or absent.
8. Stool bloody from irritation.

III. **Analysis/nursing diagnosis**
A. *Altered peripheral tissue perfusion* related to distal arterial emboli.
B. *Pain* related to pressure on lumbar nerves.
C. *Anxiety* related to risk of rupture.

IV. **Nursing care plan/implementation**
A. Goal: *provide emergency care prior to surgery for dissection or rupture.*
   1. *Vital signs*: at least every 5 min (systolic blood pressure <100 mm Hg and pulse >100 beats/ min with rupture).
   2. *IVs*: may have 2–4 sites; lactated Ringer's may be ordered.
   3. *Urine output*: monitored every 15–30 min.
   4. *O₂*: usually via nasal prongs.
   5. Medications as ordered: *antihypertensives* to prevent extension of dissection; *tranquilizers* and *narcotics* to reduce pain and anxiety.
   6. Transport to operating room quickly.
   7. See **The Perioperative Experience, p. 127-129**, for general preoperative care.
B. Goal: *prevent complications postoperatively.*
   1. *Position*: initially *flat* in bed; *avoid* sharp flexion of hip and knee, which places pressure on femoral and popliteal arteries; turn gently side to side; note erythema on back from pooled blood.
   2. *Vital signs*: CVP; hourly peripheral pulses distal to graft site, including neurovascular check of lower extremities; absent pulses for 6–12 h indicates occlusion; *Doppler blood flow* instrument; intraarterial line to monitor blood pressure and manage vasoactive medications.
   3. Urine output: hourly from indwelling catheter.
      a. Immediately report anuria or oliguria (<30 mL/h).
      b. Check color for hematuria.

   c. Monitor daily blood urea nitrogen and creatinine levels.
   4. Observe for *signs of atheroembolization* (patchy areas of ischemia); report change in color, motor ability, or sensation of lower extremities (*CSM*).
   5. Observe for *signs of bowel ischemia* (decreased/absent bowel sounds, pain, *guaiac positive* diarrhea, abdominal distention); may have *nasogastric tube.*
   6. Measure abdominal girth; increase seen with graft leakage.
C. Goal: *promote comfort.*
   1. *Position*: alignment, comfort; prevent heel ulcers.
   2. *Medication*: narcotics.
D. Goal: **health teaching.**
   1. Minimize recurrence; *avoid*: trauma, infection, smoking, *high cholesterol diet*, obesity.
   2. Regular medical supervision.

V. **Evaluation/outcome criteria**
   1. Surgical intervention before rupture.
   2. No loss of renal or neurological function.

Varicose Veins

Varicose veins are abnormally lengthened, tortuous, dilated superficial veins (saphenous) and result from incompetent valves, especially in lower extremities. The process is irreversible.

I. **Pathophysiology:** dilated vein → venous stasis → edema; fibrotic changes; pigmentation of skin; lowered resistance to trauma.

II. **Risk factors/causes:**
A. Congenital defect of venous valves.
B. Trauma.
C. Deep-vein thrombosis.
D. Pregnancy.
E. Abdominal tumors.
F. Chronic disease (heart, liver).
G. Occupations requiring long periods of standing.
H. Obesity.

III. **Assessment**
A. *Subjective data:*
   1. Dull aches; heaviness in legs.
   2. Pain; muscle cramping.
   3. Fatigue in lower extremities, increased with hot weather, high altitude; history of risk factors.
B. *Objective data:*
   1. Nodular protrusions along veins.
   2. Edema.
   3. *Diagnostic tests*: *Trendelenburg test*; venography; duplex ultrasound; *Doppler blood flow measurement.*

TABLE 2.2 COMPARISON OF ARTERIAL AND VENOUS ULCERS

	Arterial ulcers	Venous ulcers
Causes	Peripheral vascular disease	Chronic venous insufficiency, caused by: - DVT - varicose veins - valve defects - prolonged immobility - CHF
Common locations	Over bony prominences, esp. top of toes & lateral malleoli.	Calves, medial malleoli.
▶ **Assessment: signs and symptoms**	Weak or absent pulses. Capillary refill > 3 seconds. Ankle-brachial index < 0.75. No edema. No hair on legs, feet, toes. Well-defined wound margins. Minimal drainage. Pain, worse at night & at rest, when leg elevated; ulcer may or may not be painful. Dependent rubor, pallor with elevation. Skin: thin, friable, shiny, dry. Skin cool, gets cooler more distal.	Pulses present; difficult to palpate due to edema. Capillary refill < 3 seconds. Ankle-brachial index > 0.90. Edema. Hair may or may not be present. Irregular wound margins. Moderate to large amount drainage. Dull ache in calf or thigh, ulcer often painful. Brown or bronze skin. Skin: thick, hardened, indurated Skin warm.
▶ **Treatment/Nursing Implementation:**	• Keep clean & dry. • Cover with dry sterile dressing. • Wound *will not heal* until arterial flow is restored.	• Assess client for arterial sufficiency *before* applying compression dressings. • Compression: customized. support hose (*not* TEDS), Ace wraps, velcro wraps (Circaid), Unna's boot. • Other compression/topical treatment bandages. • *Elevate* leg as much as possible. • Hydrocolloid dressings may be used. DO NOT USE povidone-iodine solutions on venous ulcers.

▶ **IV. Analysis/nursing diagnosis**

    A. *Altered tissue perfusion* related to venous valve incompetence.

    B. *Pain* related to edema and muscle cramping.

    C. *Risk for activity intolerance* related to leg discomfort.

    D. *Body image disturbance* related to disfigurement of leg.

▶ **V. Nursing care plan/implementation**

    A. Goal: *promote venous return from lower extremities.*

        1. Activity: walk every hour.

        2. Discourage: prolonged sitting, standing, sitting with crossed legs.

        3. *Position*: elevate legs q2–3h; elastic stockings or Ace wraps.

    B. Goal: *provide for safety.*

        1. Assist with early ambulation.

        2. Surgical asepsis with wounds, leg ulcers (see **Table 2.2**).

        3. Observe for hemorrhage—if occurs: *elevate leg*, apply pressure, notify physician.

        4. Observe for allergic reactions if sclerosing drugs used; have *antihistamine* available

C. Goal: **health teaching.**

    1. Weight-reducing techniques, dietary approaches if indicated.

    2. Preventive measures: *leg elevation; avoid*: prolonged standing, sitting, high chairs, tight girdles, constrictive clothing; wear support hose.

    3. Expectations for *Trendelenburg test.*

        a. While client is lying down, elevate leg 65 degrees to empty veins.

        b. Apply tourniquet high on upper thigh (do not constrict deep veins).

        c. Client stands with tourniquet in place.

        d. Filling of veins is observed.

        e. Normal response is slow filling from below in 20–30 sec, with no change in rate when tourniquet is removed.

        f. Incompetent veins distend very quickly from the top down.

    4. Prepare for vein ligation and stripping.

▶ **VI. Evaluation/outcome criteria**

    A. Relief or control of symptoms.

    B. Activity without pain.

TABLE 2.3 ◄ NURSING RESPONSIBILITIES WITH ANTICOAGULANT THERAPY

	Heparin	Warfarin (Coumadin)
Monitor	⏦ aPTT (25-38 sec); therapeutic level usually 1.5-2.0 times control (50-80 sec)	⏦ PT (11-15 sec); therapeutic level—International Normalized Ratio (INR): 2-3 (sample/control)
Inspect	Ecchymosis, bleeding gums, petechiae, hematuria	Bleeding, ecchymosis
Administer	With an infusion pump, *never* mix with other drugs, *never* aspirate, *avoid* massaging site	Same time every day; PO
Avoid	⬤ Salicylates and other anticoagulants, e.g., non-steroidal anti-inflammatory agents, corticosteroids, some penicillins	Same as heparin
Antidote	⬤ Protamine sulfate	⬤ Vitamin K

Source: ©Lagerquist, SL: *Little, Brown's NCLEX-RN® Examination Review.* Boston: Little, Brown, (out of print)

Vein Ligation and Stripping

Vein ligation and stripping is the surgical intervention used for the treatment of advancing varicosities, stasis ulcerations, and cosmetic needs of client. The procedure involves ligation of the saphenous vein at the groin, where it joins the femoral vein, and saphenous stripping from the groin to the ankle. The legs are then wrapped with a pressure bandage.

I. See **Varicose veins, p. 18–19,** for **assessment data** and **nursing diagnosis** of the client requiring surgery.

◄ II. **Nursing care plan/implementation**
   ☞ A. Goal: *prevent complications.*
      1. *Position: elevate* legs 18 out of 24 h above level of heart, for 1 wk. (See **Positioning** box at end of unit.)
      2. Activity:
        a. Assist with early, frequent ambulation;
      ⬤ medicate for pain before ambulation.
        b. *No* chair sitting to prevent venous pooling, thrombus formation.
      3. Bleeding: check elastic bandages, dressings several times a day.
   🏠 B. Goal: **health teaching** to prevent recurrence.
      1. Weight reduction.
      2. *Avoid* constricting garments.
      3. Change positions frequently.
      4. Wear support hose/stockings to enhance venous return.
      5. *No* crossing legs at knees.

◄ III. **Evaluation/outcome criteria**
    A. No complications—hemorrhage, infection, nerve damage, deep-vein thrombosis.
    B. No recurrence of varicosities.
    C. Adequate circulation to legs: strong pedal pulses.
    D. Resumes daily activities; free of pain.

Thrombophlebitis

Thrombophlebitis is the formation of a blood clot in an inflamed vein, secondary to phlebitis or partial obstruction. It may lead to venous insufficiency and pulmonary embolism.

I. **Pathophysiology**: endothelial inflammation → formation of platelet plug (blood clot) → slowing of blood flow → increase in procoagulants in local area → initiation of clotting mechanisms.

II. **Risk factors/causes:**
    A. Immobility.
    B. Venous disease.
    C. Prolonged sitting—knees bent.
    D. Childbirth.
    E. Hypercoagulability of blood.
    F. Venous trauma (IVs).
    G. Fractures, orthopedic surgery.
    H. Abdominal and pelvic surgery.
    I. Oral contraceptives.
    J. Cigarette smoking.

◄ III. **Assessment**
    A. Superficial thrombophlebitis.
      1. *Subjective data:*
        a. Surrounding area: tender, red.
      2. *Objective data:*
        a. Palpable, firm subcutaneous vein.
        b. Edema may, or may not, be present.
    B. Deep vein thrombophlebitis.
      1. *Subjectve data:*
        a. Client may have no symptoms, or may have extremity pain, warm skin on extremity.
        b. Calf may be tender.
      2. *Objective data:*
        a. Client may have unilateral leg edema.
        b. Temperature 100.4° or higher.
        c. *HOMANS* sign may be positive, but is *highly unreliable.*

IV. Analysis/nursing diagnosis

A. *Altered peripheral tissue perfusion* related to venous stasis.

B. *Pain* related to inflammation.

C. *Activity intolerance* related to leg pain.

D. *Increased risk of bleeding* related to anticoagulant therapy.

V. Nursing care plan/implementation

A. Goal: *provide rest, comfort, and relief from pain.*

   1. Bedrest.

   2. *Position*: as ordered; usually extremity *elevated*; watch for pressure points.

   3. Apply warm, moist heat to affected area as prescribed (cold may also be ordered).

   4. Assess progress of affected area: swelling, pain, soreness, temperature, color.

   5. Administer *analgesics* as ordered.

B. Goal: *prevent complications.*

   1. Observe for signs of **embolism** (pain at site of *superficial* embolism; chest pain, SOB if pulmonary embolus [*DVT*]); allergic reaction (anaphylactic shock) with *streptokinase*.

   2. *Precautions*: *no* rubbing or massage of limb.

   3. Medications: *anticoagulants* (sodium heparin, enoxaparin, coumadin); streptokinase (*Streptase*); *anti-inflammatory* agents for *superficial* thrombophlebitis. (**Table 2.3**)

   4. Bleeding: hematuria, epistaxis, ecchymosis.

   5. Skin care, to relieve increased redness/maceration from hot or cold applications.

   6. Range of motion: unaffected limb.

C. Goal: **health teaching.**

   1. *Precautions*: tight garters, girdles; sitting with legs crossed; oral contraceptives.

   2. Preventive measures: walking daily, swimming several times weekly if possible, wading, rest periods—with legs *elevated*, elastic stockings (may remove at bedtime).

   3. *Medication side effects*: anticoagulants—pink toothbrush, hematuria, easily bruised.

     a. Carry MedicAlert card/bracelet.

     b. *Contraindicated drugs*, which increase or decrease anticoagulant effects—aspirin, glutethimide (*Doriden*), cefamandole, cefotetan, plicamycin, chloramphenicol (*Chloromycetin*), neomycin, phenylbutazone (*Butazolidin*), barbiturates.

   4. Prepare for surgery (thrombectomy, vein ligation).

VI. Evaluation/outcome criteria

A. No complications (e.g., embolism).

B. No recurrence of symptoms.

C. Free of pain—ambulates without discomfort.

Peripheral Embolism

A peripheral embolism is made up of fragments of thrombi, globules of fat, clumps of tissue, calcified plaques, or air that moves in the circulation and lodges in a vessel, obstructing blood flow. Thrombic emboli are the most common. They may be venous or arterial.

🔑 Summary of Key Points

1. The pain associated with **arterial disease** is provoked by exercise/activity, relieved by rest, and worsens with elevation.

2. Concepts important to understand about **maintaining adequate circulation** include: autoregulation, coagulation, hydration, vessel size (inflammation, vasoconstriction, or vasodilation), viscosity of blood, vascular resistance, and venous valve competence.

3. Prevention of **hypertension** should focus on recognizing risk factors and managing modifiable risks. For example, weight loss may be one of the most effective ways to lower blood pressure.

4. **Disorders of the peripheral vascular system** involve narrowing, obstruction, or damage to arteries or veins, resulting in ischemia, a lack of blood flow to the tissues or organs involved, or venous stasis.

5. A client with **thrombophlebitis** may be asymptomatic.

☀ Study and Memory Aids

POSTOPERATIVE POSITIONING OF CLIENT WITH VASCULAR CONDITION

Condition	Position	Purpose
Arterial insuffiency	1. Do *not* elevate legs. 2. *Avoid* hip flexion—walk or stand, but do *not* sit	1. Arterial flow is helped by gravity. 2. Flexion of the hip compresses the vessels of the extremity
Vein strippings; vein ligations	1. Keep legs elevated. 2. Do *not* stand or sit for long periods.	1. Prevents venous stasis. 2. Prevents venous pooling.

Source: Jane Vincent Corbett, RN, MS, EdD., Professor Emerita, School of Nursing, University of San Francisco. Used with permission.

Assessment of Hypertension: "ELEVATED"

E xertional SOB
L ack of activity
E arly-morning headache
V ascular changes
A nxiety increased
T ired
E pistaxis
D iastolic pressure elevated

Hypertension: Complications—4 Cs

CAD (coronary artery disease)
CHF (congestive heart failure)
CRF (chronic renal failure)
CVA (cerebrovascular accident; now called *brain attack*)

No Smoking with Hypertension

Central Venous Pressure

• Determined by vascular tone, blood volume, and the ability of the heart to receive and pump blood.
• Measured using a central venous catheter placed in the superior vena cava; normal value: 2–12 mm Hg.

Varicose Veins Assessment: "TWISTED"

T wisted
W ork posture
I rreversible process
S welling
T rendelenburg test result positive
E xtremities—lower
D ull aches

Vein Ligation and Stripping

No sitting

⋀⋁⋀ Diagnostic Study

Venography—determines patency of the tibial-popliteal, superficial femoral—common femoral, and saphenous veins. A contrast medium is injected into the superficial and/or deep veins of the involved extremity, followed by acquisition of x-ray studies, while the leg is placed in a variety of positions; *used* to detect deep-vein thrombosis and to select a vein for use in arterial bypass grafting; localized clotting may result.

🍎 Diets

Hypertension

↓ Calories
Cholesterol
Na^+
No caffeine

Arteriosclerosis Obliterans

↑ Cholesterol, fat
↓ Vitamin B & C

Aneurysms

↓ Caloric intake
Cholesterol

Drug Review

Hypertension

Adrenergic inhibitors
Atenolol (*Tenormin*): 50–150 mg qd
Clonidine (*Catapres*): 0.2–0.8 mg/day in divided doses
Methyldopa (*Aldomet*): 0.5–2 g/day in divided doses
Prazosin (*Minipress*): up to 20 mg/day in divided doses
Propranolol (*Inderal*): 80–240 mg bid
Angiotensin inhibitors
Captopril (*Capoten*): 25–15 mg bid-tid
Enalapril (*Vasotec*): 10–40 mg qd
Losartan (*Cozaar*): 25–50 mg qd
Calcium channel blockers
Nifedipine (*Procardia*): 10 mg tid or 30–60 mg sustained release qd
Verapamil (*Calan*): 80–120 mg tid
Diuretics
Furosemide (*Lasix*): 20–80 mg qd
Hydrochlorothiazide (*Hydrodiuril*): 25–100 mg qd
Spironolactone (*Aldactone*): 25–400 mg qd
Sedatives/tranquilizers
Alprazolam (*Xanax*): 0.25–0.5 mg tid
Chlordiazepoxide HCl (*Librium*): 5–10 mg PO
Diazepam (*Valium*): 2–10 mg PO
Vasodilators
Diazoxide (*Hyperstat*): 1–3 mg/kg IV q 5–15 min
Nitroprusside (*Nipride*): 0.5–8 mcg/kg/min
Note: see also Aneurysm medications

Arteriosclerosis Obliterans

Anticoagulants
Enoxaparin (*Lovenox*): 30–40 mg SC qd or bid; 1mg/kg q 12hr
Heparin sodium: IV 5,000 U. IV to start followed by 20,000–40,000 U infusion over 24 hours; SC 8000-10,000 units q8h adjusted according to partial thromboplastin time (PTT)
Warfarin (*Coumadin*): 10 mg daily adjusted according to International Normalized Ratio (INR)
Antihyperlipidemics
Atorvastatin (*Lipitor*): 10–80 mg qd
Cholestyramine (*Questran*): 4 g 1–6 times daily
Clofibrate (*Atromid S*): 2 g/d in 2–4 divided doses
Colestipol (*Colestid*): 5–30 g daily
Lovastatin (*Mevacor*): 20–80 mg qd
Niacin (*Nicobid*): 500 mg daily up to 2 g tid
Antiplatelets
Aspirin: 1–3 g daily in 2–4 divided doses
Clopidogrel (*Plavix*): 75mg qd
Dipyridamole (*Aggrenox*): 200mg + aspirin 25mg 1 tablet qd
Hemorrheologic agents
Pentoxifylline (*Trental*): 400 mg tid with meals

Aneurysms

Antihypertensive: Angiotensin-converting enzyme (ACE) inhibitor—Captopril (*Capoten*): 12.5-25 mg tid

Thrombophlebitis/Peripheral Embolism

Anticoagulants
Enoxaparin (*Lovenox*): 30–40 mg SC qd or bid; 1mg/kg q 12hr
Heparin sodium: IV 1000 units/hr; SC 8000–10,000 units q8h adjusted according to PTT
Warfarin (*Coumadin*): 10 mg daily adjusted according to INR
Thrombolytic agent
Streptokinase (*Streptase*): IV 250,000 IU loading dose followed by 100,000 IU/h for 24h
Note: Give with **no** other anticoagulants, aspirin, large doses of penicillin or penicillin-like drugs, some cephalosporins, plicamycin or valproic acid, which may increase risk of bleeding.

Questions

1. Which vital sign change is the most likely indicator of hypertension?
   1. A narrowing pulse pressure.
   2. Irregular pulse.
   3. Fluctuating systolic pressure.
   4. Diastolic pressure exceeding 90 mm Hg.
2. After a month of treatment for hypertension, a client returns for a clinical follow-up and is found to have a blood pressure of 190/130 mm Hg. The nurse should first seek information on the client's:
   1. Stress level at work.
   2. Progress with relaxation techniques.
   3. Compliance with prescribed drug therapy.
   4. Success with a weight-loss program.
3. A client is to receive atenolol (*Tenormin*) PO. Which existing condition should the nurse assess for that may be adversely affected by this drug?
   1. Diabetes mellitus.
   2. Cholecystitis.
   3. Duodenal ulcer.
   4. Diverticulosis.
4. To evaluate the effectiveness of a low sodium diet in a client with hypertension, the nurse should check:
   1. Serum sodium levels.
   2. Changes in body weight.
   3. Appearance of ankles.
   4. Breath sounds.
5. Client teaching for a client with hypertension who is receiving captopril (*Capoten*) should include which point?
   1. The need for more potassium in the diet.
   2. The need to limit fluid intake to increase drug effectiveness.
   3. The fact that taste perception may be decreased.
   4. The need to test the urine for glucose.

6. Which abnormal laboratory result would the nurse likely see in a client taking captopril (*Capoten*)?
   1. Hypokalemia.
   2. Hyperkalemia.
   3. Leukocytosis.
   4. Hypernatremia.

WBC ↓ Na⁺ ↓
platelet ↓

7. To promote optimal rest at night in a client taking a diuretic, the client should be instructed to:
   1. Restrict daytime fluid intake to prevent nocturia.
   2. Take the diuretic in the morning with food.
   3. Drink a hot beverage before bedtime to relax.
   4. Sleep with the head elevated to promote breathing.

8. A client admitted to the emergency department with a BP of 240/180 mm Hg receives diazoxide (*Hyperstat*) IV. The nurse would monitor this client for which adverse effect?
   1. Rebound hypertension.
   2. Chest pain.
   3. Reflex bradycardia.
   4. Pallor and sweating.

vasodilator
[reflex tachycardia
flushed ↑CO
hypotension

9. The nurse should advise a client who is on a salt-restricted diet to avoid eating:
   1. Eggs and milk.
   2. Potatoes and rice.
   3. Apples and plums.
   4. Carrots and spinach.

10. The activated partial thromboplastin time (aPTT) in a client on heparin is 75 seconds. The most appropriate nursing action would be to:
    1. Prepare an injection of vitamin K and notify the physician.
    2. Discuss with the MD the need to discontinue the drug.
    3. Observe for signs of bleeding during the shift.
    4. Continue treatment: as this lab result is desirable.

desired 50-80 sec.

11. The best explanation for the nurse to give a client who asks why he is receiving both heparin and warfarin sodium (*Coumadin*) to achieve anticoagulation is that:
    1. Anticoagulation occurs faster when both are taken.
    2. There is less chance of bleeding when both are taken.
    3. Heparin treatment will be stopped once the *Coumadin* is working.
    4. *Coumadin* speeds up the effects of heparin.

12. Discharge teaching for a client receiving *Coumadin* should include the need to avoid eating:
    1. Citrus fruits.
    2. Green leafy vegetables.
    3. Potatoes and rice.
    4. Dairy products.

vit. K

13. A client with thrombophlebitis must be observed closely for the occurrence of which complication?

1. Dyspnea.
2. Petechiae.
3. Hematuria.
4. Tetany.

14. Physical assessment of a client with arterial insufficiency of the lower extremities would reveal:
    1. Thickened skin on the soles of the feet.
    2. Prominent superficial blood vessels in the legs.
    3. Diminished dorsalis pedis pulses.
    4. Excessive hair on legs above ankles.

15. Which lab test finding would be abnormal in a client with deep-vein thrombosis?
    1. Red blood cell count (RBC).
    2. Prothrombin time (PT).
    3. Hematocrit value (HCT).
    4. Activated partial thromboplastin time (aPTT).

Answers/Rationale

coagulation disorders

1. **(4)** The classic blood pressure reading denoting hypertension is a systolic pressure of 140 mm Hg or greater or a diastolic pressure of 90 mm Hg or greater. The diastolic pressure increases as vascular resistance increases. A narrowing of the pulse pressure (1) occurs with hypovolemic shock, because the systolic pressure decreases initially with decreased volume. An irregular pulse (2) may occur with heart failure and electrical conduction abnormalities. Fluctuations in the systolic pressure (3) often occur with for example, stress, anxiety, and fluid volume changes. **AN, COM, 6, PhI, Physiological adaptation**

2. **(3)** The client's blood pressure indicates a poor response to pharmacotherapy. It would be important to *first* determine whether the client is taking the medication as prescribed, because drug therapy would have the most immediate effect. Job stress (1) may *then* be considered as a possible cause of increased pressure, if it is determined that the client is complying with drug therapy. Relaxation techniques (2) and weight loss (4) would be useful in reducing the BP but they would not likely be as effective as drug therapy after only 1 month. **EV, ANL, 6, PhI, Physiological adaptation**

3. **(1)** Atenolol, a beta-blocker used in the treatment of hypertension or angina, may mask the symptoms of hypoglycemia and can produce hyperglycemia. There are no known contraindications to its use in clients with gallbladder disease (2), ulcers (3), or intestinal disorders (4). **AS, APP, 6, PhI, Pharmacological and parenteral therapies**

4. **(2)** The purpose of a low sodium diet in a client with hypertension is to minimize fluid retention. The best indication of fluid status and fluid loss is a reduction in body weight. The serum sodium level (1) may be normal and would not reflect changes in the

fluid status. Ankle swelling (**3**) would indicate heart failure or venous pooling. Although the swelling should be less if the client is observing a low sodium diet, it may not reflect a true reduction in the fluid level. If breath sounds (**4**) become congested, this *may* indicate that the heart is not handling the circulating volume (which should decrease with a low sodium diet); however, the breath sounds may also be congested as a result of other causes, such as pneumonia. **EV, EVL, 6, PhI, Reduction of risk potential**

5. (**3**) The client should be advised that captopril may cause taste to be impaired, but the problem generally disappears within 8 to 12 weeks after the start of therapy. Potassium (**1**), as well as sodium, must be *avoided*, unless the MD directs otherwise, because of the risk for electrolyte imbalance. Captopril prevents the production of angiotensin II, resulting in vasodilation. Restricting fluid intake (**2**) may contribute to more severe hypotensive episodes. *Protein, not* glucose (**4**), may be found in the urine of a client taking captopril. **IMP, APP, 6, PhI, Pharmacological and parenteral therapies**

6. (**2**) The serum potassium level may be increased. The serum potassium level would *not* be decreased (**1**), and the sodium level would be decreased, *not* increased (**4**), because the drug blocks the effects of the aldosterone mechanism, which normally conserves sodium and excretes potassium. The white blood cell count would be decreased, *not* increased (**3**). **AN, EVL, 6, PhI, Reduction of risk potential**

7. (**2**) Diuretics should be taken in the morning so the client is not awakened at night by the need to urinate. Generally, fluid intake is not restricted (**1**) as long as the kidneys are working to eliminate any excess fluid. Drinking a beverage (**3**) before bedtime would only increase the likelihood of nocturia. Sleeping with the head elevated (**4**) would help a client breathe more easily if there were problems with heart failure; it would have no bearing on the effects of a diuretic. **IMP, APP, 6, PhI, Pharmacological and parenteral therapies**

8. (**2**) Diazoxide is a vasodilator that produces reflex tachycardia, increased cardiac output, and possibly angina (chest pain). The client should be monitored for hypotension, *not* hypertension (**1**), and tachycardia, *not* bradycardia (**3**). The client may appear flushed, *not* pale (**4**). **EV, ANL, 6, PhI, Pharmacological and parenteral therapies**

9. (**1**) Milk contains the most sodium of the food choices listed. By themselves eggs are not higher in sodium than spinach (**4**), but the combination of eggs and milk should be avoided. Potatoes and rice (**2**), apples and plums (**3**), and carrots (**4**) are very low in sodium. **PL, APP, 4, PhI, Basic care and comfort**

10. (**4**) The normal aPTT is 25 to 38 seconds; the desired time is 1½ to 2 times the control (usually 50 to 80 seconds). A time of 75 seconds would therefore be desired. Vitamin K (**1**) is not the antidote to heparin; protamine sulfate would be given to control excessive anticoagulation resulting from heparin therapy. Heparin treatment should *not* be discontinued (**2**). Observing for bleeding (**3**) is important, because bleeding is always a risk of anticoagulation therapy, but the best action to take in this client is to continue therapy. **EV, SYN, 6, PhI, Reduction of risk potential**

11. (**3**) Heparin is given IV or subcutaneously and is more rapid acting than *Coumadin*. *Coumadin* is taken PO, and it takes days for a therapeutic blood level of the agent to be reached. Once the prothrombin level or INR is within a therapeutic range, the client will be discharged home on a regimen of *Coumadin*. The two drugs do *not* potentiate each other's effects (**1 and 4**). Each drug affects a different clotting component, and the risk of bleeding associated with treatment with either agent alone is as great as, not less than (**2**), that associated with treatment with the two together. **IMP, COM, 6, PhI, Pharmacological and parenteral therapies**

12. (**2**) Green leafy vegetables are high in vitamin K, which would interfere with the anticoagulant effects of *Coumadin*. The other foods (**1, 3, and 4**) *may* be eaten by clients taking *Coumadin*. **IMP, APP, 4, PhI, Pharmacological and parenteral therapies**

13. (**1**) The greatest concern in a client with thrombophlebitis is that a clot may be dislodged from the vein and migrate to the lungs (pulmonary emboli), causing respiratory distress, or to the brain, causing a stroke. Dyspnea is a symptom of a pulmonary embolus. Petechiae (**2**) are pinpoint hemorrhages on the skin and mucous membranes and result from fat emboli or bleeding disorders. Hematuria (**3**), or blood in the urine, would be a side effect of anticoagulant therapy or indicate the presence of bladder or kidney disease. Tetany (**4**), or carpopedal spasms, is associated with, for example, a low calcium level resulting from hypoparathyroidism. **AS, COM, 6, PhI, Physiological adaptation**

14. (**3**) A hallmark of arterial insufficiency is decreased or absent arterial pulses; the pedal pulse is one. The toenails, *not* the soles (**1**) thicken in arterial insufficiency. The condition in option **2** is seen in venous insufficiency. The limb would be hairless, *not* hairy (**4**), in arterial insufficiency. **AS, EVL, 6, PhI, Physiological adaptation**

15. (**4**) The aPTT is an important and very sensitive way of screening for coagulation disorders. It is also used to monitor the effects of heparin therapy. The red blood cell count (**1**) and hematocrit (**3**) are *not* coagulation studies. The prothrombin time (**2**) is also used in diagnostic coagulation studies, but the aPTT is *more* sensitive. The prothrombin time is used to monitor the effects of *Coumadin* therapy. **AS, COM, 6, PhI, Reduction of risk potential**

Key to Codes

Nursing process: AS, assessment; AN, analysis; PL, planning; IMP, implementation; EV, evaluation. (See **Appendix M** for explanation of nursing process steps.)

Cognitive level: RE/KN, recall/knowledge; COM, comprehension; APP, application; ANL, analysis; EVL, evaluation; SYN, synthesis. (See **Appendix M** for explanation.)

Category of human function: 1, protective; 2, sensory-perceptual; 3, comfort, rest, activity, and mobility; 4, nutrition; 5, growth and development; 6, fluid-gas transport; 7, psychosocial-cultural; 8, elimination. (See **Appendix 0** for explanation.)

Client need: SECE, safe, effective care environment; PhI, physiological integrity; PsI, psychosocial integrity; HPM, health promotion and maintenance. (See **Appendix P** for explanation.)

Client subneed: (See **Appendix P** for explanation)

[Handwritten notes:]
LV failure leads to RV failure

Left ♡ failure - crackles, dyspnea

Right ♡ failure - edema (cor pulmonale)

Cardiac Structure Disorders

Chapter Outline

Cardiac Valvular Defects

Alteration in the structure of a valve; impedes flow of blood or permits regurgitation; often associated with an inflammatory response resulting from an infection.

I. **Pathophysiology**

   A. *Stenosis*—narrowing of valvular opening due to adherence, thickening, and rigidity of valve cusp.

   B. *Insufficiency* (incompetence)—incomplete closure of valve due to contraction of chordae tendineae, papillary muscles, or to calcification, scarring of leaflets.

   C. **Mitral stenosis:**
   1. Narrowing of mitral valve.
   2. Most common residual cardiac lesion of rheumatic fever.
   3. Affects *women* <45 yr more often than men.
   4. Interferes with filling of left ventricle.
   5. Produces pulmonary hypertension, right-ventricular failure.

   D. **Mitral insufficiency** (incompetence):
   1. Leaking/regurgitation of blood back into left atrium.
   2. Results from myocardial infarction, chronic rheumatic heart disease; bacterial endocarditis less common.
   3. Affects *men* more often.
   4. Produces pulmonary congestion, ventricular heart failure.

   E. **Aortic stenosis:**
   1. Fusion of valve flaps between left ventricle and aorta.
   2. Congenital or acquired from atherosclerosis or bacterial endocarditis; seen in *men* more often; pulmonary circulation congested, cardiac output decreased.

   F. **Aortic insufficiency:**
   1. Incomplete closure of valve between left ventricle and aorta (regurgitation).
   2. Left ventricular failure leading to right ventricular failure.

II. **Risk factors/causes:**

   A. Congenital abnormality.
   B. History of rheumatic fever.
   C. Atherosclerosis.

III. **Assessment: Table 3.1.**

IV. **Analysis/nursing diagnosis**

   A. *Decreased cardiac output* related to inadequate ventricular filling.
   B. *Fluid volume excess* related to compensatory response to decreased cardiac output.
   C. *Impaired gas exchange* related to pulmonary congestion.
   D. *Activity intolerance* related to impaired cardiac function.
   E. *Fatigue* related to poor oxygenation.

V. **Nursing care plan/implementation**

   A. Goal: *reduce cardiac workload.*
   B. Goal: *promote physical comfort and psychological support.*
   C. Goal: *prevent complications.*
   D. Goal: *prepare client for surgery* (commissurotomy, valvuloplasty, or valvular replacement, depending on defect and severity of condition).
   E. See **Cardiac Surgery, p. 30-31,** for specific nursing actions.

VI. **Evaluation/outcome criteria**

   A. Relief of symptoms.
   B. Increase in activity level.
   C. No complications following surgery.

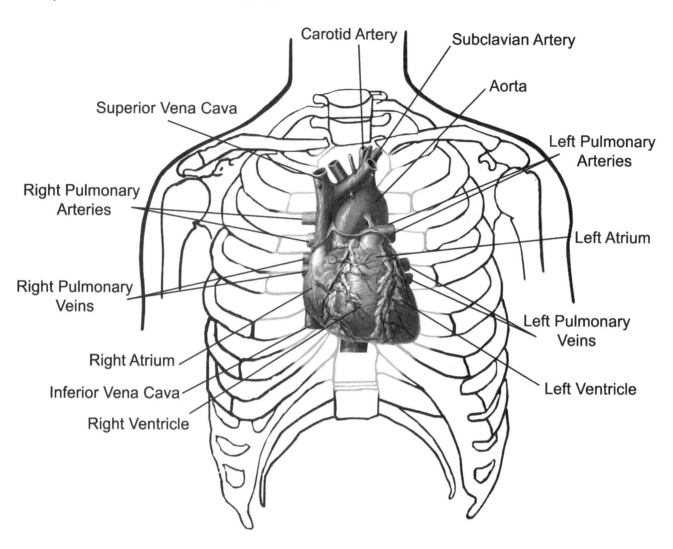

Carotid Artery

Subclavian Artery

Aorta

Superior Vena Cava

Left Pulmonary Arteries

Right Pulmonary Arteries

Left Atrium

Right Pulmonary Veins

Left Pulmonary Veins

Right Atrium

Inferior Vena Cava

Left Ventricle

Right Ventricle

Surface projection of the heart and great vessels on the anterior body wall

Cardiac Catheterization

A diagnostic procedure to evaluate cardiac status. Introduces a catheter into the heart, blood vessels; analyzes blood samples for oxygen content, cardiac output, pulmonary artery blood flow; done prior to heart surgery; frequently combined with angiography to visualize coronary arteries; also provides access for specialized cardiac techniques (e.g., internal pacing and coronary angioplasty).

I. **Approaches:**
   A. *Right-heart* catheterization—venous approach (antecubital or femoral) → right atrium → right ventricle → pulmonary artery.
   B. *Left-heart* catheterization—retrograde approach: right brachial artery or percutaneous puncture of femoral artery → ascending aorta → left ventricle.
      1. Transseptal: femoral vein → right atrium → septum → left atrium → left ventricle.

   2. *Angiography/arteriography*: done during left-heart catheterization.

II. **Precatheterization**
   A. **Assessment**
      1. *Subjective data:*
         a. Allergies: iodine, seafood.
         b. Anxiety.
      2. *Objective data:*
         a. Vital signs: baseline data.
         b. Distal pulses: mark for reference after catheterization.
   B. **Analysis/nursing diagnosis**
      1. *Anxiety* related to fear of unknown.
      2. *Knowledge deficit* related to difficulty learning or limited exposure to information.
   C. **Nursing care plan/implementation**
      1. Goal: *provide for safety, comfort.*
         a. Signed informed consent.
         b. *NPO* (except for medications 6–8 h before).

TABLE 3.1 COMPARISON OF SYMPTOMATOLOGY OF VALVULAR DEFECTS

⋈ Assessment	Mitral Stenosis	Mitral Insuffiency	Aortic Stenosis	Aortic Insuffiency
Subjective Data				
Fatigue	✓	✓	✓	✓
Shortness of breath	✓			
Orthopnea	✓		✓	✓
Paroxysmal nocturnal dyspnea (PND)	✓		✓	✓
Cough	✓	✓		
Dyspnea on exertion (DOE)		✓	✓	✓
Palpitations		✓	✓	
Syncope on exertion			✓	
Angina			✓	✓
Weight loss		✓		
Objective Data				
Vital signs *Blood pressure:*				
Low or normal	✓	✓		
Normal or elevated			✓	✓
Pulse:				
Weak, irregular	✓	✓		
Rapid, "waterhammer"				✓
Respirations: Increased, shallow	✓			
Cyanosis	✓			
Jugular vein distention	✓			
Enlarged liver	✓		✓	
Dependent edema	✓		✓	
Murmur	✓	✓	✓	✓

(handwritten note in Aortic Stenosis column: SAD: shortness of breath, angina, dyspnea)

Source: ©Lagerquist, SI,: *Little, Brown's NCLEX-RN® Examination Review.* Boston: Little, Brown, (out of print).

   c. Have client urinate before going to lab.

⊂▭ d. Give sedatives, as ordered, 30 min before procedure (e.g., midazolam HC1 [*Versed*]).

  2. Goal: **health teaching.**

   a. Procedure: duration (1–3 h).

   b. Expectations (strapped to table for safety, must be still, awake but mildly sedated).

   c. Sensations (hot, flushed feeling in head with injection of contrast medium; thudding in chest from premature beats during catheter manipulation; desire to cough, particularly with right-heart angiography and contrast medium injection).

   d. Alert physician to unusual sensations (coolness, numbness, paresthesia).

III. **Postcatheterization**

⋈ A. **Assessment** (potential complications):

  1. *Subjective data:*

   a. Puncture site: increasing pain, tenderness.

   b. Palpitations.

   c. Affected extremity: tingling numbness, pain from hematoma or nerve damage.

  2. *Objective data:*

   a. Vital signs: shock, respiratory distress (related to pulmonary emboli, allergic reaction).

   b. Puncture site: swelling, bleeding (hematoma).

〰 c. ECG: arrhythmias, signs of MI.

   d. Affected extremity: color, temperature, peripheral pulses.

⋈ B. **Analysis/nursing diagnosis**

  1. *Decreased cardiac output* related to arrhythmias or MI.

  2. *Altered tissue perfusion* related to bleeding or thrombus formation following procedure.

  3. *Pain* related to puncture site tenderness.

⋈ C. **Nursing care plan/implementation**

  1. Goal: *prevent complications.*

   a. Bed rest: 3–6 h; with femoral approach, *supine position*, 12–24 h on bed rest;

encourage ankle flexion, extension, and rotation.

   b. Vital signs: record q15 min for 1 h, q30 min for 3 h or until stable; check BP on opposite extremity.

   c. Puncture site: observe for bleeding, swelling, inflammation, or tenderness; check pulse distal to insertion site to determine patency of artery; report complaints of coolness, numbness, or paresthesia in extremity.

   d. ECG: monitor, document rhythm.

   e. Give medications as ordered: *sedatives, mild narcotics, antiarrhythmics.*

  2. Goal: *provide emotional support.*

   a. Explanations: brief, accurate; client anxious to learn results of test.

   b. Counseling: refer as indicated.

  3. Goal: **health teaching.**

   a. Late complications: infection.

   b. Prepare for surgery if indicated.

   c. Follow-up medical care.

D. **Evaluation/outcome criteria:** no complications (e.g., cardiac arrest, hematoma at insertion site).

Percutaneous Transluminal Coronary Angioplasty (PTCA)

A balloon-tipped catheter is threaded to site of coronary occlusion and inflated repeatedly until blood flow increases distal to the obstruction; a nonsurgical alternative to bypass surgery for coronary artery occlusion; recommended in clients with poorly controlled angina, mild or no symptoms, multiple- or single-vessel disease with a noncalcified, discrete, and proximal lesion that can be reached by the catheter; costs less and requires shorter hospitalization and rehabilitation period (see **Cardiac Catheterization,** for nursing process). An **intravascular stent,** a coilspring tube, may be placed in the coronary artery, and the stent acts as a mechanical scaffold to reopen the blocked artery. The client will receive *anticoagulant* and *antiplatelet* therapy following the procedure. **Excimer Laser Coronary Angioplasty (ELCA),** or laser angioplasty, uses a cool laser to dissolve blockages in the coronary arteries. **Atherectomy** also may be done. In this procedure a cutter is positioned against the blockage and mechanically debrides the plaque.

Cardiac Surgery

Done to alter the structure of the heart or vessels when the following congenital or acquired disorders interfere with cardiac functioning: septal defects; transposition of great vessels; tetralogy of Fallot; mitral/aortic stenosis; coronary artery bypass; valve replacement or repair. **Cardiopulmonary bypass** (used in open-heart

surgery): blood from cardiac chambers and great vessels is diverted into a pump oxygenator; allows full visualization of heart during surgery; maintains perfusion and body functioning.

I. **Preoperative care**

A. **Assessment**

  1. See specific conditions for preoperative signs and symptoms (i.e., valvular defects, angina, MI); see also **Preoperative Preparation, p. 127-129.**

  2. Establish complete baseline: daily weight; vital signs—integrity of all pulses, BP both arms; central venous pressure (CVP) or pulmonary artery pressures; neurologic status; emotional status; nutritional and elimination patterns.

  3. Lab values—urine, complete blood count, electrolytes, enzymes, coagulation studies.

  4. Pulmonary function studies.

B. **Analysis/nursing diagnosis** (see also **Myocardial Infarction, p. 46**)

  1. *Decreased cardiac output* related to myocardial damage.

  2. *Activity intolerance* related to poor cardiac function.

  3. *Knowledge deficit* related to insufficient time for teaching.

  4. *Anxiety* related to fear of unknown.

  5. *Fear* related to possible death.

  6. *Spiritual distress* related to possible death.

C. **Nursing care plan/implementation**

  1. Goal: *provide emotional and spiritual support.*

   a. Arrange for religious consultation if desired.

   b. Provide opportunity for family visit morning of surgery.

   c. Encourage verbalization/questions; fear, depression, despair frequently occur.

  2. Goal: **health teaching.**

   a. Diagnostic procedures, treatments, specifics for surgery (i.e., leg incision with use of saphenous vein in coronary artery bypass surgery).

   b. Postoperative regimen: turn, cough, deep breathe, ROM, equipment used, medication for pain.

   c. Tour ICU; meet personnel.

   d. Alternative method of communication while intubated.

D. Evaluation/outcome criteria

  1. Displays moderate anxiety level.

  2. Verbalizes/demonstrates postoperative expectations.

  3. Quits smoking before surgery.

II. **Postoperative care**

A. **Assessment**

  1. *Subjective data:*

   a. Pain.

b. Fatigue—sleep deprivation.
2. *Objective data:*
   a. **Neurologic**: level of consciousness; pupillary reactions; movement of limbs (purposeful, spontaneous).
   b. **Respiratory**: rate changes (*increases* occur with obstruction, pain; *decreases* occur with CO_2 retention); depth (shallow with pain, atelectasis); symmetry; skin *color; patency/drainage* from chest tubes; *sputum* (amount, color); endotracheal tube placement (bilateral breath sounds).
   c. **Cardiovascular:**
      (1) BP—*hypotension* may indicate heart failure, tamponade, hemorrhage, arrhythmias, or thrombosis; *hypertension* may indicate anxiety, hypervolemia.
      (2) Pulse: radial, apical, pedal; rate (> 100 beats/min may indicate pain, shock, fever, hypoxia, arrhythmias); rhythm, quality.
      ☞(3) CVP or pulmonary artery pressure (*elevated* in cardiac failure); temperature (normal post-op: 98.6°-101.6°F oral).
   d. **Gastrointestinal (GI)**: nausea, vomiting, distention. Check abdominal incisions if gastroepiploic or inferior epigastric artery is used for coronary artery graft.
   e. **Renal**: urine—minimum output (30 mL/h); color; specific gravity (< 1.010 occurs with *overhydration*, renal tubular damage; > 1.020 present with *dehydration*, oliguria, blood in urine).
▶ B. **Analysis/nursing diagnosis**
   1. *Decreased cardiac output* related to decreased myocardial contractility or postoperative hypothermia.
   2. *Pain* related to incision.
   3. *Ineffective airway clearance* related to effects of general anesthesia.
   4. *Altered tissue perfusion* related to postoperative bleeding or thromboemboli.
   5. *Fluid volume deficit* related to blood loss.
   6. *Risk for infection* related to wound contamination.
   7. *Altered thought processes* related to anesthesia, medications or stress.
   8. *Body image disturbance* related to incision or limitations.
   9. *Sleep pattern disturbance* related to ICU environment or pain.
▶ C. **Nursing care plan/implementation**
   1. Goal: *provide constant monitoring to prevent complications.*
      a. **Respiratory:**
         (1) Observe for respiratory distress: restlessness, nasal flaring, *Cheyne-Stokes respiration*, dusky/cyanotic skin; assisted or controlled ventilation via *endotracheal* tube common first 24 h; supplemental O_2 after extubation.
         ☞(2) *Suctioning*; cough, deep breathe.
         (3) *Elevate* head of bed.
         (4) Position chest tube to facilitate drainage; mediastinal drain maintains patency—"milking" not necessary. See also **chest tube care** in **Chap. 6, p. 86-88.**
      b. **Cardiovascular:**
         (1) *Vital signs*: BP > 80-90 mm Hg systolic; CVP: range 2–10 mm Hg unless otherwise ordered; pulmonary artery line: mean pressure 4–12 mm Hg; I&O: report <30 mL of urine/h from indwelling urinary catheter.
         〰(2) ECG; PVCs occur most frequently following aortic valve replacement and bypass surgery.
         (3) Peripheral pulses if leg veins used for grafting.
         ☞(4) Activity: turn q2h; ROM; progressive, early ambulation.
      c. Inspect dressing for bleeding.
      d. Medications according to therapeutic directives—*cardiotonics* (digoxin); *coronary vasodilators* (nitrates); *antibiotics, diuretics; analgesics; anticoagulant*s (with valve replacements); *antiarrhythmics* (quinidine, procainamide HC1 [*Pronestyl*]).
   2. Goal: *promote comfort, pain relief.*
      a. Medicate: *Demerol or morphine* sulfate, as severe pain lasts 2–3 d.
      b. Splint incision when moving or coughing.
      c. Mouth care: keep lips moist.
      d. *Position*: use pillows to prevent tension on chest tubes, incision.
   3. Goal: *maintain fluid, electrolyte, nutritional balance.*
      a. I&O (initially hourly output); urine specific gravity.
      b. Measure chest tube drainage—should not exceed 200 mL/h for first 4-6 h.
      c. Give fluids as ordered; maintain *IV patency.*
      d. *Diet*: clear fluids → solid food if no nausea, GI distention; sodium intake restricted, low fat intake.
   4. Goal: *promote emotional adjustment.*
      a. Anticipate behavior disturbances (depression, disorientation often occur

3 d postop) related to medications, fear, sleep deprivation.

    b. Calm, oriented, supportive environment, as personalized as possible.

    c. Encourage verbalization of feelings (family and client).

    d. Encourage independence to avoid cardiac-cripple role.

  5. Goal: **health teaching.**

    a. Alterations in life-style, activity, diet, work.

    b. Available community resources for cardiac rehabilitation (e.g., American Heart Association, Mended Hearts).

    c. Drug regimen: purpose, side effects.

    d. Potential complications: dyspnea, pain, palpitations common postoperatively.

D. Evaluation/outcome criteria

  1. No complications; incision heals.

  2. Activity level increases—no signs of overexertion (e.g., fatigue, dyspnea, pain).

  3. Relief of symptoms.

  4 Returns for follow-up medical care.

  5. Takes prescribed medications; knows purposes and side effects.

Pericarditis

Inflammation of parietal and/or visceral pericardium; acute or chronic condition; may occur with or without effusion.

I. Pathophysiology: fibrosis or accumulation of fluid in pericardium → compression of cardiac pumping → decreased cardiac output → increased systemic, pulmonic venous pressure.

II. Risk factors/causes:

  A. Bacterial, viral, and/or fungal infections.

  B. Tuberculosis.

  C. Collagen diseases.

  D. Uremia.

  E. Transmural MI.

  F. Trauma.

III. Assessment

  A. *Subjective data:*

    1. Pain:

      a. *Type*—sharp, moderate to severe.

      b. *Location*—wide area of pericardium, may radiate; right arm, jaw/teeth.

      c. *Precipitating factors*—movement, deep inspiration, swallowing, lying supine.

    2. Chills; sweating.

    3. Apprehension; anxiety.

    4. Fatigue.

    5. Abdominal pain.

    6. Shortness of breath.

  B. *Objective data:*

    1. *Vital signs*:

      a. BP: *decreased* pulse pressure; pulsus paradoxus—abnormal drop in systemic BP of >8–10 mm Hg during inspiration.

      b. Pulse: tachycardia.

      c. Temperature: *elevated*; erratic course; low grade.

    2. Pericardial friction rub (*hallmark finding*).

    3. *Increased* CVP, distended neck veins, dependent pitting edema, liver engorgement.

    4. Restlessness.

    5. Lab data: *elevated* AST(SGOT); WBC; chest x-ray—cardiac enlargement.

IV. Analysis/nursing diagnosis

  A. *Decreased cardiac output* related to impaired cardiac pumping ability.

  B. *Pain* related to pericardial inflammation.

  C. *Anxiety* related to unknown outcome.

  D. *Fatigue* related to inadequate oxygenation.

  E. *Ineffective breathing pattern* related to discomfort during inspiration.

V. Nursing care plan/implementation

  A. Goal: *promote physical and emotional comfort.*

    1. *Position*: semi-Fowler's (upright or sitting); bed rest.

    2. *Vital signs*: q2–4h and prn: *apical* and *radial* pulse; notify physician if heart sounds decrease in amplitude or if pulse pressure *narrows*, indicating cardiac tamponade; cooling measures as indicated.

    3. O_2 as ordered.

    4. Medications as ordered:

      a. *Analgesics*—aspirin, morphine sulfate.

      b. *Nonsteroidal anti-inflammatory drug*s (NSAIDs).

      c. *Antibiotics.*

      d. *Digitalis* and *diuretics*, if heart failure present.

    5. Assist with aspiration of pericardial sac (pericardiocentesis) if needed: medicate as ordered; *elevate head* 60 degrees; monitor ECG; have defibrillator and pacemaker available.

    6. Prepare for pericardiectomy (excision of constricting pericardium) as ordered.

    7. Continual emotional support.

    8. Enhance effects of analgesics: positioning; turning; warm drinks.

    9. Monitor for *signs of cardiac tamponade*: tachycardia; tachypnea; hypotension; pallor; narrowed pulse pressure; pulsus paradoxus; distended neck veins.

  B. Goal: *maintain fluid, electrolyte balance.*

    1. Parenteral fluids as ordered; strict I&O.

    2. Assist with feedings; *low sodium diet* may be ordered.

▶◀ **VI. Evaluation/outcome criteria**
    A. Relief of pain, dyspnea.
    B. No complications (e.g., cardiac tamponade).
    C. Return of normal cardiac functioning.

🗝 Summary of Key Points

1. Structural damage is often associated with an inflammatory response resulting from an infection.
2. A **mitral valve** defect is the most prevalent valvular disorder.
3. A **murmur** will be found on auscultation if valvular stenosis or regurgitation is present.
4. Pericardial friction rub and fever are classic signs of **acute pericarditis.**
5. Coronary arteries are assessed during **left-heart catheterization.**
6. **Normal heart sounds** (high pitched) are best heard with the diaphragm of the stethoscope, and abnormal sounds such as gallops (low pitched) are best heard with the bell.

💡 Study and Memory Aids

Prior to cardiac catheterization: ✓ for shellfish or iodine allergy.

Cardiac Surgery: Behavior Modification

⌐ Drug Review

Cardiac Valvular Defects

Aortic stenosis
    Antibiotic before invasive procedures
    Digitalis
    Diuretics
Mitral regurgitation
    Angiotensin-converting enzyme
    Nitrates
Mitral stenosis
    Anticoagulants
    Beta-blockers
    Digitalis
    Diuretics
Mitral valve prolapse
    Antibiotics
    Beta-blockers

Cardiac Catheterization

Antiarrhythmics—Procainamide (*Pronestyl*).
Local anesthesia
Sedative for relaxation before procedure.

Percutaneous Transluminal Coronary Angioplasty

Anticoagulation therapy during procedure.
Aspirin or dipyridamole (*Persantine*) for long-term use after procedure.

Pericarditis

Antibiotic therapy
Aspirin
Nonsteroidal anti-inflammatory agent

〰 Diagnostic Studies/Procedures

〰 *Noninvasive Diagnostic Procedures*
Multiple-gated acquisition scan (MUGA)—also known as *blood pool imaging*. Red blood cells are tagged with a radioactive isotope. A computer-operated camera takes sequential pictures of actual heart-wall motion; *complement* to cardiac catheterization; *used to*: determine valvular effectiveness, follow progress of heart disease, diagnose cardiac aneurysms, detect coronary artery disease, determine effects of cardiovascular drug therapy. No special preparation. Painless, except for injections. Wear *gloves* if contact with client urine occurs within 24 h after scan.

Doppler ultrasonography—*used to* measure blood flow in the major veins and arteries. The transducer of the test instrument is placed on the skin, sending out bursts of ultra-high-frequency sound. The ratio of ankle to brachial systolic pressure (API ≥ 1) provides information about vascular insufficiency. Sound varies with respiration and the Valsalva maneuver. No discomfort to the client.

〰 *Invasive Diagnostic Procedures*
Cardiac catheterization—insertion of a radiopaque catheter into a vein to study the heart and great vessels.
    Right-heart catheterization—catheter is inserted through a cutdown in the antecubital vein into the superior vena cava and through the right atrium, ventricle, and into the pulmonary artery.
    Left-heart catheterization—catheter may be passed retrogradely to the left ventricle through the brachial or femoral artery; it can be passed into the left atrium after right-heart catheterization by means of a special needle that punctures the septa; or it may be passed directly into the left ventricle by means of a posterior or anterior chest puncture.
    Cardiac catheterization is *used to*:
    • Confirm diagnosis of heart disease and determine the extent of disease.
    • Determine existence and extent of congenital abnormalities.
    • Measure pressures in the heart chambers and great vessels.

- Obtain estimate of cardiac output.
- Obtain blood samples to measure oxygen content and determine presence of cardiac shunts.

⋈ *Specific Nursing Interventions*
Preprocedure client teaching:
- Fatigue due to lying still for 3 h or more is a common complaint.
- Some fluttery sensations may be felt—occurs as catheter is passed backward into the left ventricle. Flushed, warm feeling may occur when contrast medium is injected.

☞ *Postprocedure observations*:
〰 • Monitor ECG pattern for arrhythmias.
- Check extremities for color and temperature, peripheral pulses (femoral and dorsalis pedis) for quality, puncture sites for bleeding and hematoma.

Questions

1. The nurse knows that a client understands what to expect after open-heart surgery if he says:
   1. "I won't be able to have sexual intercourse for 6 months after the surgery."
   2. "I will be on a ventilator for a while after the surgery."
   3. "I can't return to work as a carpenter after the surgery."
   4. "After the surgery I won't have to take any of my cardiac medications."

2. The nurse would expect urine output to be significantly increased in a client who undergoes cardiac catheterization because:
   1. Cardiac output would be improved.
   2. The contrast medium used has a diuretic effect.
   3. Myocardial perfusion would be restored.
   4. Fluids are given IV during the procedure.

3. A client who undergoes angioplasty and stent placement to eliminate a blockage in the left coronary artery is given one enteric-coated aspirin daily for its:
   1. Antipyretic action.
   2. Analgesic effect.
   3. Anticoagulatant action.
   4. Anti-inflammatory effect.

4. A client who has undergone a femoropopliteal bypass graft complains of pain and appears restless; nail beds and lips are slightly cyanotic, and skin is cool. What should the nurse do first?
   1. Check the vital signs.
   2. Elevate the affected leg.
   3. Assess the level of consciousness.
   4. Call the MD immediately.

Answers/Rationale

1. (2) All clients who undergo open-heart surgery are mechanically ventilated for a while after the surgery to reduce the effort of breathing and the work of the heart. The resumption of sexual activity (1), the ability to return to work (3), and the medication regimen (4) would be all "unknowns" at the time of preoperative teaching. **EV, EVL, 6, HPM, Health promotion and maintenance**

2. (2) The contrast medium, which usually has an iodine base, produces diuresis. The test is done to determine the status of cardiac function. The test does not cause cardiac output (1) or myocardial perfusion (3) to be improved. The amount of fluids infused IV during the procedure (4) is not significant enough to cause an increase in urine output. **AN, EVL, 6, PhI, Physiological adaptation**

3. (3) A low dose of aspirin is prescribed for its anticoagulant action; aspirin has this effect because it interferes with the adherence of platelets. The other actions (1, 2, and 4) are also properties of aspirin but not ones that constitute the reason for *this* client needing to take an aspirin daily. **IMP, RE/KN, 6, PhI, Pharmacological and parenteral therapies**

4. (1) These are symptoms of poor perfusion and hypoxemia. Vital signs should therefore be assessed to determine whether shock has occurred. If shock is diagnosed, the head of the client's bed should be lowered and the leg, or legs, elevated (2), as appropriate. The level of consciousness (3) has already changed. The MD should be called (4) *after* the data are gathered. **PL, ANL, 6, PhI, Physiological adaptation**

Key to Codes

Nursing process: **AS**, assessment; **AN**, analysis; **PL**, planning; **IMP**, implementation; **EV**, evaluation. (See **Appendix M** for explanation of nursing process steps.)

Cognitive level: **RE/KN**, recall/knowledge; **COM**, comprehension; **APP**, application; **ANL**, analysis; **EVL**, evaluation; **SYN**, synthesis. (See **Appendix M** for explanation.)

Category of human function: 1, protective; 2, sensory-perceptual; 3, comfort, rest, activity, and mobility; 4, nutrition; 5, growth and development; 6, fluid-gas transport; 7, psychosocial-cultural; 8, elimination. (See **Appendix 0** for explanation.)

Client need: **SECE**, safe, effective care environment; **PhI**, physiological integrity; **PsI**, psychosocial integrity; **HPM**, health promotion and maintenance. (See **Appendix P** for explanation.)

Client subneed: (See **Appendix P** for explanation)

Cardiac Function Disorders

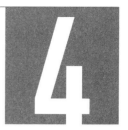

Chapter Outline

- **Cardiac Dysrhythmias**
  - Pacemaker insertion
- **Cardiac Arrest**
  - CPR
- **Angina Pectoris**
- **Myocardial Infarction**
- **Heart Failure**
- **Pulmonary Edema**
- **Summary of Key Points**
- **Study and Memory Aids**

- Diagnostic Studies and Procedures
  - ECG
  - Echocardiography
  - Phonocardiography
  - Angiocardiography
  - Angiography
  - Nuclear cardiology
- Diets
- Drug review
- **Questions**
- **Answers/Rationale**

Cardiac Dysrhythmias

Any variation in normal rate, rhythm, or configuration of waves on ECG (**Figure 4.1**).

I. **Pathophysiology**
   A. Dysfunction of SA node, atria, AV node, or ventricular conduction.
   B. Primary heart problem or secondary systemic problem.

II. **Risk factors/causes:**
   A. Myocardial infarction (MI).
   B. Drug toxicity.
   C. Stress.
   D. Cardiac surgery.
   E. Hypoxia.
   F. Conduction defects.
   G. Electrolyte imbalances.
   H. See also **Table 4.1**.

III. **Assessment:** see **Table 4.1** for specific dysrhythmias.

IV. **Analysis/nursing diagnosis**
   A. *Decreased cardiac output* related to abnormal ventricular function.
   B. *Altered tissue perfusion* related to inadequate cardiac functioning.
   C. *Risk for injury (death)* related to improper cardiac function.
   D. *Risk for activity intolerance* related to inadequate oxygenation.
   E. *Anxiety* related to dependence, fear of death.

V. **Nursing care plan/implementation**
   A. Goal: *provide for emotional and safety needs.*
   1. Obtain ECG to document dysrhythmia
   2. Encourage discussion of fears, feelings.

   3. *Bed rest*, restricted activities, quiet environment, limit visitors.
   4. Oxygen, if ordered.
   5. Check vital signs frequently for shock, heart failure (HF), drug toxicity.
   6. Prepare for cardiac emergency: CPR.
   7. Give *cardiac* medications; check lab results for digitalis and potassium levels, to prevent drug toxicity.
   B. Goal: *prevent thromboemboli.*
   1. Apply antiembolic stockings (TED hose).
   2. Give *anticoagulants* as ordered
      a. Check for bleeding—gums, urine.
      b. Monitor lab results—Lee White clotting time and activated partial thromboplastin time [aPTT] with heparin; prothrombin time [PT] and INR with *Coumadin.*
   3. Encourage flexion-extension of feet.
   C. Goal: *provide for physical and emotional needs with pacemaker insertion.*
   1. *General concerns:*
      a. Report excessive bleeding/infection at insertion site—hematoma may contribute to wound infection.
      b. Encourage verbalization of feelings.
      c. Report prolonged hiccoughs, which may indicate pacemaker failure.
      d. Know pacing mode: fixed-rate or demand (most common).
   2. **Temporary pacemaker:**
      a. *Limit excessive activity of extremity* if antecubital insertion, to prevent displacement; subclavian insertion increases catheter stability.
      b. Secure wires to chest to prevent tension on catheter.

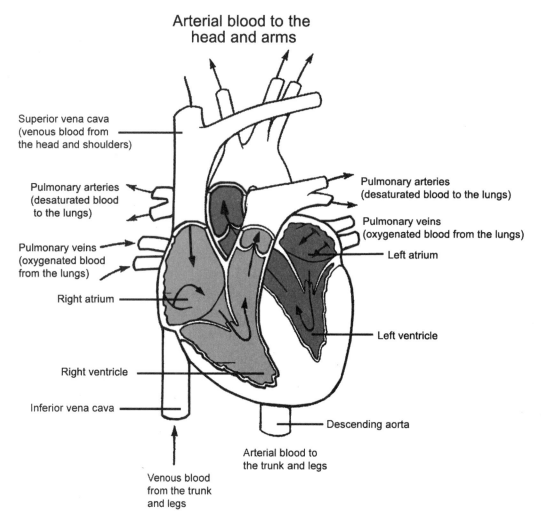

Arterial blood to the
head and arms

Superior vena cava
(venous blood from
the head and shoulders)

Pulmonary arteries
(desaturated blood
to the lungs)

Pulmonary arteries
(desaturated blood to the lungs)

Pulmonary veins
(oxygenated blood from the lungs)

Pulmonary veins
(oxygenated blood
from the lungs)

Left atrium

Right atrium

Left ventricle

Right ventricle

Inferior vena cava

Descending aorta

Arterial blood to
the trunk and legs

Venous blood
from the trunk
and legs

Blood Flow Through the Heart

c. To avoid electrical hazards, do *not* defibrillate over insertion site.

d. Electrical safety (grounding; disconnect electric beds/call lights; use battery-operated equipment; use gloves to change dressing, provide care).

e. If TCP is used, tell client to expect muscle contractions when current passes through chest wall. *Analgesics* can be used.

3. **Permanent pacemaker:**

a. *Limit activity of shoulder* for 48–72 h with transvenous catheter to prevent dislodgement.

b. Postinsertion ROM (passive) at least once per shift after 48 h to prevent frozen shoulder.

4. **Health teaching** following permanent pacemaker:

a. Explain procedure: duration, equipment, purpose, type of pacemaker.

b. MedicAlert bracelet; pacemaker information card.

c. Daily pulse-taking upon arising (report variation of ± 5 beats).

d. Signs, symptoms of: *malfunction* (vertigo, syncope, dyspnea, slowed speech, confusion, fluid retention); *infection* (fever, heat, pain, skin breakdown at insertion site).

e. *Restrictions*: contact sports, electromagnetic interferences (few)—TV/radio transmitters, improperly functioning microwave ovens, certain cautery machines; rarely triggers airport metal detector alarm.

VI. Evaluation/outcome criteria

A. Regular cardiac rhythm; monitors own radial pulse.

B. No complications (e.g., pacemaker malfunction).

C. Returns for regular follow-up of pacemaker function.

D. Tolerates physical or sexual activity.

E. Wears identification bracelet; carries pacemaker identification card.

(A)

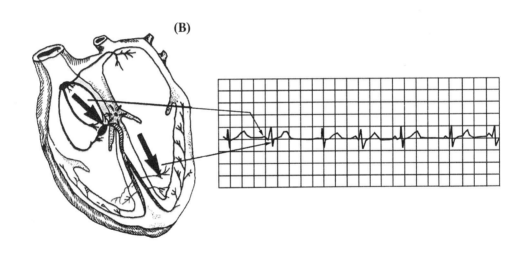

NORMAL SINUS RHYTHM

Rhythm: Regular.

Rate: 60 to 100 per minute.

P waves: Normal, preceding every QRS.

Pacemaker site: SA node.

P—R interval: Normal (0.12—0.20 sec).

QRS complexes: Normal, each preceded by a P wave.

Clinical significance: Normal rhythm.

Treatment: None.

(B)

SINUS ARRHYTHMIA

Rhythm: Regularly irregular; rate increases slightly with inspirations; decreases slightly with expiration.

Rate: Normal.

P waves: Normal, preceding every QRS.

Pacemaker site: SA node.

P—R interval: Normal (0.12—0.20 sec).

QRS complexes: Normal, each QRS preceded by a P wave.

Clinical significance: Sinus arrhythmia is a normal phenomenon, caused by the effects of the parasympathetic nervous system of breathing.

Treatment: None.

FIGURE 4.1 NORMAL SINUS RHYTHM AND ABNORMALITIES: (A) NORMAL SINUS RHYTHM, (B) SINUS ARRHYTHMIA.

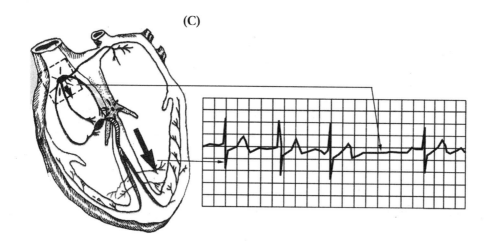

(C)

SINUS ARREST

Rhythm: Irregular.

Rate: May be normal to slow.

P waves: Normal, where present, preceding each QRS. However, if the SA node does not discharge or is blocked, the entire P—QRS—T complex is absent.

Pacemaker site: SA node.

P—R interval: Normal (0.12—0.20 sec).

QRS complexes: Normal, each preceded by a P wave.

Clinical significance: Occasional episodes are not significant; however, if the heart rate is reduced below 30 to 50 per minute, cardiac output may fall and an ectopic focus in the ventricles may take over.

Treatment:

• None necessary if the client is asymptomatic, blood pressure is well maintained, and there is no evidence of ventricular irritability.

• Treatment to increase the heart rate must be undertaken if there are signs of hypoperfusion or atrial or ventricular ectopic arrhythmias.

▭ ATROPINE SULFATE, 0.5 mg, is given by IV bolus in those instances. The dose may be repeated at 5 to 10 minute intervals until the heart rate has increased to 70 or more per minute or until a maximum dose of 2.0 mg of atropine has been given.

FIGURE 4.1 (*cont'd*) **(C) SINUS ARREST.**

Cardiac Arrest

Sudden, unexpected cessation of heartbeats and effective circulation, leading to inadequate perfusion and sudden death.

I. **Risk factors/causes:**
   A. MI.
   B. Multiple traumas.
   C. Respiratory arrest.
   D. Drowning.
   E. Electric shock.
   F. Drug reactions.
   G. Lethal arrythmia.

⋈ II. **Assessment**—*objective data*:
   A. Unresponsive to stimuli (i.e., verbal, painful).
   B. Absence of breathing, carotid pulse.
   C. Pale or bluish: lips, fingernails, skin.
   D. Pupils: dilated.

⋈ III. **Analysis/nursing diagnosis**
   A. *Decreased cardiac output* related to heart failure.
   B. *Impaired gas exchange* related to breathlessness.
   C. *Altered tissue perfusion* related to pulselessness.

⋈ IV. **Nursing care plan/implementation**
   A. Goal: *prevent irreversible cerebral anoxic damage*
   ☞initiate **CPR** within 4–6 min; continue until relieved;   document assessment factors, effectiveness of actions; presence or absence of pulse at 1 min and every 4–5 min.
   B. Goal: *establish effective circulation, respiration*: see **Emergency Nursing Procedures, Chapter 25 p. 349-350**, for complete protocols.

⋈ V. **Evaluation/outcome criteria:**
   A. Carotid pulse present; check after 1 min and every 5 minutes thereafter.
   B. Responds to verbal stimuli.
   C. Pupils constrict in response to light.
   D. Return of spontaneous respiration; adequate ventilation.

TABLE 4.1 COMPARISON OF SELECTED CARDIAC DYSRHYTHMIAS

Dysrhythmia	Description	Etiology	Symptoms/Consequences	Treatment
Dysrhythmia of Sinus Node				
Sinus dysrhythmia	Phasic shortening then lengthening of P-P and R-R interval	Respiratory variation in impulse initiation by SA node	Usually none	Usually none
	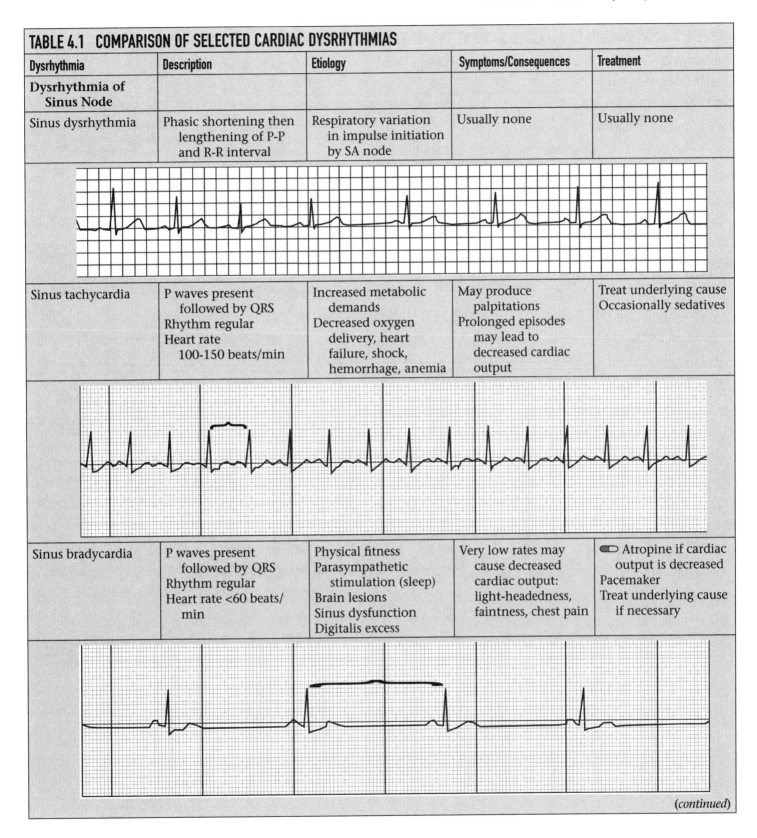			
Sinus tachycardia	P waves present followed by QRS Rhythm regular Heart rate 100-150 beats/min	Increased metabolic demands Decreased oxygen delivery, heart failure, shock, hemorrhage, anemia	May produce palpitations Prolonged episodes may lead to decreased cardiac output	Treat underlying cause Occasionally sedatives
Sinus bradycardia	P waves present followed by QRS Rhythm regular Heart rate <60 beats/min	Physical fitness Parasympathetic stimulation (sleep) Brain lesions Sinus dysfunction Digitalis excess	Very low rates may cause decreased cardiac output: light-headedness, faintness, chest pain	Atropine if cardiac output is decreased Pacemaker Treat underlying cause if necessary

(continued)

TABLE 4.1   COMPARISON OF SELECTED CARDIAC DYSRHYTHMIAS   (*continued*)

Dysrhythmia	Description	Etiology	Symptoms/Consequences	Treatment
Atrial Dysrhythmias				
Premature atrial beats	Early P wave QRS may or may not be normal Rhythm irregular	Stress Ischemia Atrial enlargement Caffeine Nicotine	May produce palpitations Frequent episodes may decrease cardiac output Is sign of chamber irritability	⬭ Sedation ⬭ Quinidine, ⬭ B-adrenergic blockers May require no other treatment

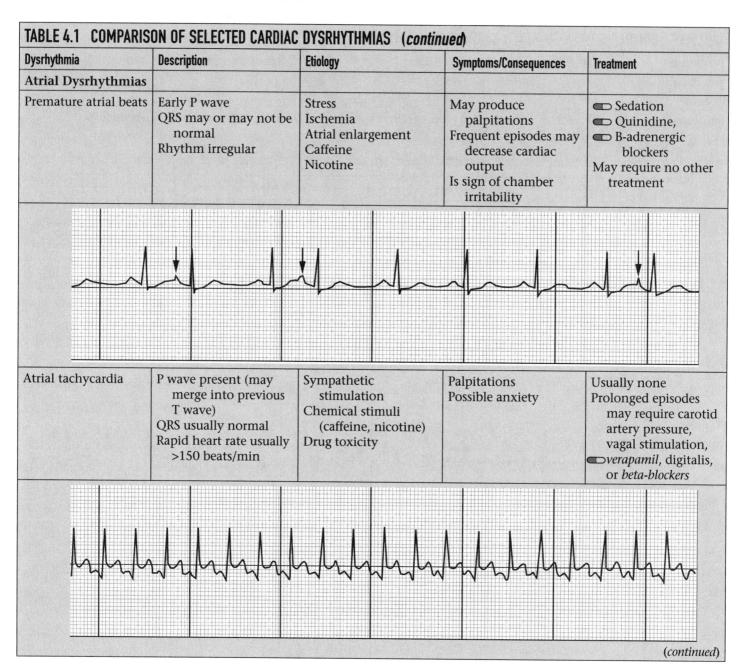

Dysrhythmia	Description	Etiology	Symptoms/Consequences	Treatment
Atrial tachycardia	P wave present (may merge into previous T wave) QRS usually normal Rapid heart rate usually >150 beats/min	Sympathetic stimulation Chemical stimuli (caffeine, nicotine) Drug toxicity	Palpitations Possible anxiety	Usually none Prolonged episodes may require carotid artery pressure, vagal stimulation, ⬭*verapamil*, digitalis, or *beta-blockers*

(*continued*)

TABLE 4.1 COMPARISON OF SELECTED CARDIAC DYSRHYTHMIAS (*continued*)

Dysrhythmia	Description	Etiology	Symptoms/Consequences	Treatment
Atrial fibrillation	No organized atrial electrical activity (>350/min). No effective atrial contraction. Ventricular rhythm irregularly irregular Ventricular rate varies from 50–180 beats/ min if untreated	Rheumatic heart disease Mitral stenosis Atrial infarction Coronary atherosclerotic heart disease Hypertensive heart disease Thyrotoxicosis	Pulse deficit Decreased cardiac output if rate is rapid Promotes thrombus formation in atria	Medications: Amiodarone B-adrenergic blockers Calcium channel blockers Digitalis Procainamide Quinidine Verapamil Cardioversion

Ventricular Dysrhythmias				
Premature ventricular beats (PVBs)	Early wide bizarre QRS, not associated with a P wave Rhythm irregular	Stress Acidosis Ventricular enlargement Electrolyte imbalance Myocardial infarction Digitalis toxicity Hypoxemia, hypercapnia	Same as for premature atrial beats	Medications: Disopyramide (*Norpace*) Lidocaine Mexiletine Potassium Procainamide Quinidine Sodium bicarbonate ☞ Oxygen Treat heart failure

(*continued*)

TABLE 4.1 COMPARISON OF SELECTED CARDIAC DYSRHYTHMIAS (*continued*)

Dysrhythmia	Description	Etiology	Symptoms/Consequences	Treatment
Ventricular tachycardia	No P wave before QRS QRS wide and bizarre Ventricular rate >100, usually 140-240 beats/min	PVB striking during vulnerable period Hypoxemia Drug toxicity Electrolyte imbalance Bradycardia	Decreased cardiac output Hypotension Loss of consciousness Respiratory arrest	Medications: Bretylium Lidocaine Mexiletine Procainamide Cardioversion

Ventricular fibrillation	Chaotic electrical activity No recognizable QRS complex	Myocardial infarction Electrocution Freshwater drowning Drug toxicity	No cardiac output Absent pulse or respiration Cardiac arrest	Defibrillation Bretylium Epinephrine Sodium bicarbonate ☞ CPR

Asystole	Can be distinguished from ventricular fibrillation only by ECG P waves may be present No QRS "Straight line"	Myocardial infarction Chronic disease of conducting system	Same as for ventricular fibrillation	☞ CPR Pacemaker Intravenous epinephrine Isoproterenol

(*continued*)

TABLE 4.1 COMPARISON OF SELECTED CARDIAC DYSRHYTHMIAS (*continued*)

Dysrhythmia	Description	Etiology	Symptoms/Consequences	Treatment
Impulse Conduction Deficits				
First-degree AV block	PR interval prolonged, > 0.20 sec	Rheumatic fever Digitalis toxicity Degenerative changes of coronary atherosclerotic heart disease Infections Decreased oxygen in AV node	Warns of impaired conduction	Usually none as long as it occurs as an isolated deficit

Second-degree AV block	P waves usually occur regularly at rates consistent with SA node initiation; not all P waves followed by QRS; PR interval may lengthen before non-conducted P wave or may be consistent; QRS may be widened.	Acute myocardial infarction	Serious dysrhythmia that may lead to decreased heart rate and cardiac output	May require temporary pacemaker ⬤▭ Atropine ⬤▭ Epinephrine

(*continued*)

TABLE 4.1 COMPARISON OF SELECTED CARDIAC DYSRHYTHMIAS (continued)

Dysrhythmia	Description	Etiology	Symptoms/Consequences	Treatment
Bundle-branch block	Same as normal sinus rhythm except QRS segment duration > 0.10 sec	Hypoxia Acute myocardial infarction Heart failure Coronary atherosclerotic heart disease Pulmonary embolus Hypertension	Same as first-degree AV block	Usually none unless severe blockage of left posterior division

| Complete third-degree AV block | Atria and ventricles beat independently
P waves have no relation to QRS
Ventricular rate may be as low as 20-40 beats/min | Digitalis toxicity
Infectious disease
Coronary artery disease
Myocardial infarction | Very low rates may cause decreased cardiac output: light-headedness, fainting, chest pain | Pacemaker
⬤ Epinephrine (if isoproterenol ineffective)
⬤ Isoproterenol to increase heart rate |

AV = atrioventricular; CPR = cardiopulmonary resuscitation; ECG = electrocardiogram; PVB = premature ventricular beat; SA = sinoatrial node.

TABLE 4.2 ◄ COMPARISON OF PHYSICAL CAUSES OF CHEST PAIN: ASSESSMENT

Characteristic	Myocardial Infarction	Pericarditis	Gastric Disorders	Angina Pectoris	Dissecting Aneurysm	Pulmonary Embolism
Onset	Gradual or sudden	Sudden	Gradual or sudden	Gradual or sudden	Abrupt, without prodromal symptoms	Gradual or sudden
Precipitating factors	Can occur at rest or after exercise or emotional stress	Breathing deeply, rotating trunk, recumbency, swallowing or yawning	Inflammation of stomach or esophagus; hypersecretion of gastric juices; some medications	Usually after: physical exertion, emotional stress, eating, exposure to cold or defecation; unstable angina occurs at rest	Hypertension	Immobility or prolonged bed rest following surgery, trauma, hip fracture, heart failure, malignancy, oral contraceptives
Location	Substernal, anterior chest, or midline; rarely back; radiates to jaw or neck	Precordial; radiates to neck or left shoulder and arm	Xiphoid to umbilicus	Substernal, anterior chest; poorly localized	Correlates with site of intimal rupture; anterior chest or back; between shoulder blades	Pleural area, retrosternal area
Quality	Crushing, burning, stabbing, squeezing or vicelike	Pleuritic, sharp	Aching, burning, cramp-like gnawing	Squeezing, feeling of heavy pressure; burning	Sharp, tearing or ripping sensation	Sharp, stabbing
Intensity	Asymptomatic to severe; increases with time	Mild to severe	Mild to severe	Mild to moderate	Severe and unbearable; maximal from onset	Aggravated by breathing
Duration	30 min to 1–2 h; may wax and wane	Continuous	Periodic	Usually 2–10 min; average 3–5 min	Continuous; does not abate once started	Variable
Relief	Narcotics	*Sitting up*, leaning forward	Physical and emotional *rest*, food, *antacids*, H₂-receptor antagonists	Nitroglycerin *rest*	Large, repeated doses of *narcotics*	O₂; *sitting up*; morphine
Associated symptoms	Nausea, fatigue, heartburn; peripheral pulses equal	Fever, dyspnea, nausea, anorexia, anxiety	Nausea, vomiting, dysphagia, anorexia, weight loss	Belching, indigestion, dizziness	Syncope, loss of sensations or pulses, oliguria, discrepancy between BP in arms; decrease in femoral or carotid pulse	Dyspnea, tachypnea, diaphoresis, hemoptysis, cough, apprehension

Source: ©Lagerquist, S. (ed) *Little Brown's NCLEX-RN® Examination Review.*

Angina Pectoris

Transient paroxysmal episodes of substernal or precordial pain.

I. **Pathophysiology**
  A. Insufficient blood flow through coronary arteries.
  B. Temporary myocardial ischemia.

II. **Risk factors/causes:**
  A. *Cardiovascular*:
    1. Atherosclerosis.
    2. Thromboangiitis obliterans.
    3. Aortic regurgitation.
    4. Hypertension.
    5. Hypercholesterolemia.
    6. Smoking.
    7. Family history of premature coronary artery disease.
  B. *Hormonal*:
    1. Hyperthyroidism.
    2. Diabetes mellitus.
  C. *Blood disorders*:
    1. Anemia.
    2. Polycythemia vera.

III. **Assessment**
  A. *Subjective data*:
    1. Pain (**Table 4.2, p. 45**).
      a. *Type*: squeezing, pressing, burning.
      b. *Location*: retrosternal, substernal, left of sternum, radiates to left arm.
      c. *Duration*: short, usually 3–5 min, <30 min.
      d. *Cause*: emotional stress, overeating, physical exertion, exposure to cold.
      e. *Relief*: rest, nitroglycerin.
    2. Dyspnea.
    3. Palpitations.
    4. Dizziness, faintness.
    5. Epigastric distress, indigestion, belching.
  B. *Objective data*:
    1. Tachycardia.
    2. Pallor.
    3. Diaphoresis.

IV. **Analysis/nursing diagnosis**
  A. *Altered cardiopulmonary tissue perfusion* related to insufficient blood flow.
  B. *Pain* related to myocardial ischemia.
  C. *Activity intolerance* related to onset of pain.

V. **Nursing care plan/implementation**
  A. Goal: *provide relief from pain.*
    1. Rest until pain subsides.
    2. Nitroglycerin or amyl nitrite, as ordered.
    3. Identify precipitating factors: large meals, heavy exercise, stimulants (coffee, smoking), sex when fatigued, cold air.
    4. Vital signs: hypotension.
    5. Assist with ambulation; dizziness, flushing occur with nitroglycerin.
  B. Goal: *provide emotional support.*
    1. Encourage verbalization of feelings, fears.
    2. Reassurance; positive self-concept.
    3. Acceptance of limitations.
  C. Goal: **health teaching.**
    1. *Pain*: alleviation, differentiation of angina from myocardial infarction, precipitating factors (see **Table 4.2**).
    2. *Medication*: frequency, expected effects (headache, flushing); carry fresh nitroglycerin; loses potency after 6 mo ("stings" under tongue when potent); may use nitroglycerin paste—instruct how to apply.
    3. *Diet*: restrict calories if weight loss indicated; restrict: fat, cholesterol, gas-producing foods; small, frequent meals.
    4. *Diagnostic tests* if ordered (e.g., cardiac catheterization; see **Chap. 3, Diagnostic Studies** box).
    5. *Exercise*: regular, graded, to promote coronary circulation.
    6. Prepare for coronary artery bypass surgery, if necessary.
    7. Behavior modification to assist with lifestyle changes, i.e., stress reduction, stop smoking).

VI. **Evaluation/outcome/criteria**
  A. Relief from pain.
  B. Fewer attacks
  C. No MI.
  D. Alters lifestyle; complies with limitations.
  E. No smoking.

Myocardial Infarction

Localized area of necrotic tissue in the myocardium from cessation of blood flow; leading cause of death in North America.

I. **Pathophysiology**
  A. Coronary occlusion due to thrombosis, embolism, or hemorrhage adjacent to atherosclerotic plaque.
  B. Insufficient blood flow from cardiac hypertrophy, hemorrhage, shock, or severe dehydration.

II. **Risk factors/causes:**
  A. Age (35–70 yr).
  B. Men more than women until menopause.
  C. Lifestyle.
  D. Stress.
  E. High cholesterol diet (specifically low-density lipoproteins).
  F. Chronic illness (diabetes, hypertension).

G. Hypertension.

H. Smoking.

I. Obesity

J. Lack of physical activity.

III. Assessment

A. *Subjective data*:

1. Pain (see **Table 4.2**).

    a. *Type*: sudden, severe, crushing, heavy tightness.

    b. *Location*: substernal; radiates to one or both arms, jaw, neck.

    c. *Duration*: >30 min.

    d. *Cause*: unrelated to exercise; frequently occurs when sleeping (REM stage).

    e. *Relief*: oxygen, narcotics; *not* relieved by rest or nitroglycerin.

    f. *Note*: MI can be painless in clients with diabetes mellitus; women may have discomfort similar to angina rather than MI; older adults may have SOB, pulmonary edema, dizziness, or altered mental status.

2. Nausea.

3. Shortness of breath.

4. Apprehension, fear of impending death.

5. History of cardiac disease (family); occupational stress.

B. *Objective data*:

1. Vital signs: shock; rapid (>100 beats/min), thready pulse; fall in blood pressure (BP); tachypnea, shallow respirations; elevated temperature within 24 h (100°–103°F).

2. Skin: cyanotic, ashen or clammy; diaphoretic.

3. Emotional: restless.

4. Lab data: *increased*—WBC (12,000–15,000/mcg/L), serum enzymes (CK-MB, LDH₁ >LDH₂ "flipped LDH", troponin, albumin cobalt-binding); *changes*—ECG (*elevated* ST segment, *inverted* T wave, arrhythmia).

IV. Analysis/nursing diagnosis

A. *Decreased cardiac output* related to myocardial damage.

B. *Impaired gas exchange* related to poor perfusion, shock.

C. *Pain* related to myocardial ischemia.

D. *Activity intolerance* related to pain or inadequate oxygenation.

E. *Fear* related to possibility of death.

V. Nursing care plan/implementation

A. Goal: *reduce pain, discomfort.*

1. *Narcotics*—morphine, note response.

2. Humidified oxygen; mouth care as oxygen is drying.

3. *Position*: semi-Fowler's to improve ventilation.

B. Goal: *maintain adequate circulation.*

1. Monitor vital signs and urine output; observe for cardiogenic shock.

2. Monitor ECG for arrhythmias.

3. Give medications as ordered:

    a. *Antiarrhythmics*—lidocaine HC1, quinidine HC1, procainamide (*Pronestyl*), bretylium (*Bretylol*); propranolol (*Inderal*); verapamil;

    b. *Anticoagulants*—heparin sodium, bishydroxycoumarin (*Dicoumarin*);

    c. *Thrombolytic agents*—streptokinase, tissue plasminogen activator(t-PA), AP-SAC/anistreplase (*Eminase*);

    d. *Vasodilator*—nitroglycerin.

4. Recognize HF: edema, cyanosis, dyspnea, cough, crackles.

5. Check lab data—normal: *serum enzymes* (CK 0–7 IU/L; LDH <115 IU/L; LDH₁, <LDH₂); Troponin T <O.1 ng/mL; Troponin I 0.1 – 3.1 ng/mL); *blood gases* (pH 7.35–7.45; PCO_2 35–45 mEq/L; PO_2 80–100 mm Hg; HCO_3, 22–26); *electrolytes* (K^+ 3.5–5.0 mEq/L); *clotting time* (aPTT 25–33 sec; PT 11–15 sec).

6. Central venous pressure (CVP)—zero level at right atrium; fluctuates with respiration; normal range 5–15 cm H_2O; note trend; *increases* with heart failure.

7. ROM of lower extremities; TED hose/anti-embolic stockings.

C. Goal: *decrease oxygen demand/promote oxygenation.*

1. Oxygen as ordered.

2. Activity: *bed rest* (24–48 h); planned rest periods; control visitors.

3. *Position*: semi-Fowler's to facilitate lung expansion and decrease venous return.

4. Anticipate needs of client: call light, water.

5. Assist with feeding, turning.

6. Environment: quiet, comfortable.

7. Reassurance; stay with anxious client.

8. Give medications as ordered: *cardiotonics, calcium channel blockers, vasodilators, vasopressors.*

D. Goal: *maintain fluid, electrolyte, nutritional status.*

1. IV (keep vein open); CVP; vital signs; urine output—30 mL/h.

2. Lab data within normal limits (Na^+ 135–145 mEq/L; K^+ 3.5–5.0 mEq/L).

3. Monitor ECG—*hyperkalemia*: *peaked* T wave; *hypokalemia*: *depressed* T wave.

4. *Diet*: progressive *low* calorie, *low* sodium, *low* cholesterol, *low* fat.

E. Goal: *facilitate fecal elimination.*

1. Medications: *stool softeners* to prevent Valsalva (straining); mouth breathing during bowel movement; recognize **complications of Valsalva**—chest pain, cyanosis, diaphoresis, arrhythmias.

2. Bedside commode if possible.

F. Goal: *provide emotional support.*

1. Recognize fear of dying: denial, anger, withdrawal.
2. Encourage expression of feelings, fears, concerns.
3. Discuss rehabilitation, life-style changes; prevent cardiac-invalid syndrome by promoting self-care activities, independence.

G. Goal: *promote sexual functioning.*

1. Encourage discussion of concerns re: activity, inadequacy, limitations, expectations—include partner (usually resume activity 5–8 wk following uncomplicated MI).
2. Identify need for referral for sexual counseling.

🏠 H. Goal: **health teaching.**

1. Diagnosis and treatment regimen.
2. *Caution* about when to *avoid* sexual activity: following heavy meal, alcohol ingestion; when fatigued, tense, under stress; with unfamiliar partners; in extreme temperatures.
3. Information about sexual activity: less fatiguing positions (side to side; noncardiac on top); *vasodilators*, if ordered, prior to intercourse; select comfortable, familiar environment.
4. Available community resources for information, support groups (e.g., American Heart Association, Stop Smoking Clinics).
5. Medications: administration, importance, untoward effects, pulse taking.
6. Control risk factors: rest, diet, exercise, no smoking, weight control, stress-reduction techniques, lipid lowering agents.
7. Need for follow-up care for regulation of medications, evaluating risk factors.
8. Prepare for coronary bypass if planned.

🔀 VI. **Evaluation/outcome criteria**

A. No complications: stable vital signs; relief of pain.
B. Adheres to prescribed medication regimen, demonstrates knowledge about medications.
C. Activity tolerance is increased, participates in program of progressive activity.
D. Reduction or modification of risk factors. Plans to alter life-style (e.g., loses weight, quits smoking).

Heart Failure

Inability of the heart to meet the peripheral circulatory demands of body; cardiac decompensation; combined right and left ventricular HF.

I. **Pathophysiology**: increased cardiac workload or decreased effective myocardial contractility → decreased cardiac output (forward effects). Left ventricular failure → pulmonary congestion; right atrial and right ventricular failure → systemic congestion → peripheral edema (backward effects). Compensatory mechanisms in HF include: tachycardia, ventricular dilatation, and hypertrophy of the myocardium; compensatory mechanisms develop in 50%–60% of heart disease clients.

II. **Risk factors/causes:**

A. Decreased myocardial contractility:
   1. Myocarditis.
   2. MI.
   3. Tachyarrhythmias.
   4. Bacterial endocarditis.
   5. Acute rheumatic fever.
   6. Congenital heart disease.

B. Increased cardiac workload:
   1. Hypertension
   2. Coronary artery disease.
   3. Elevated temperature.
   4. Physical/emotional stress.
   5. Anemia.
   6. Hyperthyroidism (thyrotoxicosis).
   7. Valvular defects.
   8. Pulmonary embolism.
   9. Pregnancy.

🔀 III. **Assessment**

A. *Subjective data*:
   1. Shortness of breath:
      a. Orthopnea (sleeps on two or more pillows).
      b. Paroxysmal nocturnal dyspnea (sudden breathlessness during sleep).
      c. Dyspnea on exertion (climbing stairs).
   2. Apprehension, anxiety, irritability.
   3. Fatigue, weakness.
   4. Reported weight gain, feeling of puffiness.

B. *Objective data*:
   1. Vital signs:
      a. BP: decreasing systolic; narrowing pulse pressure.
      b. Pulse: *pulsus alternans* (alternating strong-weak-strong cardiac contraction), increased.
      c. Respirations: crackles.
   2. Edema: dependent, pitting (1+ to 4 + mm).
   3. Liver: enlarged, tender.
   4. Neck veins: distended.
   〰 5. Chest x-ray:
      a. Cardiac enlargement.
      b. Dilated pulmonary vessels.
      c. Diffuse interstitial lung edema.

🔀 IV. **Analysis/nursing diagnosis**

A. *Decreased cardiac output* related to decreased myocardial contractility.

B. *Activity intolerance* related to generalized weakness and inadequate oxygenation.

C. *Fatigue* related to edema and poor oxygenation.

D. *Altered tissue perfusion* related to peripheral edema and inadequate blood flow.

E. *Fluid volume excess* related to compensatory mechanisms.

F. *Impaired gas exchange* related to pulmonary congestion.

G. *Anxiety* related to shortness of breath.

H. *Sleep pattern disturbance* related to paroxysmal nocturnal dyspnea.

V. Nursing care plan/implementation

A. Goal: *provide physical rest/reduce emotional stimuli.*
1. *Position*: sitting or semi-Fowler's until tachycardia, dyspnea, edema resolved; change position frequently; pillows for support.
2. Rest: planned periods; limit visitors, activity, noise.
3. Support: stay with client who is anxious; have supportive family member present; administer *sedatives/tranquilizers* as ordered.
4. Warm fluids if appropriate.

B. Goal: *provide for relief of respiratory distress; reduce cardiac workload.*
1. Oxygen: low flow rate; encourage deep breathing (5–10 min q2h); auscultate breath sounds for congestion, pulmonary edema.
2. Morphine: decreases oxygen demand and may help relieve anxiety.
3. *Position*: head of bed 20–25 cm (8–10 in.) alleviates pulmonary congestion.
4. Medications as ordered:
   a. *Digitalis* preparations.
   b. *Inotropic agents*—dobutamine, dopamine, milrinone, levosimendan.
   c. *Vasodilators*—ACE inhibitors, nitrates, calcium channel blockers.
   d. *Diuretics*—thiazides, furosemide, ethacrynic acid.
   e. *Tranquilizers*—phenobarbital, diazepam (*Valium*), chlordiazepoxide HC1 (*Librium*).
   f. *Stool softeners* to prevent Valsalva maneuver

C. Goal: *provide for special safety needs.*
1. Skin care:
   a. Inspect, lubricate bony prominences.
   b. Use foot cradle, heel protectors; sheepskin.
2. Siderails up if hypoxic (disoriented).
3. Vital signs: monitor for signs of fatigue, pulmonary emboli.
4. ROM: active, passive; thromboembolic stockings.

D. Goal: *maintain fluid and electrolyte balance, nutritional status.*

1. Urine output: 30 mL/h minimum; estimate insensible loss in client who is diaphoretic.
2. Daily weight; same time, clothes, scale.
3. IV: use microdrip to prevent circulatory overloading.
4. *Diet*:
   a. *Low* sodium as ordered.
   b. Small, frequent feedings.
   c. Discuss food preferences with patient.

E. Goal: **health teaching.**
1. Diet restrictions; meal preparation.
2. Activity restrictions, if any; planned rest periods.
3. Medications: schedule, purpose, dosage, side effects (importance of daily pulse taking, daily weights, intake of *potassium*-containing foods).
4. Available community resources for dietary assistance, weight reduction, exercise program.

VI. Evaluation/outcome criteria

A. Increase in activity level tolerance—fatigue decreased.

B. No complications—pulmonary edema, respiratory distress.

C. Reduction in dependent edema.

Pulmonary Edema

Sudden transudation of fluid from pulmonary capillaries into alveoli.

I. **Pathophysiology**: increased pulmonary capillary permeability; increased hydrostatic pressure (pulmonary hypertension); and/or decreased blood colloidal osmotic pressure; fluid accumulation in alveoli → decreased compliance → decreased diffusion of gas → hypoxia, hypercapnea.

II. **Risk factors/causes:**
A. Left ventricular HF.
B. Pulmonary embolism.
C. Drug overdose.
D. Smoke inhalation.
E. Central nervous system (CNS) damage.
F. Fluid overload.
G. High altitude.

III. **Assessment**
A. *Subjective data*:
1. Anxiety.
2. Restlessness at onset progressing to agitation.
3. Stark fear.
4. Intense dyspnea, orthopnea, fatigue.
B. *Objective data*:
1. *Vital signs*:
   a. Pulse: tachycardia, gallop rhythm.

  b. Respiration: tachypnea; moist, bubbling wheezing, use of accessory muscles.

  c. Temperature: normal to subnormal.

2. Skin: pale, cool, diaphoretic, cyanotic.

3. Auscultation: crackles, wheezes.

4. Cough: productive of large quantities of pink, frothy sputum.

5. Right ventricular HF: distended neck veins, peripheral edema, hepatomegaly, ascites. (*Note:* Left-sided failure can cause right-sided failure.)

6. Mental status: restless, confused, stuporous.

IV. Analysis/nursing diagnosis

A. *Impaired gas exchange* related to pulmonary congestion.

B. *Altered tissue perfusion* related to inadequate blood flow.

C. *Anxiety,* severe, related to difficulty breathing.

D. *Fear* related to pulmonary congestion.

V. Nursing care plan/implementation

A. Goal: *promote physical, psychological relaxation measures to relieve anxiety.*

1. Slow respirations: morphine sulfate, as ordered, to reduce respiratory rate, to sedate, and to produce vasodilation.

2. Remain with client.

3. Encourage slow, deep breathing; assist with coughing.

4. Work calmly, confidently, unhurriedly.

5. Frequent rest periods.

B. Goal: *improve cardiac function, reduce venous return, relieve hypoxia.*

1. Oxygen: 100%, preferably by demand valve to slow respiratory rate, provide uniform ventilation, reduce venous return, and inhibit "leaky capillary" syndrome.

2. IV: 5% dextrose in water via microdrip to avoid fluid overload.

3. Give aminophylline, as ordered, to lower venous pressure and increase cardiac output.

4. *Position:* high-Fowler's; extremities in dependent position to reduce venous return and facilitate breathing.

5. Medications as ordered: digitalis; diuretics furosemide (*Lasix*); inotropic agents— dobutamine (*Dobutrex*), dopamine; nitroglycerin.

6. Vital signs; auscultate breath sounds.

7. *Diet: low* sodium; fluid restriction as ordered.

C. Goal: **health teaching** (include family or significant other).

1. Medications.

  a. Side effects.

  b. Potassium supplements if indicated.

  c. Pulse taking.

2. Exercise, rest.

3. *Diet:* low sodium.

4. Signs of complications: edema; weight gain of 2–3 lb (0.9–1.4 kg) in a few days; dyspnea.

VI. Evaluation/outcome criteria

A. No complications; vital signs stable; clear breath sounds.

B. No weight gain; weight loss if indicated.

C. Alert, oriented, calm.

Summary of Key Points

1. Functional disorders of the heart are associated with coronary artery disease.

2. Cardiac pain is diffuse; a client is usually unable to point to one location, unlike respiratory pain, which is more defined or localized.

3. Establish unresponsiveness before beginning CPR. Call for help, then remember your ABCs—airway, breathing, and circulation.

4. Not all chest pain is brought on by exertion, eating, or emotion. Unstable angina occurs at rest.

5. Left ventricular failure (pulmonary edema) is a *more* severe condition than right ventricular failure.

Study and Memory Aids

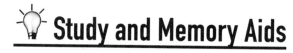

CPR – Remember the "ABCs"

AIRWAY
BREATHING
CIRCULATION

Angina: Pain Pattern

Exertion → pain
Rest + nitroglycerin → relief

Angina: Precipitating Factors—"3 E's"

E ating
E motion
E xertion (Exercise)

Myocardial Infarction: "INTENSE PAIN"

I schemia
N ecrotic cardiac tisue
T ightness in chest
E xtended duration
N ausea
S evere pain
E CG changes

P revent Valsalva maneuver
A nxiety
I ntense
N ot relieved by rest

Heart Failure: "OVERLOAD"

O rthopnea
V entricular failure
E nlarged heart
R eported weight gain
L ungs congested
O utput decreased
A pprehension
D ependent edema

Pulmonary Edema: "FOWLER'S"

F ailure—left ventricular
O rthopnea
W heezing
L ung congestion
E mergency
R estlessness
S kin—cyanotic

Review of Physiology: Blood Flow

Vena cava
↓
Right atrium
↓
Tricuspid valve
↓
Right ventricle
↓
Pulmonary valve
↓
Right and left pulmonary arteries
↓
Lung/oxygenation
↓
Pulmonary veins
↓
Left atrium
↓
Bicuspid (mitral) valve
↓
Left ventricle
↓
Aortic valve
↓
Aorta

🍎 Diets

Angina Pectoris

Calories
Cholesterol
Fat
Gas-forming foods

Heart Failure

Low sodium
Small frequent feedings

Pulmonary Edema

Fluids
Sodium

〽️ Diagnostic Studies/Procedures

Graphic Studies of Heart :

Electrocardiography—graphic record of electrical activity generated by the heart during depolarization and repolarization; *used to*: diagnose abnormal cardiac rhythms and heart disease.

Echocardiography (ultrasoundcardiography)—graphic record of motions produced by cardiac structures as high-frequency sound vibrations are echoed through chest wall into the heart; transesophageal echocardiography produces a clearer image, particularly in obese, barrel-chested, or clients with COPD; *used to*: demonstrate valvular or other structural deformities, detect pericardial effusion, diagnose tumors and cardiomegaly, or evaluate prosthetic valve function.

Phonocardiography—graphic record of heart sounds; *used to*: keep a permanent record of client's heart sounds before and after cardiac surgery.

Procedures to Evaluate the Cardiovascular System:

Angiocardiography—intravenous injection of a radiopaque solution or medium for the purpose of studying its circulation through the client's heart, lungs, and great vessels; *used to*: check the competency of heart valves, diagnose congenital septal defects, detect occlusions of coronary arteries, confirm suspected diagnoses, and study heart function and structure prior to cardiac surgery.

Angiography (arteriography)—injection of a contrast medium into the arteries to study the vascular tree; *used to*: determine obstructions or narrowing of peripheral arteries.

Nuclear Cardiology—intravenous injection of various radioactive isotopes to study myocardial perfusion and contractility, and acute cell injury.

💊 Drug Review

Cardiac Dysrhythmias

Anticholinergics: atropine
Antidysrhythmics
    Class IA Quinidine
        IB Lidocaine (xylocaine)
        IC Hecainide acetate (*Tambocor*)
        II Propranolol (*Inderal*)
        III Bretylium tosylate (*Bretylol*)
        IV Verapamil (*Calan*)
Beta-adrenergics
    Dobutamine (*Dobutrex*)
    Dopamine hydrochloride (*Intropin*)
    Epinephrine
    Isoproterenol (*Isuprel*)
    Norepinephrine (*Levophed*)

Cardiac Arrest/CPR: Medications Used, Depending on Symptoms and Response

Antiarrhythmics
Adenosine
Bretylium
Isoproterenol
Lidocaine
Procainamide hydrochloride
Anticholinergic
Atropine
Beta-adrenergic blocker
Propranolol
Calcium channel blocker
Verapamil
Cardiac glycoside
Digoxin
Cardiac stimulant
Epinephrine
Diuretic
Furosemide
Electrolyte modifiers
Calcium
Sodium bicarbonate
Inotropic agents
Dobutamine
Dopamine
Vasodilators
Nitroglycerin
Nitroprusside
Vasopressors
Dopamine
Norepinephrine

Angina Pectoris

Beta-blockers
Atenolol (*Tenormin*): 25–50 mg/d
Metoprolol (*Lopressor*): 100–450 mg/d
Propranolol (*Inderal*): 40 mg bid
Calcium channel blockers
Diltiazem (*Cardizem*): 30–120 mg 3–4 times daily.
Nifedipine (*Procardia*): 10–30 mg tid
Verapamil (*Calan*): 80–120 mg tid
Vasodilators
Isosorbide dinitrate (*Isordil*): 2.5–10 mg PO q2–3 h for acute attack
Nitroglycerin: 0.15–0.6 mg repeated q5min for 15 min for acute attacks
Nitroglycerin long-acting preparations: *ointment* 1-2 inches q8h
Nitroglycerin *patch*: 0.1–0.6 mg/h up to 0.8 mg/h worn 12–14 h/d

Acute Myocardial Infarction

Analgesic
Morphine: IV, 2.5–15 q4 h or loading dose of 15 mg with 0.8–10 mg/h, rate increased as needed; SC, 5–20 mg q4 h as needed.
Antiarrhythmics (some of the drugs used)
Bretylium (*Bretylol*): 5 mg/kg bolus over 15–30 sec, *not* to exceed 30 mg/kg/d
Lidocaine HCI: IV 50–100 mg (1 mg/kg) bolus; may be repeated in 5 min, then 1–4 mg/min infusion.
Procainamide (*Pronestyl*): 50 mg/kg/d
Propranolol (*Inderal*): 0.5–3 mg; repeat once in 2 min if needed; 180–240 mg/d in divided doses starting 5–21 days post MI.
Quinidine: 400–600 mg q2–3h, *not* to exceed 4 g/d.
Anticoagulants
Bishydroxycoumarin (*Dicumarol*): 200–300 mg to start, then 25–200 mg based on *PT*
Heparin sodium: IV, 5,000 U IV to start, followed by 20,000–40,000 U IV infusion over 24 hours; SC, 8000–10,000 U q8h, adjusted according to *aPTT*
Warfarin (*Coumadin*): 10 mg daily, adjusted according to *PT*
Calcium channel blocker: Verapamil (*Calan*): 80–120 mg tid
Cardiac glycoside: Digoxin (*Lanoxin*): digitalizing dose: IV, 10–15 mcg/kg over 24 h; or PO, 10–15 mcg/ kg over 24 h; maintenance dose, 0.1–0.375 mg/d. (Take *apical* pulse before administering drug)
Lipid-lowering:
Cholestyramine (*Questran*): 4 g 1–6 times daily
Gemfibrozil (*Lopid*): 600 mg bid 30 min *before* breakfast and dinner
Lovastatin (*Mevacor*): 20 mg qd with *evening meal*
Niacin: 10–20 mg qd
Thrombolytic agents
Alteplase (*Activase t-PA*): 100 mg over 90 min. 15 mg bolus given over 1–2 min, then, 50 mg over 30 min; then 35 mg over 60 min.
Anistreplase (*Eminase*): IV, 30 U over 2–5 min
Streptokinase (*Streptase*): 1.5 million U diluted to 45 mL infused over 60 minutes
Vasodilator: Hydralazine (*Apresoline*): 10–100 mg qid
Vasopressor: Dopamine (*Intropin*): 1–5 mcg/kg/min; gradually increase in 1–4 mcg/kg/min increments at 10–30 min intervals until optimum response. Most clients are maintained on dose of 20 mcg/kg/min or less

Heart Failure

Cardiac glycosides
Digoxin (*Lanoxin*): 0.1–0.375 mg/d
Dobutamine (*Dobutrex*): IV, 2.5–15 mcg/kg/min
Dopamine (*Intropin*): IV, 0.5–5 mcg/kg/min initially;
increase to 50 mcg/kg/min
Diuretics
Furosemide (*Lasix*): 20–80 mg/d
Hydrochlorothiazide (*HydroDIURIL, Esidrix*): 25–100
mg/d
Inotropics
Dobutamine (*Dobutrex*): IV, 2.5–15 mcg/kg/min
Dopamine (*Intropin*): IV, 0.5–5 mcg/kg/min initially;
increase to 50 mcg/kg/min
Stool softener
Docusate (*Colace*): 50–500 mg/d
Tranquilizers
Chlordiazepoxide HC1 (*Librium*): 5–25 mg 3–4 times
daily
Diazepam (*Valium*): 2–10 mg 2–4 times daily
Phenobarbital Sodium (*Luminal*): 30–120 mg/d in
divided doses.
Vasodilators
Captopril (*Capoten*): 6.25–12.5 mg 3 times daily
Isosorbide dinitrate (*Isordil*): 10–40 mg q 6h.
Nifedipine (*Procardia*): 10–30 mg 3 times daily
Verapamil (*Calan*): 80–120 mg 3 times daily

Pulmonary Edema

Aminophylline: loading dose of 500 mg followed by
250–500 mg q6–8 h. Note: monitor *theophylline levels*
Digoxin (*Lanoxin*): 0.1–0.375 mg/d
Dobutamine (*Dobutrex*): IV, 2.5–15 mcg/kg/min
Dopamine (*Intropin*): IV, 0.5–5 mcg/kg/min initially;
increase in 5–10 mcg/kg/min increments up to rate of
20–50 mcg/kg/min
Furosemide (*Lasix*): 20–80 mg/d
Morphine: IV, 2.5–15 q4h or loading dose of 15 mg with
0.8–10 mg/h, rate increased as needed; SC, 5–20 mg
q4h as needed
Nitroglycerin: 0.15–0.6 mg sublingual, repeated q5min for
15 min for acute attacks

Questions

1. When resuming activities that require physical
exertion, a client who has had a myocardial
infarction (MI) should be advised to take
nitroglycerin (NTG):
   1. When any chest pain develops.
   2. As soon as any pressure or discomfort is felt.
   3. Before engaging in activities known to involve
exertion.
   4. If the pain does not go away with rest.

2. What most common side effects would a nurse look
for in a client receiving atenolol (*Tenormin*), a beta-
blocker used to manage angina pectoris?

   1. Bradycardia and hypotension.
   2. Fatigue and weakness.
   3. Bronchospasm and wheezing.
   4. Dry eyes and blurred vision.

3. Which statement by a client scheduled for a
treadmill test would be of greatest concern to the
nurse?
   1. "I drank coffee this morning."
   2. "I took my propranolol (*Inderal*) this morning."
   3. "I slept 10 hours last night."
   4. "I've been having indigestion this morning."

4. A client has been admitted to the telemetry unit to
undergo testing to rule out an MI. The lab reports
that the CK-MB is elevated. The most appropriate
nursing action would be to:
   1. Give the client 10 mEq/L of potassium to
prevent arrhythmias.
   2. Prepare the client for transfer to the CCU.
   3. Continue to monitor the lab results.
   4. Increase the amount of O_2 being administered to
decrease the ischemia.

5. Furosemide (*Lasix*) has been given IV to treat a client
with fluid retention. The best indicator of drug
effectiveness is:
   1. Hourly urine output.
   2. Daily weight.
   3. Urine specific gravity.
   4. Serum sodium level.

6. The nurse instructs a client to take lovastatin
(*Mevacor*) with meals because taking it on an empty
stomach will:
   1. Increase gastric irritation.
   2. Decrease drug absorption.
   3. Cause constipation or diarrhea.
   4. Lead to drug toxicity.

7. Which nursing action would be most helpful in
reducing anxiety in a client being admitted for
evaluation and treatment of a possible MI?
   1. Explain the equipment being used.
   2. Pull the curtain around the bed for privacy.
   3. Offer the client literature on unit policies.
   4. Explain use of the call light, and put it within
reach.

8. Which laboratory test provides the most specific information about cardiac damage?
   1. ALT (SGPT). — liver damage
   2. CK-MB.
   3. LDH. — elevated much later
   4. AST (SGOT).

9. The nurse should assess a client with right
ventricular failure for the presence of:
   1. Orthopnea and difficulty breathing at night.
   2. Weight gain and jugular venous distention.
   3. Confusion and apathy.
   4. Chest pain and elevated temperature.

10. Which foods should the nurse suggest to a client who is on digoxin to minimize the risk of digitalis toxicity?
    1. Turkey, green beans, and French bread.
    2. Cottage cheese, cooked broccoli, and fish.
    3. Beef, green peas, and sweet corn.
    4. Whole grain cereal, orange juice, and apricots.

11. Which statement by the client would indicate an accurate understanding of the teaching regarding adverse effects of digoxin?
    1. "I will call the MD if I become nauseated."
    2. "I will report my weight to the MD daily."
    3. "My gums may get puffy."
    4. "Hives or a rash may occur."

12. Which is the correct method for checking the pulse in a client receiving digoxin?
    1. Taking the apical-radial pulses at the same time.
    2. Comparing the apical pulse with the pulse from the previous week.
    3. Counting the apical pulse for a full minute.
    4. Counting the apical pulse for 15 seconds and multiplying it by 4.

13. A client receiving digoxin has an apical pulse of 100 beats/min. The appropriate nursing response would be to:
    1. Record the rate and call the MD.
    2. Record the rate and give the next dose of digoxin.
    3. Give the medication and recheck the pulse in 15 minutes.
    4. Hold the medication and check the pulse in 30 minutes.

Answers/Rationale

1. (3) Exertion, which includes sexual activity, increases cardiac workload. Taking NTG before engaging in activities that involve exertion should prevent any ischemia. Ischemia has already occurred once pain develops (1) and pressure is felt (2). Rest (4) is important, but NTG should be taken before or during rest if chest pain arises unexpectedly with exertion. **IMP, RE/KN, 3, PhI, Pharmacological and parenteral therapies**

2. (2) All of the choices are adverse or side effects of atenolol, but the *most common* are fatigue and weakness. If the more serious (and less common) side effects (1 and 3) occurred regularly in a client, it is unlikely that treatment with the drug would be continued in that person. The visual problems (4) are also less common; a person suffering from them would be prone to have accidents, and for this reason, the drug would probably be changed. **AS, ANL, 6, PhI, Pharmacological and parenteral therapies**

3. (4) Indigestion or epigastric pain may indicate the presence of myocardial ischemia. The client should be given an antacid, and if this produces no relief, the client should be given NTG to see if this relieves the pain. The test would not be done if the client were having chest pain as the result of ischemia, even if it were relieved by NTG. Coffee (1) may cause the heart rate to increase, and the test may have to be interrupted if this should happen, but it can still be started. Clients usually take their cardiac drugs (2) the day of a treadmill test, and a restful night's sleep (3) would be desirable. **EV, EVL, 6, PhI, Reduction of risk potential**

4. (2) CK-MB is the specific isoenzyme for cardiac muscle; the normal value is 0.0 to 4.7 µg/mL, and an elevation is an indicator of an MI. The CCU is the best place for this client to receive care. A low potassium level may cause arrhythmias, but there are no data to indicate the need for potassium supplements (1) to prevent arrhythmias in clients in the acute stage of an MI. Any arrhythmias in this client would most likely be due to myocardial ischemia. Although it would not be wrong to continue to monitor (3) the client, the diagnosis is established if the CK-MB level is raised 4 to 6 hours after the infarction. The only question is the extent of damage; the level peaks in 18 to 24 hours. Oxygen (4) would be given, and most likely the client would already be receiving it. However, the deciding factor here is the priority of the action. In this instance, the most important priority is to transfer the client to a unit where closer supervision is possible until his/her condition is stable. **IMP, APP, 6, PhI, Reduction of risk potential**

5. (2) All of the choices will provide data on the hydration or fluid status of the client, but daily weight is the *best* indicator. *Lasix*, a loop diuretic, is used for the management of the acute stage of a condition such as pulmonary edema and for chronic heart failure if less potent diuretics, for example, a thiazide, have not worked. The client's weight should decrease if the drug is effective. The urine volume (1) should increase, specific gravity (3) decrease, and the serum sodium level (4) increase in a client with pulmonary edema who is receiving Lasix. **EV, EVL, 6, PhI, Pharmacological and parenteral therapies**

6. (2) Lovastatin is a lipid-lowering agent, and absorption is decreased by 30% if it is not taken *with* food. Drug side effects include numerous symptoms of GI tract irritation (1), and these occur if the drug is taken *with* food. These side effects include constipation or diarrhea (3), dyspepsia, nausea, and heartburn. These effects are less severe if lovastatin is taken on an empty stomach, and taking the agent on an empty stomach would also *lower* the risk of toxicity (4). *However, optimal absorption is the highest priority.* These other side effects, although unpleasant, can be managed by other means. **IMP, APP, 4, PhI, Pharmacological and parenteral therapies**

7. **(4)** The call light is a way for the client to get help if needed, and its availability can help allay a client's anxiety. Anxiety would impair any learning (**1** and **3**); isolating the client (**2**) would only increase the client's anxiety. **IMP, COM, 7, PsI, Psychosocial integrity**

8. **(2)** CK-MB is the cardiac-specific isoenzyme. The level is elevated 4 to 6 hours after an MI. The ALT level (**1**) is more specific to *liver* damage. The LDH level (**3**) also increases with cardiac damage, but not until *much later*. The AST level (**4**) would be elevated around the same time as the CK-MB level, but it is also elevated in other types of muscle damage. **AS, COM, 6, PhI, Reduction of risk potential**

9. **(2)** The backward flow of blood caused by right-sided (right ventricular) heart failure leads to venous distention, organomegaly, and weight gain as the result of sodium and water retention. Orthopnea and difficulty breathing at night (**1**) are symptoms of *left* ventricular failure. Confusion and apathy (**3**) are rather inconclusive findings, but electrolyte imbalance or hypoxia stemming from many different causes may produce these symptoms. Chest pain and elevated temperature (**4**) are characteristic of an MI. **AS, APP, 6, PhI, Physiological adaptation**

10. **(4)** Digitalis toxicity is likely to develop when the potassium level is low. This risk is heightened in many clients receiving digoxin because they are also taking a diuretic, which depletes the serum potassium store. Foods high in potassium include: the whole grains, citrus fruits, apricots, bananas, and potatoes. The other foods (**1, 2,** and **3**) are not sources of potassium. **IMP, APP, 4, PhI, Pharmacological and parenteral therapies**

11. **(1)** The most frequent side effects of digoxin are nausea, vomiting, fatigue, bradycardia, and anorexia most likely related to hypokalemia. Although weight gain (**2**) would indicate worsening of heart failure, weight would not be reported daily. Puffy gums (**3**), or gingival hyperplasia, is a side effect of phenytoin. Allergic reactions (**4**) are *not* common in clients taking digoxin. **EV, EVL, 6, PhI, Pharmacological and parenteral therapies**

12. **(3)** The correct method for checking the pulse of a client receiving an antiarrhythmic drug is to count the pulse for one full minute because the rhythm is usually irregular. A more accurate rate would be counted in one minute. Checking for an apical radial pulse deficit (**1**) is not done routinely. Changes in pulse rate would be noted from shift to shift, *not* from week to week (**2**). The method in option **4** is used to check the pulse in a client not receiving an antiarrhythmic drug. **AS, COM 6, HPM, Health promotion and maintenance**

13. **(2)** The next dose of digoxin should be given because the drug has not yet achieved its therapeutic effect of slowing the heart rate while also increasing cardiac contractility. If the rate slows to less than 50 beats/min, the MD should be notified (**1**). There is no reason to hold off giving the drug (**4**) or to recheck the pulse before the next scheduled assessment of the vital signs (**3** and **4**). **EV, EVL, 6, PhI, Pharmacological and parenteral therapies**

Key to Codes

Nursing process: **AS**, assessment; **AN**, analysis; **PL**, planning; **IMP**, implementation; **EV**, evaluation. (See **Appendix M** for explanation of nursing process steps.)

Cognitive level: **RE/KN**, recall/knowledge; **COM**, comprehension; **APP**, application; **ANL**, analysis; **EVL**, evaluation; **SYN**, synthesis. (See **Appendix M** for explanation.)

Category of human function: 1, protective; 2, sensory-perceptual; 3, comfort, rest, activity, and mobility; 4, nutrition; 5, growth and development; 6, fluid-gas transport; 7, psychosocial-cultural; 8, elimination. (See **Appendix 0** for explanation.)

Client need: **SECE**, safe, effective care environment; **PhI**, physiological integrity; **PsI**, psychosocial integrity; **HPM**, health promotion and maintenance. (See **Appendix P** for explanation.)

Client subneed: (See **Appendix P** for explanation)

Hematologic Disorders

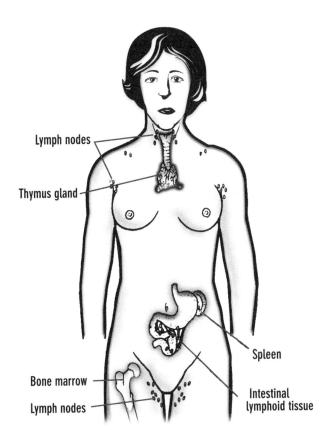

Components of the Hemapoietic System

Disseminated Intravascular Coagulation (DIC)

Diffuse or widespread coagulation initially within arterioles and capillaries with subsequent depletion of clotting factors and platelets, which leads to hemorrhage.

I. **Pathophysiology:** activation of coagulation system resulting from tissue injury → fibrin microthrombin form in brain, kidneys, lungs → microinfarcts, tissue necrosis → red blood cells (RBCs), platelets, prothrombin, other clotting factors trapped, destroyed in process → excessive clotting → release of fibrin split products → inhibition of platelet clotting → bleeding.

II. **Risk factors/causes:**
   A. Obstetric complications.
   B. Neoplastic disease.
   C. Low perfusion states.
   D. Sepsis.
   E. Severe tissue injury, e.g., burns.
   F. Transfusion reaction.

III. **Assessment**—*objective data*:
   A. Skin, mucous membranes: petechiae, ecchymosis.
   B. Extremities (fingers, toes): cyanosis.
   C. Bleeding: venipuncture sites, wound, oral, rectal, vaginal.
   D. Urine output: oliguria → anuria.
   E. Level of consciousness: convulsions, coma.
   F. Lab data: *prolonged*—prothrombin time (PT) >15 sec; *decreased*—platelets, fibrinogen level.

IV. **Analysis/nursing diagnosis**
   A. *Altered tissue perfusion* related to peripheral microthrombi.
   B. *Risk for injury*, death, related to bleeding.
   C. *Risk for impaired skin integrity* related to ischemia.
   D. *Altered urinary elimination* related to renal tubular necrosis.
   E. *Acute pain* related to bleeding into tissues.

V. **Nursing care plan/implementation**: Goal: *prevent and detect further bleeding.*
   A. Carry out nursing measures designed to alleviate underlying problem (e.g., shock, birth of fetus, surgery/irradiation for cancer).

TABLE 5.1 TRANSFUSION WITH BLOOD OR BLOOD PRODUCTS

Blood or Blood Product	Indications	▶◀ Assessment: Side Effects	▶◀ Nursing Care Plan/Implementations
Whole blood	1. Acute hemorrhage 2. Hypovolemic shock	1. Hemolytic reaction 2. Fluid overload 3. Febrile reaction 4. Pyrogenic reaction 5. Allergic reaction	1. See **Table 9.2, Postoperative Complications, p. 136** for complete discussion of nursing responsibilities 2. Protocol for checking blood before transfusion is begun varies with each institution; however, at least *two* people must verify that the unit of blood has been cross-matched for a specific client.
Red blood cells, packed	1. Acute anemia with hypoxia 2. Aplastic anemia 3. Bone marrow failure due to malignancy 4. Clients who need red blood cells but not volume	**See Whole blood**	See **Whole blood**
Red blood cells, frozen	1. See **Red blood cells, packed** 2. Clients sensitized by previous transfusions	1. Less likely to cause antigen reaction 2. Decreased possibility of transmitting hepatitis	See **Whole blood**
White blood cells (leukocytes)	Currently being used in severe leukopenia with infection (research still being done)	1. Elevated temperature 2. Graft-versus-host disease	1. Careful monitoring of temperature 2. *Must* be given as soon as collected
Platelet concentrate	1. Severe deficiency 2. Bleeding thrombocytopenic clients with platelet counts *below* 10,000 mcg/L	1. Fever, chills 2. Hives 3. Development of antibodies that will destroy platelets in future transfusions *Contraindications*: 1. Immune thrombocytopenic purpura 2. Disseminated intravascular coagulation (DIC)	Monitor temperature
Single-donor fresh plasma	1. Clotting deficiency or concentrates not available or deficiency not fully diagnosed 2. Shock (used less for shock in favor of albumin plasma expanders).	1. Side effects rare 2. Heart failure 3. Possible hepatitis	Use sterile, pyrogen-free filters
Plasma removed from whole blood (up to 5 d after expiration date, which is 21 d)	1. Shock due to loss of plasma 2. Burns 3. Peritoneal injury 4. Hemorrhage 5. While awaiting blood crossmatch results	See **Single-donor fresh plasma**	See **Single-donor fresh plasma**

(continued)

TABLE 5.1 TRANSFUSION WITH BLOOD OR BLOOD PRODUCTS (continued)

Blood or Blood Product	Indications	▶◀ Assessment: Side Effects	▶◀ Nursing Care Plan/Implementations
Freeze-dried plasma	See **Plasma removed from whole blood**	See **Single-donor fresh plasma**	Must be reconstituted with sterile water before use
Single-donor fresh-frozen plasma	1. See **Single-donor fresh plasma** 2. Inherited or acquired disorders of coagulation 3. Preoperative with hemophilia	See **Single-donor fresh plasma**	1. Notify blood bank to thaw about 30 min before administration 2. Give *immediately*
Cryoprecipitate concentrate (factor VIII—antihemophilic factor)	For hemophilia: 1. Prevention 2. Preoperatively 3. During bleeding episodes	Rare	0.55 mL of cryoprecipitate concentrate has same effect on serum level as 1600 mL of fresh frozen plasma
Factors II, VII, IX, and X compiled	Specific deficiencies	Hepatitis	Commercially prepared
Fibrinogen (factor I)	Fibrinogen deficiency	Increased risk of hepatitis since the hepatitis virus combines with fibrinogen during fractionation	1. Reconstitute with sterile water 2. Do *not* warm fibrinogen or use hot water to re-constitute 3. Do *not* shake 4. Must be given with a filter
Albumin or salt-poor albumin	1. Shock due to hemorrhage, trauma, infection, surgery, or burns 2. Treatment of cerebral edema 3. Low serum-protein levels	None; these are heat-treated products	Commercially prepared
Dextran	Hypovolemic shock	1. Rare allergic reaction 2. Clients with heart or kidney disease, susceptible to heart failure or pulmonary edema	Commercially prepared

Source: ©Lagerquist, SL: *Little, Brown's NCLEX-RN® Examination Review*. Boston: Little, Brown, (out of print).

- B. *Medications*: heparin sodium, if ordered, to reverse abnormal clotting (controversial); antithrombin III, hirudin, *Amicar* (all are controversial).
- C. IVs: blood to lessen shock; platelets, cryoprecipitate, fresh plasma to restore clotting factors, fibrinogen (**Table 5.1**).
- D. Observe: vital signs, *CVP* (normal, 5-15 mm Hg), *pulmonary artery pressure* (normal, 20-30 mm Hg systolic and 8-12 mm Hg diastolic), and intake and output for signs of shock or fluid overload from frequent infusions; specimens for *occult* blood (urine, stool).
- E. Precautions: *avoid* IM injections if possible; pressure 5 min to venipuncture sites; *no* rectal temperatures.
- F. Chronic DIC does not respond to oral anticoagulants, but may be treated with long-term *heparin* or *enoxaparin*.

▶◀ **VI. Evaluation/outcome criteria**

A. Clotting mechanism restored (increased platelets, normal PT).

B. Renal function restored (urine output >30 mL/h).

C. Circulation to fingers, toes; no cyanosis.

D. No irreversible damage from renal, cerebral, cardiac, or adrenal hemorrhage.

Iron Deficiency Anemia
(Hypochromic Microcytic Anemia)

Inadequate production of RBCs due to lack of heme (iron); common in infants, women who are pregnant, and women who are premenopausal .

I. **Pathophysiology**: decreased dietary intake, impaired absorption, or increased utilization of iron decreases the amount of iron bound to plasma transferrin and transported to bone marrow for hemoglobin synthesis; decreased hemoglobin in erythrocytes decreases amount of oxygen delivered to tissues.

II. **Risk factors/causes:**
  A. *Excessive menstruation.*
  B. *Gastrointestinal bleeding*—peptic ulcer, hookworm, tumors.
  C. *Inadequate diet*—anorexia, fad diets, cultural practices.
  D. *Poor absorption*—stomach, small intestine disease.
  E. *Young age.*

III. **Assessment**
  A. *Subjective data*:
    1. Fatigue: increasing.
    2. Headache.
    3. Change in appetite; difficulty swallowing due to pharyngeal edema/ulceration; heartburn.
    4. Shortness of breath on exercise.
    5. Extremities: numb, tingling.
    6. Flatulence (reported).
    7. Menorrhagia (reported).
  B. *Objective data*:
    1. Vital signs:
      a. *BP*—increased systolic, widened pulse pressure.
      b. *Pulse*—tachycardia.
      c. *Respirations*—tachypnea.
      d. *Temperature*—normal or subnormal.
    2. Skin/mucous membranes: pale, dry.
    3. Sclera: pearly white.
    4. Nails: brittle, spoon-shaped, flattened.
    5. Lab data: *decreased*—hemoglobin (<10 g/dL blood), serum iron (<65 mcg/dL blood); *Increased*—total iron-binding capacity.

IV. **Analysis/nursing diagnosis**
  A. *Altered nutrition, less than body requirements,* related to inadequate iron absorption.
  B. *Altered tissue perfusion* related to reduction in RBCs.
  C. *Risk for activity intolerance* related to profound weakness.
  D. *Hypoxemia* related to decreased oxygen carrying capacity.

V. **Nursing care plan/implementation**
  A. Goal: *promote physical and mental equilibrium.*
    1. *Position*: optimal for respiratory excursion; deep breathing; turn frequently to prevent skin breakdown.
    2. Rest: balance with activity, as tolerated; assist with ambulation.
    3. Medication (hematinics):
      a. Oral iron therapy (ferrous sulfate)—give *with* meals.
      b. Parenteral therapy.
        (1) Iron dextran IM—use second needle for injection after withdrawal from ampule; use **Z track method**; inject 0.5 cc of air before withdrawing needle to prevent tissue necrosis; use 2–3 in. needle; rotate sites; do *not* rub site or wear constricting garments after injection.
        (2) Erythropoietin—for certain types of anemia; 50–100U/kg SC 3x/week. May increase to 300U/kg 3x/week depending upon condition and Hct.
    4. Keep warm: *no* hot water bottles, heating pads, due to decreased sensitivity.
    5. Diet: *high* in protein, iron, vitamins (see **Appendixes B and C**); assistance with feeding, if needed.
  B. Goal: **health teaching**.
    1. Dietary regimen.
    2. Iron therapy: explain purpose, dosage, side effects (black or green stools, constipation, diarrhea); take with meals.
    3. Activity: exercise to tolerance, with planned rest periods.

VI. **Evaluation/outcome criteria**
  A. Hemoglobin level returns to normal range.
  B. Tolerates activity without fatigue.
  C. Selects foods appropriate for dietary regimen.

Hemolytic Anemia
(Normocytic Normochromic Anemia)

Unknown factor causes antibodies to destroy the body's own erythrocytes (autoimmune); most common in those over 40 yr.

I. **Risk factors/causes:**
  A. Malignant lymphoma.
  B. Ulcerative colitis.
  C. Lupus erythematosus.
  D. Drug therapy

II. **Assessment**
  A. *Subjective data*:
    1. Fatigue, physical weakness.
    2. Dizziness.
    3. Shortness of breath.
    4. Diaphoresis on slight exertion.
  B. *Objective data*:
    1. Skin: pallor, jaundice.
    2. Posture: drooping.
    3. Lab data: *decreased* hemoglobin; *increased* reticulocyte count; *Direct* Coombs test positive.

III. See **Iron Deficiency Anemia, p.59-60,** for analysis, nursing care plan/implementation, and evaluation.

Pernicious Anemia
(Hyperchromic Macrocytic Anemia)

Lack of intrinsic factor found in gastric mucosa, which is necessary for vitamin B_{12} (extrinsic factor) absorption; slowly developing, usually after age 50 yr; may be an autoimmune disorder.

I. **Pathophysiology**: atrophy or surgical removal of glandular mucosa in fundus of stomach → degenerative changes in brain, spinal cord, and peripheral nerves from lack of vitamin B_{12}.

II. **Risk factors/causes:**
    A. Partial or complete gastric resection.
    B. Prolonged iron deficiency.
    C. Heredity.
    D. Clients with Crohn's disease.
    E. Long-term uses of H_2-histamine receptor blockers.

III. **Assessment**
    A. *Subjective data*:
        1. Hands, feet: tingling, numbness.
        2. Weakness, fatigue.
        3. Sore tongue, anorexia.
        4. Difficulties with memory, balance.
        5. Irritability, mild depression.
        6. Shortness of breath.
        7. Palpitations.
    B. *Objective data*:
        1. Skin: pale, flabby, jaundiced.
        2. Sclera: icterus (yellow).
        3. Tongue: smooth, glossy, red, swollen.
        4. Vital signs:
            a. *BP*—normal or elevated.
            b. *Pulse*—tachycardia.
        5. Nervous system:
            a. Decreased vibrator sense in lower extremities.
            b. Loss of coordination.
            c. *Babinski* present (flaring of toes with stimulation of sole of foot).
            d. *Positive Romberg* (loses balance when eyes closed).
            e. Increased or diminished reflexes.
        6. Lab data:
            a. *Increased*—hemoglobin, bilirubin;
            b. *Decreased*—RBCs, platelets, gastric secretions, *Schilling test* (radioactive vitamin B_{12} urine test).

IV. **Analysis/nursing diagnosis**
    A. *Altered nutrition, less than body requirements*, related to vitamin B_{12} deficiency.
    B. *Impaired physical mobility* related to numbness of extremities.
    C. *Fatigue* related to decreased oxygen-carrying capacity.
    D. *Altered oral mucous membrane* related to changes in gastric mucosa.
    E. *Altered thought processes* related to progressive neurologic degeneration.

V. **Nursing care plan/implementation**
    A. Goal: *promote physical and emotional comfort*.
        1. Activity: bed rest or activity as tolerated—restrictions depend on neurologic or cardiac involvement.
        2. Comfort: keep extremities warm—light blankets, loose-fitting socks.
        3. Medication: vitamin B_{12} therapy as ordered.
        4. *Diet*:
            a. Six small feedings.
            b. Soft or pureed.
            c. Organ meats, fish, eggs.
        5. Mouth care: before and after meals, to increase appetite and relieve mouth discomfort.
    B. Goal: **health teaching**.
        1. Medication:
            a. Lifelong therapy.
            b. Injection techniques, rotation of sites.
        2. Diet.
        3. Rest, exercise to tolerance.

VI. **Evaluation/outcome criteria**
    A. No irreversible neurologic or cardiac complications.
    B. Takes vitamin B_{12} for the rest of life—uses safe injection technique.
    C. Returns for follow-up care.

Polycythemia Vera

Abnormal increase in circulating RBCs; considered to be a form of malignancy.

I. **Pathophysiology**: unknown causes → massive increases of erythrocytes, myelocytes (bone marrow leukocytes), and thrombocytes → increased blood viscosity/volume and tissue/organ congestion; increased peripheral vascular resistance; intravascular thrombosis usually develops in middle age, particularly in Jewish men; in contrast, *secondary* polycythemia occurs as a compensatory response to tissue hypoxia associated with prolonged exposure to high altitude, chronic lung disease, and heart disease.

II. **Assessment**
    A. *Subjective data*:
        1. Headache; dizziness; ringing in ears.
        2. Weakness; loss of interest.
        3. Feelings of abdominal fullness.
        4. Shortness of breath; orthopnea.
        5. Pruritus, especially after bathing.
        6. Pain: gouty-arthritic.

B. *Objective data*:
1. Skin: mucosal erythema, ruddy complexion (reddish purple).
2. Ecchymosis; gingival (gum) bleeding.
3. Enlarged liver, spleen.
4. Hypertension.
5. Lab data:
   a. *Increased*—hemoglobin, hematocrit, RBCs, leukocytes, platelets, uric acid;
   b. *Decreased*—bone marrow iron.

III. **Analysis/nursing diagnosis**
A. *Altered tissue perfusion* related to capillary congestion.
B. *Risk for injury* related to dizziness, weakness.
C. *Fluid volume excess* related to mass production of RBCs.
D. *Risk for impaired skin integrity* related to pruritus.
E. *Ineffective breathing pattern* related to shortness of breath, orthopnea.

IV. **Nursing care plan/implementation**
A. Goal: *promote comfort and prevent complications*.
1. Observe for signs of bleeding, thrombosis—stools, urine, gums, skin, ecchymosis.
2. Reduce occurrence: *avoid* prolonged sitting, knee gatch.
3. Assist with ambulation.
4. *Position*: *elevate* head of bed.
5. Skin care: cool-water baths to decrease pruritus; may add bicarbonate of soda to water.
6. Fluids: *force*, to reduce blood viscosity and promote urine excretion: 1500–2500 mL/24 h.
7. Diet: *avoid* foods high in iron, to reduce RBC production.
8. Assist with venesection (phlebotomy), as ordered.
B. Goal: **health teaching**.
1. *Diet*: foods to *avoid* (e.g., liver, egg yolks); fluids to be increased.
2. Signs/symptoms of complications: infections, hemorrhage.
3. *Avoid*: falls, bumps; hot baths/showers (worsens pruritus).
4. Drugs: myelosuppressive agents (busulfan [*Myleran*], cyclophosphamide [*Cytoxan*]), chlorambucil, radioactive phosphorus); purpose, side effects.
5. Procedures: venesection (phlebotomy) if ordered.

V. **Evaluation/outcome criteria**
A. Acceptance of chronic disease.
B. Reports at prescribed intervals for follow-up.
C. Remission: lab data: reduction of bone marrow activity, blood volume and viscosity (RBC <6,500,000/mcg/L; hemoglobin <18 g/dL; hematocrit <45%; white blood cell count <10,000 mcg/L).

D. No complications (e.g., thrombi, hemorrhage, gout, heart failure, leukemia).

Leukemia
(Acute and Chronic)

A neoplastic disease involving the leukopoietic tissue in either the bone marrow or lymphoid areas; acute leukemia occurs in children, young adults; chronic forms occur in later adult life.

I. **Types**:
A. Acute nonlymphocytic (ANLL) — *formerly* known as *acute myelogenous leukemia* (AML); seen generally in older age (>60 yr).
B. Acute lymphocytic (ALL)—seen most often in children 2–10 yr.
C. Chronic lymphocytic (CLL)—generally affects the elderly.
D. Chronic myelogenous (CML)—also known as *chronic granulocytic leukemia* (CGL); more likely to occur between 25 and 60 yr.

II. **Pathophysiology**: displacement of normal marrow cells by proliferating leukemic cells (abnormal, immature leukocytes) → normochromic anemia, thrombocytopenia.

III. **Risk factors/causes**:
A. Viruses.
B. Genetic abnormalities.
C. Exposure to chemicals.
D. Radiation.
E. Treatment for other types of cancer (e.g., alkylating agents).

IV. **Assessment**
A. *Subjective data*:
1. Fatigue, weakness.
2. Anorexia, nausea.
3. Pain: joints, bones (acute leukemia).
4. Night sweats, weight loss, malaise.
B. *Objective data*:
1. Skin: pallor due to anemia, *jaundice*.
2. Fever: frequent infections; mouth ulcers.
3. Bleeding: petechiae, purpura, ecchymosis, epistaxis, gingiva.
4. Organ enlargement: spleen, liver.
5. Enlarged lymph nodes; tenderness.
6. Bone marrow aspiration: *increase* in blast cells.
7. Lab data:
   a. WBC—15,000–500,000/mL.
   b. RBCs—normal to severely *decreased*;
   c. Hgb—low or normal;
   d. Platelets—low to *elevated*.

V. **Analysis/nursing diagnosis**
A. *Risk for infection* related to immature or abnormal leukocytes.

B. *Activity intolerance* related to hypoxia and weakness.

C. *Fatigue* related to anemia.

D. *Altered tissue perfusion* related to anemia.

E. *Anxiety* related to diagnosis and treatment.

F. *Altered oral mucous membrane* related to susceptibility to infection.

G. *Fear* related to diagnosis.

H. *Ineffective individual or family coping* related to potentially fatal disease.

VI. Nursing care plan/implementation

A. Goal: *prevent, control, and treat infection.*

1. Protective isolation if indicated.
2. Observe for early signs of infection:
   a. Inflammation at injection sites.
   b. Vital sign changes.
   c. Cough.
   d. Obtain cultures.
3. Give antibiotics as ordered.
4. Mouth care: clean q2h, examine for new lesions, *avoid* trauma.

B. Goal: *assess and control bleeding, anemia.*

1. Activity: *restrict* to prevent trauma.
2. Observe for hemorrhage: vital signs, body orifices, stool, urine.
3. Control localized bleeding: ice, pressure at least 3–4 min after needle sticks, positioning.
4. Use soft-bristle or foam-rubber toothbrush to prevent gingival bleeding.
5. Give blood/blood components as ordered (see **Table 5.1**); observe for transfusion reactions.

C. Goal: *provide rest, comfort, nutrition.*

1. Activity: 8 h sleep, daily nap.
2. Comfort measures: flotation mattress, bed cradle, sheepskin.
3. Analgesics: without delay.
   a. Mild pain (acetaminophen [*Tylenol*], propoxyphene HCl [*Darvon*] without aspirin).
   b. Severe pain (codeine, meperidine HCl [*Demerol*]).
4. *Diet*: bland.
   a. *High* in protein, minerals, vitamins.
   b. *Low* roughage.
   c. Small, frequent feedings.
   d. Favorite foods.
5. Fluids: 3000–4000 mL/d.

D. Goal: *reduce side effects from therapeutic regimen.*

1. Nausea: antiemetics, usually half hour *before* chemotherapy.
2. Increased uric acid level : *force* fluids; may use allopurinol.
3. Stomatitis: *antiseptic anesthetic* mouthwashes.
4. Rectal irritation: meticulous toileting, *sitz baths*, topical relief (e.g., Tucks).

E. Goal: *provide emotional/spiritual support.*

1. Contact clergy if client desires.
2. Allow, encourage client-initiated discussion of death (developmentally appropriate).
3. Allow family to be involved in care.
4. If death occurs, provide privacy, listening, sharing of grief for family.

F. Goal: **health teaching**.

1. Prevent infection.
2. Limits of activity.
3. Control bleeding.
4. Reduce nausea.
5. Mouth care.
6. Chemotherapy: regimen, side effects.

VII. Evaluation/outcome criteria

A. Alleviate symptoms; obtain remission.

B. Prevent complications (e.g., infection).

C. Ventilates emotions—accepts and deals with anger.

D. Experiences peaceful death (e.g., pain free).

Idiopathic Thrombocytopenic Purpura (ITP)

Potentially fatal disorder characterized by spontaneous increase in platelet destruction; ITP is an autoimmune disease; remissions occur spontaneously or following splenectomy; in contrast, *secondary* thrombocytopenia (STP) is caused by viral infections, drug hypersensitivity (i.e., *quinidine, sulfonamides*), lupus, or bone marrow failure; treat cause.

I. Assessment

A. *Subjective data*:

1. Spontaneous skin hemorrhages—lower extremities.
2. Menorrhagia.
3. Epistaxis.

B. *Objective data*:

1. Bleeding: gastrointestinal, urinary, nasal; following minor trauma, dental extractions.
2. Petechiae; ecchymosis.
3. Lab data:
   a. *Decreased* platelets (<100,000/mL);
   b. *Increased* bleeding time;
   c. Tourniquet test—*positive*, demonstrating increased capillary fragility.

II. Analysis/nursing diagnosis

A. *Risk for injury* related to hemorrhage.

B. *Altered tissue perfusion* related to fragile capillaries.

C. *Impaired skin integrity* related to skin hemorrhages.

III. Nursing care plan/implementation

A. Goal: *prevent complications from bleeding tendencies.*

1. Precautions:
   a. Injections—use small-bore needles; rotate sites; apply direct pressure.
   b. *Avoid* bumping, trauma.
   c. Use swabs for mouth care.
2. Observe for signs of bleeding, petechiae following BP reading, ecchymosis, purpura.
3. Administer *steroids* (e.g., prednisone) with immune thrombocytopenic purpura to increase platelet count; give platelets for count below 20,000–30,000/mcg/L with secondary thrombocytopenic purpura.

B. Goal: **health teaching.**

1. *Avoid* traumatic activities:
   a. Contact sports.
   b. Violent sneezing, coughing, nose blowing.
   c. Straining at stool.
   d. Heavy lifting.
2. *Signs of decreased platelets*—petechiae, ecchymosis, gingival bleeding, hematuria, menorrhagia.
3. Use MedicAlert tag/card.
4. Precautions: self-medication; particularly *avoid* aspirin-containing drugs.
5. Prepare for splenectomy if drug therapy unsuccessful (prednisone, cyclophosphamide, azathioprine [*Imuran*]).

IV. Evaluation/outcome criteria

A. Returns for follow-up.
B. No complications (e.g., hemorrhage).
C. Lab data: Platelet count >200,000/mcg/L.
D. Skin remains intact.
E. Resumes self-care activities.

Splenectomy

Removal of spleen following rupture due to acquired hemolytic anemia, trauma, tumor, or idiopathic thrombocytopenia purpura.

I. Assessment (see above for cause of rupture.)

II. Analysis/nursing diagnosis

A. *Risk for fluid volume deficit* related to hemorrhage.
B. *Risk for infection* related to impaired immune response.
C. *Pain* related to abdominal distention.

III. Nursing care plan/implementation

A. Goal: *prepare for surgery.*
1. Give whole blood, as ordered.
2. Insert nasogastric tube to decrease postoperative abdominal distention, as ordered.

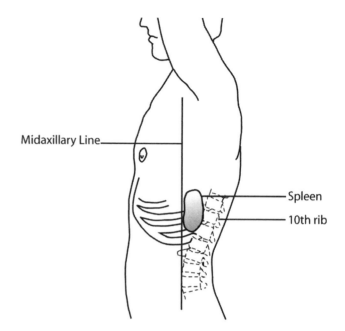

Location of Spleen

B. Goal: *prevent postoperative complications.*
1. Observe for:
   a. *Hemorrhage*—bleeding tendency with thrombocytopenia due to decreased platelet count.
   b. *Gastrointestinal distention*—removal of enlarged spleen may result in distended stomach and intestines, to fill void.
2. Recognize temperature of 101°F as normal for 10 d.
3. Incision: splint when coughing, to prevent atelectasis (frequent complication), pneumonia with upper abdominal incision.

C. Goal: **health teaching.**
1. Increased risk of infection after splenectomy.
2. Report signs of infection *immediately.*

IV. Evaluation/outcome criteria

A. No complications (e.g., respiratory, subphrenic abscess or hematoma, thromboemboli, infection).
B. Complete and permanent remission—occurs in 60-80% of clients.

🔑 Summary of Key Points

1. DIC occurs following low-perfusion states, such as shock. DIC should be suspected in a client with no prior history of a bleeding tendency.

2. All types of anemia result in a decrease in oxygen-carrying capacity.

3. Fatigue, weakness, easy bruising, and bleeding gums are frequently seen in all types of leukemia.

4. If platelet count is below normal, there will be spontaneous bleeding into any part of the body.

💡 Study and Memory Aids

Complete Blood Count

Erythrocytes
  Hematocrit
  Hemoglobin
  Red blood cells

Leukocytes

  White blood cells
    Differential count
    Granulocytes
      Basophils
      Eosinophils
      Neutrophils

  Agranulocytes
    Lymphocytes
    Monocytes

  Thrombocytes
    Platelets

🍎 Diets

Iron Deficiency Anemia

↑ Protein, iron, vitamins

Pernicious Anemia

Small pureed feedings
Organ meat, fish, eggs

Polycythemia Vera

Ø Fe⁺
↑ Fluids

Leukemia

↑ Fluids
  Minerals   ↓ Roughage
  Proteins
  Vitamins

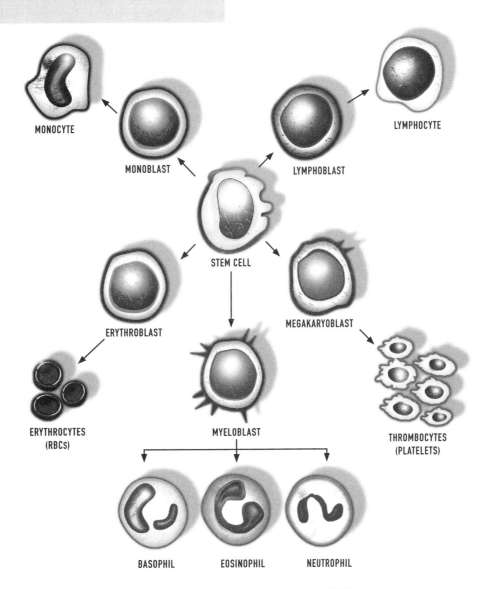

MONOCYTE

MONOBLAST

LYMPHOBLAST

LYMPHOCYTE

STEM CELL

ERYTHROBLAST

MEGAKARYOBLAST

ERYTHROCYTES
(RBCS)

MYELOBLAST

THROMBOCYTES
(PLATELETS)

BASOPHIL   EOSINOPHIL   NEUTROPHIL

Development of Blood Cells (RBC & WBC)

Drug Review

Disseminated Intravascular Coagulation

Aminocaproic acid (*Amicar*): 4–5 gm IV initially, then 1–1.25 gm/h IV for 8 h. Maximum 30 gm/24 h.
Antithrombin III in fresh frozen plasma to decrease complications
Cryoprecipitate given for depletion of factors V and VIII
Fresh frozen plasma
Heparin sodium: IV, 1000 U/h adjusted according to partial thromboplastin time (PTT)
Platelets

Iron Deficiency Anemia

Ferrous sulfate (*Fer-In-Sol*): 300 mg 2–4 times daily; give with meals
Iron dextran (*Imferon*): 100–250 mg IM via Z track method. Do *not* exceed 250 mg (5 mL).

Pernicious Anemia

Hydroxocobalamin (Vit B$_{12}$): 100–200mcg monthly, given IM, SC ("Flushing" dose for Schilling test: 1000 mcg/mL)
Vitamin derivatives to correct nutritional deficiency

Polycythemia Vera: Drug and Other Treatment

Myelosuppressive agents to produce remission: radioactive phosphorus, chlorambucil, busulfan (*Myleran*), hydroxyurea (*Hydrea*) cyclophosphamide (*Cytoxan*)
Other treatment
Phlebotomy
Radiation

Leukemia

Analgesics to relieve discomfort
Antibiotics to fight infections
Antiemetics to combat nausea and vomiting
Antineoplastic drugs
L-asparaginase
Busulfan
Cyclophosphamide
Cytarabine (*Ara-C*) in combination with other drugs
Daunorubicin
Prednisone
Vincristine

Immune Thrombocytopenic Purpura: Drug and Other Treatment

Immunosuppressive therapy:
Azathioprine (*Imuran*)
Cyclophosphamide (*Cytoxan*)
Vinblastine (*Velban*)
Vincristine (*Oncovin*)
Plasmapheresis until steroids take effect, large volumes of the client's plasma are removed and fresh plasma is administered
Steroid therapy: prednisone, danazol (*Danocrine*)

Splenectomy

Preoperative and postoperative medications, as with any surgical client.
Antibiotic therapy to decrease risk of infection.

Questions

1. Which laboratory values would necessitate a nursing action?
   1. A hematocrit (Hct) value of 40%.
   2. A hemoglobin (Hgb) level of 9 g/dL.
   3. A white blood cell count (WBC) of 9,000/mm³.
   4. A potassium (K⁺) concentration of 4.8 mEq/L.

2. The nurse would record in the client's chart the finding of large, irregular hemorrhagic areas on a client's leg as:
   1. Ecchymoses.
   2. Hematoma.
   3. Petechiae.
   4. Hemangioma.

3. Treatment for a client's leukemia has resulted in an apparent state of remission. The nurse explains to the client that *remission* means that:
   1. A complete cure has occurred.
   2. The symptoms from the disease have subsided.
   3. The blood findings are normal, but the bone marrow is still affected.
   4. The leukemia will not come back because there is no evidence of disease.

4. Which group of assessment findings would be seen in a client with acute nonlymphocytic leukemia (ANLL)?
   1. Diarrhea, nausea, and restlessness.
   2. Weakness, fever, and bleeding.
   3. Dehydration, chills, and joint pain.
   4. Tremors, lymph node tenderness, and headache.

5. As part of the preparation for a bone marrow aspiration, the nurse would:
   1. Explain the procedure to the client and have the client sign a consent form.
   2. Tell the client that no anesthetic can be given because it interferes with the quality of the sample.
   3. Show the client the location of the posterior iliac crest where the sample will be taken.
   4. Discuss the need to remain on bed rest for 6 to 8 hours after the procedure to prevent bleeding.

6. Which solution should the nurse infuse before starting a blood transfusion?
   1. 5% dextrose in water.
   2. 0.9% sodium chloride.
   3. 5% dextrose in 0.45% sodium chloride.
   4. Ringer's lactate solution.

7. The nurse finds a client crying who is undergoing chemotherapy for leukemia. The best response for the nurse to make would be:
   1. "All of these changes in your life have been difficult."
   2. "When you're done crying I'll come back."
   3. "Fortunately there are effective treatments available."
   4. "You'll feel better when you are done crying."

8. Which nursing action is most important before starting an infusion of packed red blood cells IV?
   1. Weighing the client as a baseline assessment.
   2. Finding out whether an 18-gauge needle is being used.
   3. Checking the Hgb and Hct levels.
   4. Clearing the existing tubing with 5% dextrose in water.

9. During the first 15 minutes of a blood transfusion, the nurse should set the rate of a transfusion at:
   120/hr. first 15 min
   1. 2mL/min.
   2. 5mL/min.
   3. 10mL/min.
   4. 15mL/min.

10. A client receiving a blood transfusion complains of a headache and of feeling cold and having a heaviness in the chest. The client appears flushed and is shaking; blood pressure is 100/58 mm Hg. The first nursing action would be to:
    1. Remove the IV immediately.
    2. Clamp off the blood transfusion.
    3. Continue to monitor the vital signs.
    4. Call the MD.

Answers/Rationale

1. **(2)** The Hgb level for a man or woman should be 12 g/dL or higher. A level of 9 g/dL is low and may indicate the presence of anemia or blood loss. The oxygen-carrying capacity of the blood would be reduced, and as a result, the client might be experiencing the symptoms of hypoxia, such as fatigue and shortness of breath. An Hct value of 40% **(1)** is within the normal limits of 37% or higher. The normal range of the WBC is 5000 to 10,000/mm³, so 9,000/mm³ **(3)** is normal. The normal potassium concentration ranges from 3.5 to 5.0 mEq/L, so 4.8 mEq/L **(4)** is also normal. **AN, ANL, 6, PhI, Reduction of risk potential**

2. **(1)** An ecchymosis is a discoloration of the skin resulting from the extravasation of blood into the subcutaneous tissues. A hematoma **(2)** is a circumscribed extravascular collection of blood, which is usually clotted. Petechiae **(3)** are pinpoint hemorrhages on a surface such as the skin or mucous membranes. A hemangioma **(4)** is a tumor composed of blood vessels. **IMP, RE/KN, 6, PhI, Physiological adaptation**

3. **(2)** When the signs, and hence the symptoms, of a chronic condition subside, this is called a *remission*. The client is *not* cured **(1)**. During a remission there are no symptoms **(3)**. The symptoms *often* return **(4)**, which is called an *exacerbation*. **IMP, RE/KN, 7, PhI, Physiological adaptation**

4. **(2)** The signs and symptoms of all types of leukemia are similar. (The symptoms are also characteristic of anemia and thrombocytopenia, however.) In addition to weakness, fever, and bleeding, the client often complains of generalized pain and headache. ANLL was formerly known as *acute myelogenous leukemia*. None of the symptoms in option **1** are those of ANLL. In option **3**, only joint pain is a symptom. Lymph node enlargement and tenderness in option **4** is a sign and headache a possible symptom, but not tremors. **AS, COM, 6, PhI, Physiological adaptation**

5. **(3)** The posterior iliac crest is the most common site for bone marrow aspiration. Other possible sites are the sternum and anterior iliac crest. Obtaining informed consent **(1)** is the responsibility of the MD, though the nurse should make sure the form is signed before the procedure. The skin and subcutaneous tissue down to the periosteum are anesthetized, and this does not interfere with the quality of the sample **(2)**. The site needs to be watched for bleeding, but bed rest **(4)** is not required. **IMP, COM, 1, PhI, Reduction of risk potential**

6. **(2)** If blood is mixed with any IV solution other than normal saline outside the body, it will precipitate in the tubing. The other solutions (**1, 3,** and **4**) would cause the blood to precipitate. **IMP, COM, 6, PhI, Pharmacological and parenteral therapies**

7. **(1)** The most therapeutic communication reflects what the client is expressing. Such a client needs to know the feelings are recognized and that it is okay to feel depressed and discouraged; a loss has occurred. The other responses (**2, 3,** and **4**) do not recognize the client's feelings. **IMP, APP, 7, PsI, Psychosocial integrity**

8. **(2)** The needle needs to be at least an 18-gauge one to prevent lysis of the red blood cells. Vital signs, *not* weight **(1)**, are used for the baseline assessment. Hgb and Hct values **(3)** would be checked *later* to determine the effects of the transfusion. The line is cleared with saline, *not* dextrose **(4)**. **PL, ANL, 6, PhI, Pharmacological and parenteral therapies**

9. **(1)** The rate of a blood transfusion during the first 15 minutes should be 1 to 2 mL/min because this is the time when transfusion reactions are most likely to occur. This would be enough blood to produce a reaction but not too much so that the reaction can be easily reversed. The other rates are too fast (**2, 3** and **4**) and would allow too much blood to be transfused for a reaction to be easily reversed. **IMP, APP, 6, PhI, Pharmacological and parenteral therapies**

10. (2) The client is experiencing a hemolytic transfusion reaction resulting from ABO incompatibility; the transfusion should be stopped, but the IV line left in place in case drugs need to be given in an emergency. The nurse should change the tubing immediately and infuse normal saline. If the client goes into shock, starting a new IV may be difficult (1). Vital signs would be monitored (3) and the MD notified (4) *after* the IV tubing has been changed. **PL, ANL, 6, PhI, Physiological adaptation**

Key to Codes

Nursing process: **AS**, assessment; **AN**, analysis; **PL**, planning; **IMP**, implementation; **EV**, evaluation. (See **Appendix M** for explanation of nursing process steps.)

Cognitive level: RE/KN, recall/knowledge; **COM**, comprehension; **APP**, application; **ANL**, analysis; **EVL**, evaluation; **SYN**, synthesis. (See **Appendix M** for explanation.)

Category of human function: 1, protective; **2**, sensory-perceptual; **3**, comfort, rest, activity, and mobility; **4**, nutrition; **5**, growth and development; **6**, fluid-gas transport; **7**, psychosocial-cultural; **8**, elimination. (See **Appendix 0** for explanation.)

Client need: SECE, safe, effective care environment; **PhI**, physiological integrity; **PsI**, psychosocial integrity; **HPM**, health promotion and maintenance. (See **Appendix P** for explanation.)

Client subneed: (See **Appendix P** for explanation)

Respiratory Disorders

Chapter Outline

Pneumonia

Acute inflammation of lungs with exudate accumulation in alveoli and other respiratory passages that interferes with ventilation.

I. **Types:**
   A. *Community acquired*—lower respiratory infection with onset in community or within 2 days of hospitalization; e.g.,

   Streptococcus pneumoniae
   Mycoplasma
   Haemophilus influenzae
   Respiratory viruses
   Staphylococcus aureus
   Enteric aerobic gram-negative bacteria
   Fungi
   Mycobacterium tuberculosis

   B. *Hospital acquired*—occurs 48 hours or longer after admission; e.g.,

   Pseudomonas aeruginosa
   Enterobacter
   Escherichia coli
   Proteus
   Klebsiella
   Staphylococcus aureus
   Streptococcus pneumoniae
   Oral anaerobes

   C. *Opportunistic pneumonia*—affects clients with altered immune response; e.g.,

   Pneumocystis carinii
   Cytomegalovirus

   D. *Aspiration pneumonia*:
      1. *Noninfectious*: aspiration of fluids (gastric secretions, foods, liquids, tube feedings) into the airways.
      2. *Bacterial aspiration pneumonia*: related to poor cough mechanisms due to anesthesia, coma (mixed flora of upper respiratory tract cause pneumonia).

   E. *Hematogenous pneumonia bacterial infections*: related to spread of bacteria from the bloodstream.

II. **Pathophysiology**: caused by infectious or noninfectious agents, clotting of an exudate rich in fibrin, consolidated lung tissue.

III. **Risk factors/causes:**
   A. Impaired defense mechanisms.
   B. Impaired cough and epiglottal reflexes.
   C. Impaired mucociliary escalator.
   D. Smoking.
   E. Pollution.
   F. Viral upper respiratory infection.
   G. Normal changes due to aging.
   H. Chronic or debilitating diseases such as leukemia, alcoholism, diabetes mellitus, heart disease, chronic lung disease.
   I. Prolonged bed rest/immobility.

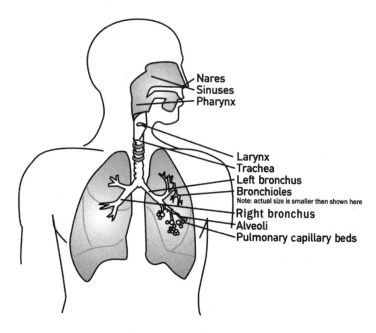

Respiratory System

Nares
Sinuses
Pharynx
Larynx
Trachea
Left bronchus
Bronchioles
Note: actual size is smaller then shown here
Right bronchus
Alveoli
Pulmonary capillary beds

IV. Assessment

A. *Subjective data*:

1. Pain location: chest (affected side), referred to abdomen, shoulder, flank.
2. Irritability, restlessness.
3. Apprehension.
4. Nausea, anorexia.
5. History of exposure.

B. *Objective data*:

1. Cough:
   a. Productive, rust (blood) or yellowish sputum (greenish with *atypical pneumonia*).
   b. Splinting of affected side when coughing.
2. Sudden increased fever, chills.
3. Nasal flaring, circumoral cyanosis.
4. Respiratory distress: tachypnea.
5. Auscultation:
   a. Decreased breath sounds on *affected* side.
   b. Exaggerated breath sounds on *unaffected* side.
   c. Crackles, bronchial breath sounds.
   d. Dullness over consolidated area.
   e. Possible pleural friction rub.
6. Chest retraction (air hunger in infants).
7. Vomiting.
8. Facial herpes simplex.
9. *Diagnostic* studies:
   a. Chest x-ray: haziness to consolidation.
   b. Sputum culture: specific organisms, usually pneumococcus.
10. Lab data:
    (1) Blood culture—organism specific except when viral;
    (2) White blood cell count (WBC)—leukocytosis;
    (3) Sedimentation rate—*elevated*.

V. Analysis/nursing diagnosis

A. *Ineffective airway clearance* related to retained secretions.
B. *Activity intolerance* related to inflammatory process.
C. *Pain* related to continued coughing.
D. *Knowledge deficit* related to proper management of symptoms.
E. *Risk for fluid volume deficit* related to tachypnea.
F. *Impaired gas exchange* related to infection in parenchyma.

VI. Nursing care plan/implementation

A. Goal: *promote adequate ventilation, patent airway*.
   1. Deep breathe, cough.
   2. Remove respiratory secretions, *suction* prn.
   3. High humidity with or without oxygen therapy.
   4. *Nebulizer treatments with bronchodilators; incentive spirometry, chest physiotherapy,* as ordered and needed to loosen secretions.
   5. Use of *expectorants*, as ordered.
   6. Supplemental O_2 as ordered.
B. Goal: *control infection*.
   1. Monitor vital signs; use methods to reduce elevated temperature.
   2. Administer *antibiotics*, as ordered to control infection—cephalexin (*Keflex*), cephalothin (*Keflin*), erythromycin, gentamicin sulfate (*Garamycin*), penicillin G. *Note*: need culture *before* starting on antibiotics.
C. Goal: *provide rest and comfort*.
   1. Planned rest periods.
   2. Adequate hydration by mouth, intake and output (I&O).
   3. *Diet*: high carbohydrate, *high* protein to meet energy demands and promote healing.
   4. *Position*: in semi-Fowler's or Fowler's to reduce work of breathing.
D. Goal: *prevent potential complications*.
   1. Cross-infection: use good handwashing technique.
   2. Hyperthermia: tepid baths, hypothermia blanket, *antipyretics*.
   3. Respiratory insufficiency and acidosis: clear airway, promote expectoration of secretions.
   4. Assess cardiac and respiratory function.
E. Goal: **health teaching**.
   1. Proper disposal of tissues, cover mouth when coughing.
   2. Expected side effects of prescribed medications.
   3. Need for rest, limited interactions, increased caloric intake.

4. Need to *avoid* future respiratory tract infections.
5. Correct dosage of antibiotics and the importance of taking entire prescription at prescribed times (times evenly distributed throughout the 24-h period to maintain blood level of antibiotic) for increased effectiveness.

VII. Evaluation/outcome criteria
  A. Adheres to medication regimen.
  B. Has improved gas exchange, as shown by improved pulmonary function test results.
  C. No acid-base or fluid imbalance: normal pH.
  D. Energy level increased.
  E. Sputum production decreased, normal color.
  F. Vital signs stable.
  G. Breath sounds clear.
  H. Culture results negative.
  I. Reports comfort level increased.

Atelectasis

Collapsed alveoli in part or all of the lung.

I. **Pathophysiology**: due to compression (tumor), airway obstruction, decreased surfactant production, or progressive regional hypoventilation.

II. **Risk factors/causes:**
  A. Shallow breathing due to pain, abdominal distention, narcotics, or sedatives.
  B. Decreased ciliary action due to anesthesia, smoking.
  C. Thickened secretions due to immobility, dehydration.
  D. Aspiration of foreign substances.
  E. Bronchospasms.

III. Assessment
  A. *Subjective data*: restlessness.
  B. *Objective data*:
    1. Tachypnea.
    2. Tachycardia.
    3. Dullness on percussion.
    4. Absent bronchial breathing.
    5. Tactile fremitus in affected area.
    6. X-ray:
      a. Patches of consolidation.
      b. Elevated diaphragm.
      c. Mediastinal shift.
    7. Breath sounds diminished in affected area.

IV. Analysis/nursing diagnosis
  A. *Impaired gas exchange* related to shallow breathing.
  B. *Pain* related to collapse of lung.
  C. *Fear* related to altered respiratory status.

V. Nursing care plan/implementation
  A. Goal: *relieve hypoxia*.
    1. Frequent respiratory assessment.
    2. Respiratory hygiene measures, cough, deep breathe.
    3. Oxygen as ordered
    4. Monitor effects of respiratory therapy, ventilators, breathing assistance measures to ensure proper gas exchange.
    5. *Position* on unaffected side to allow for lung expansion.
  B. Goal: *prevent complications*.
    1. *Antibiotics* as ordered.
    2. Sterile technique when doing tracheal bronchial suctioning to reduce risk of possible infection.
    3. Turn, cough, and deep breathe.
    4. *Increase fluid* intake to liquefy secretions.
  C. Goal: **health teaching**.
    1. Need to report signs and symptoms listed in assessment data for early recognition of problem.
    2. Importance of coughing and deep breathing to improve present condition and prevent further problems.

VI. Evaluation/outcome criteria
  A. Lung expanded on x-ray.
  B. Acid-base balance obtained and maintained.
  C. No pain on respiration.
  D. Activity level increased.

Pulmonary Embolism

Undissolved mass that travels in bloodstream and occludes a blood vessel; can be thromboemboli, fat, air, or catheter. Constitutes a **critical medical emergency**.

I. **Pathophysiology**: obstructs blood flow to lung → increased pressure on pulmonary artery and reflex constriction of pulmonary blood vessels → poor pulmonary circulation → pulmonary infarction.

II. **Risk factors/causes:**
  A. Deep vein thrombophlebitis (most common cause).
  B. Recent surgery.
  C. Invasive procedures.
  D. Immobility.
  E. Obesity.
  F. Myocardial infarction, heart failure.

III. Assessment
  A. *Subjective data*:
    1. Chest pain: substernal, localized; type—crushing, sharp, stabbing with respirations.
    2. Dyspnea.
    3. Restless, irritable, anxious.
    4. Sense of impending doom.

B. *Objective data*:
1. Respirations: either rapid, shallow or deep, gasping.
2. Elevated temperature.
☞ 3. Auscultation: friction rub, crackles, diminished breath sounds.
4. Shock:
    a. Tachycardia.
    b. Hypotension.
    c. Skin: cold, clammy.
5. Cough: hemoptysis.
〰 6. X-ray: area of density.
7. Lung scan: uses radioactive isotope intravenously and radioactive gas to evaluate pulmonary perfusion and ventilation.
8. Lab data:
    a. *Decreased* $PaCO_2$, PO_2
    b. *Elevated* WBC.

IV. **Analysis/nursing diagnosis:**
A. *Ineffective breathing pattern* related to shallow respirations.
B. *Impaired gas exchange* related to dyspnea.
C. *Pain* related to decreased tissue perfusion.
D. *Altered peripheral tissue perfusion* related to occlusion of blood vessel.
E. *Fear* related to emergency condition.
F. *Anxiety* related to sense of impending doom.

V. **Nursing care plan/implementation**
A. Goal: *prevent or minimize respiratory distress*.
1. Institute measures to prevent or treat deep vein thrombosis.
〰 2. Monitor blood coagulation studies, e.g., partial thromboplastin time (PTT).
3. Ambulate as tolerated and indicated.
▬ 4. Administer IVs, transfusions, *vasopressor* medications, anticoagulant therapy (*Heparin*).
5. Fluids, by mouth, when able.
6. Monitor signs: *Homans'* (unreliable), acidosis.
7. Prepare for surgery if peripheral embolectomy indicated.
B. Goal: **health teaching**.
1. Prevent recurrence.
2. Decrease stasis.
3. If history of thrombophlebitis, *avoid* birth control pills.
4. Need to continue medication.
5. Follow-up care.

VI. **Evaluation/outcome criteria**
A. No complications; no further incidence of emboli.
B. Respiratory rate returns to normal.
C. Coagulation studies within normal limits (aPTT) 25–38 sec).
D. Reports comfort achieved.

Histoplasmosis

Infection found mostly in central United States. *Not transmitted from human to human but from dust and contaminated soil*. Progressive histoplasmosis, seen most frequently in middle-aged white men who have COPD, is often seen in house painters, and is characterized by cavity formation, fibrosis, and emphysema.

I. **Pathophysiology**: spores of *Histoplasma capsulatum* (from droppings of infected birds and bats) are inhaled, multiply, and cause fungal infections of respiratory tract. Leads to necrosis and healing by encapsulation.

II. **Assessment**
A. *Subjective data*:
1. Malaise.
2. Chest pain, dyspnea.
B. *Objective data*:
1. Weight loss.
2. Nonproductive cough.
3. Fever.
〰 4. Positive skin test for histoplasmosis.
5. Benign acute pneumonitis.
〰 6. Chest x-ray: nodular infiltrate.
〰 7. Sputum culture shows *H. capsulatum*.
8. Hepatomegaly, splenomegaly.

III. **Analysis/nursing diagnosis**
A. *Ineffective airway clearance* related to pneumonitis.
B. *Ineffective breathing pattern* related to dyspnea.
C. *Pain* related to infectious process.
D. *Risk for infection* related to repeated exposure to fungal spores.
E. *Impaired gas exchange* related to chronic pulmonary disease.
F. *Knowledge deficit* related to prevention of disease.

IV. **Nursing care plan/implementation**
A. Goal: *relieve symptoms of the disease*:
▬ 1. Administer medications as ordered.
    a. Amphotericin B (IV) and ketoconazole.
        (1) Monitor for drug side effects: local phlebitis, renal toxicity, hypokalemia, anemia, anaphylaxis, bone marrow depression.
        (2) *Azotemia* (presence of nitrogen-containing compounds in blood) is monitored by biweekly blood urea nitrogen (BUN) or creatinine levels BUN >40 mg/dL or creatinine 3.0 mg/dL necessitate stopping amphotericin B until values return to within normal limits.
    b. *Aspirin*, diphenhydramine HC1 [*Benadryl*], promethazine HCl [*Phenergan*], prochlorperazine [*Compazine*]: used to decrease systemic toxicity of chills, fever, aching, nausea, and vomiting.

🏠 B. Goal: **health teaching**.

1. Desired effects and side effects of prescribed medications; importance of taking medications for entire course of therapy (usually from 2 wk to 3 mo).
2. Importance of follow-up laboratory tests to monitor toxic effects of drug.
3. Identify source of contamination if possible and avoid future contact if possible.
4. Importance of deep breathing, pursed-lip breathing, coughing (see **Emphysema, p. 74**, for specific care).
5. Signs and symptoms of chronic histoplasmosis, COPD, drug toxicity, and drug side effects, as in **IV.A.1**.

◄► V. **Evaluation/outcome criteria**

A. Complies with treatment plan.
B. Respiratory complications avoided.
C. Symptoms of illness decreased.
D. No further spread of disease.
E. Source of contamination identified and eliminated.

Tuberculosis

Inflammatory, communicable disease that commonly attacks the lungs, although may occur in other parts of body.

I. **Pathophysiology**: exposure to causative organism (*Mycobacterium tuberculosis*) in the alveoli in susceptible person leads to inflammation. Infection spreads by lymphatics to hilus; antibodies are released, leading to fibrosis, calcification, or inflammation. Exudate formation leads to caseous necrosis, then liquefaction of caseous material leads to cavitation.

II. **Risk factors/causes:**

A. Persons who have been exposed to tubercle bacillus, e.g., health care workers.
B. Persons who have diseases or are undergoing therapies known to suppress the immune system.
C. Immigrants from Latin America, Africa, Asia, and Oceania living in the United States for less than a year.
D. Americans living in the above regions for a prolonged time.
E. Residents of overcrowded metropolitan cities.
F. Men >65 yr.
G. Women between 25–44 yr and >65 yr.
H. Children <5 yr.
I. People who are homeless.
J. Persons in institutions, e.g., long-term care facilities and prisons.

◄► III. **Assessment**

A. *Subjective data*:

1. Loss of appetite, weight loss.
2. Weakness, loss of energy.
3. Pain: knifelike, chest.
4. Though client may be symptom free, the disease is found on screening.

B. *Objective data*:

1. Night sweats.
2. Fever: low grade, late afternoon.
3. Pulse: increased.
4. *Respiratory* assessment:
   a. Productive cough, hemoptysis.
   b. Respirations: normal, increased depth.
   c. Asymmetric lung expansion.
   d. Increased tactile fremitus.
   e. Dullness to percussion.
   f. Crackles following short cough.

〰️ 5. *Diagnostic* tests:
   a. *Positive tuberculin test* (*Mantoux*—reaction to test begins approximately 12 h after administration with area of redness and a central area of induration. The peak time is 48 h. Determination of positive or negative is made. A reaction is positive when it measures 10 mm. Contacts reacting from 5–10 mm may need to be treated prophylactically.
   b. *Sputum*: positive for acid-fast bacilli (smear and culture).
   c. X-ray: infiltration, cavitation.

6. Lab data: blood: *decreased* RBCs, *increased* sedimentation rate.

7. **Classification of tuberculosis:**
   Class Description
   0 No TB exposure, not infected.
   1 TB exposure, no evidence of infection.
   2 TB infection, no disease.
   3 TB: current disease (persons with completed diagnostic evidence of TB—both a significant reaction to tuberculin skin test and clinical and/or x-ray evidence of disease).
   4 TB: no current disease (persons with previous history of TB or with abnormal x-ray films but no significant tuberculin skin test reaction or clinical evidence).
   5 TB: suspect (diagnosis pending; used during diagnostic testing period of suspected persons, for no longer than a 3-mo period).

◄► IV. **Analysis/nursing diagnosis**

A. *Ineffective airway clearance* related to productive cough.
B. *Impaired gas exchange* related to asymmetric lung expansion.
C. *Pain* related to unresolved disease process.

D. *Body image disturbance* related to feelings about tuberculosis.

E. *Social isolation* related to fear of spreading infection.

F. *Non-compliance* related to lack of knowledge and long-term nature of treatment regimen.

V. Nursing care plan/implementation

A. Goal: *reduce spread of disease.*

1. Administer medications: isoniazid (*INH*), rifampin—most commonly used.

2. The following may need to take 300 mg of *INH* daily for 1 yr as *prophylactic* measure: positive skin test reactors, including contacts; persons who have diseases or are receiving therapies that affect the immune system; persons who have leukemia, lymphoma, or uncontrolled diabetes or who have had a gastrectomy.

3. *Avoid direct contact with sputum.*

   a. Use good handwashing technique after contact with client, personal articles.

   b. Have client cover mouth and nose when coughing and sneezing, and use disposable tissues to collect sputum.

4. *Provide good circulation of fresh air* (Changes of air dilute the number of organisms. This plus chemotherapy provide protection needed to prevent spread of disease).

5. Implement respiratory isolation procedure (**Table 6.1**).

B. Goal: *promote nutrition.*

1. *Increase protein, calories* to aid in tissue repair and healing.

2. Small, frequent feedings.

3. *Increase* fluids, to liquefy secretions so they can be expectorated.

C. Goal: *promote increased self-esteem.*

1. Encourage client and family to express concerns regarding long-term illness and treatment.

2. Encourage client to maintain role in family

while home treatment is ongoing and to return to work and social contacts as soon as it is determined safe for progress of treatment.

D. Goal: **health teaching**.

1. Desired effects and side effects of medications:

   a. *INH* may affect memory and ability to concentrate. May result in peripheral neuritis, hepatitis, rash, or fever.

   b. *Streptomycin* may cause eighth cranial nerve damage and vestibular ototoxicity, causing hearing loss; may cause labyrinth damage, manifested by vertigo and staggering; also may cause skin rashes, itching, and fever.

   c. Important for client to know that medication regimen must be adhered to for entire course of treatment.

   d. Discontinuation of therapy may allow organism to flourish and make the disease more difficult to treat.

2. Explain methods of disease prevention, encourage contacts to be tested and treated if necessary.

3. Need for follow-up, long-term care.

4. Importance of nutritious diet, rest, avoidance of respiratory infections.

5. Identify community agencies for support and follow-up.

6. Inform that this communicable disease must be reported.

VI. Evaluation/outcome criteria

A. Complies with medication regimen.

B. Lists desired effects and side effects of medications prescribed.

C. Gains weight, eats food *high* in protein and carbohydrates.

D. Sputum culture result becomes negative.

E. Retains role in family.

F. No complications (i.e., no hemorrhage, bacillus not spread to others).

TABLE 6.1 ⚡ RESPIRATORY ISOLATION

When used:
For infectious diseases that are contracted through airborne droplet transmission (e.g., tuberculosis).
Precautions:
Isolate in private room (clients infected with same disease can be placed in same room).
Client should wear mask if out of room for testing, etc.
HEPA masks to be worn by personnel when working within 3 ft of client.
Gowns *not* necessary.
Contaminated articles need to be labeled before being sent for decontamination.
Provide adequate ventilation in the client's room.
Careful handwashing.

Source: ©Lagerquist, SL: *NCLEX-RN® Examination Review.* Boston: Little, Brown.

Emphysema

Chronic disease with excessive inflation of the air spaces distal to the terminal bronchioles, alveolar ducts, and alveoli; characterized by increased airway resistance and decreased diffusing capacity. *Emphysema* and *chronic bronchitis* are examples of *chronic obstructive pulmonary disease* (COPD).

I. **Pathophysiology**: increased airway resistance during expiration results in air trapping and hyperinflation → increased residual volumes. Increased dead space → unequal ventilation → perfusion of poorly ventilated alveoli → hypoxia and carbon dioxide retention (hypercapnia).

Chronic hypercapnia reduces sensitivity of respiratory center; chemoreceptors in aortic arch and carotid sinus become principal regulators of respiratory drive (respond to hypoxia).

II. **Risk factors/causes:**
   A. Smoking.
   B. Air pollution: fumes, dust.
   C. Antienzymes and *alpha-1/antitrypsin* deficiencies.
   D. Destruction of lung parenchyma.
   E. Family history and increased age.

III. **Assessment**
   A. *Subjective data*:
      1. Weakness, lethargy.
      2. History of repeated respiratory infections.
      3. History of long-term smoking.
      4. Irritability.
      5. Inability to accept medical diagnosis and treatment plan.
      6. Refusal to stop smoking.
      7. Dyspnea on exertion and at rest.
   B. *Objective data*:
      1. Increased blood pressure (BP).
      2. Increased pulse.
      3. Nostrils: flaring.
      4. Cough: chronic, productive.
      5. Episodes of wheezing, crackles.
      6. Increased anteroposterior diameter of chest (barrel chest).
      7. Use of accessory respiratory muscles, abdominal and neck.
      8. Asymmetric thoracic movements, decreased diaphragmatic excursion.
      9. *Position*: sits up, leans forward to compress abdomen and push up diaphragm, increasing intrathoracic pressure, producing more efficient expiration
      10. Pursed lips for greater expiratory breathing phase ("*pink puffer*").
      11. Weight loss due to hypoxia.
      12. Skin: ruddy color, nail clubbing; when combined with bronchitis: cyanosis (*blue bloater*).
      13. Respiratory: *early* disease—alkalosis; *late* disease—acidosis, respiratory failure.
      14. Spontaneous pneumothorax.
      15. Cor pulmonale (**emergency cardiac condition** involving right ventricular failure due to increased pressure within pulmonary artery).
      16. X-ray: hyperinflation of lung, flattened diaphragm.
      17. *Pulmonary function tests*:
         a. Prolonged, rapid, forced exhalation.
         b. *Decreased*: vital capacity (<4000 mL); forced expiratory volume.
         c. *Increased*: residual volume (may be 200%); total lung capacity.
      18. Lab data:
         a. PO_2 <80 mm Hg; pH <7.35;
         b. PCO_2 >45 mm Hg.
      Note: In clients whose compensatory mechanisms are functioning, lab values may be out of the normal range, but if a 20:1 ratio of bicarbonate to carbonic acid is maintained, then appropriate acid-base balance also will be maintained. (Carbonic acid value can be obtained by multiplying the PCO_2 value by 0.003.)

IV. **Analysis/nursing diagnosis**
   A. *Impaired gas exchange* related to thick pulmonary secretions.
   B. *Ineffective breathing pattern* related to hyperinflated alveoli.
   C. *Altered nutrition, less than body requirements,* related to weight loss due to poor appetite, low energy level, shortness of breath.
   D. *Activity intolerance* related to increased energy demands used for breathing.
   E. *Sleep pattern disturbance* related to changes in body positions necessary for breathing.
   F. *Anxiety* related to disease progression.
   G. *Risk for infection* related to impaired pulmonary function.

V. **Nursing care plan/implementation**
   A. Goal: *promote optimal ventilation.*
      1. Institute measures designed to decrease airway resistance and enhance gas exchange.
      2. *Position*: Fowler's or leaning forward to encourage expiratory phase.
      3. *Oxygen* with humidification, as ordered—no more than 2 L/min to prevent depression of hypoxic respiratory drive (see **Oxygen Therapy, p. 86-90**).
      4. *Nebulizer* treatments as ordered.
      5. Assisted ventilation.
      6. *Postural drainage, chest physiotherapy.*
      7. Medications, as ordered:
         a. *Bronchodilators* to increase air flow through bronchial tree: albuterol, aminophylline, theophylline, terbutaline, ipratropium, isoproterenol (*Isuprel*).
         b. *Antimicrobials* to treat infection (determined by sputum cultures and sensitivity): tetracycline and ampicillin most common (condition deteriorates with respiratory infections).
         c. *Steroids* used when bronchodilators are ineffective or for short-term therapy in acute episodes: prednisone, methylprednisolone sodium succinate (*Solu-Medrol*), dexamethasone (*Decadron*).
         d. *Expectorants* (*increase water intake* to achieve desired effect): glyceryl guaiacolate (*Robitussin*), guaifenesin.

e. *Bronchial detergents*/liquefying agents (*Mucomyst*).

B. Goal: *employ comfort measures and support other body systems.*

☞ 1. Oral hygiene prn; frequently; (client is mouth breather).

☞ 2. Skin care: water bed, air mattress, foam pads to prevent skin breakdown.

☞ 3. Active and passive range of motion (ROM) exercises to prevent thrombus formation; antiembolic stocking or woven elastic (Ace) bandages may be applied.

4. Increase activities to tolerance.

5. Adequate rest and sleep periods to prevent mental disturbances due to sleep deprivation and to reduce metabolic rate.

C. Goal: *improve nutritional intake.*

1. *High protein, high calorie diet* to prevent negative nitrogen balance.

2. *Small, frequent* meals.

3. Supplement diet with high calorie drinks.

4. *Push fluids* to 3000 mL/d, unless contraindicated—helps moisten secretions.

D. Goal: *provide emotional support for client and family.*

1. Identify factors that increase anxiety:

a. Fears related to mechanical equipment.

b. Loss of body image.

c. Fear of dying.

2. Assist family coping:

a. Do not reinforce denial or encourage overconcern.

b. Give accurate, up-to-date information on client's condition.

c. Be open to questioning.

d. Encourage client-family communication.

e. Provide appropriate diversional activities.

E. Goal: **health teaching.**

1. Breathing exercises, such as pursed-lip breathing and diaphragmatic breathing.

2. Stress-management techniques.

3. Methods to stop smoking.

4. Importance of preventing respiratory infections.

5. Desired effects and side effects of prescribed medications, possible interactions with over-the-counter drugs, correct use of metered dose inhalers.

6. Purposes and techniques for effective bronchial hygiene therapy.

7. Rest/activity schedule that increases with ability.

8. Food selection for high protein, high calorie diet.

9. Importance of taking 2500–3000 mL fluid per d (unless contraindicated by another medical problem).

10. Importance of medical follow-up.

VI. **Evaluation/outcome criteria**

A. Takes prescribed medication.

B. Participates in rest/activity schedule.

C. Improves nutritional intake, gains appropriate weight for body size.

D. No complications of respiratory failure, cor pulmonale.

E. No respiratory tract infections.

Asthma

Increased responsiveness of the trachea and bronchi to various stimuli, with difficulty breathing; caused by narrowing of the airways. *Immunologic* asthma occurs in childhood and follows other allergic disease. *Nonimmunologic* asthma occurs in adulthood and is associated with history of recurrent respiratory tract infections. Asthma was previously classified with emphysema and chronic bronchitis as an *obstructive* pulmonary disease. However, the distinguishing feature of asthma is *inflammation* of the airways, and it is now separately classified.

I. **Pathophysiology**: bronchial smooth muscle constricts, bronchial secretions increase, mucosa swells, and there is a significant narrowing of air passages. Histamine is produced by the lung. Bronchospasm, production of large amounts of thick mucus, and inflammatory response all contribute to the condition.

A. *Immunologic*, or allergic, asthma in persons who are atopic (hypersensitivity state that is subject to hereditary influences); immunoglobulin E usually elevated.

B. *Nonimmunologic*, or nonallergic, asthma in persons who have a history of repeated respiratory tract infections; age usually >35 yr.

C. *Mixed*, combined immunologic and nonimmunologic; any age, allergen, or nonspecific stimuli.

II. **Risk factors/causes:**

A. History of allergies to identified or unidentified irritants; seasonal and environmental inhalants.

B. Recurrent respiratory tract infection.

C. Decreased ability to effectively cope with emotional stress.

D. Genetic predisposition.

E. Tobacco exposure.

F. Gastroesophageal reflux disease (GERD).

III. **Assessment**

A. *Subjective data*:

1. History: upper respiratory tract infections, rhinitis, allergies, family history of asthma.

2. Increasing tightness of the chest → dyspnea.

3. Anxiety, restlessness.

4. Attack history:

a. *Immunologic*: contact with allergen to which person is sensitive; seen most often in children and young adults.

b. *Nonimmunologic*: develops in adults >35 yrs; aggravated by infections of the sinuses and respiratory tract.

B. *Objective data*:

1. Tachycardia, tachypnea.

2. Cough: dry, hacking, persistent.

☞ 3. Respiratory assessment: audible expiratory wheeze (also inspiratory) on auscultation; crackles, rib retraction, use of accessory muscles on inspiration.

4. General appearance: pallor, cyanosis, diaphoresis, chronic barrel chest, elevated shoulders, flattened molar bones, narrow nose, prominent upper teeth, dark circles under eyes, distended neck veins, orthopnea.

5. Expectoration of tenacious mucoid sputum.

〰 6. *Pulmonary function diagnostic* tests:

a. Vital capacity: *reduced*.

b. Forced expiratory volume: *decreased*.

c. Residual volume: *increased*.

d. Peak expiratory flow rate: *decreased*.

7. Lab data: Blood gases: *elevated* PCO_2; *decreased* PO_2, pH.

Emergency Note: Persons severely affected may suffer *status asthmaticus*, a life-threatening asthmatic attack in which symptoms of asthma persist and do not respond to usual treatment. Could lead to respiratory failure and hypoxemia.

▶ IV. **Analysis/nursing diagnosis**

A. *Ineffective airway clearance* related to bronchospasm, ineffective cough, copious and tenacious secretions.

B. *Impaired gas exchange* related to constricted bronchioles.

C. *Anxiety* related to breathlessness.

D. *Activity intolerance* related to persistent cough.

E. *Knowledge deficit* related to causal factors.

▶ V. **Nursing care plan/implementation**

A. Goal: *promote pulmonary ventilation*.

1. *Position*: high-Fowler's for comfort.

⬤ 2. Medications as ordered:

a. *Bronchodilators* and expectorants to improve ventilation (monitor for alterations in BP and tachycardia).

b. *Antibiotics* to control infection.

c. *Steroids* to reduce inflammatory response.

☞ 3. Oxygen therapy with increased humidity as ordered.

4. Frequent monitoring for respiratory distress.

5. Rest periods and gradual increase in activity.

B. Goal: *facilitate expectoration*.

1. High humidity.

2. *Increase fluid* intake.

3. Monitor for dehydration.

☞ 4. Respiratory therapy: nebulizer treatments.

⌂ C. Goal: **health teaching** to *prevent further attack*.

1. Identify and avoid allergens.

2. Encourage compliance with medication regimen.

3. Medication side effects, withdrawals. Correct use of metered dose inhalers.

☞ 4. Show *postural drainage*, *percussion* techniques to family

☞ 5. Breathing techniques to increase expiratory phase.

6. Teach effective stress-management techniques.

7. Recognition of precipitating factors.

▶ VI. **Evaluation/outcome criteria**

A. No complications.

B. Has fewer attacks.

C. Takes prescribed medications, avoids infections.

D. Adjusts life-style.

Bronchitis

Acute or chronic inflammation of bronchus resulting as a complication from colds and flu. *Acute bronchitis* is caused by an extension of upper respiratory tract infection, such as a cold, and can be transmitted to others. It can also result from an irritation from physical or chemical agents. *Chronic bronchitis* is characterized by hypersecretion of mucus and chronic cough for 3 mo a year for 2 consecutive years.

I. **Pathophysiology**: bronchial walls are infiltrated with lymphocytes and macrophages; lumen becomes obstructed due to decreased ciliary action and repeated bronchospasms. Hyperventilation of alveolar sacs occurs. Long-term condition results in respiratory acidosis, recurrent pneumonitis, emphysema, or cor pulmonale.

II. **Risk factors/causes:**

A. Smoking.

B. Repeated respiratory tract infections.

C. History of living in area where there is much air pollution.

▶ III. **Assessment**

A. *Subjective data*:

1. History: recurrent, chronic cough, especially when arising in the morning.

2. Anorexia.

B. *Objective data*:

1. Respiratory:

a. Shortness of breath.

b. Use of accessory muscles.

c. Cyanosis, dusky complexion ("blue bloater").

d. Sputum: excessive, nonpurulent.

e. Vesicular and bronchovesicular breath sounds, wheezing.
2. Weight loss.
3. Fever.
4. *Pulmonary function* tests:
   a. *Decreased* forced expiratory volume.
   b. Lab data: PO_2 <90 mm Hg; PCO_2 >40 mm Hg.
5. Lab data.
   a. RBC—*elevated* to compensate for hypoxia (polycythemia);
   b. WBC—*elevated* to fight infection.

IV. **Analysis/nursing diagnosis**
   A. *Ineffective airway clearance* related to excessive sputum.
   B. *Ineffective breathing pattern* related to need to use accessory muscles for breathing.
   C. *Impaired gas exchange* related to shortness of breath.
   D. *Activity intolerance* related to increased energy used for breathing.

V. **Nursing care plan/implementation**
   A. Goal: *assist in optimal respirations.*
      1. *Increase fluid* intake.
      2. Nebulizer treatments, chest physiotherapy.
      3. Administer medications as ordered:
         a. *Bronchodilators.*
         b. *Antibiotics.*
         c. *Bronchial detergents,* liquefying agents.
   B. Goal: *minimize bronchial irritation.*
      1. *Avoid* respiratory irritants—for example, smoke, dust, cold air, allergens.
      2. Environment: air-conditioned, increased humidity.
      3. Encourage nostril breathing rather than mouth breathing.
   C. Goal: *improve nutritional status.*
      1. *Diet*: soft, high calorie.
      2. *Small, frequent* feedings.
   D. Goal: *prevent secondary infections.*
      1. Administer *antibiotics* as ordered.
      2. *Avoid* exposure to infections, crowds.
   E. Goal: **health teaching.**
      1. *Avoid* respiratory tract infections.
      2. Medications: desired effects and side effects, correct use of metered dose inhalers.
      3. Methods to stop smoking.
      4. Rest and activity balance.
      5. Stress management.

VI. **Evaluation/outcome criteria**
   A. Stops smoking.
   B. Acid-base balance maintained.
   C. Respiratory tract infections less frequent.

Acute Respiratory Distress Syndrome (ARDS)

Noncardiogenic pulmonary infiltrations resulting in stiff, wet lungs and refractory hypoxemia in adults who were previously healthy. Acute hypoxemic respiratory failure without hypercapnia. (formerly called by other names, including *shock lung*):

I. **Pathophysiology**: damage to alveolar capillary membrane, increased vascular permeability → pulmonary edema, and impaired gas exchange; decreased surfactant production and potential atelectasis; severe hypoxia → death.

II. **Risk factors/causes:**
   A. *Primary*:
      1. Shock, multiple trauma.
      2. Infections, sepsis
      3. Aspiration, inhalation of chemical toxins.
      4. Drug overdose.
      5. DIC.
      6. Emboli, especially fat emboli.
   B. *Secondary*:
      1. Overaggressive fluid administration.
      2. Oxygen toxicity.

III. **Assessment**
   A. *Subjective data*:
      1. Restlessness, anxiety.
      2. History of risk factors.
      3. Severe dyspnea (**Table 6.2**).
      4. Onset may be insidious over 1-2 days.
   B. *Objective data*:
      1. Cyanosis.
      2. Tachycardia.
      3. Hypotension.
      4. Hypoxemia, acidosis.
      5. Crackles.
      6. Chest x-ray—widespread consolidation and infiltrates (white lung).
      7. Death if untreated (50% mortality with treatment).

IV. **Analysis/nursing diagnosis**
   A. *Anxiety* related to serious physical condition.
   B. *Ineffective breathing pattern* related to severe dyspnea.
   C. *Impaired gas exchange* related to alveolar damage.
   D. *Altered tissue perfusion* related to hypoxia.

V. **Nursing care plan/implementation**
   A. Goal: *assist in respirations.*
      1. May require mechanical ventilatory support to maintain respirations.
      2. May need to be transferred to ICU.
      3. May need *oxygen* to combat hypoxia.
      4. *Suction* prn.
      5. Monitor blood gas results to detect early signs of acidosis/alkalosis.

TABLE 6.2 DIFFERENTIAL DIAGNOSIS OF DYSPNEA

⋈ Assessment	Pulmonary Edema	COPD	Spontaneous Pneumothorax	Pulmonary Emboli	Asthma
Possible *history*	Symptoms of acute myocardial infarction "Water pills" *Sudden* weight gain Cough, watery sputum Orthopnea	Emphysema, bronchitis Heavy smoking Recent cold *Chronic* dyspnea "Breathing pills" or inhalers	*Sudden*, sharp chest pain *Sudden* dyspnea, brought on by strenuous exertion, coughing, air travel Client often young, tall, thin, man	*Sudden*, sharp chest pain *Sudden* dyspnea Prolonged immobilization, recent surgery or trauma to lower extremities Thrombophlebitis Sickle cell anemia Birth control pills	Acute, episode dyspnea Often younger client Allergic history Relieved by shots in the past Cold or flu may have preceded attack
Possible *physical* findings	Distended neck veins Crackles S_3 gallop	↑ Anteroposterior diameter of chest Pursed-lip breathing Wheezing, crackles Prolonged expiratory phase of respiration Use of accessory muscles to breathe	↓ Breath sounds and ↑ resonance on side of collapsed lung Tracheal deviation	Tachypnea Tachycardia Hypotension Pleural rub Phlebitis in legs	Wheezing Hyperresonance If bronchospasm severe, chest may be silent

Source: Caroline NL. Adapted from *Emergency Care in the Streets* (5th ed). Boston: Little, Brown (out of print).

6. If not on ventilator, assess vital signs and respiratory status every 15 min.
7. Cough, deep breathe every hour.
8. May need:
    ☞ a. *Chest percussion, vibration*.
    ☞ b. *Postural drainage*, suction.
    ⬤ c. *Bronchodilator* medications.
B. Goal: *prevent complications*.
    1. Decrease anxiety and provide psychological care:
        a. Maintain a calm atmosphere.
        b. Encourage rest to conserve energy.
        c. Emotional support.
    2. Obtain fluid balance:
        a. Slow IV flow rate.
        ⬤ b. *Diuretics*: rapid acting, low dose.
    3. Monitor:
        ⟿ a. Pulmonary artery and capillary wedge pressure.
        ⟿ b. Central venous pressure, cardiac output, peripheral perfusion.
        c. I&O
        d. Assess for bleeding tendencies, potential for DIC
    4. Protect from infection:
        ▲ a. Strict *aseptic* technique.
        ⬤ b. *Antibiotic* therapy.

5. Provide physiologic support:
    ⬤ a. *Inotropic/vasopressor* medications to maintain cardiac function and BP.
    b. Maintain nutrition.
    c. Skin care.
🏠 C. Goal: **health teaching**.
    1. Briefly explain procedures as they are happening (emergency situation can frighten client).
    2. Give rationale for follow-up care.
    3. Identify risk factors as appropriate for prevention of recurrence.
⋈ VI. **Evaluation/outcome criteria**
    A. Client survives and is alert.
    B. Skin warm to touch.
    C. Respiratory rate within normal limits.
    D. Lab values and pressures within normal limits.
    E. Urinary output >30 mL/h.

Chest Trauma

Flail Chest

Multiple rib fractures resulting in instability of the chest wall, with subsequent paradoxical breathing (portion of lung under injured chest wall moves in on inspiration while remaining lung expands; on expiration the injured portion of the chest wall expands while unaffected lung tissue contracts).

Sucking Chest Wound

Penetrating wound of chest wall with hemothorax and pneumothorax, resulting in lung collapse and mediastinal shift toward unaffected lung.

- I. **Assessment**
  - A. *Subjective data*:
    1. Severe, sudden, sharp pain.
    2. Dyspnea.
    3. Anxiety, restlessness, fear, weakness.
  - B. *Objective data*:
    1. Vital signs:
       - a. Pulse: tachycardia, weak.
       - b. BP: hypotension.
       - c. Respirations: shallow, decreased expiratory force, tachypnea, stridor, accessory muscle breathing.
    2. Skin color: cyanosis, pallor.
    3. Chest:
       - a. Asymmetric chest expansion (*paradoxical movement*).
       - b. Chest wound, rush of air through trauma site.
       - c. Crepitus over trauma site (from air escaping into surrounding tissues).
       - d. Lateral deviation of trachea, mediastinal shift toward *unaffected* side.
    4. Pneumothorax: documented by absence of breath sounds, x-ray examination.
    5. Hemothorax: documented by needle aspiration by physician, x-ray examination.
    6. Shock; blood and fluid loss.
    7. Hemoptysis.
    8. Distended neck veins.
- II. **Analysis/nursing diagnosis**
  - A. *Ineffective airway clearance* related to shallow respirations.
  - B. *Impaired gas exchange* related to asymmetric chest expansion.
  - C. *Pain* related to chest trauma.
  - D. *Fear* related to emergency situation.
  - E. *Risk for trauma* related to fractured ribs.
  - F. *Risk for infection* related to open chest wound.
- III. **Nursing care plan/implementation**
  - A. Goal: r*estore adequate ventilation and prevent further air from entering pleural cavity*: **MEDICAL EMERGENCY**.
    1. In emergency situation: place air-occlusive dressing or hand over open wound as client exhales forcefully against glottis (*Valsalva maneuver* helps expand collapsed lung by creating positive intrapulmonary pressures); or place client's weight onto *affected* side. Administer *oxygen*.

    2. Assist with *endotracheal tube* insertion; client will be placed on volume-controlled *ventilator*. (See discussion of ventilators under **Oxygen Therapy**, p. 89.)
    3. Assist with *thoracentesis* and insertion of chest tubes with connection to water-seal drainage as ordered. (see **Tubes** box, **p. 86, 87, 88**.)
    4. Monitor vital signs to determine early shock.
    5. Monitor *blood gases* to determine early acid-base imbalances.
    6. Pain medications given with caution (small, frequent doses), so as not to depress respiratory center.
- IV. **Evaluation/outcome criteria**
  - A. Respiratory status stabilizes, lung reexpands.
  - B. Shock and hemorrhage are prevented.
  - C. No further damage done to surrounding tissues.
  - D. Pain is controlled.

Pneumothorax

Presence of air within the pleural cavity; occurs spontaneously or as a result of trauma (**Table 6.3**).

- I. **Types:**
  - A. *Closed*: rupture of a subpleural bulla, tuberculous focus, carcinoma, lung abscess, pulmonary infarction, severe coughing attack, or blunt trauma.
  - B. *Open*: communication between atmosphere and pleural space because of opening in chest wall.
  - C. *Tension*: positive pressure within chest cavity resulting from accumulated air that cannot escape during expiration. Leads to collapse of lung, mediastinal shift, and compression of the heart and great vessels.
- II. **Pathophysiology**: pressure builds up in the pleural space, lung on the affected side collapses, and the heart and mediastinum shift toward the unaffected lung.
- III. **Assessment**
  - A. *Subjective data*:
    1. Pain:
       - a. Sharp, aggravated by activity.
       - b. Location—chest; may be referred to shoulder, arm on affected side.
    2. Restlessness, anxiety.
    3. Dyspnea.
  - B. *Objective data*:
    1. Cough.
    2. Cessation of normal movements on affected side.
    3. Absence of breath sounds on affected side.
    4. Pallor, cyanosis.
    5. Shock.
    6. Tracheal deviation to unaffected side

TABLE 6.3 DIFFERENTIATING AMONG TENSION PNEUMOTHORAX, HEMOTHORAX, AND CARDIAC TAMPONADE

Assessment	Tension Pneumothorax	Massive Hemothorax	Cardiac Tamponade
Presenting sign or symptom	Respiratory distress	Shock	Shock
Neck veins	Distended	Flat	Distended
Trachea	Deviated	Midline	Midline
Breath sounds	Decreased or absent on side of injury	Decreased or absent on side of injury	Equal on both sides
Percussion of chest	Hyperresonant on side of injury	Dull on side of injury	Normal
Heart sounds	Normal	Normal	Muffled

Source: Adapted from Caroline NL. *Emergency Care in the Streets* (5th ed). Boston: Little, Brown (out of print).

7. X-ray: air in pleural space.

IV. Analysis/nursing diagnosis

A. *Ineffective breathing pattern* related to collapse of lung.

B. *Impaired gas exchange* related to abnormal thoracic movement.

C. *Pain* related to trauma to chest area.

D. *Fear* related to emergency situation.

V. Nursing care plan/implementation

A. Goal: *protect against injury during thoracentesis.*
1. Provide sterile equipment.
2. Explain procedure.
3. Monitor vital signs for shock.
4. Monitor for respiratory distress, mediastinal shift.

B. Goal: *promote respirations.*
1. *Position*: Fowler's.
2. Oxygen therapy as ordered.
3. Encourage slow breathing to improve gas exchange.
4. Careful administration of *narcotics* to prevent respiratory depression (*avoid* morphine).

C. Goal: *prepare client for closed-chest drainage, physically and psychologically.*
1. Explain purpose of the procedure—to provide means for evacuation of air and fluid from pleural cavity; to reestablish negative pressure in pleural space; to promote lung reexpansion.
2. Explain procedure and apparatus (see **chest tubes** in box, **p. 85, 86, 87, 88**).
3. Cleanse skin at tube insertion site, place client in *sitting* position, ensuring safety by having locked over-bed table for client to lean on, or have a nurse stay with client so appropriate position is maintained throughout the procedure.

D. Goal: *prevent complications with chest tubes.*
1. Observe for and immediately report: crepitations (air under skin, also called *subcutaneous emphysema*), labored or shallow breathing, tachypnea, cyanosis, tracheal deviation, or signs of hemorrhage.
2. Monitor for signs of infection.
3. Ensure that tubing stays intact; tape all connections.
4. Monitor for proper tube function (*fluctuation or oscillation* of water seal chamber will occur with respirations; water level will *rise* when client inhales or coughs; water level will *lower* during exhalation). If *no bubbling in water*, check tubing for kinks or lack of patency. Manipulation of chest tube done only according to specific physician order.
5. Monitor for air leaks (*continuous bubbling* in water seal chamber).
6. Arm and shoulder ROM.
7. Maintain air-occlusive dressing over insertion site.

E. Goal: **health teaching.**
1. How to prevent recurrence by *avoiding* overexertion; *avoid* holding breath.
2. Signs and symptoms of condition.
3. Methods to stop smoking.
4. Encourage follow-up care.

VI. Evaluation/outcome criteria

A. No complications noted.

B. Closed system remains intact until chest tubes are removed.

C. Lung reexpands, breath sounds heard, pain diminished, symmetric thoracic movements.

Hemothorax

Presence of blood in pleural cavity related to trauma or rup-tured aortic aneurysm. See **Pneumothorax, p. 80-81** for assessment, analysis/nursing diagnosis, nursing care plan/implementation, and evaluation/outcome criteria; see also **Table 6.3.**

Thoracic Surgery

Performed for bronchogenic and lung carcinomas, lung abscesses, tuberculosis, bronchiectasis, emphysematous blebs, and benign tumors.

I. **Types:**

A. *Thoracotomy*—incision in the chest wall, pleura is entered, lung tissue examined, biopsy specimen secured. *Chest tube is needed postoperatively.*

B. *Lobectomy*—removal of a lobe of the lung. *Chest tube is needed postoperatively.*

C. *Pneumonectomy*—removal of an entire lung. *No chest tube is needed postoperatively.*

II. **Analysis/nursing diagnosis**

A. *Risk for injury* related to chest wound.

B. *Impaired gas exchange* related to pain from surgical procedure.

C. *Ineffective airway clearance* related to decreased willingness to cough due to pain.

D. *Pain* related to surgical incision.

E. *Impaired physical mobility* related to large surgical incision and chest tube drainage apparatus.

F. *Knowledge deficit* related to importance of coughing and deep breathing to prevent complications

III. **Nursing care plan/implementation**

A. **Preoperative care:**

1. Goal: *minimize pulmonary secretions.*
   a. *Humidify* air to moisten secretions.
   b. Cough and deep breathe, as ordered, to improve ventilation.
   c. Administer *bronchodilators, expectorants,* and *antibiotics,* as ordered.
   d. Use *postural drainage, cupping,* and *vibration* to mobilize secretions.

2. Goal: **preoperative teaching.**
   a. Teach client to cough against a closed glottis to increase intrapulmonary pressure for improved expiratory phase.
   b. Instruct in diaphragmatic breathing and coughing.
   c. Encourage to stop smoking.
   d. Instruct and supervise practice of postoperative arm exercises—flexion, abduction, and rotation of shoulder—to prevent ankylosis.
   e. Explain postoperative use of chest tubes, IV, and oxygen therapy.

B. **Postoperative care:**

1. Goal: *maintain patent airway.*
   a. Auscultate chest for breath sounds; report diminished or absent breath sounds on unaffected side (indicates decreased ventilation → respiratory embarrassment).
   b. Turn, cough, and deep breathe, every 15 min to 1 h first 24 h and prn according to pulmonary congestion heard on auscultation.

2. Goal: *promote gas exchange.*
   a. Splint chest during coughing—support incision to help *cough up sputum (most important activity postoperatively).*

b. *Position:* high-Fowler's.
   (1) Turn client who has had a *pneumonectomy* to *operative side* (*avoid* extreme lateral positioning and mediastinal shift) to allow unaffected lung expansion and drainage of secretions; can also be turned onto back.
   (2) Client who has had a *lobectomy* or *thoracotomy* can be turned on *either* side or back because chest tubes will be in place.

3. Goal: *reduce incisional stress and discomfort*—pad area around chest tube when turning on operative side to maintain tube patency and promote comfort.

4. Goal: *prevent complications related to respiratory function.*
   a. Maintain chest tubes to water-seal drainage system.
   b. See **Chest tubes** section in **Tubes** box **p. 86, 87, 88.**
   c. Observe for *mediastinal shift* (trachea should always be midline; movement toward either side indicates shift).
      (1) Move client onto back or toward opposite side.
      (2) **MEDICAL EMERGENCY:** Notify physician immediately.

5. Goal: *maintain fluid and electrolyte balance*
   administer parenteral infusion *slowly* (risk of pulmonary edema due to decrease in pulmonary vasculature with removal of lung lobe or whole lung).

6. Goal: **postoperative teaching.**
   a. Prevent ankylosis of shoulder—teach *passive* and *active ROM* exercises of operative arm.
   b. Importance of early ambulation, as condition permits.
   c. Importance of stopping smoking.
   d. Dietary instructions—nutritious diet to promote healing.
   e. Importance of deep breathing, coughing exercises to prevent stasis of respiratory secretions.
   f. Importance of *increased fluids* in diet to liquefy secretions.
   g. Desired effects and side effects of prescribed medications.
   h. Importance of rest, avoidance of heavy lifting and work during healing.
   i. Importance of follow-up care; give names of referral agencies where client and family can obtain assistance.
   j. Signs and symptoms of complications

IV. **Evaluation/outcome criteria**

A. Client and/or significant other will be able to:

1. Give rationale for activity restriction and demonstrate prescribed exercises.
2. Identify name, route, frequency, dosage, and side effects of prescribed medications.
3. State plans for necessary modifications in lifestyle, home.
4. Identify support systems.
B. Wound heals without complications.
C. Obtains ROM in affected shoulder.
D. No complications of thoracotomy:
   1. *Respiratory*—pulmonary insufficiency, respiratory acidosis, pneumonitis, atelectasis, pulmonary edema.
   2. *Circulatory*—hemorrhage, hypovolemia, shock, myocardial infarction.
   3. *Mediastinal shift.*
   4. *Renal failure.*
   5. *Gastric distention.*

Tracheostomy

Opening into trachea, temporary or permanent. *Rationale*: airway obstruction due to: foreign body, edema, tumor, excessive tracheobronchial secretions, respiratory depression, decreased gaseous diffusion at alveolar membrane, or increased dead space (e.g., severe emphysema).

I. Analysis/nursing diagnosis
   A. *Ineffective airway clearance* related to increased secretions and decreased ability to cough effectively.
   B. *Ineffective breathing pattern* related to physical condition that necessitated tracheostomy.
   C. *Impaired verbal communication* related to inability to speak when tracheostomy tube cuff inflated.
   D. *Fear* related to need for specialized equipment to breathe.

II. Nursing care plan/implementation
   A. **Preoperative care:**
      1. Goal: *relieve anxiety and fear.*
         a. Explain purpose of procedure and equipment.
         ☞ b. Demonstrate suctioning procedure.
         c. Establish means of postoperative communication, e.g., paper and pencil, magic slate, picture cards, and call bell. Specialized tubes such as a fenestrated tracheostomy tube or a tracheostomy button allow the client to talk when the external opening is plugged.
         d. Remain with client as much as possible.
   B. **Postoperative care:**
      ☞ 1. Goal: *maintain patent airway* (**Table 6.4**).
      2. Goal: *alleviate apprehension.*
         a. Remain with client as much as possible.

TABLE 6.4 ☞ TRACHEOSTOMY SUCTIONING PROCEDURE

1. Suction as necessary to facilitate respirations.
2. *Position*: semi-Fowler's to prevent forward flexion of neck, facilitate respiration, promote drainage, and minimize edema.
3. Administer *mist* to tracheostomy since natural humidifying of oropharynx pathways has been eliminated.
4. Auscultate for moist, noisy respirations, as nonproductive coughing may indicate need for suctioning.
5. Prevent hypoxia by administering *100% oxygen before suctioning* (unless contraindicated).
6. Use *strict aseptic technique* and sterile suctioning catheters with each aspiration; use sterile saline to clear catheter of secretions. Keep dominant hand gloved with sterile glove, nondominant hand with nonsterile glove to control thumb control of suction. Suction tracheostomy *before* nose or mouth.
7. *Do not apply suction when inserting* suction catheter to prevent injury to respiratory tract and loss of oxygen.
8. If client coughs during suctioning, gently remove catheter to permit ejection and suction of mucus.
9. Apply suction intermittently for *no longer* than 10 to 15 sec, as prolonged suction decreases arterial oxygen concentrations. Do *not* suction for more than 3-5 min.
10. *Cuff pressure*: tracheal cuff pressure should *not* exceed 20 mm Hg or 25 cm H_2O.
11. Use caution not to dislodge tube when changing dressing or ties that secure tube. Best practice is for two nurses to change ties.

Source: ©Lagerquist, SL: *NCLEX-RN® Examination Review*. Boston: Little, Brown, (out of print).

      b. Encourage client to communicate feelings using preestablished communication system.
   🍎 3. Goal: *improve nutritional status.*
      a. Nutritious foods/liquids the client can swallow.
      b. Supplemental drinks to maintain necessary calories.
   📖 4. Goal: **health teaching.**
      a. Explain all procedures.
      b. Teach alternative methods of communication (best if done before the tracheostomy if it is not an emergency situation).
      c. Teach self-care of tracheostomy as soon as possible.

III. Evaluation/outcome criteria
   A. Airway patent.
   B. Acid-base balance maintained.
   C. No respiratory infection/obstruction.

Laryngectomy

Radical Neck Dissection

Removal of entire larynx, lymph nodes, sternomastoid muscle, and jugular vein for cancer of the larynx that extends beyond the vocal cords. Permanent tracheostomy; new methods of speech will have to be learned.

Partial laryngectomy: removal of lesion on larynx. Client will be able to speak after operation, but quality of voice may be altered.

I. **Assessment**
- A. *Subjective data*:
  1. Feeling of lump in throat.
  2. Pain: Adam's apple; may radiate to ear.
  3. Dysphagia.
- B. *Objective data*:
  1. Hoarseness: persistent, progressive.
  2. Lymphadenopathy: cervical.
  3. Breath odor: foul.

II. **Analysis/nursing diagnosis**
- A. *Impaired verbal communication* related to removal of larynx.
- B. *Body image disturbance* related to radical neck dissection.
- C. *Ineffective airway clearance* related to copious amounts of mucus.
- D. *Fear* related to diagnosis of cancer.
- E. *Impaired swallowing* related to edema.
- F. *Impaired social interaction* related to altered speech.

III. **Nursing care plan/implementation**
- A. **Preoperative care:**
  1. Goal: *provide emotional support and optimal physical preparation.*
     - a. Encourage verbalization of fears; answer all questions honestly, particularly about having no voice after surgery.
     - b. Visit from person with laryngectomy (contact International Association of Laryngectomees, www.larynxlink.com).
  2. Goal: **health teaching.**
     - a. Prepare for tracheostomy.
     - b. Other means to speak (esophageal "burp" speech).
- B. **Postoperative care:**
  1. Goal: *maintain patent airway and prevent aspiration.*
     - a. *Position*: semi-Fowler's, preventing forward flexion of neck to reduce edema and keep airway open.
     - b. Observe for hypoxia:
       - (1) *Early signs*: increased respiratory and pulse rates, apprehension, restlessness.
       - (2) *Late signs*: dyspnea, cyanosis, swallowing difficulties—client should chew food well and swallow with water.
     - c. *Laryngectomy* tube care:
       - (1) Observe for stridor (coarse, high-pitched inspiratory sound)—**report immediately**.
       - (2) Have extra laryngectomy tube at bedside.
       - (3) Suction with sterile equipment; instill 2–3 mL of sterile saline into stoma to loosen secretions.
  2. Goal: *promote optimal physical and psychological function*
     - a. Frequent mouth care.
     - b. Dressings: may be pressure type; note color and amount of drainage; reinforce as ordered.
     - c. *Tubes: Hemovac* (**Figure 6.1**); expect 80–120 mL of serosanguineous drainage first postoperative day; drainage should decrease daily; observe patency.
     - d. *Post-Hemovac removal*—observe: skin flaps down, adherent to underlying tissue; may have to "roll" flaps to prevent drainage buildup.
     - e. Use surgical asepsis.
     - f. Answer call bell *immediately*; use preestablished means of communication.
     - g. Reexplain all procedures while giving care.
     - h. Support head when lifting.
  3. Goal: **health teaching.**
     - a. Speech rehabilitation as soon as esophageal suture is healed.
       - (1) Information on laryngeal speech (International Association of Laryngectomees, American Cancer Society, American Speech and Hearing Association).
       - (2) *Esophageal speech* best learned in speech clinic—learn to burp column of air needed for speech; new voice sounds are natural but hoarse.
     - b. *Stoma* care:
       - (1) Cover with scarf or shirt made of a porous material (material substitutes for nasal passage—warms and filters out particles).
       - (2) Use source of humidification ("mister" or commercial humidifier).
       - (3) Caution while bathing or showering, to decrease likelihood of aspiration.
       - (4) Swimming and boating permitted only with snorkel device.

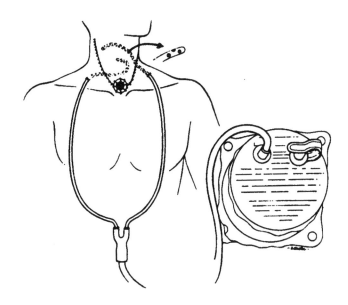

FIGURE 6.1 HEMOVAC APPARATUS FOR CONSTANT CLOSED SUCTION.

In this system of wound drainage, suction is maintained by a plastic container with a spring inside that tries to force apart the lids and thereby produces suction that is transmitted through the plastic tubing. The neck skin is pulled down tight, and no external dressing is required. The container serves as both suction source and receptable for blood. It is emptied as required, and drainage tubes are left in the neck for 3 days.

(Adapted from DeWeese DD, Saunders WH. *Textbook of Otolaryngoloty* [6th ed]. St. Louis: Mosby, out of print)

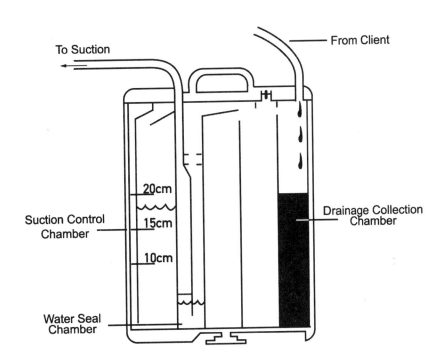

FIGURE 6.2 CLOSED CHEST DRAINAGE SYSTEM

REVIEW OF THE USE OF COMMON TUBES

Tube or Apparatus	Purpose	Examples of Use	⋈ Key Points for Nursing Implementation
Chest tubes	1. *Anterior tube* drains mostly air from pleural space 2. *Posterior tube* drains mostly fluid from pleural space 3. Removal of fluid and air from pleural space is necessary to reestablish negative intrapleural pressure	1. *Thoracotomy* 2. *Open-heart surgery* 3. *Spontaneous pneumothorax* 4. *Traumatic pneumothorax* 5. *Hemothorax*	1. See **Key Points** for each of the three entries under **Drainage System**, below 2. Sterile technique is used when changing dressings around the tube insertions 3. Fowler's *position* to facilitate air and fluid removal 4. Cough, deep breathe, q1h; splint chest; medicate for pain 5. Manage pain carefully in order *not* to depress respirations 6. Prepare for removal when there is little or no drainage, air leak disappears, or fluctuations stop in water seal; have suture set, petrolatum gauze (or other ointment), 4 X 4s, and sturdy elastic tape ready; medicate for pain before removal; monitor breathing after removal (breath sounds, rate, chest pain)
Drainage system (see **Figure 6.2, p. 85**) #1: **drainage compartment**	Collects drainage		1. Mark level in drainage chamber each shift to keep accurate record—*not* routinely emptied; replace when full 2. *Never* raise container above the level of the chest; otherwise back flow will occur

(continued)

(5) Procedure for suctioning if cough ineffective.
☞ c. Simple ROM of neck; how to support head.
d. Possible *contraindications*: use of talcum powder, tissues.

⋈ **IV. Evaluation/outcome criteria**
A. No surgical complications (e.g., airway obstruction, infection, hemorrhage).
B. Learns alternative speech 60–90 d after surgery.
C. Demonstrates proper stoma care.
D. Resumes productive life-style (work, family).
E. Normal response to change in body image (e.g., anger, grief, denial).

Oxygen Therapy

I. **Purpose**—to relieve hypoxia and provide adequate tissue oxygenation.

II. **Clinical indications:**
A. Any client likely to have significant *shunt* from:
1. Fluid in the alveoli:
a. Pulmonary edema.
b. Pneumonia.
c. Near drowning.
d. Chest trauma.
2. Collapsed alveoli (atelectasis).
a. Airway obstruction:
(1) Any client who is unconscious.
(2) Choking.
b. Failure to take deep breaths:
(1) Pain (rib fracture).
(2) Paralysis of the respiratory muscles (spine injury).
(3) Depression of the respiratory center (head injury, drug overdose, post-anesthesia).
c. Collapse of an entire lung (pneumothorax).
3. Other gases in the alveoli:
a. Smoke inhalation.
b. Toxic inhalations.
c. Carbon monoxide poisoning.
4. Respiratory arrest.
B. Cardiac arrest.
C. Shock.
D. Shortness of breath.
E. Signs of respiratory insufficiency.
F. Breathing fewer than 10 breaths/min.
G. Chest pain.
H. Stroke.
I. Anemia.
J. Fetal decelerations during labor.

III. **Precautions:**
A. Clients with COPD should receive oxygen at *low* flow rates, to prevent inhibition of hypoxic respiratory drive.

REVIEW OF THE USE OF COMMON TUBES (*continued*)

Tube or Apparatus	Purpose	Examples of Use	▶◀ Key Points for Nursing Implementation
#2: water-seal chamber	Water seal prevents flow of atmospheric air into pleural space; essential to prevent recollapse of the lung		1. Air bubbles from postoperative residual air *will* continue for 24–48 h 2. *Persistent* large amounts of air bubbles in this compartment indicate an *air leak* between the alveoli and the pleural space ☞ 3. Clamp tube(s) only to verify a leak; replace a broken, cracked, or full drainage unit, or verify readiness of client for tube removal; *not* necessary to clamp when ambulating if water seal intact ☞ 4. If tube becomes disconnected, clean off tubing ends and reconnect; if dislodged from chest, seal insertion site ***immediately*** on expiration if possible; use sterile petrolatum gauze and adhesive tape to form *air-occlusive* dressing 5. If air leak is present, clamping the tube for very long may cause a tension pneumothorax 6. Fluctuation of the fluid level in this chamber is *expected* (when the suction is turned off) because respiration changes the pleural pressure; if there is *no fluctuation* of the fluid in the tube of this chamber (when the suction is turned off), then either the lung is fully expanded or the tube is blocked by kinking or by a clot ☞ 7. Although not routinely used, milking (gently squeezing) the tubes, if ordered, will prevent blockage from clots or debris; otherwise gravity drainage is sufficient to maintain patency 8. Drainage of >100 mL in 1 h should be ***reported*** to physician

(continued)

B. *Excessive* (>40%) amounts of oxygen for prolonged periods will cause retrolental fibroplasia and blindness in premature infants, or possibly ARDS in adults.

C. Oxygen delivered *without* humidification will result in drying and irritation of respiratory mucosa, decreased ciliary action, and thickening of respiratory secretions.

D. Oxygen supports combustion, and *fire* is a potential hazard during its administration.
1. Ground electrical equipment.
2. Prohibit smoking.
3. Institute measures to decrease static electricity.

E. *High* flow rates of oxygen delivered by ventilator or cuffed tracheostomy and endotracheal tubes can produce signs of oxygen toxicity in 24–48 h.
1. Signs and symptoms: cough, sore throat, decreased vital capacity, and substernal discomfort.
2. Pulmonary manifestations due to:
   a. Atelectasis.
   b. Exudation of protein fluids into alveoli.
   c. Damage to pulmonary capillaries.
   d. Interstitial hemorrhage.

IV. **Oxygen administration**

A. Oxygen is dispensed from cylinder or piped-in system.

B. Methods of delivering oxygen:
1. **Nasal catheter:**
   a. Effective and comfortable.
   b. Delivers 30%–50% oxygen at flow rates of 6–8 L/min.
   c. Can produce excoriation of nares.
   d. Do *not* use in client who is comatose.
2. **Nasal prongs/cannula:**
   a. Comfortable and simple, and allows client to move about in bed.
   b. Delivers 25%–40% oxygen at flow rates of 4–6 L/min.
   c. Difficult to keep in position unless client is alert and cooperative.
3. **Venturi mask:**
   a. Allows for accurate delivery of prescribed concentration of oxygen.

REVIEW OF THE USE OF COMMON TUBES (*continued*)

Tube or Apparatus	Purpose	Examples of Use	▶ Key Points for Nursing Implementation
#3: suction control— connected to wall suction	Level of the column of water (i.e.; 15-20 cm) is used to control the amount of suction applied to the chest tube—if the water evaporates to only *10 cm* depth, then this will be the *maximum* suction generated by the wall suction		1. Air *should continuously bubble* through this compartment when the suction is on; the bubbles are from the atmosphere—*not* the client; when the wall suction is turned higher, the bubbling will increase, but the increased pulling of air is from the atmosphere and *not* from the pleural space 2. Since the level of H_2O determines the maximum negative pressure that can be obtained, make sure the water does *not* evaporate—keep filling the chamber to keep the ordered level; if there is *no* bubbling of air through this container, the wall suction is *too low*
Heimlich flutter valve	1. Has a one-way valve so fluids and air can drain out of the pleural space but cannot flow back 2. Eliminates the need for a water seal—no danger when tube is unclamped below the valve	Same as for other chest tubes	1. Can be connected to suction if ordered 2. Sometimes can just drain into portable bag, so client is more mobile 3. Client is occasionally sent home with Heimlich valve in place
Tracheostomy tube	1. Maintains patent airway and promotes better O_2-CO_2 exchange 2. Makes removal of secretions by suctioning easier 3. Cuff on tracheostomy tube is necessary if an airtight fit for assisted ventilation is needed	1. *Acute respiratory distress* due to poor ventilation 2. *Severe burns of head and neck* 3. *Laryngectomy* (tracheostomy is permanent)	☞ 1. Use oxygen *before* and *after* each suctioning 2. Humidify oxygen ☞ 3. Sterile technique in suctioning 4. Disposable inner cannula is used—only leave out *5-10 min* 5. Hemostat handy if outer cannula is expelled—have obturator taped to bed and another tracheostomy set handy 6. Cuff pressure should *not* exceed 20 mm Hg or 25 cm H_2O.

Note: This review focuses on care of the tubes, not on total client care.

Source: Jane Vincent Corbett, RN, MS, EdD, Professor Emerita, School of Nursing, University of San Francisco. Used with permission.

b. Delivers 24%–40% oxygen at flow rates of 4–8 L/min.

c. Useful in long-term treatment of COPD.

4. **Face mask:**

   a. Poorly tolerated—utilized for short periods; feeling of "suffocation."

   b. Delivers 50%–60% oxygen at flow rates of 8–12 L/min.

   c. Significant rebreathing of carbon dioxide at low oxygen flow rates.

   d. Hot—may produce pressure sores around nose and mouth.

5. **Partial rebreathing mask:**

   a. About one-third of exhaled air is rebreathed.

   b. Reservoir contains mostly oxygen inspired during previous inhalation.

   c. Delivers 35%-60% oxygen at flow rates of 6–10 L/min.

6. **Nonrebreathing mask:**

   a. Reservoir bag has one-way valve preventing the client from exhaling back into the bag.

   b. Oxygen flow rate prevents collapse of bag during inhalation.

   c. Delivers 100% oxygen at flow rates of 10–12 L/min.

d. Ideal for severe hypoxia, but client may complain of feelings of suffocation.

7. T tube:
   a. Provides humidification and enriched oxygen mixtures to tracheostomy or endotracheal tube.
   b. Delivers 40%–60% oxygen at flow rates of 4–12 L/min.

V. **Ventilators**
A. *Indications*:
   1. Hypoventilation.
   2. Hypoxia.
   3. Counteract pulmonary edema by changing pressure gradient.
   4. Decrease work of breathing.
B. *Contraindications*:
   1. Tuberculosis—may rupture tubercular bleb.
   2. Hypovolemia—increased intrathoracic pressures decrease venous return.
   3. Air trapping—increased because adequate exhalation is not allowed.
C. *Complications*:
   1. Decreased BP; impaired venous return.
   2. Atelectasis.
   3. Infection.
   4. Oxygen toxicity.
   5. Difficulties weaning.
   6. Gastric dilatation.
   7. Pneumothorax.
   8. Hyperventilation or hypoventilation.
   9. Tracheal injury.
   10. Sodium/water imbalance.
   11. Increased intra-cranial pressure.
   12. Stress ulcers.
D. *Types of ventilators*:
   1. **Oscillating** or **rocking bed**:
      a. Indirectly aids respirations by using weight and gravity of abdominal contents to change position of diaphragm.
      b. *Used with* paralytic disease, as an aid in weaning.
   2. **Iron lung, Curass,** and **negative pressure ventilators**:
      a. Driven by motors that create negative pressure within tank or shell and thus allow air to enter client's lungs.
      b. *Used for* neuromuscular disease.
      c. *Not* used extensively for clients who are *acutely* ill.
   3. **Intermittent positive-pressure breathing** (*IPPB*):
      a. Produces greater-than-atmospheric pressures, intermittently.
      b. Improves tidal volume and minute volume and aids in overcoming respiratory insufficiency.
      c. Produces more uniform distribution of alveolar aeration and reduces work of breathing.
      d. *Used to:* deliver both oxygen and medications during treatment and rehabilitative pulmonary therapy, particularly if client has decreased tidal volume.
      e. *Contraindicated* in pneumothorax, active tuberculosis, and history of recent hemoptysis.
   4. **Pressure-constant ventilators**:
      a. *Bird*—Mark VII:
         (1) Pressure cycled, pneumatic powered.
         (2) When preset pressure is reached, valve closes, terminating inspiration.
         (3) Flow rate, sensitivity, and pressure limit are all adjustable.
         (4) Adjustable flow rate allows for increasing tidal volume.
         (5) *Disadvantage*—changes in compliance or airway resistance can affect oxygen concentration and tidal volume.
      b. *Bennett*—PR II:
         (1) Positive-pressure cycled, time cycled, flow sensitive.
         (2) May be triggered by client's inspiration or controlled by pressure or time setting.
         (3) Oxygen delivery variable, so frequent monitoring is *essential*.
   5. **Volume-constant ventilators**:
      a. *Bennett*—MA 1:
         (1) Delivers preset tidal volume.
         (2) Oxygen concentration adjusted by lighter flow being fed into machine.
         (3) Sophisticated alarms.
         (4) Has a sigh mechanism and positive end-expiratory pressure (*PEEP*), which maintains lung inflation.
         (5) *Used for* decreased compliance (stiff lungs).
         (6) Excellent humidification system.
   6. **Minute volume ventilators**—Servo 990 C:
      a. Delivers preset inspiratory minute volume.
      b. Has PEEP, continuous positive airway pressure (*CPAP*), spontaneous intermittent mandatory ventilation (*SIMV*), and inverse ratio ventilation (*IRV*) capabilities.
      c. *Used for:* clients with ARDS who have not responded to conventional treatment (PEEP, IMV) and need the advantage of IRV and prolonged inspiratory ventilation.

🔑 Summary of Key Points

1. Normal breath sounds over the peripheral lung fields are called *vesicular breath sounds.*

2. *Dyspnea,* difficulty breathing, is a subjective symptom and one of the most common complaints with any respiratory disorder.

3. Airways are narrowest on expiration, thus *expiratory wheezing* is heard most often.

4. *Chest pain* resulting from a respiratory disorder is frequently related to breathing and may be more localized then cardiac pain. The client may be able to point to a specific location.

5. *Crackles,* formerly called *rales,* are usually heard on inspiration and do not clear with coughing. *Wheezing* and *rhonchi* are used interchangeably; both result from narrowing of airways. If the term *rhonchi* is used, it means fluid is the cause of the narrowing, and the sound often clears with coughing.

6. A client who is experiencing *difficulty breathing:* will not tolerate activity, has a poor appetite, fatigues easily, speaks in broken phrases ("staccato" speech), may breathe through pursed lips (obstructive disorder), and will not be receptive to client teaching.

7. Giving *high levels of oxygen* to a client with *emphysema* (carbon dioxide retainer) will *interfere* with the *hypoxic drive* to breathe.

8. *Obstructive* respiratory disorders trap air, and total lung capacity is *increased*; while clients with *restrictive* disorders have a *decreased* total lung capacity and have difficulty taking in a breath.

💡 Study and Memory Aids

Pneumonia—Signs, Sx, Tx: "FRAPPÉ"

F ever
R espiratory distress
A ntibiotics after culture
P ain, affected side
P roductive cough
E valuate effectiveness of treatment

Atelectasis—Characteristics and Tx: "COLLAPSE"

C hest tubes not necessary
O xygen
L azy breathing habits
L ung reexpansion necessary
A lveoli collapsed
P osition on unaffected side
S uction, liquefy secretions
E ncourage cough and deep breathing

Pulmonary Embolism—Signs, Dx: "SUDDEN"

S ense of doom
U ntreated → death
D yspnea
D ensity on x-ray
E mergency condition
N ew symptoms

Histoplasmosis—Characteristics: "SOIL"

S pores
O bstructive pulmonary disease
I nhaled from bird droppings
L ocation: endemic to central United States

Tuberculosis—Cause, Dx, Sx, Tx: "SPREAD"

S putum positive for acid-fast bacilli
P ositive Mantoux test
R espiratory symptoms
E xposure to *M. tuberculosis*
A ppetite decreased
D rug regimen crucial

Asthma—Sx, Cause, Dx, Tx: "WHISTLE"

W heeze
H istory of respiratory tract infections
I nflammatory response
S easonal allergies
T reat early with bronchodilators
L ab data show blood gas abnormalities
E xpectoration—facilitate

Bronchitis—Sx, Tx: "COUGH"

C yanosis
O bstructed lumen
U pper respiratory tract problem
G ive medications as ordered
H elp to stop smoking

⌇ Diagnostic Studies/Procedures

Pulmonary Function Studies

1. **Ventilatory studies**—utilization of a spirometer to determine how well the lung is ventilating.
   a. *Vital capacity* (VC)—largest amount of air that can be expelled after maximal inspiration.
      (1) *Normally* 4000–5000 mL.
      (2) *Decreased* in restrictive lung disease.
      (3) May be normal, slightly increased, or decreased in COPD.
   b. *Forced expiratory volume* (FEV)—percentage of vital capacity that can be forcibly expired in 1, 2, or 3 sec.
      (1) *Normally* 81%–83% in 1 sec, 90%–94% in 2 sec, and 95%–97% in 3 sec.
      (2) *Decreased* values indicate expiratory airway obstruction.
   c. *Maximum breathing capacity* (MBC)—maximum amount of air that can be breathed in and out in 1 min with maximal rates and depths of respiration.
      (1) Best overall measurement of ventilatory ability.
      (2) *Reduced* in restrictive and chronic obstructive lung disease.
2. **Diffusion studies**—measure the rate of exchange of gases across alveolar membrane. Carbon monoxide single-breath, rebreathing, and steady-state techniques—utilized because of special affinity of hemoglobin for carbon monoxide; *decreased* when fluid is present in alveoli or when alveolar membranes are thick or fibrosed.

Sputum Studies

1. **Gross sputum evaluations**—collection of sputum samples to ascertain quantity, consistency, color, and odor.
2. **Sputum smear**—sputum is smeared thinly on a slide so that it can be studied microscopically; *used to:* determine cytologic changes (malignant cell) or presence of pathogenic bacteria, e.g., tubercle bacilli.
3. **Sputum culture**—sputum samples are implanted or inoculated into special media; *used to:* diagnose pulmonary infections.
4. **Gastric lavage or analysis**—insertion of a nasogastric tube into the stomach to siphon out swallowed pulmonary secretions; *used to:* detect organisms causing pulmonary infections; especially useful for detecting tubercle bacilli in children.

Procedures to Evaluate the Respiratory System

1. **Pulmonary circulation studies**—*used to:* determine regional distribution of pulmonary blood flow.
   a. *Lung scan*—injection of radioactive isotope into the body, followed by lung scintigraphy, which produces a graphic record of gamma rays emitted by the isotope in lung tissues; *used to:* determine lung perfusion when space-occupying lesions or pulmonary emboli and infarct are suspected.
   b. *Pulmonary angiography*—x-ray visualization of the pulmonary vasculature after the injection of a radiopaque contrast medium; *used to:* evaluate pulmonary disorders, e.g., pulmonary embolism, lung tumors, aneurysms, and changes in the pulmonary vasculature due to such conditions as emphysema or congenital defects.
2. **Bronchoscopy**—introduction of a special lighted instrument (bronchoscope) into the trachea and bronchi; *used to:* inspect tracheobronchial tree for pathologic changes, remove tissue for cytologic and bacteriologic studies, remove foreign bodies or mucous plugs causing airway obstruction, assess functional residual capacity of diseased lung, and apply chemotherapeutic agents.

☞ *Prebronchoscopy nursing actions*:
   Oral hygiene.
   Postural drainage is indicated.
   ▭ Sedatives, if ordered.

☞ *Postbronchoscopy nursing actions*:
   Instruct client *not* to swallow oral secretions but to let saliva run from side of mouth.
   Save expectorated sputum for lab analysis, and observe for frank bleeding.
   NPO until gag reflex returns.
   Observe for subcutaneous emphysema and dyspnea.
   Apply ice collar to reduce throat discomfort.

3. **Thoracentesis**—needle puncture through the chest wall and into the pleura; *used to:* remove fluid and, occasionally, air from the pleural space.

☞ *Nursing responsibilities before thoracentesis:*
   Position: high-Fowler's position or sitting up on edge of bed, with feet supported on chair to facilitate accumulation of fluid in the base of the chest. If client is unable to sit up, turn on unaffected side.

☞ *After procedure*:
   Evaluate continually for signs of shock, pain, cyanosis, increased respiratory rate, and pallor.

Roentgenologic studies (X-ray)

Chest—*used to:* determine size, contour, and position of the heart; size, location, and nature of pulmonary lesions; disorders of thoracic bones or soft tissue; diaphragmatic contour and excursion; pleural thickening or effusions; and gross changes in the caliber or distribution of pulmonary vasculature

Diets

Pneumonia

↑ Carbohydrate
↓ Protein

Pulmonary Tuberculosis

↑ Calories
↑ Protein

Emphysema

↑ Calories (3000/d)
↑ Fluids
↑ Protein

Bronchitis

↑ Calories
↑ Feedings
↑ Fluids

Acute Respiratory Distress Syndrome

IV maintenance while client is on ventilator

Thoracic Surgery

↑ Fluids
Nutritious diet to promote healing

Drug Review

Pneumonia

Antibiotics (to control infection)
Cephalexin (*Keflex*): 250–500 mg q6h
Cephalothin (*Keflin*): IV, 0.5–2 g q4-6h
Erythromycin: 250–500 mg q6–12h
Gentamicin (*Garamycin*): 3–5 mg/kg/d in divided doses
Penicillin G procaine (*Wycillin*): 1.2 million U, single IM dose
Antipyretics (to reduce fever):
Acetaminophen: 325–650 mg PO/RECT q4h prn; max 4G/day;
Aspirin: 325–1000 mg q4–6h, *not* to exceed 4 g/d
Expectorant:
Guaifenesin (*Robitussin*): 100–400 mg q4h to clear airway

Atelectasis

Acetylcysteine (*Mucomyst*) 3-5 mL 3–4 times via nebulizer; inhalation lowers viscosity of mucus, allowing easier mobilization and expectoration

Pulmonary Embolism

Anticoagulants
Heparin sodium: IV, 5,000 U IV to start, followed by 20,000– 40,000 U infusion over 24 hours; SC 8000
10,000 U q8h, adjusted according to *PTT*;
Warfarin (*Coumadin*): 10 mg/d, adjusted according to *INR*.
Pain control
Morphine: IV, 2.5–15 q4h or loading dose of 15 mg with 0.8–10 mg/h, rate increased as needed; SC, 5–20 mg q4h as needed
Note: *Avoid* birth control pills after pulmonary embolism.

Histoplasmosis

Antiemetic
Promethazine (*Phenergan*): 10–25 mg q4h
Antifungals
Amphotericin B: after 1 mg test dose, 0.25 mg/kg, increase to 0.50 mg/kg twice daily
Ketoconazole (*Nizoral*): 200–400 mg/d, single dose
Antipyretics (to reduce fever):
Acetaminophen: 325–650 mg PO/RECT q4h prn; max 4G/day
Aspirin: 325–1000 mg q4–6h, *not* to exceed 4 g/d

Pulmonary Tuberculosis

Ethambutol: 2.5 g/d
Isoniazid: 5–10 mg/kg to 300 mg with pyridoxine (10 mg/d) to prevent neuritis
Rifampin: 600 mg/d
Streptomycin: 1 g/d (*Caution*: may cause eighth cranial nerve damage, nephrotoxicity)

Emphysema

Antimicrobials
Ampicillin: 1–2 g/d q6–12h
Tetracycline: 1–2 g/d q6–12h
Bronchial detergent
Acetylcysteine (*Mucomyst*) inhalation 3–5 mL 3 to 4 times daily via nebulizer
Bronchodilators
Albuterol (*Proventil, Ventolin*): via metered-dose inhaler (MDI) 2 puffs q4h.
Aminophylline: loading dose, 500 mg, followed by 250–500 mg q6-8h. *Note*: monitor theophylline level
Ipratropium (*Atrovent*): MDI 2 puffs 4X/day
Isoproterenol (*Isuprel*): 1–2 inhalations 4–6 times daily
Terbutaline sulfate (*Bricanyl*): 2 inhalations q4–6h
Theophylline: 5 mg/kg initially then 3 mg/kg q8h
Expectorant
Guaifenesin (*Robitussin*): 100–400 mg q4h to clear airway
Steroids: Should **never** be abruptly discontinued; gradually taper dosage to prevent complications
Dexamethasone (*Decadron*): 0.5–9 mg/d in single or divided doses
Methylprednisolone (*Medrol*): 4–48 mg/d
Prednisone: 5–60 mg/d.

Asthma

Antibiotics
   Ampicillin: 1–2 g/d q6–12h
   Tetracycline: 1–2 g/d q6–12h
Bronchodilators
   Albuterol (*Ventolin*): via metered-dose inhaler, 2
      inhalations q4-6h or 2 inhalations before exercise
   Aminophylline: loading dose, 500 mg, followed by
   ⌇⌇ 250–500 mg q6-8 h. *Note*: monitor theophylline levels.
   Ipratropium (*Atrovent*): MDI 2 puffs 4X/day
   Isoproterenol (*Isuprel*): 1–2 inhalations 4–6 times daily
   Theophylline: 5 mg/kg initially then 3 mg/kg q8h
Expectorant
   Guaifenesin (*Robitussin*): 100–400 mg q4h to clear airway
Steroids: Should **never** be abruptly discontinued;
      gradually taper dosage to prevent complications
   Dexamethasone (*Decadron*): 0.5–9 mg/d in single or
      divided doses
   Methylprednisolone (*Medrol*): 4–48 mg/d
   Prednisone: 5–60 mg/d
   Triamcinolone (*Azmacort*): 2 sprays 3–4/d

Bronchitis

Antibiotics
   Ampicillin: 1–2 g/d q6–12h
   Cefixime (*Suprax*): 20 mg/d
   Tetracycline: 1–2 g/d q6–12h
Bronchial detergent
   Acetylcysteine (*Mucomyst*) inhalation 3–5 mL 3 to 4
      times daily via nebulizer
Bronchodilators
   Albuterol (*Ventolin*): via metered-dose inhaler, 2
      inhalations q4–6h
   Aminophylline: loading dose, 500 mg, followed by
   ⌇⌇ 250–500 mg q6–8h. *Note*: monitor theophylline levels
   Ipratropium (*Atrovent*): MDI 2 puffs 4X/day
   Isoproterenol (*Isuprel*): 1–2 inhalations 4–6 times daily
   Theophylline: 5mg/kg initially then 3 mg/kg q8h
Expectorant
   Guaifenesin (*Robitussin*): 100–400 mg q4h to clear airway

Adult Respiratory Distress Syndrome

Antibiotics (to control infection)
   Cephalexin (*Keflex*): 250–500 mg q6h
   Cephalothin (*Keflin*): IV, 0.5-2 g q4–6h
   Erythromycin: 250–500 mg g6–12h
   Gentamicin (*Garamycin*): 3–5 mg/kg/d in divided doses
   Penicillin G Procaine (*Wycillin*): 1.2 million U single IM
      dose
Bronchodilator
   Aminophylline: loading dose, 500 mg, followed by
   ⌇⌇ 250–500 mg q6-8h. *Note*: monitor theophylline levels.
Diuretic
   Furosemide (*Lasix*): 20–80 mg/d
Pharmacologic paralysis
   (Pancuronium bromide, curare) if respirations are out of
      phase with mechanical ventilation
Sedation to reduce anxiety and restlessness

Hemothorax and Pneumothorax

Pain control
   Must not depress respirations
   Small, frequent doses
   Other medications according to health status

Thoracic Surgery

Antibiotics
   Cephalexin (*Keflex*): 250–500 mg q6h
   Cephalothin (*Keflin*): IV, 0.5–2 g q4–6h
   Erythromycin: 250–500 mg q6-12h
   Gentamicin (*Garamycin*): 3–5 mg/kg/d in divided doses
Bronchodilators
   Albuterol (*Ventolin*): via metered-dose inhaler, 2
      inhalations q4–6h
   Aminophylline: loading dose, 500 mg, followed by
   ⌇⌇ 250–500 mg q6–8h. *Note*: monitor theophylline levels
   Isoproterenol (*Isuprel*): 1–2 inhalations 4–6 times daily
   Theophylline: 5 mg/kg initially then 3 mg/kg q8h
Expectorant
   Guaifenesin (*Robitussin*): 100–400 mg q4h to clear
      airway
Pain control
   Must not depress respirations
   Small, frequent doses

Laryngectomy

Antibiotics to prevent infection
Pain control without respiratory depression
Ultrasonic nebulization to facilitate expectoration

Questions

1. The nurse would conclude that a client with
   emphysema is experiencing respiratory acidosis if,
   on assessment, he/she observes:
   1. A change in respiratory rate from 18 to 26
      breaths/ min.
   2. An increasing rate and depth of respirations.
   3. A change in heart rate from 86 to 60 beats/min.
   4. A decreasing level of consciousness.
2. The breath sounds heard during a physical
   assessment in a client with emphysema would be
   described as:
   1. Bronchovesicular.
   2. Vesicular.
   3. Bronchial.
   4. Diminished.
3. Which infection control technique is unnecessary
   when caring for a client with tuberculosis (TB)?
   1. Washing hands before and after contact.
   2. Putting on isolation gown, mask, and gloves. *not necess.*
   3. Avoiding face-to-face contact.
   4. Careful disposal of soiled tissues.

4. The nurse would tell a client with TB that the drug treatment for TB frequently consists of:
   1. Rifampin and ethambutol.
   2. Isoniazid and rifampin.
   3. Streptomycin and ethambutol.
   4. Isoniazid and streptomycin.

5. If a client experiences cardiac irregularities during suctioning, the best action for the nurse to take would be to:
   1. Give an antiarrhythmic drug before suctioning.
   2. Suction no longer than 10 to 15 seconds at a time.
   3. Give additional O_2 before suctioning.
   4. Use a smaller suction catheter to reduce O_2 loss.

6. The nurse would know that an important aspect of proper tracheostomy care is to:
   1. Secure the twill ties at the back of the client's neck.
   2. Clean the inner cannula at least once a shift.
   3. Inflate the tracheostomy cuff before tracheostomy care.
   4. Use hydrogen peroxide to clean around the stoma.

7. The nurse would know that the client's chest tubes are functioning properly if which condition were noted?
   1. Continuous bubbling in the water seal chamber.
   2. The tubing hanging in a dependent loop to facilitate drainage.
   3. Fluid fluctuating in the water seal tube during respirations.
   4. A minimum drainage of 100 mL/h for 24 hours after insertion.

8. In what position should the nurse place a client during thoracentesis?
   1. Supine, head elevated.
   2. Side-lying, affected lung up.
   3. Sitting up, leaning forward.
   4. Prone, affected lung down.

9. The client with emphysema is feeling short of breath and asks the nurse to increase the oxygen flow rate. The nurse explains that if the level is increased the following may occur:
   1. More alveoli will be destroyed and breathing will become more difficult.
   2. Cilia will be destroyed and congestion will increase.
   3. Breathing will become shallow and slow and eventually stop.
   4. The serum CO_2 level will drop, causing hypocapnia.

10. A client's pulmonary function tests show an increase in the residual volume and a reduction in vital capacity. Which nursing diagnosis would best apply to this client?
    1. Altered health maintenance.
    2. Risk for activity intolerance.
    3. Risk for fluid volume excess.
    4. Impaired physical mobility.

11. For what expected therapeutic effect of *Theo-Dur* should the nurse watch a client?
    1. Dilatation of the bronchioles.
    2. Improved alveolar gas exchange.
    3. Increase in pulmonary compliance.
    4. Decrease in pulmonary friction.

12. The client has been receiving cefixime (*Suprax*) and theophylline (*Theo-Vent*) for the treatment of acute bronchitis. He complains of feeling nervous, anxious, and nauseated. The most appropriate action for the nurse to take would be to:
    1. Encourage the client to use relaxation techniques.
    2. Call the MD to get an order for an antiemetic.
    3. Check the client's most recent theophylline level.
    4. Institute a breathing treatment immediately.

13. A client is observed using pursed-lip breathing. If the technique is working, the greatest change in the client's pulmonary function the nurse would see would be in the:
    1. Tidal volume.
    2. Expiratory capacity.
    3. Inspiratory reserve.
    4. Vital capacity.

14. A client with emphysema is being discharged. Discharge teaching regarding diet should include instructions to:
    1. Eat three full-size meals each day.
    2. Restrict fluid intake with meals.
    3. Increase intake of calories and protein.
    4. Limit intake of foods high in sodium.

15. Which personal factor revealed during a nursing history would be the most likely contributory cause of a client's emphysema?
    1. Family history of diabetes.
    2. History of alcohol abuse.
    3. No regular exercise plan.
    4. Job working for highway maintenance department.

16. On assessment, the nurse should recognize which symptom as a characteristic of emphysema?
    1. Barrel chest.
    2. Dusky skin color around mouth.
    3. Vesicular breath sounds.
    4. Frequent dry cough.

17. The nurse knows that the most positive evidence of active TB is:
    1. A positive skin test result.
    2. A raised WBC.
    3. Positive sputum culture findings.
    4. Positive chest x-ray study findings.

18. Which assessment finding would be consistent with a pneumothorax secondary to a ruptured emphysematous bleb?
    1. Paradoxical chest motion.
    2. Chest pain on the affected side.
    3. Mediastinal shift toward the affected side.
    4. Hematemesis.

    tension pneumo *unaffected*

19. Client teaching about INH therapy would include:
    1. Taking the drug on an empty stomach for best absorption.
    2. Expecting concentrated and dark urine.
    3. Avoiding the consumption of alcohol, to prevent drug toxicity.
    4. Taking an antacid to relieve the gastric distress which occurs.

20. To prevent the peripheral neuropathy INH treatment can cause, the nurse should anticipate that the client will most likely be started on a regimen of:
    1. Thiamine.
    2. Pyridoxine.
    3. Calcium.
    4. Potassium chloride.

21. After arriving at the clinic for an appointment, the client has an asthma attack. Which event would most likely have precipitated the attack?
    1. Weeding in the yard the day before.
    2. Only 4 hours of sleep the night before.
    3. Running from the bus to the clinic for the appointment.
    4. Jogging earlier in the day.

22. For what side effect of an epinephrine inhaler should the nurse assess?
    1. Dry mouth.
    2. Tachycardia.
    3. Apnea.
    4. Hypotension.

    HTN

23. Which symptom would a client most likely complain of after an asthma attack?
    1. Dry cough.
    2. Sore chest.
    3. Restlessness.
    4. Profuse perspiration.

24. Which factor identified during a nursing history would be the most likely contributory cause of a client's emphysema?
    1. A recent episode of pneumonia.
    2. A two–pack per day history of smoking.
    3. Client was raised and is currently living in an industrial area.
    4. A diet high in saturated fat and cholesterol.

25. On assessment, the nurse observes that the client with emphysema is mouth breathing and the secretions are tenacious. The first nursing action would be to:
    1. Elevate the head of the client's bed.
    2. Increase the client's oral fluid intake.

    ↑ fluids to liquefy secretions

    3. Encourage the client to breathe slowly and deeply.
    4. Check the breath sounds for wheezes.

26. Which breathing-enhancing strategy should the nurse teach the client with emphysema?
    1. Diaphragmatic breathing and pursed-lip breathing during inspiration.
    2. Diaphragmatic breathing and pursed-lip breathing during exhalation.
    3. Use of upper chest and neck muscles during inhalation.
    4. Orthopnea and pursed-lip breathing during exhalation.

27. Which signs and symptoms would the nurse recognize to be side effects of aminophylline?
    1. BP 90/60 mmHg., P–120, insomnia, and headache.
    2. BP 120/70 mmHg., P–78, tremors, and lethargy.
    3. BP 140/90 mmHg., P–78, anxiety, and nausea.
    4. BP 90/50 mmHg., P–56, insomnia, and vomiting.

Answers/Rationale

1. **(4)** As the CO_2 level rises during respiratory acidosis, the client would become more somnolent and, if breathing is not improved, would eventually lose consciousness. The client with emphysema *normally* has a rapid respiratory rate (**1**) to compensate for the hypoxia which is present. As the CO_2 level rises, the respiratory rate would slow. Because of the disease process, the client is unable to breathe deeply (**2**); the client with emphysema hypoventilates. The heart rate would most likely increase, *not* decrease (**3**). **AS, APP, 6, PhI, Physiological adaptation**

2. **(4)** In emphysema the alveoli (the site of gas exchange) are hyperinflated or destroyed, resulting in diminished or absent breath sounds. Bronchovesicular (**1**) or bronchial (**3**) breath sounds would be abnormal if heard over the lung fields, but in emphysema there is little to no air movement to produce these sounds. Vesicular (**2**) breath sounds are *normal* sounds and would *not* be heard over the diseased lung. **AS, COM, 6, PhI, Physiological adaptation**

3. **(2)** Because TB is an airborne disease, a mask would be appropriate but the gown and gloves are *not* necessary. The mask is often put on the client, and staff or visitors may also wear masks. It *is* necessary to use the techniques in options **1**, **3**, and **4** to prevent cross-contamination. **IMP, APP, 6, SECE, Safety and infection control**

4. **(2)** All of the drugs in the options are used in the treatment of TB, but isoniazid (INH) and rifampin are the *most commonly* used first-line drugs and are given in combination. INH is low in toxicity and a drug of choice. Rifampin is always given in combination with another agent. Ethambutol (**1** and

3) would be the third drug of choice. Streptomycin (**3** and **4**) is used only if resistance to the other drugs occurs. **IMP, RE/KN, 6, PhI, Pharmacological and parenteral therapies**

5. (**2**) Prolonged suctioning will cause hypoxia and may also produce an arrhythmia; bradycardia frequently occurs during suctioning as the result of vagal stimulation. Suctioning no longer than 10 to 15 seconds at a time decreases the likelihood of arrhythmias. Drugs (**1**) are not needed because the cause of the problem is *not* cardiac in origin. Hyperoxygenation (**3**) may be induced *if* limiting the duration of suctioning is not effective. A smaller catheter (**4**) would probably be ineffective in removing the secretions, thus necessitating more frequent suctioning. **IMP, APP, 6, PhI, Physiological adaptation**

6. (**2**) The cannula must be cleaned at least once a shift to remove any mucus buildup. The ties (**1**) are secured at the *side* of the client's neck. Although option **3** is an important aspect of tracheostomy care, not all tracheostomies have an inflatable cuff (**3**). The correct choice must be applicable to all types of tracheostomies. Saline *not* hydrogen peroxide (**4**), is used to clean around the stoma. **PL, COM, 6, PhI, Reduction of risk potential**

7. (**3**) The fluid level will fluctuate with the changes in intrapleural pressure during respiration. On inspiration the fluid rises up the tube; on expiration the fluid goes down the tube. Continuous bubbling (**1**) indicates a leak in the drainage system or the pleural cavity. A dependent loop (**2**) would impair gravity drainage. Drainage of 100 mL/h (**4**) is normal only during the first 2 hours; after that, such an amount would be excessive. The total normal drainage for 24h is 500 to 1000 mL. **AS, EVL, 6, PhI, Reduction of risk potential**

8. (**3**) Having the client sit up and lean forward with his/her arms on the lap or a bedside table exposes the area where the needle is to be inserted. The other positions (**1, 2,** and **4**) would make it more difficult to get into the pleural space without puncturing the lung. **IMP, APP, 3, PhI, Basic care and comfort**

Key to Codes

Nursing process: **AS**, assessment; **AN**, analysis; **PL**, planning; **IMP**, implementation; **EV**, evaluation. (See **Appendix M** for explanation of nursing process steps.)

Cognitive level: **RE/KN**, recall/knowledge; **COM**, comprehension; **APP**, application; **ANL**, analysis; **EVL**, evaluation; **SYN**, synthesis. (See **Appendix M** for explanation.)

Category of human function: 1, protective; 2, sensory-perceptual; 3, comfort, rest, activity, and mobility; 4, nutrition; 5, growth and development; 6, fluid-gas transport; 7, psychosocial-cultural; 8, elimination. (See **Appendix 0** for explanation.)

Client need: **SECE**, safe, effective care environment; **PhI**, physiological integrity; **PsI**, psychosocial integrity; **HPM**, health promotion and maintenance. (See **Appendix P** for explanation.)

Client subneed: (See **Appendix P** for explanation)

9. (**3**) The stimulus for the client with emphysema to breathe is the low partial pressure of oxygen in the blood; increasing the O_2 level without the support of mechanical ventilation may actually suppress ventilation. The disease has already destroyed alveoli (**1**) and cilia (**2**), contributing to the breathing difficulty and congestion. The CO_2 level will decrease (**4**) only if ventilation improves, but supplemental O_2 will not improve ventilation. **IMP, COM, 6, PhI, Physiological adaptation**

10. (**2**) The client will experience dyspnea on exertion and activity intolerance as the result of the trapped air and reduced vital capacity. Even activities of daily living are difficult for a client with severe respiratory disease. Health maintenance (**1**) is not specific enough. Fluid volume excess (**3**) is not causing the pulmonary function problems; the abnormalities are consistent with chronic obstructive pulmonary disease. Physical mobility (**4**) is impaired only because the client cannot tolerate activity. The client is able to move but tires easily as a result of the hypoxia. **AN, APP, 6, SECE, Management of care**

11. (**1**) *Theo-Dur,* an extended release theophylline, is a bronchodilator. A *secondary* effect would be an improvement in gas exchange (**2**) as a result of the improved flow of air in and out of the bronchioles. Pulmonary compliance may actually already be increased (**3**) in some clients with broncho-constriction, such as that caused by emphysema. Anti-inflammatory agents or antibiotics would cause pulmonary friction (**4**) to be decreased. **EV, EVL, 6, PhI, Pharmacological and parenteral therapies**

12. (**3**) These are the symptoms of a theophylline excess. The therapeutic level is 10 to 20 mcg/mL; any level over 20 mcg/mL is considered toxic. If theophylline toxicity is ruled out, the symptoms might indicate anxiety, and relaxation techniques (**1**) would help. An antiemetic (**2**) treats the symptom, not the problem. Breathing treatment (**4**) would be indicated if the symptoms were due to hypoxia. **IMP, APP, 6, PhI, Pharmacological and parenteral therapies**

13. (**2**) Pursed-lip breathing keeps the airways from collapsing on expiration, allowing more air to be exhaled; therefore the greatest change would occur in the expiratory capacity. With an increase in exhalation, there would be an improvement in inspiratory volume, which would then cause a change in all the other components of pulmonary function (**1, 3,** and **4**). However, the *greatest* effect would be on expiratory capacity. **EV, EVL, 6, PhI, Physiological adaptation**

14. (**3**) There is more work involved in breathing, as well as hypoxemia, in a client with a chronic obstructive pulmonary disease such as emphysema. High calorie foods and protein provide the energy needed. It is not necessary to consume full-size meals to meet energy needs (**1**). Fluid intake (**2**) should be increased, *not* decreased, to help liquefy secretions. There is no indication of the need to restrict sodium

intake (**4**), however, if fluid retention occurred, breathing and circulation would be further impaired. **IMP, APP, 4, PhI, Basic care and comfort**

15. (**4**) Constant exposure to automobile exhaust may cause lung damage. The regular inhalation of fumes, such as may occur on the job, is potentially harmful to the lungs. The conditions in the other options (**1, 2**, and **3**) are *not* known to contribute to the development of lung disease. **AN, COM, 6, SECE, Safety and infection control**

16. (**1**) The increase in the anteroposterior diameter of the chest, the barrel appearance, is a consequence of the alveolar hyperinflation and trapped air that occur in emphysema. These cause the client to be unable to exhale fully and eventually to lose the elasticity of the lung. Circumoral cyanosis (**2**) may be seen with hypoxia, which is not the primary problem in emphysema. Vesicular breath sounds (**3**) are normal sounds; in emphysema the breath sounds are diminished or absent. The cough is not dry (**4**) but is often productive of thick, tenacious secretions. **AS, COM, 6, PhI, Physiological adaptation**

17. (**3**) A diagnosis of TB can only be established when *Mycobacterium tuberculosis* is cultured from secretions or tissue. The specimen can be from the lung or it can be gastric contents if sputum is swallowed. A skin test (**1**) may confirm the presence of TB, but false-positive results can occur. Other diseases can assume the same appearance as that of TB on an x-ray study (**4**). An elevated WBC (**2**) indicates the presence of an infection but is not a definitive characteristic of TB. **EV, ANL, 6, PhI, Reduction of risk potential**

18. (**2**) A tension pneumothorax exerts pressure on the heart and the unaffected lung, causing the client to experience severe pain, difficulty breathing, and a mediastinal shift toward the unaffected side. The pressure must be relieved immediately or cardiac function will be severely compromised. The mediastinal shift is *not* toward the affected side (**3**). Paradoxical chest motion (**1**) is seen in a client with a flail chest. Hemoptysis, *not* hematemesis (**4**), might be present in a client with a pneumothorax. **AS, ANL, 6, PhI, Physiological adaptation**

19. (**3**) Regular alcohol consumption increases the risk of INH toxicity and hepatic injury or hepatitis, another drug side effect. Taking the drug on an empty stomach (**1**) is not necessary because drug absorption is not delayed when the drug is taken with food. If urine is concentrated and dark (**2**), the MD should be notified, because this would indicate liver impairment. An antacid (**4**) would delay absorption; the drug should be taken with food or milk to minimize the nausea and other forms of gastric distress that are side effects of the agent. **IMP, COM, 6, PhI, Pharmacological and parenteral therapies**

20. (**2**) Pyridoxine, vitamin B_6, increases neuro-transmitter formation to prevent peripheral neuropathy. Thiamine (**1**), calcium (**3**), and potassium chloride (**4**) will not prevent this drug side effect. **PL, COM, 1, PhI, Pharmacological and parenteral therapies**

21. (**3**) There are two types of asthma—allergic and nonallergic; this attack appears to be nonallergic in origin. Precipitating factors include *recent* exercise, stress, emotion and strong odors. The nurse would look for the precipitant closest in time to the attack. The attack was immediately preceded by running. The other events (**1, 2**, and **4**) occurred several hours to a day *before* the attack and for this reason are unlikely causes. **AN, ANL, 6, HPM, Health promotion and maintenance**

22. (**1**) The client should be instructed to rinse the mouth after each use of the inhaler to prevent dryness from vasoconstriction. Other side effects of epinephrine include restlessness, insomnia, arrhythmias, bronchial irritation, and hypertension. Tachycardia (**2**), apnea (**3**), and hypotension (**4**) are *not* side effects of epinephrine. **AS, COM, 6, PhI, Pharmacological and parenteral therapies**

23. (**2**) There is dyspnea and use of the accessory muscles during an asthma attack and this results in fatigue and a sore chest. During the attack the cough would be nonproductive (**1**), but after the bronchospasms are relieved, the client will generally cough up a mucous plug. During the attack the client is hypoxic, restless, and anxious (**3**); afterward the client is usually calm and fatigued. Perspiration (**4**), or diaphoresis, occurs *during* the attack. **AS, ANL, 6, PhI, Physiological adaptation**

24. (**2**) A major contributory cause of emphysema is smoking which destroys lung tissue. Pneumonia (**1**) would not cause emphysema but would destroy more lung tissue. Environmental irritants (**3**) may be associated with lung disease, but not as consistently so as smoking. A high fat and cholesterol diet (**4**) would contribute to the development of *heart* disease. **AN, COM, 1, HPM, Health promotion and maintenance**

25. (**2**) The best action for the nurse to take is to increase the client's oral fluid intake to liquefy tenacious secretions. Mouth breathing may be pursed-lip breathing, which does not indicate the presence of respiratory distress, so the head of the bed does *not* have to be elevated (**1**). The client will be *unable* to breathe deeply (**3**) until secretions are liquefied and mobilized. The assessment would not include the checking of breath sounds (**4**). **PL, ANL, 6, PhI, Reduction of risk potential**

26. (**2**) Diaphragmatic (abdominal) breathing is done during both inhalation and exhalation, and pursed-lip breathing is done during exhalation only. Diaphragmatic breathing is more effective than the use of accessory muscles, such as the shoulder muscles; it can increase the tidal volume, exercise tolerance, and alveolar ventilation and decrease the respiratory rate. Pursed-lip breathing slows the

flow of exhaled air, creating a back pressure, which keeps the airway open and prevents collapse; as a result, there is more complete emptying of the lungs. Pursed lip breathing is *not* done on *inspiration* (**1**). Use of the accessory muscles (**3**) is *ineffective* and more fatiguing. Orthopnea (**4**) is dyspnea that is relieved by assuming the upright *position*; it is *not* a breathing technique. **IMP, COM, 6, HPM, Health promotion and maintenance**

27. (**1**) A key side effect of aminophylline is tachycardia from the chronotropic effects of the drug. If the agent is given too rapidly, hypotension will occur. In addition to complaining of insomnia and headache, the client may appear nervous or anxious. Tremors (**2**), nausea (**3**), and vomiting (**4**) are also side effects; but in all of these options the pulse rate is normal or low, rather than rapid. **AN, APP, 6, PhI, Pharmacological and parenteral therapies**

Fluid and Electrolyte Imbalances

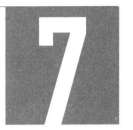

Chapter Outline

Imbalances in fluid and electrolytes may be due to changes in the total quantity of either substance (deficit or excess), protein deficiencies, and/or extracellular fluid volume shifts. Older clients and very young clients are particularly susceptible.

Fluid Volume Deficits

Decreased quantities of fluid and electrolytes may be caused by *deficient intake* (poor dietary habits, anorexia, and nausea), *excessive output* (vomiting, nasogastric suction, and prolonged diarrhea), or *failure of regulatory mechanism*.

I. **Pathophysiology:** water moves out of the cells to replace a significant water loss; cells eventually become unable to compensate for the lost fluid, and cellular dehydration begins, leading to circulatory collapse.

II. **Risk factors/causes:**
   A. No fluids available, or fluids not drinkable.
   B. Inability to take fluids independently.
   C. No response to thirst; does not recognize the need for fluids.
   D. Inability to communicate need; does not speak same language.
   E. Aphasia.
   F. Weakness, comatose.
   G. Inability to swallow.
   H. Psychological alterations.

III. **Assessment**
   A. *Subjective data:*
      1. Thirst.

   2. Behavioral changes: apprehension, apathy, lethargy, confusion, restlessness.
   3. Dizziness.
   4. Numbness and tingling of hands and feet.
   5. Anorexia, nausea.
   6. Abdominal cramps.
   B. *Objective data:*
      1. Sudden weight loss of 5%.
      2. Vital signs:
         a. *Decreased* blood pressure (BP); postural changes.
         b. *Increased* temperature.
         c. *Irregular*, weak, rapid pulse.
         d. *Increased* rate and depth of respirations.
      3. Skin: cool and pale in absence of infection; decreased turgor.
      4. Urine: oliguria to anuria, high specific gravity
      5. Eyes: soft, sunken.
      6. Tongue: furrows.
      7. Lab data:
         (1) Blood—*increased* hematocrit and blood urea nitrogen (BUN).
         (2) Urine—*decreased* 17–ketosteroids.

IV. **Analysis/nursing diagnosis:** *Fluid volume deficit* related to inadequate fluid intake.

V. **Nursing care plan/implementation**
   A. Goal: *restore fluid and electrolyte balance*—increase fluid intake to hydrate client.
      1. IVs as ordered; small, frequent drinks by mouth.
      2. Daily weights (same time of day) to monitor progress of fluid replacement.

3. Intake & output (I&O), *hourly* outputs (when in *acute* state).

4. *Avoid* hypertonic solutions (may cause fluid shift when compensatory mechanisms begin to function).

B. Goal: *promote comfort.*

1. Frequent skin care (lack of hydration causes dry skin, which may increase risk for skin breakdown).

2. *Position*: change every hour to relieve pressure.

3. Medications, as ordered: *antiemetics, antidiarrheals.*

C. Goal: *prevent physical injury.*

1. Frequent mouth care (mucous membrane dries due to dehydration; therefore, client is at risk for breaks in mucous membrane, halitosis).

2. Monitor *IV* flow rate—observe for circulatory overload, pulmonary edema related to potential fluid shift when compensatory mechanisms begin, or client's inability to tolerate rate of fluid replacement.

3. Monitor vital signs, including *level of consciousness* (*decreasing* BP and level of consciousness indicate continuation of fluid loss).

4. Prepare for surgery if hemorrhage present (internal bleeding can only be controlled by surgical intervention).

VI. Evaluation/outcome criteria

A. Mentally alert.

B. Moist, intact mucous membranes.

C. Urinary output approximately equal to intake.

D. No further weight loss.

E. Gradual weight gain.

Fluid Volume Excess

Excessive quantities of fluid and electrolytes may be due to *increased ingestion*, tube feedings, intravenous infusions, multiple tap-water enemas, or a *failure of regulatory systems*, resulting in inability to excrete excesses.

I. **Pathophysiology**: hypo-osmolar water excess in extracellular compartment leads to intracellular water excess because the concentration of solutes in the intracellular fluid is greater than that in the extracellular fluid. Water moves to equalize concentration, causing swelling of the cells.

II. **Risk factors/causes:**

A. Excessive intake of electrolyte-free fluids, e.g., water.

B. Increased secretion of antidiuretic hormone in response to stress, drugs, anesthetics.

C. Decreased or inadequate output of urine.

D. Psychogenic polydipsia.

E. Certain medical conditions: tuberculosis; encephalitis; meningitis; endocrine disturbances; tumors of lung, pancreas, duodenum.

F. Inadequate kidney function or kidney failure.

III. Assessment

A. *Subjective data*:

1. Behavioral changes: irritability, apathy, confusion, disorientation.

2. Headache.

3. Anorexia, nausea, cramping.

4. Fatigue.

5. Dyspnea.

B. *Objective data*:

1. Vital signs: *elevated* BP.

2. Skin: warm, moist; edema—eyelids, facial, dependent, pitting.

3. Sudden weight gain of *5%.*

4. Pink, frothy sputum; productive.

5. Urine: polyuria, nocturia.

6. Lab data:
   (1) Blood—*decreasing* hematocrit, BUN;
   (2) Urine—*decreasing* specific gravity.

IV. Analysis/nursing diagnosis: *Fluid volume excess* related to excessive fluid intake or decreased fluid output.

V. Nursing care plan/implementation

A. Goal: *maintain oxygen to all cells.*

1. *Position*: semi-Fowler's or Fowler's to facilitate improved gas exchange.

2. Vital signs: q4h.

3. Fluid *restriction.*

4. Possible *rotating tourniquets* as needed (especially for interstitial-to-plasma shift).

B. Goal: *promote excretion of excess fluid.*

1. Medications, as ordered: *diuretics.*

2. If in kidney failure, may need dialysis; explain procedure.

3. Assist client during paracentesis, thoracentesis, phlebotomy.

   a. Monitor vital signs to detect shock.

   b. Prevent injury by monitoring sterile technique.

   c. Prevent falling by stabilizing appropriate position during procedure.

   d. Support client psychologically.

C. Goal: *obtain/maintain fluid balance.*

1. Daily weights; 1 kg = 1000 mL of fluid.

2. Measure all edematous parts, abdominal girth, I&O.

3. *Limit*: fluids by mouth, IVs, sodium.

4. Strict monitoring of IV fluids.

D. Goal: *prevent tissue injury.*

1. Skin and mouth care as needed.

2. Evaluate feet for edema and discoloration when client is out of bed.

3. Observe suture line on surgical clients (potential for evisceration due to excess fluid retention).

4. IV route preferred for parenteral

☞ medications; *Z track* if medications are to be given IM (otherwise injected liquid will escape through injection site).

🏠 E. Goal: **health teaching.**

🍎 1. Improve nutritional status with *low sodium diet.*

2. Identify cause of imbalance, methods to avoid this situation in the future.

3. Desired effects and side effects of diuretics and other prescribed medications.

4. Monitor urinary output, ankle edema; report to health care manager when fluid retention is noticed.

5. Limit fluid intake when kidney/cardiac function impaired.

⋈ VI. **Evaluation/outcome criteria**
A. Fluid balance obtained.
B. No respiratory, cardiac complications.
C. Vital signs within normal limits.
D. Urinary output improved, no evidence of edema.

Common Electrolyte Imbalances

Electrolytes are taken into the body in foods and fluids; normally lost through sweat and urine. May also be lost through hemorrhage, vomiting, and diarrhea. Clinically important electrolytes are:

I. **Sodium** (Na⁺): normal 135–145 mEq/L. Most prevalent cation in extracellular fluid. Controls osmotic pressure; essential for neuromuscular functioning and intracellular chemical reactions. Aids in maintenance of acid-base balance.
A. *Hyponatremia*—sodium *deficit,* resulting from either a sodium loss or water excess. Serum sodium level *below* 135 mEq/L; symptoms usually do not occur *until* below 120 mEq/L unless rapid drop.
B. *Hypernatremia*—*excess* sodium in the blood, resulting from either high sodium intake, water loss, or low water intake. Serum sodium level *above* 145 mEq/L.

II. **Potassium** (K⁺): normal 3.5–5.0 mEq/L. Direct effect on excitability of nerves and muscles. Contributes to intracellular osmotic pressure and influences acid-base balance. Major cation of the cell. Required for storage of nitrogen as muscle protein.
A. *Hypokalemia*—potassium *deficit* related to: dehydration, starvation, vomiting, diarrhea, diuretics. Serum potassium level *below* 3.5 mEq/L; symptoms may not occur *until* below 2.5 mEq/L.

B. *Hyperkalemia*—potassium *excess* related to: severe tissue damage, renal disease, excess administration of oral or IV potassium. Serum potassium level *above* 5 mEq/L; symptoms usually occur when *above* 6.5 mEq/L.

III. **Calcium** (Ca²⁺): normal 4.5–5.5 mEq/L. Essential to muscle metabolism, cardiac function, and bone health. Controlled by parathyroid hormone; *reciprocal* relationship between calcium and phosphorus.
A. *Hypocalcemia*—loss of calcium related to: inadequate intake, vitamin D deficiency, hypoparathyroidism, damage to the parathyroid gland, decreased absorption in the gastrointestinal (GI) tract, excess loss through kidneys. Serum calcium level *below* 4.5 mEq/L.
B. *Hypercalcemia*—calcium excess related to: hyperparathyroidism, immobility, bone tumors, renal failure, excess intake of calcium or vitamin D. Serum calcium level *above* 5.5 mEq/L.

IV. **Magnesium** (Mg²⁺): normal 1.5–2.5 mEq/L. Essential to cellular metabolism of carbohydrates and proteins.
A. *Hypomagnesemia*—magnesium deficit related to: impaired absorption from GI tract, excess loss through kidneys, and prolonged periods of poor nutritional intake. Hypomagnesemia leads to neuromuscular irritability. Serum magnesium level *below* 1.5 mEq/L.
B. *Hypermagnesemia*—magnesium excess related to: renal insufficiency, overdose during replacement therapy, severe dehydration, repeated enemas with magnesium sulfate (Epsom salts). Serum magnesium level *above* 2.5 mEq/L.

V. **Table 7.1** provides *assessment, analysis, nursing care plan/implementation, and evaluation/outcome* criteria information for the various electrolyte imbalances.

VI. **See Table 7.8** for *electrolyte composition of fluid compartments*

Acid-Base Imbalances

Concentration of hydrogen ions in extracellular fluid is determined by the ratio of bicarbonate to carbonic acid. The normal ratio is 20:1. Even when arterial blood gas values are abnormal, if the ratio remains at 20:1, no imbalance will occur. **Table 7.2** shows *blood gas variations with acid-base imbalances.*

I. **Causes of blood gas abnormalities: Table 7.3.**

II. **Types of acid-base imbalance:**
A. *Acidosis*: hydrogen ion concentration *increases* and pH *decreases.*
B. *Alkalosis*: hydrogen ion concentration *decreases* and pH *increases.*

TABLE 7.1 ELECTROLYTE IMBALANCES

Disorder and Related Condition	⧗ Assessment Subjective Data	Objective Data	⧗ Analysis/Nursing Diagnosis	⧗ Nursing Care Plan/Implementation	⧗ Evaluation/Outcome Criteria
Hyponatremia Addison's disease Starvation GI suction ⊂▪ Thiazide diuretics Excess water intake, enemas Fever Fluid shifts Ascites Burns Small-bowel obstruction Profuse perspiration	Apathy, apprehension, mental confusion, delirium Fatigue Vertigo, headache Anorexia, nausea Abdominal and muscle cramps	*Pulse:* rapid and weak *BP:* postural hypotension Shock, coma *GI:* weight loss, diarrhea, loss through NG tubes *Muscle:* weakness	*Diarrhea* *Fluid volume deficit* *Altered nutrition, less than body requirements* *Sensory/perceptual alteration (kinesthetic)*	*Obtain normal sodium level:* identify cause of deficit, *increase sodium intake* PO (salty foods), IVs— ⊂▪ hypertonic solutions *Prevent further sodium loss:* irrigate ☞ NG tubes with saline; hourly I&O to monitor kidney output *Prevent injury* related to shock, dizziness, decreased sensorium; dangle before ambulation *Skin care*	Na⁺ 135–145 mEq/L No complications of shock present Return of muscle strength Alert, oriented Limits intake of plain water
Hypernatremia High sodium intake Low water intake Diarrhea High fever with rapid respirations Impaired renal functions Acute tracheobronchitis	Lethargy Restlessness, agitation Confusion	*BP and temperature:* elevated *Neuromuscular:* diminished reflexes *Skin:* flushed; firm turgor *GI:* mucous membrane dry, sticky *GU:* decreased output	*Fluid volume deficit* *Fluid volume excess* *Altered nutrition: less than body requirements* *Sensory/perceptual alteration (kinesthetic)*	*Obtain normal sodium level: decrease sodium intake* I&O to recognize signs and symptoms of complications, e.g., heart failure, pulmonary edema	Na⁺ 135–145 mEq/L No complaint of thirst Alert, oriented Relaxed in appearance Identifies high sodium foods to avoid

(Continued)

TABLE 7.1 ELECTROLYTE IMBALANCES (continued)

Disorder and Related Condition	⧗ Assessment — Subjective Data	Objective Data	⧗ Analysis/Nursing Diagnosis	⧗ Nursing Care Plan/Implementation	⧗ Evaluation/Outcome Criteria
Hypokalemia *Decreased intake:* Poor potassium food intake Excessive dieting Nausea Alcoholism IV fluids without added potassium *Increased loss:* GI suctioning, vomiting, diarrhea Ulcerative colitis Drainage: ostomy, fistulas ⟠ Medications: potassium-losing diuretics, digoxin, cathartics Increased aldosterone production Renal disorders	Apathy, lethargy, fatigue, weakness Irritability, mental confusion Anorexia, nausea Leg cramps	*Muscles:* weakness, paralysis, paresthesia, hyporeflexia *Respirations:* shallow to respiratory arrest *Cardiac:* decreased BP; *elevated*, weak, irregular pulse; arrhythmias 〰 *ECG:* low, flat T waves; prolonged ST segment; elevated U wave; potential arrest *GI:* vomiting, flatulence, constipation; decreased motility → distention → paralytic ileus *GU:* urine not concentrated; polyuria, nocturia; kidney damage *Speech*—slow	*Decreased cardiac output* *Fatigue* *Altered cardiopulmonary tissue perfusion* *Ineffective breathing patterns* *Constipation* *Bathing/hygiene self-care deficit* *Impaired home maintenance management* *Sensory/perceptual alteration (gustatory)*	*Replace lost potassium* ✊ *increase potassium* in diet (see **Appendix B**); liquid PO potassium ⟠ medications—dilute in juice to aid taste; give potassium *only if* kidneys functioning *Prevent injury to tissues:* prevent infiltration, pain, tissue damage *Prevent potassium loss:* ☞ irrigate NG tubes with saline, *not water*	K⁺ 3.5–5.0 mEq/L Identifies cause of imbalance Lists foods to include in diet Lists signs and symptoms of imbalance Return of muscle strength No cardiac arrhythmias
Hyperkalemia Burns Crushing injuries Kidney disease Excessive infusion or ingestion of K⁺ Adrenal insufficiency Mercurial poisoning	Irritability Weakness, muscle cramps Nausea, intestinal cramps	*Muscles:* paresthesia, flaccid muscle paralysis (later) *Cardiac:* irregular pulse; arrhythmias; bradycardia → asystole 〰 *ECG:* high T waves; depressed ST segment; widened QRS complex; diminished or absent P waves; ventricular fibrillation *GI:* explosive diarrhea; hyperactive bowel sounds *Kidney:* scant to no urine	*Decreased cardiac output* *Altered urinary elimination* *Activity intolerance* *Ineffective breathing patterns* *Diarrhea* *Impaired home maintenance management*	*Decrease amount of potassium in body;* identify, and treat cause of imbalance; give foods *low in K⁺; avoid* drugs or IV fluids containing K⁺ If kidney failure present, may need to prepare for dialysis	K⁺ 3.5–5.0 mEq/L No complications (e.g., arrhythmias, acidosis, respiratory failure)

(Continued)

TABLE 7.1 ELECTROLYTE IMBALANCES (continued)

Disorder and Related Condition	Assessment — Subjective Data	Objective Data	Analysis/Nursing Diagnosis	Nursing Care Plan/Implementation	Evaluation/Outcome Criteria
Hypocalcemia Acute pancreatitis Diarrhea Peritonitis Damage to parathyroid during thyroidectomy Hypothyroidism Burns Pregnancy and lactation Low vitamin D intake Multiple blood transfusions Renal disorders Massive infection	Fatigue Tingling/numbness: fingers and circumoral Abdominal cramps Palpitations Dyspnea	*Muscles:* spasms: tonic muscles, carpopedal, laryngeal; tetany → convulsions *Neuromuscular:* grimacing: hyper-irritable facial nerves *Cardiac:* arrhythmias → arrest *GI:* diarrhea *Ortho:* osteoporosis → fractures	*Pain* *Diarrhea* *Altered nutrition: less than body requirements* *Risk for injury* *Sensory/perceptual alteration (gustatory)*	*Prevent tetany (medical emergency):* calcium gluconate IV, 2.5–5.0 mL 10% solution; repeated q10 min to maximum dose of 30 mL *Prevent tissue injury* due to hypoxia and sloughing; administer *slowly; avoid infiltration* *Prevent injury related to medication administration. Caution:* drug interaction with carbonate, phosphate, digitalis; *avoid hypercalcemia. In less acute condition:* increase calcium intake—calcium gluconate or lactate	Ca²⁺ 4.5–5.5 mEq/L No signs of tetany Absent *Trousseau's* and *Chvostek's* signs Lists foods high in vitamin D and calcium
Hypercalcemia Parathyroid glands: overactive, tumor Increased immobility Decreased renal function Bone cancer Increased vitamin D and calcium intake *Milk-alkali syndrome*—self-administration of antacids; increased milk in diet to relieve GI symptoms	*Pain:* flank, deep bone, shin splints *Muscle:* weakness, fatigue *GI:* anorexia, nausea *Neuro:* headache Thirst → polyuria	*Muscles:* relaxed *GU:* kidney stones *GI:* increased milk intake; constipation; dehydration *Neuro:* stupor → coma	*Decreased cardiac output* *Constipation* *Activity intolerance* *Altered urinary elimination* *Pain*	*Reduce calcium intake: decrease* foods high in *calcium;* identify cause of imbalance; *give steroids, diuretics,* as ordered; isotonic saline IV *Prevent injury:* prevent pathologic fractures, (e.g., advanced cancer): prevent renal calculi by *increasing fluid intake*	Ca²⁺ 4.5–5.5 mEq/L No pain reported No fractures/calculi seen on x-ray

(Continued)

TABLE 7.1 ELECTROLYTE IMBALANCES (continued)

Disorder and Related Condition	Assessment		Analysis/Nursing Diagnosis	Nursing Care Plan/ Implementation	Evaluation/Outcome Criteria
	Subjective Data	Objective Data			
Hypomagnesemia Impaired GI absorption Prolonged malnutrition or starvation Alcoholism Excess loss of magnesium through kidneys related to increased aldosterone production Prolonged diarrhea Draining GI fistulas	Agitation Depression Confusion Paresthesia	*Muscles:* irritable tremors, spasticity, tetany → convulsions *Cardiac:* arrhythmias, tachycardia	*Risk for injury related to seizure activity* *Decreased cardiac output*	*Provide safety:* prevent injury to disoriented client; administer magnesium salts PO or IV **Health teaching:** prevention; diet *high magnesium* foods: fruits, green vegetables, whole grain cereals, milk, meats, nuts	Mg²⁺ 1.5–2.5 mEq/L
Hypermagnesemia Renal failure Diabetic ketoacidosis Severe dehydration Antacid therapy	Drowsiness, lethargy	*Neuromuscular:* loss of deep-tendon reflexes *Respiratory:* depression *Cardiac:* hypotension; cardiac arrest	*Ineffective breathing pattern* *Decreased cardiac output* *Fluid volume deficit* *Fluid volume excess* *Altered cardiopulmonary tissue perfusion*	*Obtain normal magnesium level* IV calcium; fluids; possible dialysis	Mg²⁺ 1.5–2.5 mEq/L No complications (e.g., respiratory depression, arrhythmias) Identifies magnesium-based antacids (e.g., *Gelusil*) Deep-tendon reflexes 2+

BP = blood pressure GI = gastrointestinal; NG = nasogastric; I&O = intake & output; GU = genitourinary; ECG = electrocardiogram.

Source: ©Lagerquist, SL: *Little, Brown's NCLEX-RN® Examination Review.* Boston: Little, Brown, (out of print)

TABLE 7.2 BLOOD GAS VARIATIONS WITH ACID–BASE IMBALANCES

Blood Gas Feature	Normal Value	Value with:			
		Respiratory Acidosis	Respiratory Alkalosis	Metabolic Acidosis	Metabolic Alkalosis
HCO_3 (bicarbonate)	22–26 mm Hg	Normal or ↑	Normal or ↓	↓	↑
PCO_2 (carbonic acid*)	35–45 mm Hg (1.05–1.35)	↑ ↑	↓ ↓	Normal or ↓ Normal or ↓	Normal or ↑ Normal or ↑
pH	7.35–7.45	↓	↑	↓	↑

↑ = increased; ↓ = decreased.

*To obtain carbonic acid level, multiply PCO_2 value by 0.03.

Source: ©Lagerquist, SL: *Little. Brown's NCLEX-RN® Examination Review*. Boston: Little, Brown, (out of print)

C. *Metabolic imbalances: bicarbonate* is the problem. In primary conditions, the level of bicarbonate is directly *proportional* to pH.
  1. *Metabolic acidosis*: excessive acid is pro-duced or added to the body; bicarbonate is lost or acid is retained due to poorly functioning kidneys. *Deficit* of bicarbonate.
  2. *Metabolic alkalosis*: excessive acid is lost or bicarbonate or alkali is retained. *Excess* of bicarbonate.
  3. As compensatory mechanism, PCO_2 will be *low in metabolic acidosis*, as the body attempts to eliminate excess carbonic acid and elevate pH. PCO_2 will become *elevated in metabolic alkalosis*.
D. *Respiratory imbalances: carbonic acid* is the problem. In primary conditions, PCO_2 is *inversely* proportional to the pH.
  1. *Respiratory acidosis*: pulmonary ventilation decreases, causing an *elevation* in the level of carbon dioxide or carbonic acid. *Excess* of PCO_2.
  2. *Respiratory alkalosis*: pulmonary ventilation increases, causing a *decrease* in the level of carbon dioxide or carbonic acid. *Deficit* of PCO_2.
  3. As a compensatory mechanism, the level of bicarbonate will *increase in respiratory acidosis* and *decrease in respiratory alkalosis*.

III. **Assessment: Table 7.4 Acid-Base Imbalances**
IV. **Analysis/nursing diagnosis**
  A. *Impaired gas exchange* related to hyperventilation.
  B. *Ineffective breathing pattern* related to decreased thoracic movements.
  C. *Ineffective airway clearance* related to retained secretions.
  D. *Risk for injury* related to poorly functioning kidneys.
  E. *Altered renal tissue perfusion* related to dehydration.
  F. *Altered urinary elimination* related to renal failure.
  G. *Fluid volume excess* related to altered kidney function.
  H. *Fluid volume deficit* related to diarrhea or dehydration.
  I. *Knowledge deficit* related to self-administration of antacid medications.
V. **Nursing care plan/implementation**: see Table 7.4.
VI. **Evaluation/outcome criteria**: see Table 7.4.

Intravenous Therapy

I. **Infusion systems**
  A. Plastic bag:
    1. Contains no vacuum—needs no air to replace fluid as it flows from container.
    2. Medication can be added with syringe and needle through a resealable latex port.
      a. During infusion, administration set should be completely clamped before medications are added.
      b. Prevents undiluted, and perhaps toxic, dose from entering administration set.
  B. Closed system:
    1. Requires partial vacuum—however, only fil-tered air enters container.
    2. Medication may be added during infusion through air vent in administration set.
  C. Administration sets:
    1. *Standard*—deliver 10–15 gtt/mL.
    2. *Pediatric or minidrop sets*—deliver 60 gtt/mL.
    3. *Controlled-volume sets*—permit accurate infusion of measured volumes of fluids.
      a. Particularly valuable when piggybacked into primary infusion.
      b. Solutions containing drugs can then be administered intermittently.
    4. *Y-type administration sets*—allow for simulta-neous or alternate infusion of two fluids.
      a. May contain filter and pressure unit for blood transfusions.
      b. *Air embolism* significant hazard with this type of administration set.

TABLE 7.3 CAUSES OF BLOOD GAS ABNORMALITIES

Blood Gas Abnormality	Cause

Elevated PCO$_2$ (hypercarbia, hypercapnia)	■ *Increased* CO$_2$ production:
	1. Fever
	2. Muscular exertion
	3. Anaerobic metabolism
	■ *Decreased* CO$_2$ elimination (hypoventilation):
	1. *Decreased* tidal volume
	  a. Pain (rib fractures, pleurisy)
	  b. Weakness (myasthenia gravis)
	  c. Paralysis (spinal cord injury, polio)
	2. *Decreased* respiratory rate:
	  a. Head injury
	  b. Depressant drugs
	  c. Brain attack (stroke)

Decreased PO$_2$ (hypoxemia, shunt)	■ *Fluid in the alveoli:*
	1. Pulmonary edema
	2. Pneumonia
	3. Near-drowning
	4. Chest trauma
	■ *Collapsed alveoli* (atelectasis):
	1. Airway obstruction:
	  a. By the tongue
	  b. By a foreign body
	2. Failure to take deep breaths:
	  a. Pain (rib fracture, pleurisy)
	  b. Paralysis of respiratory muscles (spinal cord injury, polio)
	  c. Depression of the respiratory center (head injury, drug overdose)
	3. Collapse of the whole lung (pneumothorax)
	■ *Other gases in the alveoli:*
	1. Smoke inhalation
	2. Inhalation of toxic chemicals
	3. Carbon monoxide poisoning
	■ *Respiratory arrest*

Source: adapted from Caroline NL. *Emergency Care in the Streets* (5th ed.) Boston. Little, Brown, (out of print).

5. *Positive-pressure sets*—designed for rapid infusion of replacement fluids.
   a. In emergency, built-in pressure chamber increases rate of blood administration.
   b. Pump chamber *must* be filled at all times to prevent air embolism.
   c. Application of positive pressure to infusion fluids is responsibility of *physician*.
6. *Infusion pumps*—utilized to deliver small volumes of fluid or doses of high-potency drugs.
   a. Used widely in all acute settings.
   b. Have increased the safety of parenteral therapy and reduced nursing time.

II. **Fluid administration**
   A. Factors influencing rate:
      1. Client's size.
      2. Client's physical condition.
      3. Client's age.
      4. Type of fluid
      5. Client's tolerance of fluid.
   B. Flow rates for parenteral infusions can be computed using the following **formula**:

$$\frac{gtt/mL \text{ of given set}}{60 \text{ min/h}} \times \text{total volume/h} = gtt/min$$

Example:
   If 1000 mL is to be infused in an 8-h (125 mL/h) period and the administration set delivers 15 gtt/mL, the rate is 31.2 gtt/min:

$$\frac{15}{60} \times 125 = \frac{1}{4} \times 125 = 31.2 \text{ gtt/min or } 31 \text{ gtt/min}$$

   C. Generally the type of fluid administration set determines its rate of flow.
      1. *Fluid* administration sets—10–20 gtt/min.
      2. *Blood* administration sets—approximately 10 gtt/min.
      3. *Pediatric* administration sets—approximately 60 gtt/min.
      4. Always check information on the administration set box to determine the number of gtt/mL before calculating; varies with manufacturer.
   D. Factors influencing flow rates:
      1. *Gravity*—a change in the height of the infusion bottle will increase or decrease the rate of flow; for example, raising the bottle will increase the rate of flow, and vice versa.
      2. *Blood clot* in needle—stopping the infusion for any reason or an increase in venous pressure may result in partial or total obstruction of needle by clot due to:
         a. *Delay* in changing infusion bottle.
         b. Blood pressure cuff on, or restraints *on* or *above* infusion needle.
         c. Client *lying on arm* in which infusion is being made.
      3. Change in *needle position*—against or away from vein wall.

TABLE 7.4 ACID-BASE IMBALANCES

Disorder and Related Conditions	Assessment		Nursing Care Plan/ Implementation	Evaluation/Outcome Criteria
	Subjective Data	Objective Data		
Respiratory Acidosis Acute bronchitis Emphysema Respiratory obstruction Atelectasis Damage to respiratory center Pneumonia Asthmatic attack Drug overdose	Headache Irritability Disorientation Weakness Dyspnea on exertion Nausea	Increased respirations Cyanosis Tachycardia Diaphoresis Dehydration Coma (CO_2 narcosis Hyperventilation to compensate if no pulmonary abnormality present HCO_3 normal, PCO_2 elevated, pH < 7.35	*Assist with normal breathing:* encourage coughing; *suction* ☞ airway; *postural drainage;* pursed-lip breathing; *raise* HOB *Protect from injury* ☞ *oxygen* at 2 L; encourage *fluids; avoid* sedation; ⊂⊃ medications as ordered— *bicarbonates, antibiotics, bronchial dilators, detergent* 🏠 **Health teaching:** identify cause, prevent future episodes; increase awareness re-garding risk factors and early signs of impending imbalance; encour-age compliance	Normal acid-base balance obtained Respiratory rate slows, <30 breaths/min No signs of pulmonary infection (e.g., sputum colorless, breath sounds clear) Demonstrates breathing exercises (e.g., diaphragmatic breathing)
Metabolic Acidosis Diabetic ketoacidosis Hyperthyroidism Severe infections Lactic acidosis in shock Renal failure → uremia Prolonged starvation diet; low protein diet Diarrhea, dehydration Hepatitis Burns	Headache Restlessness Apathy, weakness Disorientation Thirst Nausea, abdominal pain	*Kussmaul's* respirations: deep, rapid air hunger; ↑ Temperature Vomiting, diarrhea Dehydration Stupor → convulsions → coma HCO_3 below normal PCO_2 normal, K^+ > 5 mEq/L; pH <7.35	*Restore normal metabolism:* correct underlying problem; sodium ⊂⊃ bicarbonate PO/IV; sodium lactate; fluid replacement, Ringer's solution; 🍎 *diet:* high calorie *Prevent complications* ⊂⊃ regular *insulin* for ketoacidosis; hourly outputs; prepare for dialysis if in kidney failure 🏠 **Health teaching:** identify signs and symptoms of primary illness; prevent complications, cardiac arrest; diet instructions	Normal acid-base balance obtained No rebound respiratory alkalosis following therapy No tetany following return of normal pH Alert, oriented No signs of K^+ excess

(continued)

TABLE 7.4 ACID-BASE IMBALANCES (*continued*)

Disorder and Related Conditions	Assessment		Nursing Care Plan/ Implementation	Evaluation/Outcome Criteria
	Subjective Data	Objective Data		
Respiratory Alkalosis Hyperventilation— CO_2 loss Fever Metabolic acidosis Increased ICP Encephalitis Salicylate poisoning After intense exercise Hypoxia, high altitudes	Circumoral paresthesia Weakness Apprehension	Increased respirations Increased neuromuscular irritability; hyperreflexia, muscle twitching, tetany, positive *Chvostek's* sign Convulsions Unconsciousness Hypokalemia HCO_3 normal; PCO_2 *decreased*; pH > 7.45	*Increase carbon dioxide level*: rebreathing into a paper bag; adjusting respirator for CO_2 retention and oxygen inspired *Prevent injury*: safety measures for those who are unconscious; hypothermia for elevated temperature ☞ **Health teaching**: recognize stressful events; counseling if problem is hysteria	Normal acid-base balance obtained Recognizes psychological and environmental factors causing condition Respiratory rate returns to normal limits No cardiac arrhythmias Alert, oriented
Metabolic Alkalosis Potassium deficiencies Vomiting GI suctioning Intestinal fistulas Inadequate electrolyte replacement Increased use of antacids Diuretic therapy, steroids Increased ingestion/ injection of bicarbonates	Lethargy Irritability Disorientation Nausea	*Respirations*: shallow; apnea, decreased thoracic movement; cyanosis *Pulse*: irregular → cardiac arrest *Muscle*: twitching → tetany, convulsions *GI*: vomiting, diarrhea, paralytic ileus HCO_3 *elevated* above 26; PCO_2 normal; K+ <3.5 mEq/L; pH > 7.45	*Obtain, maintain acid-base balance*: irrigate NG *tubes* with saline; monitor I&O; IV saline, potassium added; isotonic solutions PO; monitor vital signs *Prevent physical injury*: monitor for potassium loss, side effects of medications ☞ **Health teaching**: increase sodium when loss expected; instructions regarding self-administration of medications (e.g., baking soda)	Normal acid-base balance obtained No signs of potassium deficit Respiratory rate 16–20 breaths/min No arrhythmias–pulse regular Lists food sources *high* in *potassium*

COPD = chronic obstructive pulmonary disease; HOB = head of bed; 1CP = intracranial pressure; GI = gastrointestinal; NG= nasogastric; I&O= intake & output.

Source: ©Lagerquist SL: *Little, Brown's NCLEX-RN® Examination Review*. Boston: Little, Brown,. (out of print)

4. *Venous spasm*—due to cold blood or irritating solution.
5. *Plugged vent*—causes infusion to stop.

III. Fluid and electrolyte therapy

A. Types of therapy:
   1. *Maintenance* therapy—provides water, electrolytes, glucose, vitamins, and in some instances, protein to meet daily requirements.
   2. *Restoration* of deficits—in addition to maintenance therapy, fluid and electrolytes are added to replace *previous* losses.
   3. *Replacement* therapy—infusions to replace *current* losses of fluid and electrolytes.

B. Types of intravenous fluids (**Table 7.5**):
   1. **Isotonic solutions**—fluids that approximate the osmolarity (290 mOsm/L) of normal blood plasma.
      a. *Sodium chloride* (0.9%)—normal saline.
         (1) *Indications*:
            (a) Extracellular fluid replacement when C1- loss is equal to or greater than Na+ loss.
            (b) Treatment of metabolic alkalosis.

TABLE 7.5 COMMONLY USED INTRAVENOUS FLUIDS

Solution	Glucose (g/L)	Calories	Tonicity	Electrolytes (mEq/L)				
				Na+	K+	Ca++	Cl-	Lactate
D5/W	50	170/L	Isotonic	0	0	0	0	0
D10	100	340/L	Hypertonic	0	0	0	0	0
0.45% NaCl	0	0	Hypotonic	77	0	0	77	0
0.9% NaCl	0	0	Isotonic	154	0	0	154	0
Ringer's lactate	0	0	Isotonic	130	4	3	109	28
D5/0.45% NaCl	50	170/L	Hypertonic	77	0	0	77	0
D5/0.9% NaCl	50	170/L	Hypertonic	154	0	0	154	0

(c) Na^+ depletion.
(d) Initiating and terminating blood transfusions.
(2) Possible *side effects*:
  (a) Hypernatremia.
  (b) Acidosis.
  (c) Hypokalemia.
  (d) Circulatory overload.
b. *5% dextrose in water* (5% D/W):
(1) *Provides minimal calories* for energy, *sparing body protein* and preventing ketosis resulting from fat breakdown. Provides total body water.
  (a) 3.75 calories are provided per gram of glucose.
  (b) USP standards require use of monohydrated glucose, so only 91% is actually glucose.
  (c) 5% D/W yields 170.6 calories; 5% D/W means 5 g glucose/L.

> 50 X 3.75 = 187.5 calories
> 0.91 X 187.5 = 170.6 calories

(2) *Indications*:
  (a) Dehydration.
  (b) Hypernatremia.
  (c) Drug administration.
(3) Possible *side effects*:
  (a) Hypokalemia.
  (b) Osmotic diuresis—dehydration.
  (c) Transient hyperinsulinism.
  (d) Water intoxication.
c. *5% dextrose in normal saline*:
(1) *Prevents* ketone formation and *loss* of potassium and intracellular water.
(2) *Indications*:
  (a) Hypovolemic shock—temporary measure.
  (b) Burns.
  (c) Acute adrenocortical insufficiency.
(3) Same *side effects* as those of normal saline.

d. *Isotonic multiple-electrolyte fluids*—utilized for replacement therapy; ionic composition approximates that of blood plasma.
(1) Types—*Plasmanate, Polysol*, and lactated Ringer's.
(2) *Indicated in*: vomiting, diarrhea, excessive diuresis, and burns.
(3) Possible *side effect*—circulatory overload.
(4) Lactated Ringer's is *contraindicated* in lactic acidosis and/or alkalosis and liver disease.
(5) Same *side effects* as those of normal saline.
2. **Hypertonic solutions**—fluids with an osmolarity much higher than 290 mOsm (+ 50 mOsm); increase osmotic pressure of blood plasma, thereby drawing fluid from the cells.
a. *10% dextrose in normal saline*.
(1) Administered in large vein to dilute and prevent venous trauma.
(2) *Used* for nutrition and to replenish Na^+ and Cl^-.
(3) Possible *side effects*:
  (a) Hypernatremia (excess Na^+).
  (b) Acidosis (excess Cl^-).
  (c) Circulatory overload.
b. *3% and 5% sodium chloride* solutions.
(1) Slow administration essential to prevent overload (100 mL/h).
(2) *Indicated in* water intoxication and severe sodium depletion.
3. **Hypotonic solution**—fluids whose osmolarity is significantly less than that of blood plasma (– 50 mOsm); these fluids lower plasma osmotic pressures, causing fluid to enter cells.
a. *0.45% sodium chloride*—utilized for replacement when requirement for Na^+ is questionable.
b. *5% dextrose in 0.2% saline*
(1) *Indications*:

(a) Fluid replacement when some Na⁺ replacement is also necessary.

(b) Promote diuresis in clients who are dehydrated.

(c) Evaluate kidney status before instituting electrolyte infusions.

(2) Possible *side effects*:

(a) Hypernatremia.

(b) Circulatory overload.

(c) Use with *caution* in clients who are edematous with cardiac, renal, or hepatic disease.

(d) After adequate renal function is established, appropriate electrolytes should be given to prevent hypokalemia.

4. **Alkalizing agents**—fluids used in the treatment of *metabolic acidosis*:

a. *Ringer's lactate*

(1) Administration—rate usually not more than 300 mL/h.

(2) *Side effects*—observe carefully for signs of alkalosis.

b. *Sodium bicarbonate*:

(1) *Indications*:

(a) Replace excessive loss of bicarbonate ion.

(b) **Emergency treatment of life-threatening acidosis.**

(2) Administration:

(a) Depends on client's weight, condition, and carbon dioxide level.

(b) Usual dose is 500 mL of a 1.5% solution (89 mEq).

(3) *Side effects*:

(a) Alkalosis.

(b) Hypocalcemic tetany.

(c) Rapid infusion may induce cellular acidity and death.

5. **Acidifying solutions**—fluids used in treatment of *metabolic alkalosis*.

a. Types:

(1) Normal saline (see *Isotonic solutions*, **p. 109-110**).

(2) Ammonium chloride.

b. Administration—dosage depends on client's condition and serum lab values.

c. *Side effects*:

(1) Hepatic encephalopathy in presence of decreased liver function since ammonia is metabolized by liver.

(2) Toxic effects of irregular respirations, twitching, and bradycardia.

(3) *Contraindicated* in renal failure.

6. **Blood** and **blood products** (Table 5.1, p. 58).

a. *Indications*:

(1) Maintenance of blood volume.

(2) Supply red blood cells to maintain oxygen-carrying capacity.

(3) Supply clotting factors to maintain coagulation properties.

(4) Exchange transfusion.

IV. **Intravenous cancer chemotherapy**

A. Usual sites: forearm, dorsum of hand, wrist, antecubital fossa.

☞ B. *Procedure*:

1. Normal saline infusion usually started first, to verify vein patency, position of needle. Chemotherapy "piggybacked" into IV line that is running.

2. Rate: usually 1 mL/min. Running slowly decreases nausea, vomiting, and the degree of vein damage.

3. Check vein patency every 3–5 min.

4. If more than one drug is to be infused, normal saline should be infused *between* drugs.

5. *Never* infuse against resistance.

6. Stop treatment if client reports pain at needle site. *Extravasation* (infiltration of toxic drugs into tissue surrounding vessel) may be present.

☞ 7. If extravasation present, begin protocol appropriate to drug administered (e.g., flushing of line with saline, applying ice or heat, local injection of site with antidote drugs, topical application of *steroid* creams).

8. Once treatment is completed, remove needle, apply Bandaid, exert pressure to prevent hematoma formation.

V. **Complications of IV therapy: Table 7.6.**

⬤ Total Parenteral Nutrition

Provides nutrition through a central venous line to clients who are in a catabolic state; are malnourished and cannot tolerate food by mouth; are in negative nitrogen balance; or have conditions that interfere with protein ingestion, digestion, and absorption, e.g., Crohn's disease, major burns, and side effects of radiation therapy of abdomen.

I. **Types of solutions**

A. Hydrolyzed proteins (*Hyprotein, Amigen*).

B. Synthetic amino acids (*FreAmine*).

C. Usual components:

1. 3%–8% amino acid.

2. 10%–25% glucose.

3. Multivitamins.

4. Electrolytes.

D. Supplements that can be added:

1. Fructose.

(continued on p. 113)

TABLE 7.6 COMPLICATIONS OF IV THERAPY

Complication	⋈ Assessment		⋈ Nursing Care Plan/Implementation
	Subjective Data	Objective Data	
Infiltration—fluid infusion into surrounding tissue rather than into vessel	Pain around needle insertion	1. Infusion rate slow 2. Swelling, hardness, coolness, blanching of tissue at site of needle 3. Blood does not return into tubing when bag/bottle lowered 4. Puffiness under surface of arm	1. Stop IV ☞ 2. Apply warm towel to area 3. Restart at another site 4. Record
Thrombophlebitis—inflammatory changes in vessel, **thromboemboli**— the development of venous clots within the inflamed vessel	Pain along the vein	Redness, swelling around affected area (red line), warmth	1. Stop IV 2. Notify physician ☞ 3. Cold compresses or warm towel, as ordered 4. Restart at another site 5. *Rest affected limb; do not rub* 6. See nursing care of **thrombophlebitis, Chap. 2**
Pyrogenic reaction—contaminated equipment/solution	1. Headache 2. Backache 3. Nausea 4. Anxiety	1. ↑Temperature 2. Chills 3. Face flushed 4. Vomiting 5. ↓BP 6. Cyanosis	1. Discontinue IV; restart IV in new location 2. Vital signs 3. Send equipment for culture/analysis ⊂⊃ 4. *Antibiotic* ointment, as ordered, at injection site ☞ 5. *Prevention*: change tubing q24-48h; *meticulous sterile* technique; check for: precipitation, expiration dates, damage to containers, tubings, etc.; refrigerate hyperalimentation fluids, discard hyperalimentation fluids that have been at room temperature *8–12 h* and use new bag regardless of amount left in first bag (change, to prevent infection—excellent medium for bacterial growth)
Fluid overload—excessive amount of fluid infused; infants/ elderly at risk	1. Headache 2. Shortness of breath 3. Syncope 4. Edema	1. ↑Pulse, venous pressure 2. Venous distention 3. Flushed skin 4. Coughing 5. ↑Respiration 6. Cyanosis, pulmonary edema 7. Shock	1. Slow IV to keep vein open (KVO), or saline lock it 2. Semi-Fowler's *position* 3. Notify physician ⊂⊃ 4. Be prepared for *diuretic* therapy 5. *Preventive measures*: monitor flow rate and client's response to IV therapy (see **Fluid Volume Excess, p. 100**, for subjective and objective data)
Air emboli—air in circulatory system	Loss of consciousness Chest pain	1. Hypotension, cyanosis 2. Tachycardia 3. ↑Venous pressure 4. Tachypnea	☞ 1. Turn on *left* side, with head *down* 2. Administer oxygen therapy 3. **Medical emergency—call physician**

(continued)

TABLE 7.6 COMPLICATIONS OF IV THERAPY (continued)

Complication	⋈ Assessment		⋈ Nursing Care Plan/Implementation
	Subjective Data	Objective Data	
Nerve damage—improper position of limb during infusion or *tying* limb down too tight during infusion → damage to nerve	Numbness; fingers, hands	Unusual position for limb	1. Untie ☞ 2. Passive ROM exercise 3. Monitor closely for return of function 4. Record limb status
Pulmonary embolism—blood clot enters pulmonary circulation and obstructs pulmonary artery	Dyspnea Chest pain	1. Orthopnea 2. Signs of circulatory and cardiac collapse	⬤ 1. Slow IV to keep vein open (rate: 5-6 gtt/min) 2. Notify physician 3. **Medical emergency** 4. Be prepared for life-saving ⬤　measures and *anticoagulation* therapy

Source: ©Lagerquist SL: *Little, Brown's NCLEX-RN® Examination Review.* Boston: Little, Brown, (out of print)

　　2. Alcohol.
　　3. Minerals: iron, copper, calcium.
　　4. Trace elements: iodine, zinc, magnesium.
　　5. Vitamins: A, B, C.
　　6. Androgen.
　　7. Insulin.
II. **Administration**
　A. Dosage varies with clinical condition; 1 L q5–8h; rate of flow must be constant.
　B. Solution prepared under laminar flow hood (usually in pharmacy); solution must be *refrigerated*; when refrigerated, *expires in 24 h*; once removed from refrigerator, *expires in 12 h.*
　C. **No** meds or other IVs should be combined with TPN solution.
　D. Route: catheter inserted in a central vein (e.g., subclavian) by physician; placement confirmed by x-ray before beginning infusion (**Figure 7.1**).
　E. *Side effects*:
　　1. Hyperosmolar coma.
　　2. Hyperglycemia >130 mg/100 mL
　　3. Septicemia.
　　4. Thrombosis/sclerosis of vein.
　　5. Air embolus.
　　6. Pneumothorax.
　F. *Prolonged use*: >10d, fat needed; intralipids piggy-backed close to insertion site or mixed with TPN solution; do *not* give through filter; observe for hypersensitivity (e.g., tachypnea, tachycardia, nausea, urticaria).
⋈ III. **Analysis/nursing diagnosis**
　A. *Risk for fluid volume excess* related to inability to tolerate amount and consistency of solution.
　B. *Fluid volume deficit* related to state of malnutrition.
　C. *Risk for injury* related to possible complications.
　D. *Altered nutrition, more or less than body requirements,* related to ability to tolerate parenteral nutrition.

⋈ IV. **Nursing care plan/implementation**
　A. Goal: *prevent infection.*
☞　1. Dressing change:
　　a. Strict *aseptic* technique.
⚠　b. Nurse and client wear mask during dressing change.
　　c. Cleanse skin with solution, as ordered:
　　　(1) Acetone to defat the skin, destroy the bacterial wall.
　　　(2) 1% iodine solution as antiseptic agent.
　　d. Dressing changed q48–72h; transparent polyurethane dressings may be changed weekly.
　　e. Mark with nurse's initials, date and time of change.
　　f. Air-occlusive dressing.
☞　2. Attach final filter on tubing setup, to prevent air embolism.
　3. Solution: change q12h to prevent infection.
　4. Culture wound and catheter tip if signs of infection appear.
　5. Monitor temperature q4h.
　6. Use lumen line for feeding only (*not* for CVP or medications).
　B. Goal: *prevent fluid and electrolyte imbalance.*
　1. Daily weights.
　2. I&O.
〰　3. Blood glucose measured q4h using glucometer; may need insulin coverage.
　4. Specific gravity q8h to determine hydration status; normal serum osmolality 275–295 mOsm, total parenteral nutrition (TPN) 600–1400 mOsm.
　5. Infusion pump to maintain constant infusion rate.
　C. Goal: *prevent complications.*
　1. Warm TPN solution to room temperature to prevent chills.

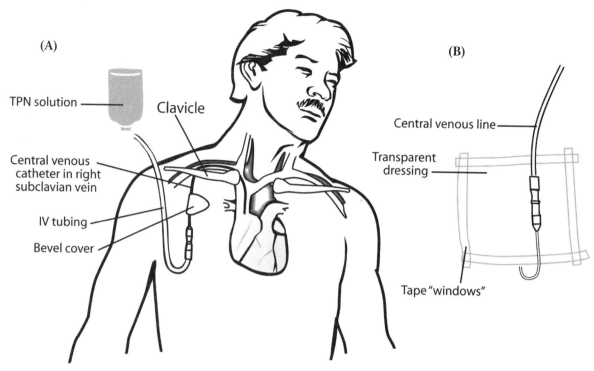

FIGURE 7.1 **(A) CLIENT WITH SUBCLAVIAN CENTRAL VENOUS LINE.**
(B) DRESSING CENTRAL VENOUS LINE.

2. Monitor for signs of complications (**Table 7.7**).
   a. Infiltration.
   b. Thrombophlebitis.
   c. Fever.
   d. Hyperglycemia.
   e. Fluid imbalance.
3. Have client perform *Valsalva maneuver*, or apply a plastic coated clamp when changing tubing to prevent air embolism.
4. Tape tubings together to prevent accidental separation.

V. Evaluation/outcome criteria
1. No signs of infection.
2. No complications
3. Blood sugar <130 mg/100 mL.
4. Specific gravity between 1.010–1.020.
5. Wounds begin to heal.
6. Weight: no further loss, begins to gain

🔑 Summary of Key Points

1. Thirst is a *poor* indicator of fluid status.
2. Rapid change in body weight is the *best* indication of hydration status.
3. An *inverse* relationship exists between calcium and potassium. Many of the signs and symptoms of an *elevation in one* are similar to the signs and symptoms of a *decrease in the other*. For example, tingling sensations and increased peristalsis are present in low calcium or high potassium state because each disorder causes increased excitability.
4. Fluid imbalances are *most critical* in *older* adults because the amount of body water is naturally reduced with age. Fluid reserves are decreased, and reduced heart and kidney function make rapid fluid replacement by IV difficult.
5. *Extracellular* fluid excess results primarily from increased sodium and H_2O and produces increased intravascular and interstitial fluid volumes. *Intracellular* fluid excess (water intoxication) results from increased H_2O or decreased solutes and leads to increased cerebral edema.
6. Dysrhythmias and muscle weakness occur with *both* high and low potassium levels. However, a low potassium level reduces cell excitability and a high level increases excitability initially.
7. If acid-base compensation has occurred, the pH will be in the normal range.
8. Although tissue oxygenation (PaO_2) is separate from acid-base regulation, the release of oxygen to the tissues is affected by carbon dioxide.

TABLE 7.7 COMPLICATIONS OF TOTAL PARENTERAL NUTRITION (TPN)

Complication	⋈ Nursing Intervention
Infection Local infection (pain, redness, edema) Generalized, systemic infection (elevated temperature, WBC)	⋈ Sterile dressings ⬤ Administer *antibiotics* as ordered General comfort measures Remove catheter and send for culture
Arterial Puncture Artery is punctured instead of vein Physician aspirates bright red blood that is pulsating strongly	Needle is withdrawn and pressure is applied
Air Embolus Air enters venous system during catheter insertion or tubing changes; or catheter/tubing pull apart Chest pain, dizziness, cyanosis, confusion	⌇⌇ Stat ABGs, chest x-ray, ECG ☞ Connect catheter to sterile syringe and aspirate air Clean catheter tip, connect to new tubing *Place client on left side with head lowered* (left Trendelenburg prevents air from going into pulmonary artery) ☞ *Prevent: have client perform Valsalva maneuver or use plastic-coated clamp on catheter at insertion or tubing changes*
Catheter Embolus ⌇⌇Catheter must be checked for placement by *x-ray* and observed when removed to be sure it is intact	Careful observation of catheter Monitor for signs of distress
Pneumothorax If needle punctures pleura, client reports dyspnea, chest pain	May seal off or may need chest tubes

Source: ©Lagerquist SL: *Little, Brown's NCLEX-RN® Examination Review.* Boston Little, Brown, (out of print)

TABLE 7.8 ELECTROLYTE COMPOSITION OF FLUID COMPARTMENTS

Electrolyte	Intracellular Compartment	Extracellular Compartment	
		Intravascular	*Interstitial*
Sodium (Na⁺)	10 mEq/L	142 mEq/L	145 mEq/L
Potassium (K⁺)	140 mEq/L	4 mEq/L	4 mEq/L
Calcium (Ca²⁺)	0.0001 mEq/L	5 mEq/L	3 mEq/L
Magnesium (Mg²⁺)	35 mEq/L	3 mEq/L	2 mEq/L
Chloride (Cl⁻)	2 mEq/L	103 mEq/L	115 mEq/L
Bicarbonate (HCO₃⁻)	10 mEq/L	27 mEq/L	30 mEq/L
Phosphate (PO₄)	140 mEq/L	2 mEq/L	2 mEq/L
Protein	55 mEq/L	16 mEq/L	1 mEq/L

💡 Study and Memory Aids

Acid–Base Balance: "RAMS" (Respiratory: Alternate, Metabolic: Same)

	Respiratory (alternate)	Metabolic (same)
Acidosis	↓ pH ↑ PCO_2	↓ pH ↓ HCO_3
Alkalosis	↑ pH ↓ PCO_2	↑ pH ↑ HCO_3

🍎 Diets

Fluid Volume Deficit

Force fluids

Fluid Volume Excess

↓ Fluids
↓ Sodium

⊂Drug Review

Fluid Volume Deficits

Antidiarrheals
Diphenoxylate (*Lomotil*): 2.5 mg to 5 mg 4 times
Kaolin/pectin: 60–20 mL after each loose bowel
   movement
Loperamide (*Imodium*): 4 mg initially, then 2 mg after
   each unformed stool

Antiemetics
Prochlorperazine (*Compazine*): 5–10 mg, repeat once in
   30 minutes as needed
Promethazine (*Phenergan*): 12.5–25 mg q4–6h
Trimethobenzamide (*Tigan*): 200 mg 3–4 times a day

Antipyretic (to reduce fever): Aspirin: 325-1000 mg q4–6h
not to exceed 4 g/d
See Intravenous Therapy, **p. 106-107, 109-111.**

Fluid Volume Excess

Diuretics
Furosemide (*Lasix*): 20–80 mg/d
Hydrochlorothiazide: 25–100 mg/d

Questions

1. The nurse would recognize the need for additional teaching if a client made which statement about a low sodium diet?
   1. "Cooking lowers the sodium content of food."
   2. "It is important to check labels for the sodium content."
   3. "Canned vegetables have more sodium than fresh vegetables."
   4. "A good rule is 'no added salt' at the table."

2. Which entree should the nurse advise a client who is on a low sodium diet to avoid eating?
   1. Barbecued salmon fillet.
   2. Baked chicken breast.
   3. Sliced smoked turkey.
   4. Beef tenderloin.

3. The client has the following vital signs: pulse, 120 beats/min; respiration, 30 breaths/min; temperature, 100.4° F; blood pressure, 90/60 mm Hg. The nurse knows that these findings most likely indicate the presence of: *hypovolemic shock*
   1. Severe dehydration. *↑ pulse*
   2. Increased intracranial pressure. *↓ BP*
   3. Digitalis toxicity.
   4. Cardiogenic shock.

4. Interventions to correct respiratory acidosis would first include:
   1. Administering morphine sulfate prn.
   2. Giving sodium bicarbonate in an IV push.
   3. Increasing supplemental O_2 levels.
   4. Correcting the cause of hypoventilation.

5. Which assessment finding would be expected in a client with respiratory alkalosis?
   1. Oversedation.
   2. Heart rate of less than 60 beats/min.
   3. Intractable pain.
   4. High arterial partial pressure of O_2 (PO_2).

6. A client has had a peripherally inserted central venous catheter in place for about 16 hours. The nurse notices erythema along the catheterized vein. What should the nurse's first action be?
   1. To apply ice to the extremity immediately.
   2. To apply warm packs, as ordered, for 24 hours.
   3. To remove the line and have it reinserted.
   4. To replace the dressing, because it is too tight.

7. Which nursing intervention will help prevent occlusion of a peripherally inserted central catheter (PICC)?
   1. Application of a proper dressing to prevent kinking of the line.
   2. Regular irrigation with streptokinase.
   3. Flushing with an equal amount of saline after drawing a blood sample. *20 mL*
   4. Infusion of a 1% hydrochloric acid solution prn.

8. The correct technique for removal of a peripherally inserted central catheter (PICC) from the right cephalic vein includes:
   1. Putting the client in semi-Fowler's position with the arm placed on the over-bed table.
   2. Wearing a gown, sterile gloves, and mask.
   3. Using a hand-over-hand technique and pulling slowly without too much tension.
   4. Placing the client flat with the arm next to his/her side to straighten the line.

9. To administer 1000 mL of IV fluid in 8 hours (15 gtt/mL), the nurse should make sure that the drops per minute will be:
   1. 25.
   2. 31.
   3. 38.
   4. 45.

10. Which arterial blood gas findings indicate the presence of acute uncompensated respiratory acidosis?
    1. PCO_2 increased, HCO_3^- normal. *pH ↓*
    2. PCO_2 decreased, HCO_3^- normal.
    3. PCO_2 decreased, HCO_3^- decreased.
    4. PCO_2 increased, HCO_3^- increased.

11. Which finding would indicate to the nurse that a client is recovering from respiratory acidosis?
    1. Increased respiratory rate.
    2. Increased serum creatinine level.
    3. Increased heart rate.
    4. Increased HCO_3^-, concentration.

12. Which arterial blood gas finding would the nurse view as a sign of metabolic acidosis?
    1. Increased PCO_2.
    2. Decreased PCO_2.
    3. Increased HCO_3^- concentration.
    4. Decreased HCO_3^- concentration. *(circled)*

    (handwritten: ↓ pH, ↓ HCO3)

13. The blood gas values in a client with emphysema are as follows: PCO_2, 60 mm Hg; HCO_3^-, 30 mEq/L; pH, 7.30. The nurse would know the client is suffering from:
    1. Metabolic acidosis.
    2. Metabolic alkalosis.
    3. Respiratory acidosis. *(circled)*
    4. Respiratory alkalosis.

14. A client becomes diaphoretic, weak, and confused while receiving total parenteral nutrition (TPN). The initial nursing action would be to:
    1. Slow the rate of the TPN infusion.
    2. Increase the rate of the TPN infusion.
    3. Check the client's blood glucose level. *(circled)*
    4. Notify the MD of the client's symptoms.

15. A client with diabetes mellitus is becoming lethargic. For what additional change should the nurse assess that would indicate developing metabolic acidosis?
    1. Blood pressure decrease from 128/80 to 96/40 mm Hg.
    2. Pulse rate change from 94 to 72 beats/min.
    3. Muscle weakness. *(circled)*
    4. Slow, shallow breathing.

    (handwritten: DM ↓ acidosis ↓)

16. When changing the TPN line and dressing, the nurse knows that a critical element in TPN care is to:
    1. Change the dressing every shift, using a strict aseptic technique.
    2. Stop the infusion briefly to prevent contamination. *(circled)*
    3. Have the client perform the Valsalva maneuver during the line change. *(circled)*
    4. Use vaseline gauze as the dressing.

    (handwritten: hyper-kalemia ↓ weakness, paralysis)

17. A client is to be given 50 mL of cefazolin (*Kefzol*) IV over 30 minutes (10 gtt/mL). How many drops should be delivered per minute?
    1. 9.
    2. 12.
    3. 14.
    4. 17.

18. When the nurse arrives for an 8-hour shift, a client is receiving 5% dextrose in water (D5W) at the rate of 30 gtt/min (15 gtt/mL). The IV is interrupted for 3 hours so that 650 mL of blood can be transfused. How much D5W will the client receive during this shift?
    1. 600 mL.
    2. 900 mL.
    3. 1250 mL.
    4. 1500 mL.

19. If a client is to receive D5W and lactated Ringer's solution at a rate of 125 mL/h, what should the rate be for a drop factor of 15 gtt/mL?
    1. 28 gtt/min.
    2. 29 gtt/min.
    3. 30 gtt/min.
    4. 31 gtt/min.

20. Which foods would the nurse recommend as the best source of calcium?
    1. Spinach and mustard greens. *(circled)*
    2. Lentils and green beans.
    3. Strawberries and cantaloupe.
    4. White beans and spinach.

21. The nurse would best assess the adequacy of fluid volume replacement in a client with hypovolemia by monitoring:
    1. Vital signs and daily weight. *(circled)*
    2. Oral intake and vital signs.
    3. Hemoglobin and hematocrit values.
    4. Serum electrolyte levels and urinary output.

22. Muscular twitching and hyperirritability of the nervous system indicate tetany. The nurse would identify these as symptoms of which electrolyte imbalance?
    1. Low sodium level.
    2. High potassium level.
    3. Low calcium level. *(circled)*
    4. High magnesium level.

23. The most applicable nursing diagnosis for a client experiencing hypercalcemia would be:
    1. Risk for injury related to muscle weakness and confusion. *(circled)*
    2. Risk for injury related to spasm or tetany.
    3. Diarrhea related to decreased gastrointestinal absorption.
    4. Fluid volume excess related to impaired kidney function.

24. Hyperglycemia may occur in a client receiving TPN. How often should the blood glucose level be checked?
    1. Hourly.
    2. Every 6 hours. *(circled)*
    3. Every shift.
    4. Every 24 hours.

25. During insertion of a subclavian central line, the client suddenly experiences sharp pain. Which complication of insertion would the nurse suspect?
    1. Air embolism.
    2. Hemothorax.
    3. Pneumothorax. *(circled)*
    4. Pleural effusion.

Answers/Rationale

1. **(1)** Cooking reduces the vitamin content of food, but if the food is high in sodium, the sodium content will not change significantly with cooking. Checking labels to find out the salt content (2), avoiding canned and processed foods (3), and not adding salt to food at the table (4) *are* all *effective* ways to maintain a low sodium diet. **EV, EVL, 4, PhI, Basic care and comfort**

2. **(3)** Smoked meats are restricted in a low sodium diet because the preparation includes curing with salt. Fish (1), chicken (2), and beef (4), cooked by barbecuing, baking, or broiling and carefully seasoned, would *all be included* in a low sodium diet. **IMP, ANL, 4, PhI, Basic care and comfort**

3. **(1)** Tachycardia and low blood pressure are signs of low blood volume (hypovolemic shock), which could occur with severe dehydration. The fever is also a sign of dehydration. Vital signs in the presence of increased intracranial pressure (2) are the opposite of those of hypovolemic shock. The pulse would be slow in digitalis toxicity (3). Cardiogenic shock (4) is a possible choice, but if the heart is failing, the pulse rate would not likely be as high because the heart would not be able to compensate. **AN, SYN, 6, PhI, Physiological adaptation**

4. **(3)** In respiratory acidosis, there is an increase in the CO_2 level as a result of inadequate ventilation. There is also hypoxemia in most cases. Even in a client with emphysema who has a hypoxic drive, ventilation should be supported by giving the client O_2 first. Giving the client morphine sulfate (1) would only further decrease the respiratory rate and depth and would also likely cause the respiratory acidosis to worsen. Sodium bicarbonate (2) is given to correct acidosis; however, the nurse would first support the client's ventilation by increasing the flow of O_2. It would also be important to determine the cause of the hypoventilation (4), but supplemental O_2 should be administered while diagnostic tests are being conducted. **IMP, ANL, 6, PhI, Physiological adaptation**

Key to Codes

Nursing process: **AS,** assessment; **AN,** analysis; **PL,** planning; **IMP,** implementation; **EV,** evaluation. (See **Appendix M** for explanation of nursing process steps.)

Cognitive level: **RE/KN,** recall/knowledge; **COM,** comprehension; **APP,** application; **ANL,** analysis; **EVL,** evaluation; **SYN,** synthesis. (See **Appendix M** for explanation.)

Category of human function: 1, protective; 2, sensory-perceptual; 3, comfort, rest, activity, and mobility; 4, nutrition; 5, growth and development; 6, fluid-gas transport; 7, psychosocial-cultural; 8, elimination. (See **Appendix 0** for explanation.)

Client need: **SECE,** safe, effective care environment; **PhI,** physiological integrity; **PsI,** psychosocial integrity; **HPM,** health promotion and maintenance. (See **Appendix P** for explanation.)

Client subneed: (See **Appendix P** for explanation)

5. **(3)** Clients with intractable pain will most likely breathe rapidly and excessively rid themselves of CO_2, resulting in respiratory alkalosis. Oversedation (1) will depress respirations and lead to *respiratory acidosis*. A slow heart rate (2) will result in poor perfusion and *metabolic acidosis*. Hypoxemia (low O_2 level), *not* a high O_2 level (4), is usually seen in acidosis. **AS, EVL, 6, PhI, Physiological adaptation**

6. **(2)** Erythema along the catheterized vein does not necessarily indicate phlebitis. During the first 24 hours after insertion, the vein's epithelial lining may show irritation resulting from the insertion process. Before ordering removal of the line (3), the physician would mostly likely order the application of warm packs, *not* ice (1), for 24 hours to see whether this resolves the problem. During that time, the nurse should observe not only for a decrease in redness but also for other indicators of infection, such as a fever. As long as there is good blood return, the line flushes easily, and the client does not feel any discomfort, the line is considered patent. The dressing, which may only be changed every 7 days, does not encircle the limb, so there would not be any tightness (4) to cause the redness. **IMP, ANL, 6, PhI, Pharmacological and parenteral therapies**

7. **(1)** The most common cause of occlusion is kinked tubing, and a proper dressing technique will *prevent* such a problem. Sterile adhesive strips or sutures may be used to secure the line at the insertion site and a transparent occlusive dressing applied over the site. The PICC can be looped loosely under the dressing to prevent kinking and tugging on the line. Streptokinase (2) or urokinase are administered according to hospital policy to clear an occlusion caused by a suspected clot or fibrin plugs. After drawing a sample of blood (3), the line is flushed with 20 mL of saline regardless of the amount of blood drawn. If a drug has precipitated in the line, a 1% hydrochloric acid solution is instilled (4) to open up the line, which has *already* occluded. **IMP, APP, 6, PhI, Reduction of risk potential**

8. **(3)** The PICC should be removed in about 30 seconds, using a gentle, slow, and a hand-over-hand technique, and without exerting too much tension. The client should be supine with the arm placed at a 45-to 90-degree angle to the body to ensure a straight pull; the techniques named in options 1 and 4 are therefore incorrect. This prevents bending, kinking or possible breakage. Unless hospital policy states otherwise or a catheter-related infection is suspected, it is only necessary for the nurse to wear clean gloves during removal (2). **IMP, APP, 6, PhI, Reduction of risk potential**

9. **(2)** The rate is calculated using the following formula: (mL/h X the drop factor)/60. Using this formula, the correct rate in this instance is calculated as follows: (125 mL/h X 15 gtt/mL)/60 = 31.25, or 31 gtt/min. The number of drops named in the other options (1, 3, and 4) are incorrect according to this formula. **IMP, APP, 6, PhI, Pharmacological and parenteral therapies**

10. **(1)** The PCO_2 is *increased* in respiratory acidosis, and the HCO_3^- concentration would be normal in an uncompensated state. (The arterial PO_2, has no bearing on the acid-base status.) Option 2 is incorrect because the CO_2 level is decreased. Option 3 is incorrect because both the CO_2 level and the HCO_3^- concentration are decreased. Option 4 is incorrect because the HCO_3^- concentration is increased, which would be seen in the presence of *compensated* respiratory acidosis. **AN, ANL, 6, PhI, Physiological adaptation**

11. **(4)** An increase in the HCO_3^- concentration and an increase in the CO_2 level in a client suffering from respiratory acidosis indicate the occurrence of renal compensation. The relationship is *direct*: when one goes up, the other goes up. An increased respiratory rate **(1)** is a *symptom* of respiratory acidosis. An increased serum creatinine level **(2)** would be more likely to occur in metabolic acidosis resulting from renal failure. An increased heart rate **(3)** is a *symptom* of respiratory acidosis, and the heart rate should decrease if the client's condition is improving. **EV, EVL, 6, PhI, Physiological adaptation**

12. **(4)** When there is a metabolic disorder, there is a decrease in the HCO_3^-. concentration. Metabolic problems (acid-base) are regulated by the kidneys which excrete or retain HCO_3^-, depending on the disorder. An increased PCO_2 **(1)** would be seen with respiratory acidosis. A decreased PCO_2 **(2)** occurs with respiratory alkalosis. An increased HCO_3^- concentration **(3)** indicates metabolic alkalosis. **AN, ANL, 6, PhI, Physiological adaptation**

13. **(3)** The CO_2 level is elevated in respiratory acidosis; the normal level is 35 to 45 mm Hg. The HCO_3^- concentration is also elevated to compensate for the raised CO_2 level; the normal concentration is 22 to 26 mEq/L. The client's pH is below the normal range of 7.35 to 7.45, also indicating acidosis. In metabolic acidosis **(1)**, the HCO_3^- concentration and the pH are decreased. An elevated HCO_3^- concentration and pH would occur in metabolic alkalosis **(2)**. In respiratory alkalosis **(4)**, the CO_2 level is decreased and the pH increased. **EV, SYN, 6, PhI, Physiological adaptation**

14. **(3)** The client is showing the symptoms of hypoglycemia, but additional data are needed to confirm this suspicion. Changing the rate **(1 and 2)** is not an independent nursing action. Transferring the decision to the MD **(4)** is not the best choice. The best choice is a *nursing* action. **AN, ANL, 4, PhI, Pharmacological and parenteral therapies**

15. **(3)** Metabolic acidosis in a client with diabetes is due to ketoacidosis and hyperglycemia. As the acidosis develops, potassium leaves the cell, resulting in hyperkalemia. The client will experience weakness, paralysis, and paresthesia. If the metabolic acidosis goes undetected, the client will continue to lose fluids through oliguria, leading to clinical manifestations similar to those of shock.

Hypotension **(1)** would occur, but as a late sign. The pulse rate should increase, *not* decrease **(2)**, as a result of shock. The breathing pattern that occurs in order to eliminate the excess CO_2 is called *Kussmaul's breathing*, and it is rapid and deep, *not* slow and shallow **(4)**. **AS, ANL, 4, PhI, Physiological adaptation**

16. **(3)** To prevent an air embolus from developing, the client should hold his/her breath or bear down (the *Valsalva maneuver*) as the old tubing is disconnected and new tubing is reconnected. This prevents air from being sucked in. Although a strict aseptic technique is used, the dressing is *not* changed every shift **(1)**, because the more often the dressing is changed, the greater the chance of contamination. The infusion should *not* be stopped **(2)**, because this may cause the line to occlude. The dressing should be air occlusive, but vaseline is *not* used **(4)**. **IMP, APP, 4, PhI, Pharmacological and parenteral therapies**

17. **(4)** The same formula used to calculate any IV rate is used to determine the rate in this instance: (cc or mL/h X the drop factor)/60, or (100 mL X 10 gtt/mL)/60 = 16.6, or about 17 gtt/min. The number of drops in the other options **(1, 2, and 3)** are incorrect. **IMP, APP, 6, PhI, Pharmacological and parenteral therapies**

18. **(1)** At 30 gtt/min the client will receive 2 mL/min and 120 mL/h. If the D5W is infused for only 5 hours, the client will receive a total of 600 mL. The amounts in options **2** and **4** are mathematically incorrect. The amount in option **3** is the total of the D5W and the blood; the amount of blood transfused would be recorded separately. **IMP, APP, 6, PhI, Pharmacological and parenteral therapies**

19. **(4)** Using the formula mL (h X the drop factor)/60, (125 X 15)/60 = 31.25, or about 31 drops per minute. The rates in options **1, 2,** and **3** are incorrect calculations. **IMP, APP, 6, PhI, Pharmacological and parenteral therapies**

20. **(1)** Leafy green vegetables are the best sources of calcium, as well as of iron. Of the foods named in options **2** and **4**, only one of the foods in each, green beans and spinach, is a source of calcium. Strawberries and cantaloupe **(3)** are high in vitamin C and potassium, respectively. **IMP, COM, 4, PhI, Basic care and comfort**

21. **(1)** Daily weight is the best indicator of volume status. Vital signs—rapid pulse and low blood pressure—can also indicate the presence of hypovolemia. Option 2, oral intake and vital signs, is not the best choice; vital signs can be used to assess adequacy, but because fluid replacement is usually accomplished by the IV routes oral intake would not be an accurate indicator. The hematocrit value **(3)** is used to assess the status of volume, hemodilution, or hemoconcentration, but the hemoglobin level does not accurately reflect the status of these. The serum electrolyte levels, particularly that of sodium,

and urinary output (4) are also affected by volume but are not the best indicators of improvement. **AS, ANL, 6, PhI, Reduction of risk potential**

22. **(3)** When the serum calcium level drops, nerve fibers become increasingly excitable and discharge spontaneously, causing muscles to twitch and go into spasms, or tetany. Sodium (1) does not interfere with the action potential of muscles. A high potassium level (2) causes muscle cramping, but *not* tetany. Tetany can also occur when the magnesium level is low, but *not* when it is high (4). **AN, APP, 6, PhI, Physiological adaptation**

23. **(1)** In the presence of high levels of calcium, smooth muscle activity decreases and there is neurologic depression, resulting in muscle weakness and confusion. The other nursing diagnoses (2, 3, and 4) would be appropriate for a client with *hypocalcemia*. **AN, ANL, 6, SECE, Management of care**

24. **(2)** Every 6 hours is the best choice. Hourly (1) is *too often* and daily (4) is *not* often enough. Checking it during every shift (3) is *not specific* enough because shifts may be 8, 10, or 12 hours long. **PL, RE/KN, 4, PhI, Pharmacological and parenteral therapies**

25. **(3)** The most common complication of insertion of a subclavian central line is pneumothorax from puncture of the lung by the needle. Breathing in this instance would be difficult, chest movements may be asymmetrical, and breath sounds would be absent. An x-ray study is needed to confirm the extent of the collapse. Air embolism (1) is a possible complication, but *not* the *most common* one and can be prevented by having the client do the Valsalva maneuver (during insertion). Hemothorax (2) is another possible complication but, again, *not* the *most common* one. Pleural effusion (4) is *not* a complication of subclavian insertion. **AN, ANL, 6, PhI, Physiological adaptation**

Shock

Shock

A critically severe deficiency in nutrients, oxygen, and electrolytes delivered to body tissues, plus deficiency in removal of cellular wastes; results from cardiac failure, insufficient blood volume, and/or increased vascular bed size.

I. Types, pathophysiology, and risk factors:

  A. **Hypovolemic** (hemorrhagic, hematogenic)—markedly decreased **volume** of blood (hemorrhage or plasma loss from intestinal obstruction, burns, physical trauma, or dehydration) → decreased venous return, cardiac output → decreased tissue perfusion.

  B. **Cardiogenic**—failure of cardiac muscle **pump** (myocardial infarction) → generally decreased cardiac output → pulmonary congestion, hypoxia → inadequate circulation; high mortality.

  C. **Distributive:**

    1. **Neurogenic**—massive **vasodilatation** from reduced vasomotor, vasoconstrictor tone (e.g., **spinal shock**, head injuries, anesthesia, pain); interruption of sympathetic nervous system; blood volume that is normal but inadequate for vessels → decreased venous return → tissue hypoxia.

    2. **Vasogenic** (*anaphylactic, septic, endotoxic*)—severe reaction to foreign protein (insect bites; drugs; toxic substances; aerobic, *gram-negative* organisms) → histamine release → **vasodilatation**, venous stasis → diminished venous return.

  D. **Systemic Inflammatory Response Syndrome** (SIRS) —systemic inflammatory response to various insults, e.g., burns, crush injuries, abscesses, myocardial infarction, microbial infection, and post-cardiac resuscitation.

  E. **Multi Organ Dysfunction Syndrome** (MODS)—failure of multiple organ systems; homeostasis cannot be maintained without intervention; consequence of SIRS; 90-95% mortality rate.

II. Assessment: varies, depending on degree and type of shock (**Table 8.1**).

  A. *Subjective data*:

    1. Anxiety, restlessness.

    2. Dizziness, fainting.

    3. Thirst.

    4. Nausea.

  B. *Objective data*:

    1. Vital signs:

      a. *Blood pressure* (BP)—hypotension (postural changes in *early* shock; systolic <70 mm Hg in *late* shock).

      b. *Pulse*—tachycardia; thready, irregular (**cardiogenic shock**); could be slow if conduction system of heart is damaged.

      c. *Respirations*—increased depth, rate; wheezing (**anaphylactic shock**).

      d. *Temperature*—decreased (elevated in **septic shock**).

    2. Skin:

      a. Pale (or mottled), cool, clammy (warm to touch in **septic shock**).

      b. Urticaria (**anaphylactic shock**).

    3. Level of consciousness: alert, oriented → unresponsive.

    4. Central venous pressure (*CVP*):

      a. *Below 5 cm* H_2O with **hypovolemic shock**.

      b. *Above* 15 cm H_2O with **cardiogenic, possibly septic shock**.

    5. Urine output: decreased (<30 mL/h).

    6. Capillary refill: slowed (**Figure 8.1**).

III. Analysis/nursing diagnosis

  A. *Altered tissue perfusion* related to vasoconstriction or decreased myocardial contractility.

  B. *Impaired gas exchange* related to ventilation-perfusion imbalance.

  C. *Decreased cardiac output* related to loss of circulating blood volume or diminished cardiac contractility.

  D. *Altered urinary elimination* related to decreased renal perfusion.

  E. *Fluid volume deficit* related to blood loss.

  F. *Anxiety* related to severity of condition.

  G. *Risk for injury* related to death.

▶◀ **IV. Nursing care plan/implementation**

  A. Goal: *promote venous return, circulatory perfusion.*

  1. *Position*: foot of bed *elevated* 20 degrees (12–16 in.), knees straight, trunk horizontal, head slightly elevated; *avoid* Trendelenburg position.

  ☞ 2. Ventilation: monitor respiratory effort, loosen restrictive clothing; *oxygen* as ordered.

  ⬭ 3. Fluids: maintain IV infusions; give *blood, plasma expanders* as ordered (exception—*stop* blood transfusion immediately in anaphylactic shock).

  4. Vital signs:

  〰 a. *CVP* (↓ with hypovolemia) arterial line, pulmonary artery catheter (↑ pulmonary artery wedge pressure, indicating cardiac failure).

  ☞ b. Urine output (insert *catheter* for hourly output).

  〰 c. Monitor *electrocardiogram* (↑ rate, arrhythmias).

  ⬭ 5. Medications as ordered (depending on type of shock):

  a. *Antihypotensives*—epinephrine (*Adrenalin*), norepinephrine (*Levophed*), isoproterenol (*Isuprel*), dopamine (*Intropin*).

  b. *Antiarrhythmics.*

  c. *Cardiac glycosides.*

  d. *Adrenocorticoids.*

  e. *Antibiotics.*

  f. *Vasodilators* (nitroprusside).

  g. *Beta-blockers* (dobutamine).

  ☞ 6. Mechanical support: military antishock trousers (*MAST*) or pneumatic antishock garment (*PASG*); used to promote internal autotransfusion of blood from legs and abdomen to central circulation; at lower pressures may control bleeding and promote hemostasis; *do not* remove (deflate) suddenly to examine underlying areas or BP will drop precipitously; *compartment syndrome* may result with prolonged use and high pressure; controversial.

☞ **V. Evaluation/outcome criteria**

  A. Vital signs stable, within normal limits.

  B. Alert, oriented.

  C. Urine output >30 mL/h.

TABLE 8.1 SIGNS AND SYMPTOMS OF HYPOVOLEMIC SHOCK	
Blood Loss	▶◀ **Assessment Parameters**
<800 mL	Usually none (equivalent to donating one unit of blood)
800–1500 mL (15%-30%)	Anxiety and restlessness Pulse >100 beats/min* Systolic pressure unchanged Diastolic pressure ↑ Urine output ↓
2000 mL (30%–40%)	Pulse >120 beats/min* Respirations > 30 breaths/min Systolic pressure ↓ Mental status ↓
<2500 mL (>40%)	Pulse > 120 beats/min* Respirations > 30 breaths min Narrow pulse pressure (= systolic – diastolic) Cold, clammy skin

*In some cases of abdominal trauma, there is a shock without a rapid pulse.

Adapted from Caroline NL, *Emergency Care in the Streets* (5th ed) Boston: Little, Brown (out of print)

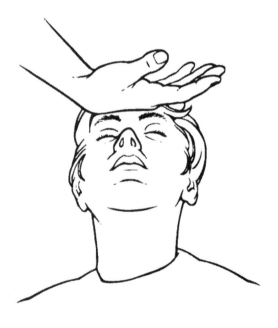

Clinical Signs of Shock—skin pale, mottled, cold, and sweaty

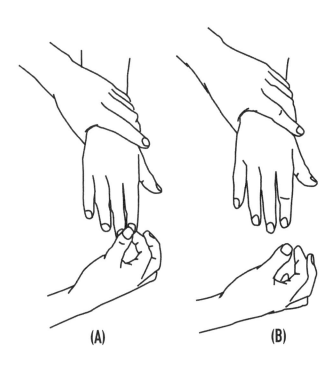

Figure 8.1 Capillary Refill Test. (A) Press on the fingernail until it blanches. (B) then release the pressure. The skin under the nail should "pink up" within 2 seconds if the client is normally perfused. *Modified by ATI*

🔑 Summary of Key Points

1. All types of shock alter tissue perfusion.

2. The three basic types of shock have *different causes—hypovolemic shock* is due to a decrease in circulatory volume; *cardiogenic shock* occurs from pump (heart) failure; and *distributive shock* results from inadequate vascular tone.

3. Urine output is an important indicator of perfusion (circulation) through the vital organs. Normal hourly output is 60 mL. A decrease below 30 mL/h should be reported.

4. Trendelenburg positioning in shock is *contraindicated*. A head-down position actually interferes with pulmonary function and may cause cerebral edema.

💡 Study and Memory Aids

💊 Drug Review

Shock

Antiarrhythmics (some of the drugs used)
  Bretylium (*Bretylol*): 5mg/kg bolus over 15–30 sec, *not* to exceed 30 mg/kg/d
  Lidocaine HCl: IV, 50–100 mg (1 mg/kg) bolus; may be repeated in 5 min, then 1–4 mg/kg/min infusion (*no more than 200–300 mg/h*)
  Procainamide (*Pronestyl*): 100 mg IV q 5 m until arrhythmia suppressed
  Quinidine: 100–600 mg PO q2–3h, *not* to exceed 4g/d

Antibiotics (to control infection)
  Cephalexin (*Keflex*): 250–500 mg PO q6h
  Cephalothin (*Keflin*): IV, 0.5–2 g q4–6h
  Erythromycin: 250–500 mg PO q6–12h
  Gentamicin (*Garamycin*): 3–5 mg/kg/d in divided doses
  Penicillin G: 1.2 million U in single IM dose

Antihypotensives
  Dopamine (*Intropin*): IV, 2–5 mcg/kg/min; titrate to client response
  Epinephrine (*Adrenalin*); 0.1–1 mg IV (1–10 mL of 1:10,000 concentration); may repeat q5–15 min
  Isoproterenol (*Isuprel*): IV, 0.5–5 mcg/min (0.25–2.5 mL of 1:500,000 dilution)
  Norepinephrine (*Levophed*): 8–12 mcg/min IV; adjust rate of flow to maintain BP

Beta-blockers
  Atenolol (*Tenormin*): 25–50 mg/d
  Dobutamine (*Dobutrex*): IV, 2.5–15 mcg/kg/min
  Metoprolol (*Lopressor*): 100–450 mg/d
  Propranolol (*Inderal*): 40 mg bid

Cardiac glycosides
  Digoxin (*Lanoxin*): digitalizing dose—IV, 0.6–1 mg over 24 h, or PO, 10–15 mcg/kg over 24 h; maintenance dose, 0.125–03.75 mg/d (*take apical pulse before administering drug*)

Glucocorticoids
  Cortisone (*Cortone*): 20–300 mg/d
  Dexamethasone (*Decadron*): 0.75–9 mg/d in single or divided doses
  Methylprednisolone (*Medrol*): 4–48 mg/d
  Prednisone (*Deltasone*): 5–60 mg/d

Vasodilators
  Hydralazine (*Apresoline*): 10 mg (qid for 2–4d); increase to 25 mg qid. for first week; 50 mg qid maintenance dose.
  Nitroprusside (*Nitropress*); IV. 0.3-10 mcg/kg/min, *not* to exceed 10 min of therapy at 10 mcg/kg/ min

Questions

1. A client is experiencing a hemolytic transfusion reaction. Which planned nursing action should be questioned?
    1. Hanging new tubing and infusing saline.
    2. Raising the head and foot of the bed.
    3. Inserting an indwelling urinary catheter.
    4. Drawing a blood sample from the IV site.

2. What desired effects of subcutaneously administered epinephrine should the nurse watch for in a client given this agent to manage an anaphylactic reaction?
    1. Vasodilatation and bronchodilatation.
    2. Vasodilatation and bronchoconstriction.
    3. Vasoconstriction and bronchodilatation.
    4. Vasoconstriction and bronchoconstriction.

    ↑ BP by vasoconstriction

3. Which change in a vital sign observed after surgery would require further assessment for indications of hypovolemic shock?
    1. Heart rate of 110 beats/min.
    2. Increasing diastolic pressure.
    3. Widening pulse pressure.
    4. Respiratory rate of 10 breaths/min.

4. Blood and fluid loss resulting from frequent diarrhea may cause hypovolemia. The fastest way for a nurse to assess for volume depletion is to:
    1. Measure the quantity and specific gravity of urine.
    2. Take the client's blood pressure with the client supine, then sitting, and noting the resultant change.
    3. Compare the client's present weight with the weight 6 months ago.
    4. Administer the oral water test.

5. Four hours after coronary artery bypass surgery, a client's blood pressure is 90/46 mm Hg and the central venous pressure is 6 cm H_2O; 300 mL of bloody fluid has drained from the mediastinal chest tube in the past hour. The nurse knows the client would most likely need which measure?
    1. Milking of the mediastinal chest tube.
    2. A transfusion to replace blood loss.
    3. Premedication for a pericardiocentesis.
    4. A sodium nitroprusside (*Nipride*) IV push, as ordered.

    for hypertension

Answers/Rationale

1. **(4)** A hemolytic transfusion reaction occurs as the result of the infusion of ABO incompatible blood, and any blood obtained from the IV site will be hemolyzed; that is, the red blood cells will be destroyed. The results of any laboratory test or such a blood sample would be abnormal. The extent of hemolysis will need to be determined using a sample drawn from *another* large peripheral vein with a large (19)–gauge needle. The tubing needs to be changed completely and a saline infusion *should* be started **(1)** to prevent any additional incompatible blood from being infused. Symptoms of the transfusion reaction usually include hypotension and respiratory distress, so elevation of the client's head and feet **(2)** *will* help relieve the symptoms. A catheter *should* be inserted, if it is not already in place, to assess for any renal damage stemming from the reaction **(3)**. **PL, ANL, 6, PhI, Pharmacological and parenteral therapies**

2. **(3)** Anaphylaxis causes bronchospasm and hypotension. By means of its adrenergic effects, epinephrine produces bronchodilation, which will relieve the breathing difficulty, and increases the blood pressure through vasoconstriction. Options **1**, **2**, and **4** are incorrect because they include *vasodilatation* or *bronchoconstriction*, neither of which would be desirable in a client in anaphylactic shock. **EV, EVL, 6, PhI, Pharmacological and parenteral therapies**

3. **(1)** Tachycardia occurring postoperatively may indicate the development of hypovolemic shock and hypoxia, though it can also occur with pain. It would be important to look for a drop in the systolic pressure initially indicating decreased volume, followed by a decrease, not an increase, in the diastolic pressure **(2)**. The pulse pressure will initially narrow in hypovolemic shock. A widening pulse pressure **(3)** is seen in the presence of increased intracranial pressure. If the client is experiencing hypovolemic shock and hypoxia, the respiratory rate would exceed the normal rate of 12 to 16 breaths/min. A rate of 10 breaths/min **(4)** is a slow normal one. **AN, EVL, 6, PhI, Physiological adaptation**

4. **(2)** Taking a client's vital signs supine, then sitting, will reveal the presence of postural blood pressure changes. If the client is hypovolemic, the pressure will drop by 20 to 30 mm Hg systolic when the client sits up. If the client is volume depleted, the urine output **(1)** will most likely be diminished and *less frequent*, so urine output would not be a rapid way to assess volume status. Although body weight **(3)** is an excellent indicator of hydration status, it would take time to find out the prior weight. The oral water test **(4)** is a test for Addison's disease that involves the rapid intake of a large quantity of water. A normal diuresis does not occur in clients with the disease. **AS, ANL, 6, PhI, Reduction of risk potential**

5. **(2)** The vital signs are indicative of hypovolemia, and the chest tube drainage is excessive for 1 hour. Judging by the large amount of fluid that has drained, the tube appears to be draining. Milking **(1)** is done if the tube is *not* draining and usually is *not* needed with mediastinal chest tubes. Pericardiocentesis **(3)** is done to remove blood that is collecting in the pericardium; this is not necessary in this client because blood is draining profusely.

Nipride (**4**) is a potent vasodilator and is used to treat malignant hypertension; this client is *hypotensive*.
AN, ANL, 6, PhI, Physiological adaptation

Key to Codes

Nursing process: AS, assessment; **AN**, analysis; **PL**, planning; **IMP**, implementation; **EV**, evaluation. (See **Appendix M** for explanation of nursing process steps.)

Cognitive level: RE/KN, Recall/Knowledge; **COM**, comprehension; **APP**, application; **ANL**, analysis; **EVL**, evaluation; **SYN**, synthesis. (See **Appendix M** for explanation.)

Category of human function: 1, protective; **2**, sensory-perceptual; **3**, comfort, rest, activity, and mobility; **4**, nutrition; **5**, growth and development; **6**, fluid-gas transport; **7**, psychosocial-cultural; **8**, elimination. (See **Appendix O** for explanation.)

Client need: SECE, safe, effective care environment; **PhI**, physiologic integrity; **Psl**, psychosocial integrity; **HPM**, health promotion and maintenance. (See **Appendix P** for explanation.)

Client subneed: (See **Appendix P** for explanation).

Perioperative Nursing

Chapter Outline

- Preoperative Preparation
  - Teaching
  - Skin preparation
  - Gastrointestinal tract preparation
  - Day of surgery
- Intraoperative Preparation
  - Regional anesthesia
  - General anesthesia
  - Muscle relaxant
  - Hypothermia
- Postoperative Experience

- Immediate post anesthesia nursing care
- General postoperative nursing care
- Postoperative complications
- Review of Use of Common Tubes
- Positioning the Client for Specific Surgical Conditions
- Summary of Key Points
- Study and Memory Aids
  - Drug review
- Questions
- Answers/Rationale

Preoperative Preparation

I. Assessment
   A. *Subjective data*:
   1. Understanding of proposed surgery—site, type, extent of hospitalization.
   2. Previous experiences with hospitalization.
   3. Concerns or feelings about surgery:
      a. Exaggerated ideas of surgical risk (e.g., fear of colostomy when none is being considered).
      b. Nature of anesthesia, e.g., fears of going to sleep and not waking up, saying or revealing things of a personal nature.
      c. Degree of pain, e.g., may be incapacitating.
      d. Misunderstandings regarding prognosis.
   4. Identification of significant others as a source of client support and/or care responsibilities after discharge.
   B. *Objective data*:
   1. Speech patterns indicating anxiety—repetition, changing topics, avoiding talking about feelings.
   2. Interactions with others—withdrawn or involved.
   3. Physical signs of anxiety, i.e., increased pulse, respirations; clammy palms; restlessness.
   4. *Baseline physiologic status*: vital signs, breath sounds, peripheral circulation, weight, hydration status (hematocrit, skin turgor, urine output), degree of mobility, muscle strength.
   5. Allergies.
   6. Medication history–date/time of last dose.
   7. Previous surgical history.
   8. Presence of chronic conditions, e.g. diabetes.

II. Analysis/nursing diagnosis
   A. *Anxiety* related to proposed surgery.
   B. *Knowledge deficit* related to incomplete teaching or lack of understanding.
   C. *Fear* related to threat of death or disfigurement.
   D. *Risk for injury* related to surgical complications.
   E. *Ineffective* individual coping related to anticipatory stress.

III. Nursing care plan/implementation
   A. Goal: *reduce preoperative and intraoperative anxiety and prevent postoperative* complications.
      1. *Preoperative* teaching:
         a. Provide information about hospital and nursing routines to reduce fear of unknown.
         b. Explain purpose of diagnostic procedures to enhance ability to cooperate and tolerate procedure.
         c. What will occur and what will be expected in the postoperative period:
            (1) Will return to room, recovery room, or intensive care unit.
            (2) Special equipment—monitors, tubes, suction equipment.
   B. Goal: *instruct in exercises to reduce complications.*
      1. **Diaphragmatic breathing**—refers to flattening of diaphragm during inspiration, which results in enlargement of upper abdomen; during expiration the abdominal muscles are contracted, along with the diaphragm.
         a. The client should be in a *flat, semi-Fowler's,* or *side* position, with knees flexed and hands on the midabdomen.

b. Have the client take a deep breath through nose and mouth, letting the abdomen rise.

c. Have client exhale through nose and mouth, squeezing out all air by contracting the abdominal muscles.

d. Repeat 10–15 times, with a short rest after each five to prevent hyperventilation.

e. Inform client that this exercise will be repeated 5–10 times every hour postoperatively.

2. **Coughing**—helps clear chest of secretions and, although uncomfortable, will not harm incision.

a. Have client lean forward slightly from a sitting position, and place client's hands over incisional site or have client hold a pillow over incision; this acts as a splint during coughing.

b. Have client inhale and exhale several times.

c. Have client inhale deeply and cough sharply three times as exhaling—client's mouth should be slightly open.

d. Tell client to inhale again and to cough deeply once or twice.

3. **Turning and leg exercises**—help prevent circulatory stasis, which may lead to thrombus formation and postoperative flatus, or "gas pains," as well as respiratory' problems.

a. Tell client to turn on one *side* with uppermost leg flexed; use siderails to facilitate the movement.

b. In a *supine position*, have client bend the knee and lift the foot; this position should be held for a few seconds, then the leg should be extended and lowered; repeat five times, and do the same with the other leg.

c. Teach client to move each foot through full range of motion (ROM).

C. Goal: *reduce the number of bacteria on the skin to eliminate incision contamination.*

☞ **Skin preparation**:

1. Prepare area of skin wider and longer than proposed incision in case a larger incision is necessary.

2. Gently scrub with an antiseptic agent such as povidone-iodine (*Betadine*). Note possibility of allergy to iodine.

a. Hexachlorophene should be left on the skin for 5–10 min.

b. If benzalkonium chloride (*Zephiran*) solution is ordered, do *not* soap skin prior to use; soap reduces effectiveness of benzalkonium by causing it to precipitate.

3. Note any nicks, cuts, or irritations, potential infection sites.

4. Opinions differ on hair removal—may leave hair.

5. Clipping of hair or electric razor may be ordered; lower rate of infection.

6. Skin preparation may be done in surgery.

D. Goal: *reduce the risk of vomiting and aspiration during anesthesia; prevent contamination of abdominal operative sites by fecal material.*

Gastrointestinal tract preparation:

1. *No* food or fluid for at least 6–8 h before surgery.

2. Remove food and water from bedside.

3. Place NPO signs on bed or door.

4. Inform kitchen and oncoming nursing staff that client is NPO for surgery.

5. Give IV infusions up to time of surgery if dehydrated or malnourished.

☞ 6. *Enemas*: two or three may be given the evening prior to intestinal, colon, or pelvic surgeries; 3 d of cleansing with large intestine procedures.

7. Possible *antibiotic* therapy to reduce colonic flora with large bowel surgery.

☞ 8. Gastric or intestinal intubation may be done the evening prior to major abdominal surgery.

a. Types of tubes:

(1) *Levin*: single lumen; sufficient to remove fluids and gas from stomach; suction may damage mucosa.

(2) *Salem sump*: large lumen with a sump lumen to prevent tissue-wall adherence.

(3) *Miller-Abbott*: long single or double lumen; required to remove the contents of jejunum or ileum.

b. Pressures: low, *intermittent* setting with Levin and intestinal tubes, *low, continuous* setting with Salem sump; excessive pressures will result in injury to mucosal lining of intestine or stomach.

E. Goal: *promote rest and reduce apprehension.*

1. Medications as ordered: evening prior to surgery may give *barbiturate*—pentobarbital (*Nembutal*), secobarbital (*Seconal*).

2. Quiet environment: eliminate noises, distractions.

3. *Position*: reduce muscle tension.

4. Back rub.

5. Report client verbalization of feeling of impending doom to physician.

F. Goal: *protect from injury; ensure final preparation for surgery.*
Day of surgery:
1. Operative permit signed and on chart; physician responsible for obtaining informed consent.
2. Shower or bathe.
   a. Dress: hospital gown.
   b. Remove: hair pins (cover hair); nail polish, to facilitate observation of peripheral circulation;   jewelry (tape wedding bands securely); pierced earrings; contact lenses; dentures (store and give mouth care); if client objects, remove in OR; give valuable personal items to family; chart disposition of items. (see **Table 9.1** for **care of dentures**.)
3. Proper identification—check band for secureness and legibility.
4. Make sure "Allergy" band is attached to client's wrist and front of chart is marked.
5. Vital signs—baseline data.
6. Void, to prevent distention and possible injury to bladder.
7. Give preoperative medication, to ensure smooth induction and maintenance of anesthesia:
   a. Administered 45–75 min before anesthetic induction.
   b. Siderails up (client will begin to feel drowsy and light-headed).
   c. Expect complaint of dry mouth if atropine sulfate given.
   d. Observe for side effects—morphine sulfate and meperidine HCl (*Demerol*) may cause nausea and vomiting or drop in blood pressure.
   e. Quiet environment until transported to operating room.

TABLE 9.1 ☞ CARE OF DENTURES

Wear gloves.
If client cannot remove own dentures, grasp upper plate at the front teeth and move up and down gently to release suction.
Lift the lower plate up one side at a time.
Use extreme care not to damage dentures while cleaning.
Use tepid, *not* hot, water to clean.
Avoid soaking for long periods.
Inspect for sharp edges.
Do oral cavity assessment.
Replace moistened dentures in client's mouth.
Use appropriately labeled container for storage when dentures are to remain out of client's mouth.

Source: Lagerquist SL: *Little, Brown's NCLEX-RN® Examination Review*. Boston: Little, Brown, (out of print)

---

8. Note completeness of chart:
   a. Surgical checklist and consent completed.
   b. Vital signs recorded.
   c. Routine laboratory reports present.
   d. Preoperative medications given.
   e. Significant client observations.
   f. Medical history and physical exam results are in chart.
9. Assist client's family in finding proper waiting room.
   a. Inform them that the surgeon will contact them after the procedure is over.
   b. Explain length of time client is expected to be in post-anesthesia recovery room.
   c. Prepare family for any special equipment or devices that may be needed to care for client postoperatively—oxygen, monitoring equipment, ventilator, or blood transfusions.

Intraoperative Preparation

Anesthesia: blocks transmission of nerve impulses, suppresses reflexes, promotes muscle relaxation, and depending upon the type of anesthesia used, achieves reversible unconsciousness.

I. **Regional anesthesia**—purpose is to block pain reception and transmission in a specified area. Commonly used drugs are lidocaine HCl, tetracaine HCl, cocaine HCl and procaine HCl. Types of regional anesthetics:
   A. *Topical*—applied to mucous membranes or skin; drug anesthetizes the nerves immediately *below* the area. May be used for bronchoscopic or laryngoscopic examinations. *Side effects:* rare anaphylaxis.
   B. *Local infiltration*—used for minor procedures; anesthetic drug is injected directly into the area to be incised, manipulated, or sutured. *Side effects:* rare anaphylaxis.
   C. *Peripheral nerve block*—regional anesthesia is achieved by injecting drug into or around a nerve after it passes from vertebral column; procedure is named for nerve involved, such as *brachial plexus block*. Requires a high degree of anatomic knowledge. *Side effects:* may be absorbed into bloodstream. Observe for signs of excitability, twitching, changes in vital signs, or respiratory difficulties.
   D. *Field block*—a group of nerves is injected with anesthetic as the nerves branch from a major or main nerve trunk. May be used for dental procedures, plastic surgery. *Side effects:* rare.

E. *Epidural anesthesia*—anesthetic is injected into the epidural space of vertebral canal; produces a bandlike anesthesia around body. Frequently used in obstetrics. Rare complications.

F. *Spinal anesthesia*—anesthetic is injected into the subarachnoid space and mixes with spinal fluid; drug acts on the nerves as they emerge from the spinal cord, thereby inhibiting conduction in the autonomic, sensory, and motor systems.

  1. *Advantages*: rapid onset; produces excellent muscle relaxation.
  2. Utilization: surgery on lower limbs, perineum, and lower abdomen.
  3. *Disadvantages*:
    a. Loss of sensation below point of injection for 2–8 h—watch for signs of *bladder distention;* prevent injuries by maintaining alignment, keeping bedclothes straightened.
    b. Client awake during surgical procedure—*avoid* light or upsetting conversations.
    c. Leakage of spinal fluid from puncture site—keep *flat in bed* for 8 h to prevent headache. Keep well hydrated to promote spinal fluid replacement.
    d. Depression of vasomotor responses—frequent checks of vital signs.

G. *Intravenous regional anesthesia*—used in an extremity whose circulation has been interrupted by a tourniquet; the anesthetic is injected into vein, and blockage is presumed to be achieved from extravascular leakage of anesthetic near a major nerve trunk. *Precautions:* same as for peripheral nerve block.

II. General anesthesia—a reversible state in which the client loses consciousness due to the inhibition of neuronal impulses in the brain by a variety of chemical agents; may be given intravenously, by inhalation, or rectally.

A. *Side effects:*
  1. Respiratory depression.
  2. Nausea, vomiting.
  3. Excitement.
  4. Restlessness.
  5. Laryngospasm.
  6. Hypotension.

B. **Nursing care plan/implementation**—Goal: *prevent hazardous drug interactions.*
  1. *Notify anesthesiologist* if client is taking any of the following drugs:
    a. *Antibiotics*, such as neomycin sulfate, streptomycin sulfate, polymyxin A and B sulfate, colistin sulfate, and kanamycin sulfate—when mixed with curariform muscle relaxant, they interrupt nerve transmission and may cause *respiratory paralysis and apnea.*

    b. *Antidepressants*—particularly MAO (monoamine oxidase) inhibitors, which increase *hypotensive* effects of anesthetic agents.
    c. *Diuretics*—particularly thiazide diuretics, which may induce *potassium depletion;* a potassium deficit may lead to *respiratory depression* during anesthesia.
    d. *Antihypertensives*, such as reserpine, hydralazine, and methyldopa—*potentiate* the hypotensive effects of anesthetic agents.
    e. *Anticoagulants*, such as heparin, warfarin (*Coumadin*)—increase bleeding times, which may result in excessive *blood loss* and/or hemorrhage.
    f. *Aspirin*—decreases platelet aggregation and may result in increased *bleeding*.
    g. *Steroids*, such as cortisone—anti-inflammatory effect may delay wound healing.

  2. *Stages of inhalation anesthesia and nursing goals:*
    a. *Stage I*—extends from beginning of induction to loss of consciousness. *Nursing goal: reduce external stimuli,* as all movement and noises are exaggerated for the client and can be highly distressing.
    b. *Stage II*—extends from loss of consciousness to relaxation; stage of delirium and excitement. *Nursing goal: prevent injury* by helping anesthesiologist *restrain* client if necessary; maintain a quiet, nonstimulating environment.
    c. *Stage III*—extends from loss of lid reflex to cessation of voluntary respirations. *Nursing goal: reduce risk of untoward effects* by preparing the operative site, assisting with procedures, and observing for signs of complications.
    d. *Stage IV*—indicates overdose and consists of respiratory arrest and vasomotor collapse due to medullary paralysis. *Nursing goal:promote restoration of ventilation and vasomotor tone* by assisting with cardiac arrest procedures and by administering cardiac stimulants or narcotic antagonists as ordered.

III. Muscle relaxants—given to supplement general anesthetic agents, i.e., curare, succinyl choline (*Anectine*).
A. **Actions:**
  1. Facilitates endotracheal intubation.
  2. Relaxes abdominal muscles.
  3. Facilitates the administration of lower doses of potent general anesthetic.

B. **Nursing care plan/implementation**
1. Goal: *observe for respiratory depression*—respiratory rate >30 breaths/min, shallow, quiet, use of accessory muscles.
2. Goal: *document observations*.

IV. **Hypothermia**—a specialized procedure in which the client's body temperature is lowered to 28°–30°C (82°-86°F).
   A. Reduces tissue metabolism and oxygen requirements.
   B. Used in heart surgery, brain surgery, and surgery on major blood vessels.
   C. **Nursing care plan/implementation**
   1. Goal: *prevent complications:*
      a. Monitor vital signs for shock.
      b. Note levels of consciousness.
      c. Record intake and output (I&O) accurately.
      d. Maintain good body alignment; reposition to prevent edema, pressure, or discoloration of skin.
      e. Maintain patent IV.
   2. Goal: *promote comfort*.
      a. Apply blankets to rewarm and prevent shivering.
      b. Mouth care.

V. **General evaluation/outcome criteria:** complete reversal of anesthetic effects (e.g., spontaneous respirations, pupils react to light).

Postoperative Experience

I. **Assessment**
   A. *Subjective data*:
   1. Pain: location, onset, intensity.
   2. Nausea.
   B. *Objective data*:
   1. Operative summary:
      a. Type of operation performed.
      b. Pathologic findings, if known.
      c. Anesthesia and medications received.
      d. Problems during surgery that will affect recovery, (e.g., arrhythmias, bleeding [estimated blood loss]).
      e. Fluids received: type, amount.
      f. Need for drainage or suction apparatus.
   2. Observations:
      a. Patency of airway.
      b. Vital signs.
      c. Skin color and dryness.
      d. Level of consciousness.
      e. Status of reflexes.
      f. Dressings.
      g. Type and rate of IV infusion and blood transfusion.

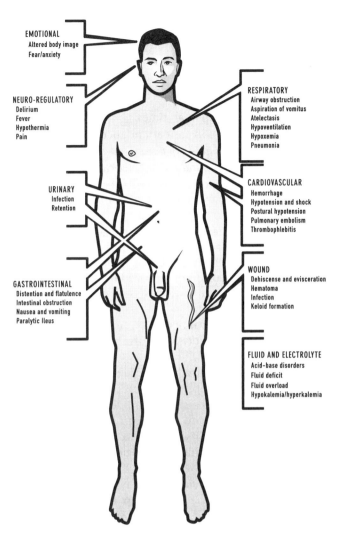

EMOTIONAL
Altered body image
Fear/anxiety

NEURO-REGULATORY
Delirium
Fever
Hypothermia
Pain

URINARY
Infection
Retention

GASTROINTESTINAL
Distention and flatulence
Intestinal obstruction
Nausea and vomiting
Paralytic Ileus

RESPIRATORY
Airway obstruction
Aspiration of vomitus
Atelectasis
Hypoventilation
Hypoxemia
Pneumonia

CARDIOVASCULAR
Hemorrhage
Hypotension and shock
Postural hypotension
Pulmonary embolism
Thrombophlebitis

WOUND
Dehiscense and evisceration
Hematoma
Infection
Keloid formation

FLUID AND ELECTROLYTE
Acid–base disorders
Fluid deficit
Fluid overload
Hypokalemia/hyperkalemia

Common Potential Problems in the Postoperative Period

      h. Tubes/drains: urinary, chest, Penrose, Hemovac; note color and amount of drainage.

II. **Analysis/nursing diagnosis**
   A. *Ineffective breathing pattern* related to general anesthesia.
   B. *Ineffective airway clearance* related to absent or weak cough.
   C. *Risk* for aspiration related to vomiting.
   D. *Pain* related to surgical incision.
   E. *Altered tissue perfusion* related to hypotensive effects of medications.
   F. *Risk for fluid volume deficit* related to blood loss.
   G. *Risk for injury* related to disorientation.
   H. *Risk for infection* related to disruption of skin integrity.
   I. *Urinary retention* related to anesthetic effects.
   J. *Constipation* related to decreased peristalsis.

III. Nursing care plan/implementation—immediate postanesthesia nursing care: refers to time following surgery that is usually spent in the recovery room (1–2 h).

A. Goal: *promote a safe, quiet, nonstressful environment.*
   1. Siderails up at all times.
   2. Nurse in constant attendance.

B. Goal: *promote lung expansion and gas exchange.*

C. Goal: *prevent aspiration and atelectasis.*
   1. *Position:* side or back, with head turned to side to prevent obstruction of airway by tongue; allows for drainage from mouth.
   2. *Airway:* leave the oropharyngeal or nasopharyngeal airway in place until client awakens and begins to eject; gagging and vomiting may occur if not removed before pharyngeal reflex returns. Snoring is obstructed breathing.
   3. After removal of airway: turn on side in a *lateral position;* support upper arm with pillow.
   4. *Suction:* remove excessive secretions from mouth and pharynx.
   5. Encourage coughing and deep breathing: aids in upward movement of secretions.
   6. Give humidified *oxygen* as necessary: reduces respiratory irritation and keeps bronchotracheal secretions soft and moist.
   7. *Mechanical ventilation:* if needed (see **Ventilators** in **Chap. 6, p. 89**).

D. Goal: *promote and maintain cardiovascular function.*
   1. *Vital signs,* as ordered: usually q15min until stable.
      a. Compare with preoperative vital signs.
      b. **Immediately report:** systolic blood pressure that *drops 20* mm Hg or more, a pressure *below 80* mm Hg, or a pressure that continually drops 5–10 mm Hg over several readings; pulse rates *under 60* or *over 110* beats/min, or irregularities; respirations *over 30* breaths/min; becoming shallow, quiet, slow; use of neck and diaphragm muscles (symptoms of *respiratory depression* or distress).
      2. Observe for other alterations in circulatory function—pallor; thready pulse; cold, moist skin; decreased urine output; restlessness.
         a. **Immediately report** to physician.
         b. Initiate *oxygen* therapy.
         c. Place client in *shock position* unless contraindicated—feet elevated 20 degrees, legs/knees straight, head *slightly* elevated to increase venous return.
   3. *Intravenous* infusions: time, rate, orders for added medications.
   4. Monitor blood transfusions, if ordered: observe for signs of *reaction* (chills, elevated temperature, urticaria, laryngeal edema, wheezing); usually first 15–20 min. **Table 9.2, p. 136,** summarizes the nursing care plan/implementation.
   5. If reaction occurs, **immediately** stop transfusion and notify physician. Send **STAT** urine to lab.

E. Goal: *promote psychological equilibrium.*
   1. Reassure on awakening—orient frequently.
   2. Explain procedures even though client does not appear alert.
   3. Answer client's questions briefly and accurately.
   4. Maintain quiet, restful environment.
   5. Comfort measures:
      a. Good body alignment.
      b. Support dependent extremities to *avoid* pressure areas and possible nerve damage.
      c. Check for constriction: dressings, clothing, bedding.
      d. Check IV sites frequently for patency and signs of infiltration (swelling, blanching, cool to touch).

F. Goal: *maintain proper function of tubes and apparatus.* (See **Review of Use of Common Tubes p. 138**).

IV. General postoperative nursing care: refers to period from admission to the general nursing unit until anticipated recovery and discharge from the hospital. See **Table 9.2:** Review of **Postoperative Complications** and **Positioning** the Client for Specific Surgical Indications (see **Positioning** box p. 140-141).

A. Goal: *promote lung expansion, gaseous exchange, and elimination of bronchotracheal secretions.*
   1. Turn, cough, and deep breathe q2h.
   2. Use *incentive spirometer* as ordered to enable client to observe depth of ventilation.
   3. Administer nebulization as ordered to help mobilize secretions.
   4. Encourage hydration to thin mucous secretions.
   5. Assist in ambulation as soon as allowed.

B. Goal: *provide relief of pain.*
   1. Assess type, location, intensity, and duration; possible causative factors, such as poor body alignment or restrictive bandages.
   2. Observe and evaluate reaction to discomfort.
   3. Utilize comfort measures, such as back rubs and proper ventilation, staying with client and encouraging verbalization.
   4. Reduce incidence of pain: change position frequently; support dependent extremities with pillows, sandbags, foot cradle, and footboards; keep bedding dry and straight.
   5. Give *analgesics* or *tranquilizers* as ordered; assure client that they will help.
   6. Observe for desired and untoward effects of medication. (*continued on p.137*)

TABLE 9.2 POSTOPERATIVE COMPLICATIONS

Condition and Etiology	◄ Assessment: Signs and Symptoms	◄ Nursing Care Plan/Implementation
RESPIRATORY COMPLICATIONS—Most common are Airway Obstruction, Atelectasis, Pneumonias (Lobar, Bronchial, and Hypostatic), and Pleuritis; other complications are Hemothorax and Pneumothorax.		
Airway Obstruction—decreased level of consciousness due to anesthetic medications causes tongue to fall backward and obstruct airway. Obstruction may be less commonly caused by secretions, laryngospasm, or laryngeal edema.	Use of accessory muscles; snoring or noisy respirations; stridor, *acute* respiratory distress, sternal retractions; decreased O_2 saturation.	☞ 1. Oxygen 2. Stimulate client. 3. Jaw thrust maneuver, chin lift. 4. Artifical airway. ☞ 5. Suctioning ☞ 6. Chest physiotherapy. 7. Intubation and mechanical ventilation if needed.
Atelectasis—undetected preoperative upper respiratory tract infections, aspiration of vomitus; irritation of the tracheobronchial tree with increased mucous secretions due to intubation and inhalation anesthesia; a history of heavy smoking, or chronic obstructive pulmonary disease; severe postoperative pain or high abdominal or thoracic surgery, which inhibits deep breathing; and debilitation or old age, which lowers the client's resistance.	Dyspnea; ↑ temperature; absent or diminished breath sounds over affected area; asymmetric chest expansion; ↑ respirations and pulse rate; anxiety and restlessness.	1. *Position*: unaffected side. 2. Turn, cough, and deep breathe. ☞ 3. Postural drainage. ☞ 4. Nebulization 5. *Force* fluids, if not contraindicated.
Pneumonia—see **Atelectasis** for etiology.	Rapid, shallow, painful respirations; crackles; diminished or absent breath sounds; asymmetric lung expansion; chills and fever; productive cough, rust-colored sputum; circumoral and nailbed cyanosis.	1. *Position* of comfort—semi- to high-Fowler's. 2. *Force* fluids to 3000 mL/d. ☞ 3. Humidification of air and *oxygen* therapy. ☞ 4. Oropharyngeal *suction* prn. 5. Assist during coughing. ▭ 6. Administer *antibiotics* and *analgesics*, as ordered. 🍎 7. *Diet*: high calorie, as tolerated. ☞ 8. Cautious disposal of secretions; proper oral hygiene.
Pleuritis—see **Atelectasis** for etiology.	Knifelike chest pain on inspiration; intercostal tenderness; splinting of chest by client; rapid, shallow respirations; pleural friction rub; ↑ temperature; malaise.	1. *Position: affected* side to splint the chest. ☞ 2. Manually splint client's chest during cough. ☞ 3. Apply binder or adhesive strapping, as ordered. ▭ 4. Administer *analgesics*, as ordered.
Hemothorax—chest surgery, gunshot or knife wounds, and multiple fractures of the chest wall.	Chest pain, increased respiratory rate, dyspnea; decreased or absent breath sounds; decreased blood pressure; tachycardia; *mediastinal shift* may occur (heart, trachea, esophagus, and great vessels are pushed toward unaffected side).	1. Observe vital signs closely for signs of shock and respiratory distress. 2. Assist with *thoracentesis* (needle aspiration of fluid). ☞ 3. Assist with insertion of thoracotomy tube to closed-chest drainage (see care of *water-sealed drainage* system **Chap. 6**).

(continued)

TABLE 9.2 POSTOPERATIVE COMPLICATIONS (*continued*)

Condition and Etiology	►◄ Assessment: Signs and Symptoms	►◄ Nursing Care Plan/Implementation
Pneumothorax, *closed* or *tension* —thoracentesis (needle nicks the lung), rupture of alveoli or bronchi due to accidental injury, and chronic obstructive lung disease.	Marked dyspnea, *sudden sharp* chest pain, subcutaneous emphysema (air in chest wall. tissue); cyanosis; tracheal shift to unaffected side; hyperresonance on percussion, decreased or absent breath sounds; increased respiratory rate, tachycardia; asymmetric chest expansion, feeling of pressure within chest; *mediastinal shift*—severe dyspnea and cyanosis, deviation of larynx and trachea toward unaffected side, deviation either medially or laterally of apex of heart, decreased blood pressure; distended neck veins; increased pulse and respirations.	1. Remain with client—keep as calm and quiet as possible. 2. *Position*: high-Fowler's (sitting). 3. Notify physician through another nurse, and have thoracentesis equipment brought to bedside. ☞ 4. Administer *oxygen* as necessary. 5. Take vital signs to evaluate respiratory and cardiac function. 6. Assist with *thoracentesis*. ☞ 7. Assist with initiation and maintenance of *closed-chest* drainage.

CIRCULATORY COMPLICATIONS

Condition and Etiology	►◄ Assessment: Signs and Symptoms	►◄ Nursing Care Plan/Implementation
Shock—hemorrhage, sepsis, decreased cardiac contractility (myocardial infarction, cardiac failure, tamponade), drug sensitivities, transfusion reactions, pulmonary embolism, and emotional reaction to pain or deep fear.	Dizziness, fainting, restlessness; anxiety. *Blood pressure*: ↓ or falling. *Pulse*: weak, thready. *Respirations*: ↑, shallow. *Skin*: pale, cool, clammy, cyanotic. *Temperature*: ↓ *GU*: oliguria $CVP < 5$ cm/H_2O Thirst	1. *Position*: foot of bed raised 20 degrees, knees straight, trunk horizontal, head slightly elevated; *avoid* Trendelenburg position. ⊂⊃ 2. Administer *blood* transfusions, plasma expanders, and *intravenous infusions* as ordered; medications specific to type of shock. ☞ 3. Check: vital signs, *CVP*, temperature. ☞ 4. Insert urinary *catheter* to monitor hourly urine output. ☞ 5. Administer *oxygen*, as ordered.
Thrombophlebitis—injury to vein wall by tight leg straps or leg holders during gynecologic surgery; hemoconcentration due to dehydration or fluid loss; stasis of blood in extremities due to postoperative circulatory depression (see **Chap. 2, Peripheral Vascular Disorders, p. 20, 21**).	Calf pain or cramping, redness and swelling (the left leg is affected more frequently than the right), extremity warmth, *Homan's* sign is *unreliable*, slight fever, chills, , tenderness over the anteromedian surface of thigh.	1. Maintain complete bed rest, *avoiding positions* that restrict venous return. ☞ 2. Apply elastic stockings or wrap from legs from toes to groin with elastic bandages to prevent swelling and pooling of venous blood. ☞ 3. Apply warm, moist soaks to area, as ordered. ⊂⊃ 4. Administer *anticoagulants*, as ordered. ☞ 5. Use bed cradle over affected limb. ☞ 6. Perform active and passive ROM exercises on unaffected limb.
Pulmonary embolism—obstruction of a pulmonary artery by a foreign body in bloodstream, usually a blood clot that has been dislodged from its original site. (See **Respiratory Disorders, Chap. 6**)	*Sudden*, severe stabbing chest pain; *severe* dyspnea; cyanosis; *rapid* pulse; anxiety and apprehension; pupillary dilation; *profuse diaphoresis*; *loss* of consciousness.	☞ 1. Administer *oxygen* and *inhalants* while client is *sitting upright*. 2. Maintain *bed rest* and frequent reassurance. ⊂⊃ 3. Administer heparin sodium, as ordered. ⊂⊃ 4. Administer *analgesics*, such as morphine sulfate, to reduce pain and apprehension.

(*continued*)

TABLE 9.2 POSTOPERATIVE COMPLICATIONS (continued)

Condition and Etiology	▶ Assessment: Signs and Symptoms	▶ Nursing Care Plan/Implementation
WOUND COMPLICATIONS		
Wound infection—*obesity* or *undernutrition*, particularly protein and vitamin deficiencies; *decreased* antibody production in aged; *decreased* phagocytosis in newborn; metabolic disorder, such as diabetes mellitus, Cushing's syndrome, malignancies, and shock; break-down in aseptic technique.	Redness, tenderness, and heat in area of incision; purulent wound drainage; ↑temperature; ↑ pulse rate.	☞ 1. Assist in *cleansing* and irrigation of *wound* and insertion of a drain. ☞ 2. Perform dressing changes as ordered. Record amount and characteristics of drainage. ▬ 3. Give *antibiotics* as ordered; observe responses.
Wound dehiscence and evisceration—obesity and undernutrition, particularly protein and vitamin C deficiencies; immunosuppression; metabolic disorders; cancer; liver disease; common site is midline abdominal incision, frequently about 7 d postoperatively; precipitating factors include: abdominal distention, vomiting, coughing, hiccups, and uncontrolled motor activity.	Slow parting of wound edges with a gush of pinkish serous drainage or rapid parting with coils of intestines escaping onto the abdominal wall, the latter accompanied by pain and often by vomiting.	1. *Position*: bed rest, low-Fowler's or horizontal position; knees flexed. 2. Notify physician **STAT**. ☞ 3. Cover exposed coils of intestines with sterile towels or dressing and keep moist with sterile normal saline. 4. Monitor vital signs frequently. 5. Remain with client, reassure that physician is coming. ☞ 6. Prepare for physician's arrival: set up IV, suction equipment, and NG tube; obtain sterile gown, mask, gloves, towels, and warmed normal saline. 7. Notify surgery that client will be returning to operating room.
URINARY COMPLICATIONS		
Urinary retention—obstruction in bladder or urethra; neurologic disease, mechanical trauma as in childbirth or gynecologic surgery; psychological conditioning that inhibits voiding in bed; prolonged bed rest; pain with lower abdominal surgery; effects of anesthesia and intraoperative medications.	Inability to void *10–18 h* after surgery, despite adequate fluid replacement; palpable bladder; frequent voiding of small amounts of urine or dribbling; suprapubic pain.	1. Assist client to stand or use bedside commode, if not contraindicated. 2. Provide privacy. 3. Reduce tension, provide support. 4. Use warm bedpan. 5. Run tap water. 6. Place client's feet in warm water. 7. Pour warm water over perineum. ☞ 8. Catheterize if conservative measures fail.
Urinary tract infections—urinary retention, bladder distention, repeated or prolonged catheterization.	*Urinary*: burning and frequency. *Pain*: low back or flank. Pyuria, hematuria; ↑ temperature, chills; anorexia; positive urine 〰 culture.	1. *Push fluids* to 3000 mL daily, unless contraindicated. 2. *Avoid* stimulants such as caffeine. ▬ 3. Give *antibiotics, sulfonamides*, or *acidifying agents*, as ordered. ☞ 4. Give perineal care after each bowel movement.
GASTROINTESTINAL COMPLICATIONS		
Gastric distention—depressed gastric motility due to sympathoadrenal stress response; idiosyncrasy to drugs; emotions, pain, shock; fluid and electrolyte imbalances.	Feeling of fullness; hiccups; overflow vomiting of dark, foul-smelling liquid; severe retention leads to decreased blood pressure (due to pressure on vagus nerve) and other symptoms of shock syndrome.	1. Report signs to physician **immediately**. ☞ 2. Insert or assist in insertion of NG tube; attach to intermittent suction. ☞ 3. Irrigate NG tube with *saline* (water will deplete electrolytes and result in metabolic alkalosis). ▬ 4. Administer IV infusions with electrolytes, as ordered.

(continued)

TABLE 9.2 POSTOPERATIVE COMPLICATIONS   (*continued*)

Condition and Etiology	►◄ Assessment: Signs and Symptoms	►◄ Nursing Care Plan/Implementation
Paralytic ileus–see Gastric distention	Greatly decreased or absent bowel sounds; failure of either gas or feces to be passed by rectum; nausea and vomiting; abdominal tenderness, and distention; fever; dehydration.	1. Notify physician. 2. Insert or assist with insertion of *NG* tube; attach to low, intermittent suction. 3. Administer IV infusion with electrolytes, as ordered. 4. Irrigate NG tube with saline. 5. *Assist* with insertion of *Miller-Abbott* tube, if indicated. 6. Administer medications to increase peristalsis, as ordered.
Intestinal obstruction—due to poorly functioning anastomosis, hernia, adhesions, fecal impaction.	Severe, colicky abdominal pains; mild to severe abdominal distention; nausea and vomiting; anorexia and malaise; fever; lack of bowel movement; electrolyte imbalance; high-pitched tinkling bowel sounds.	1. Assist with insertion of *nasoenteric* tube and attach to intermittent *suction*. 2. Maintain IV infusions with electrolytes. 3. Encourage nasal breathing to *avoid* air swallowing. 4. Check abdomen for distention and bowel sounds every 2 h. 5. Encourage verbalization. 6. Plan rest periods for client. 7. Administer oral hygiene frequently.

TRANSFUSION REACTIONS

Condition and Etiology	►◄ Assessment: Signs and Symptoms	►◄ Nursing Care Plan/Implementation
Allergic and febrile reactions— unidentified antigen or antigens in donor blood or transfusion equipment; previous reaction to transfusions; small thrombi; bacteria; lysed red blood cells.	Fever to 103°F, may have *sudden* onset; chills; itching; erythema; urticaria; nausea; vomiting; dyspnea and wheezing, occasionally.	1. *Stop* transfusion, take vital signs and notify physician. 2. Administer *antihistamines*, as ordered. 3. Send **STAT** urine to lab for analysis. 4. Institute *cooling* measures, if indicated. 5. Maintain *strict* input and output records. 6. Send remaining blood to lab for analysis, and order recipient blood sample for analysis.
Hemolytic reaction—infusion of incompatible blood (less common, more serious).	*Early*—chills and fever; throbbing headache, feeling of burning in face; hypotension; tachycardia; chest, back, or flank pain; nausea, vomiting; feeling of doom; *Later*—spontaneous and diffuse bleeding; icterus; urine: oliguria; anuria; hemoglobinuria.	1. *Stop* infusion immediately; take vital signs and notify physician. 2. Send client blood sample and unused blood to lab for analysis. 3. Send **STAT** urine to lab. 4. Save *all* urine for observation of discoloration. 5. Administer parenteral infusions to shock, as ordered. 6. Administer medications, as ordered—*diuretics, sodium bicarbonate, hydrocortisone, and vasopressors.*

(continued)

TABLE 9.2 POSTOPERATIVE COMPLICATIONS (*continued*)

Condition and Etiology	◄ Assessment: Signs and Symptoms	◄ Nursing Care Plan/Implementation
EMOTIONAL COMPLICATIONS		
Emotional disturbances—grief associated with loss of body part or loss of body image; previous emotional problems; decreased sensory and perceptual input; sensory overload; fear and pain; decreased resistance to stress as a result of age, exhaustion, or debilitation.	Restlessness, insomnia, depression, hallucinations, delusions, agitation, suicidal thoughts.	1. Report symptoms to physician. 2. Encourage verbalization of feelings; give realistic assurance. 3. Orient to time and place, as necessary. 4. Provide safety measures, such as siderails. 5. Keep room lit, to reduce likelihood of visual hallucinations. 6. Administer tranquilizers, as ordered. 7. Use restraints as a *last* resort.

CVP = central venous pressure; NG = nasogastric; ROM = range of motion.

Source: ©Lagerquist SL: *Little, Brown's NCLEX-RN® Examination Review*. Boston: Little, Brown, (out of print).

(continued from p. 132)

C. Goal: *promote adequate nutrition and fluid and electrolyte balance.*

    1. Parenteral fluids, as ordered.

    2. Monitor blood pressure, I&O to assess adequate, deficient, or excessive extracellular fluid volume.

    3. *Diet*: liquid when nausea and vomiting stop and bowel sounds are established; progress as ordered.

D. Goal: *assist client with elimination.*

    1. Encourage voiding within 8–10 h after surgery.

      a. Allow client to stand or use commode, if not contraindicated.

      b. Run tap water or soak feet in warm water to promote micturition.

      c. Catheterization if bladder is distended and conservative treatments have failed.

    2. Maintain accurate I&O records.

    3. Expect bowel function to return in 2–3 d.

E. Goal: *facilitate wound healing and prevent infection.*

    1. *Incision* care: *avoid* pressure to enhance venous drainage and prevent edema.

    2. *Elevate* injured extremities to reduce swelling and promote venous return.

    3. Support or *splint* incision when coughing.

    4. Check *dressings* q2h for drainage.

    5. Change dressings on draining wounds prn; *aseptic technique*; protective ointments to reduce skin irritation may be ordered.

    6. Carefully observe wound suction (e.g., *Jackson-Pratt*), if applied, for kinking or twisting of the tubes.

F. Goal: *promote comfort and rest.*

    1. Recognize factors that may cause restlessness—fear, anxiety, pain, lack of oxygen, wet dressings.

    2. Comfort measures: *analgesics* or *barbiturates*; apply *oxygen* as indicated; change positions; encourage deep breathing; massage back to reduce restlessness.

    3. Group care activites to allow rest periods.

    4. Give *antiemetic* for relief of nausea and vomiting, as ordered.

    5. Vigorous oral hygiene (brushing) to prevent "surgical mumps" or parotitis from atropine given preoperatively or general anesthesia.

G. Goal: *encourage early movement and ambulation to prevent complications of immobilization.*

    1. Turn or reposition q2h.

    2. ROM: passive and active exercises.

    3. Encourage leg exercises.

    4. Assist with standing or use of commode, if allowed.

    5. Encourage resumption of personal care as soon as possible.

    6. Assist with ambulation in room as soon as allowed. *Avoid* chair-sitting, as it enhances venous pooling and may predispose to thrombophlebitis.

◄ V. **Evaluation/outcome criteria**

A. Incision heals without infection.

B. No complications, (e.g., atelectasis, pneumonia, thrombophlebitis).

C. Normal bowel and bladder functions resume.

D. Carries out activities of daily living, self-care.

E. Accepts possible limitations: dietary, activity, body image (e.g., no depression, complies with treatment regimen).

REVIEW OF THE USE OF COMMON TUBES

Tube or Apparatus	Purpose	Examples of Use	⋈ Key Points for Nursing Implementation
Penrose drain	Soft collapsible latex rubber drain inserted to *drain serosanguineous fluid* from a surgical site; usually brought out to the skin via a stab wound.	Bowel resection.	1. Expect drainage to progress from serosanguineous to more serous. ⚠ 2. *Sterile* technique when changing dressing—do often. 3. Physician will advance tube a little each day.
Nasogastric (NG) tubes:			
Levin tube and small-bore feeding tubes	1. Inserted into stomach to *decompress* by removing gastric contents and air—prevents any buildup of gastric secretions, which are continuous. 2. Used when stomach needs to be washed out (*lavage*). 3. Used for feedings when client is unable to swallow (*gavage*).	1. *Any abdominal or other surgery where peristalsis is absent* for a few days. 2. *Overdoses.* 3. *Gastrointestinal hemorrhage.* 4. *Cancer of the esophagus.* 5. *Early postoperative laryngectomy or radical neck dissection.*	☞ 1. Connect to *low* intermittent suction. ☞ 2. Irrigate prn with normal saline or puffs of air. 3. Clean, but *not* sterile, procedure. 4. Mouth care needed. 5. Report "*coffee ground*" material (digested blood). 6. For overdose: stomach is pumped out as *rapidly* as possible. 7. For hemorrhage: iced normal saline may be used to lavage. 8. Critical to make sure tube still in stomach *before* beginning feeding; *listen* for air passing into stomach and if possible *aspirate* gastric contents; small-bore tubes need placement check by *x-ray*. 9. Follow feeding with some water to rinse out the tube. 10. Clamp tube when ambulating ☞ 11. With larger-bore tubes, determine residuals and withhold feeding if large residuals obtained.
Miller-Abbot tube **Cantor** tube	Longer than **Levin** tube—has mercury or air in bags so tube can be used to *decompress the lower intestinal tract.*	1. *Small-bowel obstructions.* 2. *Intussusception.* 3. *Volvulus.*	1. Care similar to that for **Levin** tube—irrigated. ☞ 2. Connected to suction, *not* sterile technique. 3. Orders will be written on how to advance the tube, gently pushing tube a few inches each hour; client position may affect advancement of tube. 4. X-rays determine the desired location of tube.
Salem sump	Double-lumen tube with vent to *protect gastric mucosa* from trauma of suctioning.	Same as **Levin** tube.	☞ 1. Irrigate vent (blue tubing) with air *only.* 2. See **Levin** tube.

(continued)

REVIEW OF THE USE OF COMMON TUBES (*continued*)

Tube or Apparatus	Purpose	Examples of Use	►◄ Key Points for Nursing Implementation
Gastrostomy tube	1. Inserted into stomach via abdominal wall. 2. May be used for *decompression*. 3. Used *long term for feedings*.	Conditions affecting *esophagus* where it is impossible to insert a nasogastric tube.	1. Principles of tube feedings same as with **Levin** nasogastric tube, *except* no danger that tube is in trachea. 2. If permanent, tube may be replaceable.
T-tube	To *drain bile* from the common bile duct *until* edema has subsided.	*Cholecystectomy* when a common duct exploration or choledochostomy was also done.	1. Bile drainage is influenced by *position* of the drainage bag. ☞ 2. Clamp tube as ordered to see if bile will flow into duodenum normally.
Hemovac	A type of closed-wound drainage system connected to suction—used to *drain a large amount* of serosanguineous fluid from under an incision.	1. *Mastectomy*. 2. *Total hip procedures*. 3. *Total knee procedures*.	1. May compress unit to create portable vacuum or connect to wall suction. 2. Small drainage tubes may get clogged—physician may irrigate these at times.
Jackson-Pratt	1. A method of *closed-wound suction* drainage—indicated when tissue displacement and tissue trauma may occur with rigid drain tubes (i.e., **Hemovac**). 2. See **Hemovac**.	1. *Neurosurgery*. 2. *Neck surgery*. 3. *Mastectomy*. 4. *Total knee and hip replacement*. 5. *Abdominal surgery*. 6. *Urologic procedures*.	☞ 1. Empty reservoir when full, to prevent loss of wound drainage and back-contamination. 2. See **Hemovac**.
Three-way Foley	To provide avenues for *constant irrigation and constant drainage* of the urinary bladder.	1. *Transurethral resection prostatectomy (TURP)* 2. *Bladder infections*.	1. Watch for blocking by clots—causes bladder spasms. 2. Irrigant solution often has *antibiotic* added to normal saline or sterile water. 3. *Sterile water* rather than normal saline may be used for lysis of clots.
Suprapubic catheter	To *drain bladder* via an opening through the abdominal wall above the pubic bone.	*Suprapubic* prostatectomy.	☞ 1. May have orders to *irrigate* prn or continuously.
Ureteral catheter	To *drain urine* from the pelvis of one kidney, or for *splinting* ureter.	1. *Cystoscopy* for diagnostic workups. 2. *Ureteral surgery*. 3. *Pyelotomy*.	1. **Never** clamp the tube—pelvis of kidney only holds 4–8 mL. ☞ 2. Use *only* 5 mL of sterile normal saline if ordered to irrigate.

Note: This review focuses on care of the tubes, not on total client care.

Source: Jane Vincent Corbett, RN, MS, EdD, Professor Emerita, School of Nursing, University of San Francisco. Used with permission.

POSITIONING THE CLIENT FOR SPECIFIC SURGICAL CONDITIONS

Surgical Condition	▶ Key Points for Nursing Implementation	Rationale
Amputation: lower extremity	*No* pillows under stump after first 24 h. Turn client *prone* several times a day.	Prevents contracture of hip flexors.
Appendicitis: ruptured	Keep in *Fowler's* position—*not* flat in bed.	Keeps infection from spreading upward in the peritoneal cavity.
Burns (extensive)	Usually *flat* for first 24 h.	Potential problem is hypovolemia, which will be more symptomatic in a sitting position.
Cast, extremity	Keep extremity *elevated.*	Prevents edema.
Coronary surgery	May be ordered *flat* on back for 24 h.	Important to prevent possible hypotension, which may occur if head of bed raised.
Craniotomy	Head *elevated* with supratentorial incision; *flat* with cerebellar or brainstem incision.	Prevents collection of fluid in surgical area, which might contribute to increased intracranial pressure.
Flail chest	Position on *affected* side.	Reduces the instability of the chest wall that is causing the paradoxical respiratory movements.
Gastric resection	*Lie down after* meals.	May be useful in preventing dumping syndrome.
Hiatal hernia (*before* repaired)	Head of bed *elevated* on 6 inch blocks.	Prevents esophageal irritation from gastric regurgitation.
Hip prosthesis	1. Keep affected leg in *abduction* (splint or pillow between legs). 2. *Avoid* adduction and flexion of the hip. 3. Use trochanter roll along outside of femur anterior joint capsule incision to keep affected leg turned slightly *inward; no* trochanter roll with posterior joint capsule incision as leg is turned slightly *outward.*	If affected leg is flexed and allowed to adduct and internally rotate, the head of the femur may be displaced from the socket.
Iliofemoral bypass; arterial insuffiency	1. Do *not* elevate legs. 2. *Avoid* hip flexion—walk or stand, but do *not* sit.	1. Arterial flow is helped by gravity. 2. Flexion of the hip compresses the vessels of the extremity.
Laminectomy, fusion	*Avoid* twisting motion when getting out of bed, ambulating.	Prevents any bending of the spine.
Liver biopsy	Place on *right* side, and position pillow for pressure.	Prevents bleeding.
Lobectomy	Do *not* put in Trendelenburg position. Position of comfort—sides, back.	Pushes abdominal contents against diaphragm; may cause respiratory embarrassment.
Mastectomy	1. Do *not* abduct arm first few days. 2. Elevate hand and arm *higher* than shoulder if lymph glands removed.	1. Puts tension on suture line. 2. Prevents lymphedema.
Pneumonectomy	Turn *only* toward *operative* side for short periods; *no* extreme lateral positioning.	1. Gives unaffected lung room for full expansion. 2. Prevents mediastinal shift. 3. In case of bleeding there will be no drainage into the unaffected bronchi.
Radium implantation in cervix	Bedrest—usually *elevate head* to *30 degrees.*	*Must* keep radium insert positioned correctly.
Respiratory distress	*Orthopnea* position usually desirable.	Allows for maximum expansion of lungs.

(continued)

POSITIONING THE CLIENT FOR SPECIFIC SURGICAL CONDITIONS *(continued)*

Surgical Condition	▶ Key Points for Nursing Implementation	Rationale
Retinal detachment	1. Affected area toward bed—*complete* bed rest. 2. No *sudden* movements of head	1. Gravity may help retina fall in place. 2. Any sudden increase in intraocular pressure may further dislodge retina. 3. Necessary to cover both eyes to reduce ocular movements.
Traction, straight	Check specific orders about how much head may be elevated.	Body is used as the countertraction—this must *not* be *less* than the pull of the traction.
Traction, balanced suspension	May give client more freedom to move about than in straight traction.	In balanced suspension, additional weights supply countertraction.
Unconscious client	Turn on side with head slightly *lowered*—"coma" position.	1. Important to let secretions drain out by gravity. 2. *Must* prevent aspiration.
Vein strippings; vein ligations	1. Keep legs *elevated*. 2. Do *not* stand or sit for long periods.	1. Prevents venous stasis. 2. Prevents venous pooling.

Source: Jane Vincent Corbett, RN, MS, EdD, Professor Emerita, School of Nursing, University of San Francisco. Used with permission.

🦴 Summary of Key Points

1. Assess client carefully for factors that increase the risk of surgery associated with general anesthesia, such as *hypoventilation, low perfusion,* and potential for *infection.*

2. Document all prescribed and over-the-counter medications the client is taking. Drugs may interact with the anesthesia, producing respiratory depression and hypotension, masking infection, or increasing bleeding.

3. Increased preoperative anxiety increases postoperative pain, nausea, and vomiting.

4. Explaining the surgical procedure and the risks to the client is the *surgeon's* responsibility' (*informed consent*).

5. Preoperative teaching is important to ensure effective postoperative coughing and use of the incentive spirometer.

6. Any noisy breathing or snoring after general anesthesia is indicative of obstructed breathing.

7. After general anesthesia, complications will most likely develop in the following order: *lung congestion* during the first 48 hours; *wound infection* or *dehiscence and evisceration* 3–5 d after surgery; symptoms of a *urinary tract infection* within 5–7d; and indications of *thrombophlebitis* 7–14 d after surgery.

💡 Study and Memory Aids

Postoperative Complications: "4 W's"

Wind—prevent respiratory complications
Wound—prevent infection
Water—prevent dehydration/urinary tract infection
Walk—prevent thrombophlebitis

Check for Circulation: "4 P's"

Pain
Pallor
Paresthesia
Pulse

💊 Drug Review

Perioperative Nursing

Atropine sulfate: 0.4–0.6 mg SC 30–60 min before anesthesia
Meperidine HCl (*Demerol*): 50–150 mg IM or SC
Midazolam HCl (*Versed*): 70–80 mcg/kg 1h before surgery to induce desired sleepiness and decrease anxiety
Morphine sulfate: 5–20 mg IM or SC q4h
Other drugs used according to client's medical history and anticipated health status

Questions

1. What position should the nurse place a client in if wound evisceration occurs after abdominal surgery?
   1. Supine, with knees flexed.
   2. A semi-Fowler's position, with the feet elevated.
   3. A side-lying position, with the client's knees drawn up to the chest.
   4. A position of comfort.

2. Which nursing action is the proper technique for emptying a Jackson-Pratt suction drain?
   1. Opening the spout on the reservoir without gloves.
   2. Disconnecting the bulb from the wound catheter.
   3. Compressing the reservoir bulb with the spout open.
   4. Rinsing the bulb reservoir with sterile water.

3. Which symptom would the nurse tell a client is normal after a laparoscopy?
   1. Shortness of breath.
   2. Dizziness.
   3. Referred shoulder pain.
   4. Abdominal gas pains.

4. The effectiveness of preoperative teaching will be most negatively influenced by:
   1. The presence of a significant other during the teaching session.
   2. Concern regarding the amount of insurance reimbursement.
   3. Prior experience with surgery in family members.
   4. Abdominal pain unrelieved by medication.

5. What is the best way for the nurse to respond to a client who refuses to remove her dentures before surgery?
   1. Tell the client that hospital policy requires that dentures must be removed.
   2. Notify the operating room nurse that the dentures are still in place.
   3. Leave the dentures in place and inform the anesthesiologist of this.
   4. Ask the surgeon to speak to the client.

6. A client's comprehension of and compliance with client teaching for same-day (outpatient) surgery will be most enhanced by:
   1. Verbally giving the client instruction during an office visit before the surgery.
   2. Providing the client with essential instructions in writing.
   3. Telephoning the client after the surgery to review instructions.
   4. Showing the client a movie regarding the procedure to reinforce verbal instructions.

Answers/Rationale

1. **(1)** A flat position with the knees bent will return the intestines to the abdominal cavity and keep them there, as well as relax the abdominal muscles. Elevating the client's feet (2) may help, but having the client sit up would *not* keep the bowel in the abdominal cavity. Side-lying (3) would still allow the bowel to fall forward. A position of comfort (4) may *not* use gravity to return the protruding bowel to the abdomen. **IMP, APP, 1, PhI, Basic care and comfort**

2. **(3)** During emptying of a Jackson-Pratt suction drain, the reservoir bulb must be compressed, but only when the spout is open, so that air is not forced into the surgical area. All of the other actions (1, 2, and 4) will *increase* the likelihood of drain *contamination.* **IMP, APP, 1, PhI, Reduction of risk potential**

3. **(3)** Laparoscopy involves direct visualization of the abdominal or pelvic organs using a fiberoptic light inserted into the abdomen; this causes nerve irritation that leads to shoulder pain. Shortness of breath (1) and dizziness (2) are *not* expected side effects. Although gas is used during the procedure, any abdominal gas pains (4) would occur as a result of bowel distention. **AS, COM, 1, PhI, Reduction of risk potential**

4. **(4)** A client in pain will not be able to focus on teaching. In Maslow's hierarchy of need theory, it is hypothesized that lower-level physiologic needs, such as air, food, and comfort, must be met before a person seeks to get higher-level needs met. All of the other options (1, 2, and 3) would influence a client's receptivity to teaching, but they are related to *higher-level needs* and will have less effect. **EV, ANL, 1, PhI, Reduction of risk potential**

5. **(2)** The dentures can be removed after the client is in the operating room and anesthetized. It is unnecessary to upset a client before surgery (1). The best approach is for a nurse to take action, rather than calling upon the anesthesiologist (3) or the surgeon (4) to do so. **IMP, COM, 7, PsI, Psychosocial integrity**

6. **(2)** Written information that the client can refer to after the surgery is the most effective teaching tool. Client teaching is frequently done in the MD's office (1), *but* the information needs to be *reinforced later* with written material. Follow-up contact (3) is also important, but the effects of anesthesia or pain medication may interfere with retention. A video regarding the procedure can be played for the client while in the MD's office (4) but may not be available to the client at home. **PL, RE/KN, 1, HPM, Health promotion and maintenance**

Key to Codes

Nursing process: **AS**, assessment; **AN**, analysis; **PL**, planning; **IMP**, implementation; **EV**, evaluation. (See **Appendix M** for explanation of nursing process steps.)

Cognitive level: **RE/KN**, recall/knowledge; **COM**, comprehension; **APP**, application; **ANL**, analysis; **EVL**, evaluation; **SYN**, synthesis. (See **Appendix M** for explanation.)

Category of human function: **1**, protective; **2**, sensory-perceptual; **3**, comfort, rest, activity, and mobility; **4**, nutrition; **5**, growth and development; **6**, fluid-gas transport; **7**, psychosocial-cultural; **8**, elimination. (See **Appendix 0** for explanation.)

Client need: **SECE**, safe, effective care environment; **PhI**, physiological integrity; **PsI**, psychosocial integrity; **HPM**, health promotion and maintenance. (See **Appendix P** for explanation.)

Client subneed: (See **Appendix P** for explanation)

Pain

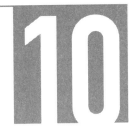

Chapter Outline

- Pain
- Summary of Key Points
- Study and Memory Aid
- Questions
- Answers/Rationale

Pain

Pain is complex, involving physiological, psychosocial, and behavioral components. Pain is experienced differently by different individuals.

I. **Types of pain**:
- A. *Superficial somatic tissues*—skin, subcutaneous or fibrous tissue, and ligaments have pain receptors, and thus pain is localized.
- B. *Deep somatic tissues and viscera*—pain may be diffuse and radiating because these do not have direct connection with sensory-discriminative system.
- C. *Neurogenic pain*—results from damage to peripheral or central nervous system; any sensation may be perceived as pain due to abnormal processing of afferent impulses or paroxysmal activity.
- D. *Psychogenic pain*—due to fantasies and psychological need for injury or punishment (called *conversion*).
- E. *Referred pain*—see also **Figure 10.1** for examples.

Organ	Area of Referred Pain
Heart	Neck, (L) jaw, (L) arm, upper back
Lungs	(L) shoulder
Liver	(R) shoulder, (R) side
Spleen	(R) side, back pain
Stomach	middle back, epigastric
Kidney	(R) (L) flank pain, thigh
Pancreas	LUQ
Gallbladder	Umbilical region
Appendix	RLQ
Bladder	Superpubic, posterior gluteus/thigh

- F. *Acute and chronic pain*—see **Table 10.1**.

II. **Components of pain experience**—pain related to:
- A. *Stimuli*—sources: chemical, ischemic, mechanical trauma; extremes of heat/cold.
- B. *Perception*—viewed with fear by children; can be altered by level of consciousness; interpreted and influenced by previous and current experience; is more severe when alone at night or immobilized.
- C. *Response*—variations in physiologic, *cultural*, and learned responses; anxiety is created; pain seen as justified punishment, witchcraft, fate, lifestyle; pain used as means for attention-getting; cultural groups express pain in different ways (stoic, demonstrative).

III. **Assessment**
- A. *Subjective data*:
  1. *Site*—medial, lateral, proximal, distal.
  2. *Strength*:
     - a. Certain tissues are more sensitive.
     - b. Changes in intensity.
     - c. Based on expectations.
     - d. Affected by distraction or concentration, state of consciousness.
     - e. Described as slight, medium, severe, excruciating.
  3. *Quality*—aching, burning, crushing, dull, piercing, shifting, throbbing, tingling.

TABLE 10.1 COMPARISON OF ACUTE AND CHRONIC PAIN

	Acute Pain	Chronic Pain
Onset	Sudden	Gradual or sudden
Duration	< 3 months, or expected period of recovery	> 3 months, or longer than expected period of recovery
Severity	Mild-severe	Mild-severe
Cause	Usually an indentifiable cause	Cause may or may not be identifiable
Signs/ Symptoms	Predominantly sympathetic nervous system: ↑ heart rate, respirations, BP Diaphoresis, pallor Anxiety, agitation, confusion Urine retention	Predominantly behavioral: ↓Physical activity Fatigue Social withdrawal

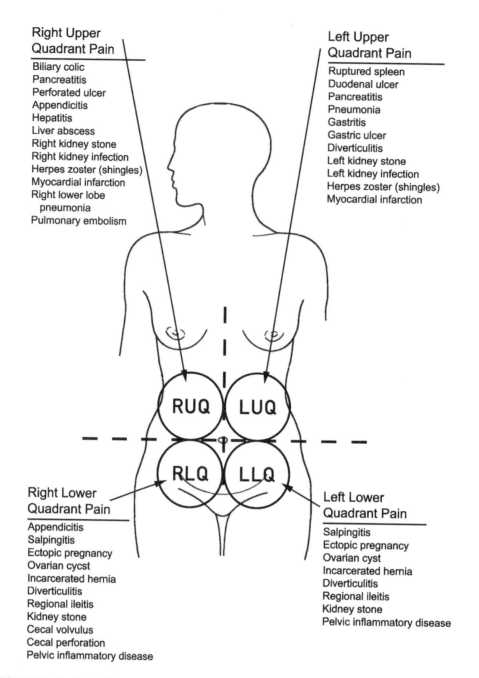

Right Upper Quadrant Pain

Biliary colic
Pancreatitis
Perforated ulcer
Appendicitis
Hepatitis
Liver abscess
Right kidney stone
Right kidney infection
Herpes zoster (shingles)
Myocardial infarction
Right lower lobe
   pneumonia
Pulmonary embolism

Left Upper Quadrant Pain

Ruptured spleen
Duodenal ulcer
Pancreatitis
Pneumonia
Gastritis
Gastric ulcer
Diverticulitis
Left kidney stone
Left kidney infection
Herpes zoster (shingles)
Myocardial infarction

Right Lower Quadrant Pain

Appendicitis
Salpingitis
Ectopic pregnancy
Ovarian cycst
Incarcerated hernia
Diverticulitis
Regional ileitis
Kidney stone
Cecal volvulus
Cecal perforation
Pelvic inflammatory disease

Left Lower Quadrant Pain

Salpingitis
Ectopic pregnancy
Ovarian cyst
Incarcerated hernia
Diverticulitis
Regional ileitis
Kidney stone
Pelvic inflammatory disease

FIGURE 10.1 POSSIBLE CAUSES OF ABDOMINAL PAIN ACCORDING TO LOCATION

4. *Antecedent factors*—physical exertion, eating, extreme temperatures, physical and emotional stressors (e.g., fear).
5. *Previous experience*—influences reaction to pain.
6. *Behavioral clues*—demanding, worried, irritable, restless, difficult to distract, sleepless.

B. *Objective data*:
   1. *Verbal clues*—moaning, groaning, crying.
   2. *Nonverbal clues*—clenching teeth, grimacing, splinting of body parts, body position, knees drawn up, involuntary reflex movements, tossing/turning, rhythmic rubbing movements, voice pitch and speed, eyes shut.
   3. *Physical clues*—breathing irregularities, abdominal distention, skin color changes, skin temperature changes, excessive salivation, perspiration.
   4. *Time/duration*—onset, duration, recurrence, interval, last occurrence. See **Table 10.2**.

▶ IV. **Analysis/nursing diagnosis**
   A. *Pain*, acute or chronic, related to specific client condition.
   B. *Activity intolerance* related to discomfort.
   C. *Sleep pattern disturbance* related to pain.
   D. *Fatigue* related to state of discomfort or emotional stress.
   E. *Ineffective individual coping* related to chronic pain.

TABLE 10.2 P²QR²S²T FORMAT FOR ASSESSING PAIN

P²   What **P**rovokes the pain? Did something in particular bring it on? Does anything make it worse? Does anything make it better? **P**oint to where the pain is?

Q   What is the **Q**uality of the pain? Dull? Sharp? Cutting? Throbbing? Crushing? Squeezing? Achy?

R²   Does the pain **R**adiate to any other area, or does it stay in one place? **R**elief: what makes it better?

S²   What is the **S**everity of the pain? Ask the client to grade it on a scale of 0 (no pain) to 10 (worst pain). **S**igns/symptoms: N/V, dizzy, SOB, diaphoresis, pallor.

T   What is the **T**iming of the pain? When did it start? What has happened to it over time (constant? intermittent? sudden? gradual? how often? gotten worse? gotten better?)? If there are associated symptoms, what is their relative timing (e.g., did the pain come on before or after the nausea?)?

Source: Adapted from Caroline NL, *Emergency Care in the Streets* [5th ed.]. Boston: Little Brown (out of print)

V. Nursing care plan/implementation

  A. Goal: *provide relief of pain.*

    1. Assess level of pain; ask client to rate on a scale of 0–10 (0 = no pain; 10 = worst pain). (**Table 10.1** and **Table 10.2**).

    2. Determine cause (see **Figure 10-1**):

      a. *Environmental factors*: noise, light, odors, motion.

      b. *Physiologic needs*: elimination, hunger, thirst, fatigue, circulatory impairment, muscle tension, ventilation, pressure on nerves.

      c. *Emotional*: fear of unknown, helplessness, loneliness (especially at night).

    3. Determine pain reactions; explore meaning of "pain" (how much, when, how long, where, why, what it feels like).

    4. *Relieve*: anger, anxiety, boredom, loneliness.

    5. Report: **sudden**, **severe**, **new** pain; pain **not** relieved by medications or comfort measures; pain associated with **casts or traction**.

    6. Try nursing comfort measures (non-drug): back rub, reassurance, reposition, relaxation techniques.

    7. *Remove pain stimulus*:

      a. Administer pain medication (**e.g.,** *analgesic, antispasmodic*) at appropriate time intervals; do *not* withhold due to overestimated danger of addiction.

      b. *Avoid* cold (to reduce immediate tissue reaction to trauma).

      c. Apply heat (to relieve ischemia).

      d. Change activity (e.g., restrict activity with cardiac pain).

      e. Change, loosen dressing.

      f. Comfort (e.g., reposition, smooth wrinkled sheets, change wet dressing).

      g. Give food (e.g., for ulcer).

    8. *Reduce pain receptor reaction.*

      a. Ointment (use as coating).

      b. Local *anesthetics*.

      c. Padding (of bony prominences).

    9. Assist with medical/surgical procedures and interventions to *block pain impulse transmission*:

      a. Injection of local anesthetic into nerve (e.g., dental).

      b. Cordotomy—sever the anterolateral spinal cord nerve tracts.

      c. Electrical stimulation—transcutaneous (skin surface), percutaneous (peripheral nerve).

      d. Peripheral nerve implant—electrode to major sensory nerve.

      e. Dorsal column stimulator—electrode to dorsal column.

    10. *Avoid causes of inadequate pain control*:

      a. Incorrect assessment.

      b. Insufficient knowledge of pharmacologic effects.

      c. Personal attitudes, e.g., concern about addiction.

      d. Fear of respiratory depression.

      e. Reluctance to accept subjective data.

    11. *Document response to pain-relief measures.*

  B. Goal: *alter pain perception* by raising pain threshold.

    1. *Distraction*, e.g., TV (cerebral cortical activity blocks impulses from thalamus).

    2. *Analgesics*—give *prior* to occurrence of severe pain; give routinely for chronic/terminal pain.

    3. *Hypnosis*—assess appropriateness of use for psychogenic pain and of anesthesia; client needs to be open to suggestion.

    4. *Acupuncture*—assess client's emotional readiness and belief in it.

  C. Goal: *alter interpretation and response to pain.*

    1. Administer *narcotics*—result: no longer sees pain as disturbing.

    2. Administer *hypnotics*—result: changes perception and decreases reaction.

    3. Help client obtain interpersonal satisfaction from ways other than attention received when in pain.

  D. Goal: *promote client control of pain and analgesia: use client-controlled analgesia* (PCA), an *analgesic* administration system designed to maintain optimal serum analgesic levels; safely delivers intermittent bolus doses of a narcotic analgesic; preset to maximum hourly dose.

1. *Advantages*: decreased client anxiety; improved pulmonary function; fewer side effects.
2. *Limitations*: requires an indwelling intravenous line; analgesic targets *central* pain, may *not relieve peripheral* discomfort; cost of PCA unit.

E. Goal: **health teaching**.
   1. Explain causes of pain and how to describe pain.
   2. Explain that it is acceptable to admit existence of pain.
   3. Relaxation exercises.
   4. Biofeedback methods of pain perception and control.
   5. Proper medication administration, when necessary, for self-care.

VI. **Evaluation/outcome criteria**
   A. Verbalizes comfort, decreased awareness of pain.
   B. Knows source of pain, how to reduce stimulus and perception.
   C. Uses alternative measures for pain relief.
   D. Able to cope with pain, e.g., remains active, relaxed appearance; verbal and nonverbal clues to pain being absent.

Summary of Key Points

1. Pain is subjective and individualized. The client knows best what pain is and whether a particular treatment has worked. Pain should be assessed without a preconceived idea of what the pain should or should not be.

2. Pain can be: acute, chronic, superficial, deep somatic, visceral, or referred.

3. Lack of predictable signs or expressions of pain does *not* mean lack of pain.

4. Clients should *not* have to tolerate pain for any reason.

5. Just because a client is sleeping, it does *not* mean the client is *not* in pain.

6. A pain assessment tool helps quantify the pain and effectiveness of treatment.

7. Anxiety *increases* pain and the need for higher doses of analgesics.

8. Pain medications should be used in combination with *nondrug interventions* such as repositioning, reassurance, a back rub, or relaxation techniques.

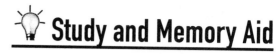

Study and Memory Aid

Pain: Management—"ABC's"

Assess by *asking* client about the pain.
Believe the client's pain is real.
Choices—let clients know their choices.
Do what you *can, when* you *said* you *would*.
Enable clients to have control over their pain.

Questions

1. Meperidine (*Demerol*) has been ordered for a client for the relief of postoperative pain. Which assessment finding is a side effect of the agent?
   1. Respiratory rate of 10 breaths/min.
   2. Blood pressure of 150/90 mm Hg.
   3. Pinpoint pupils.
   4. Urine output of 20 mL/h.

2. Which nonverbal signs observed during an admitting history would indicate a client is experiencing physical discomfort?
   1. Hesitancy in answering questions.
   2. Clenching fist and wrinkling brow.
   3. Smiling after each answer.
   4. Leaving to go to the bathroom.

3. While in the emergency department, a client receives 4 mg of morphine sulfate IV for the relief of chest pain. Soon after admission to the unit the client again complains of substernal chest pain. What should the nurse do first?
   1. Give the client another dose of morphine sulfate IV.
   2. Increase the nasal oxygen flow rate to 5 L/min.
   3. Notify the physician of the resistance to pain medication.
   4. Place the client in a high-Fowler's position.

4. The client complains of severe pain after suffering rib, arm, and leg fractures. Which pain medication would the nurse expect to provide the greatest relief?
   1. Diazepam (*Valium*) IV.
   2. Morphine sulfate IV.
   3. Meperidine hydrochloride (*Demerol*) IM.
   4. Methocarbamol (*Robaxin*) IM.

Answers/Rationale

1. **(1)** *Demerol* depresses both the rate and depth of respirations. *Demerol*, a CNS depressant, would tend to lower blood pressure, *not* cause borderline hypertension **(2)**. Pinpoint pupils **(3)** can occur in clients receiving morphine. A urine output of 20 mL/h **(4)** is inadequate and would stem from decreased renal perfusion or renal failure; *Demerol*-induced changes in vital signs would not normally lead to such an impairment of renal function. **AS, COM, 3, PhI, Pharmacological and parenteral therapies**

2. **(2)** The members of some cultures and ethnic groups are reluctant to complain of pain. Nonverbal clues to tension, such as grimacing or tight fists, may be the only indication of pain. Hesitancy **(1)** may indicate fear, shyness, or lack of understanding. Smiling **(3)** after each answer may be due to uneasiness or an attempt to be cooperative. The need to go to the bathroom during the history-taking **(4)** may be prompted by urinary frequency, urgency, or nervousness. **AS, COM, 3, PsI, Psychosocial integrity**

3. **(2)** The pain may be due to hypoxia, so the O_2 flow rate should be increased, unless a high O_2 flow rate is contraindicated (e.g. emphysema). The other actions listed may be appropriate, but this is a *priority* question. If ordered, the client could be given more morphine sulfate **(1)**, but nondrug interventions should be tried *first*. Notifying the MD **(3)** would not usually be the *first* action. Positioning **(4)** is an independent nursing action that facilitates and thereby improves breathing or lowers blood pressure but is not used for *pain* management. (The client's baseline vital signs should be assessed before positioning.) **IMP, ANL, 6, PhI, Physiological adaptation**

4. **(2)** Bone pain is considered acute pain, and an opiate such as morphine should be used for the relief of moderate to severe bone pain. It is very unlikely that tolerance and dependence will develop during such shortterm use as that necessitated by fractures. The opiates work by modifying the perception of the pain. *Valium* **(1)** and *Robaxin* **(4)** are not analgesics; they relieve pain by relaxing the muscles. Although an opiate, *Demerol* **(3)** is shorter acting than morphine sulfate and forms a toxic metabolite that stimulates the central nervous system. *Demerol* is not the drug of choice for the management of acute or chronic pain. **IMP, APP, 3, PhI, Pharmacological and parenteral therapies**

Key to Codes

Nursing process: **AS**, assessment; **AN**, analysis; **PL**, planning; **IMP**, implementation; **EV**, evaluation. (See **Appendix M** for explanation of nursing process steps.)

Cognitive level: **RE/KN**, recall/knowledge; **COM**, comprehension; **APP**, application; **ANL**, analysis; **EVL**, evaluation; **SYN**, synthesis. (See **Appendix M** for explanation.)

Category of human function: **1**, protective; **2**, sensory-perceptual; **3**, comfort, rest, activity, and mobility; **4**, nutrition; **5**, growth and development; **6**, fluid-gas transport; **7**, psychosocial-cultural; **8**, elimination. (See **Appendix 0** for explanation.)

Client need: **SECE**, safe, effective care environment; **PhI**, physiological integrity; **PsI**, psychosocial integrity; **HPM**, health promotion and maintenance. (See **Appendix P** for explanation.)

Client subneed: (See **Appendix P** for explanation)

Altered Immune System Disorders

Chapter Outline

- Acquired Immune Deficiency Syndrome (AIDS)
- Isolation Precautions
- Summary of Key Points

- Study and Memory Aids
  — Diet
  — Drug review
- Questions
- Answers/Rationale

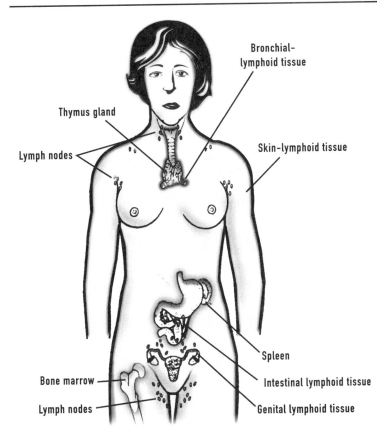

Organs of the Immune System

Acquired Immune Deficiency Syndrome (AIDS)

The terminal stage of the disease continuum caused by the human immunodeficiency virus (HIV), a retrovirus; typically progresses from asymptomatic seronegative status to asymptomatic seropositive status to subclinical immune deficiency to lymphadenopathy (*early* AIDS) to AIDS-related complex (*middle* stage with combination of symptoms) to AIDS; hallmarks of HIV infection include opportunistic infections: *Pneumocystis carinii* pneumonia (PCP), cytomegalovirus (CMV), *Mycobacterium tuberculosis*,

hepatitis B, herpes simplex or zoster, candidiasis; may take 7–10 yr before signs and symptoms occur.

I. High-risk populations
- A. Men, homosexual or bisexual (52%).
- B. Intravenous drug users (IDU) (25%).
- C. IDU/homosexual (5%).
- D. Hemophiliacs and multiple transfusion recipients (2%).
- E. Heterosexual (9%).
- F. Undetermined/other (7%).
- G. Rapidly increasing in women.

II. Pathophysiology: abnormal response to foreign antigen stimulation (acquired immunity) → deficiency in cell-mediated immunity—T lymphocytes, specifically helper cells (T4 cells) and hyperactivity of the humoral system (B cells).

III. Assessment
- A. *Subjective data:*
  1. Fatigue: prolonged; associated with headache or light-headedness.
  2. Unexplained weight loss: >10%.
- B. *Objective data:*
  1. Fever: prolonged or night sweats >2 wk.
  2. Lymphadenopathy.
  3. Skin or mucous membrane lesions: purplish red nodules (*Kaposi's sarcoma*).
  4. Cough: persistent, heavy, dry.
  5. Diarrhea: persistent.
  6. Tongue/mouth "thrush"; oral hairy leukoplakia.
  7. Lab data. *decreased*—CD4 (T4) lymphocytes, hematocrit, white blood cell count, platelets. *seropositive*—syphilis, hepatitis B; ELISA—*positive;* Western blot test—*positive* (mean time for seroconversion is 6 wk after infection) (client permission needed for ELISA and Western blot).

IV. Analysis/nursing diagnosis
- A. *Risk for infection* related to immunocompromised state.

B. *Fatigue* related to anemia.

C. *Altered nutrition, less than body requirements,* related to anorexia.

D. *Impaired skin integrity* related to nonhealing viral lesions, Kaposi's sarcoma.

E. *Diarrhea* related to infection or parasites.

F. *Risk for activity intolerance* related to shortness of breath.

G. *Ineffective airway clearance* related to pneumonia.

H. *Visual/sensory/perception alteration* related to retinitis.

I. *Risk for altered body temperature* (fever) related to opportunistic infections.

J. *Social isolation* related to stigma attached to AIDS.

K. *Powerlessness* related to inability to control disease progression.

L. *Altered thought processes* related to dementia.

M. *Ineffective individual coping* related to poor prognosis.

N. *Risk for violence, self-directed,* related to anger, panic, or depression.

V. Nursing care plan/implementation

A. Goal: *reduce risk of infection; slow disease progression.*

1. Observe for signs of opportunistic infections: weight loss, diarrhea, skin lesions, sore throat.

2. Monitor vital signs (including temperature).

3. Note secretions and excretions: changes in color, consistency, or odor indicating infection.

4. *Diet*: monitor fluid and electrolytes; strict measurement; encourage adequate dietary intake (*high calorie, high nutrient, low bulk*); 5–10 times recommended daily allowance of water-soluble vitamins (B complex, C); favorite foods from home; enteral feedings.

5. *Protective isolation,* if indicated, for severe immunocompromise.

6. Medications, as ordered: trimethoprim-sulfamethoxazole (*Septra*), acyclovir (*Zovirax*), and/or pentamidine; do *not* give at mealtime; may need antinauseants or antiemetics to control side effects.

   a. *Reverse transcriptase inhibitors*—blocks the conversion of HIV RNA to HIV DNA.
      (1) Zidovudine (*Ribovir*).
      (2) Combination drug *Trivir.*

   b. *Protease inhibitors*—interferes with activity of enzyme protease.
      (1) Ritonavir (*Norvir*).
      (2) Saquinavir (*Fortovase*).
      (3) Nelfinavir (*Viracept*).

   c. *Fusion inhibitors*—prevents binding of HIV to cell.
      (1) Enfuvirtide (*Fuzeon*).

B. Goal: *prevent the spread of disease.*

1. Frequent handwashing, even after wearing gloves.

2. *Avoid* exposure to blood, body fluids of client; wear gloves, gowns; proper disposal of needles, IV catheters (**Table 11.1**)

C. Goal: *provide physical and psychological support.*

1. Oral care: frequent.

2. Cooling bath: tepid water; *avoid* plastic-backed pads with night sweats.

3. Encourage verbalization of fears, concerns without condemnation; may suffer loss of job, life-style, significant other.

4. Determine status of support network: arrange contact with support group.

5. Observe for severe emotional symptoms (suicidal tendencies).

6. Address issues surrounding death to ensure quality of life: designation of durable power of attorney for health care, code blue status, reassurance of comfort and pain control.

D. Goal: **health teaching.**

1. Avoidance of environmental sources of infection (kitty litter, bird cages, tub bathing).

2. Precautions following discharge: risk-reducing behaviors—condoms (latex), limit number of sexual partners, *avoid* exposure to blood or semen during intercourse.

3. Family counseling, availability of community resources.

4. Information on disease progression and life span.

5. Stress reduction techniques: visualization, guided imagery, meditation.

6. Expected side effects with drug therapy, importance of compliance.

VI. Evaluation/outcome criteria

A. Relief of symptoms (e.g., afebrile, gains weight).

B. Resumes self-care activities, returns to work, improved quality of life.

C. Accepts diagnosis, participates in support group.

D. Progression of disease slows, improved survival probability.

E. Retains autonomy, self-worth.

F. Permitted to die with dignity.

TABLE 11.1 SUMMARY OF CDC GUIDELINES FOR ISOLATION PRECAUTIONS IN HEALTH CARE FACILITIES

	Standard Precautions	Transmission-based Precautions		
		Airborne Precautions	**Droplet Precautions**	**Contact Precautions**
When to use	Use with all clients	• Use, in addition to **Standard Precautions**, in clients known to be or suspected of illness with pathogens transmitted by airborne droplet (< 5 microns). Examples: Measles Tuberculosis Varicella	• Use, in addition to **Standard Precautions**, in clients known to be or suspected of illness with pathogens transmitted by airborne droplet (> 5 microns). Examples: *Haemophilus influenzae*, type b Diphtheria *Mycoplasma* pneumonia *Neisseria* meningitis Pertussis Pneumonic plague *Streptococcal* group A Adenovirus Influenza Mumps Rubella Parvovirus B19	• Use, in addition to **Standard Precautions**, in clients known to be or suspected of illness with pathogens transmitted by direct client contact or contact with items in the client's environment. Examples: *Clostridium difficile* *Escherichia coli* *Shigella* Hepatitis A Respiratory syncytial virus, parainfluenza virus, enteroviral infections in infants and young children Cutaneous diphtheria Herpes simplex virus Impetigo Major abscesses, cellulitis, or decubiti Pediculosis Scabies Staphylococcal furunculosis in infants and young children Zoster Viral hemorrhagic conjunctivitis Viral hemorrhagic infections (Ebola, Lassa, Marburg)

(continued)

TABLE 11.1 SUMMARY OF CDC GUIDELINES FOR ISOLATION PRECAUTIONS IN HEALTH CARE FACILITIES (*continued*)

	Standard Precautions	Transmission-based Precautions		
		Airborne Precautions	Droplet Precautions	Contact Precautions
Hand washing	• Wash hands promptly and thoroughly between client contacts and after contact with blood, body fluids, secretions, excretions, and equipment or articles contaminated by them. • Wash hands after gloves are removed	Same as **Standard Precautions**	Same as **Standard Precautions**	Same as **Standard Precautions**
Gloves	Wear gloves when touching: blood, body fluids, secretions, excretions, mucous membranes, and nonintact skin; to prevent the transmission of microorganisms on the hands of personnel to clients *during invasive* or other procedures that involve touching a client's mucous membranes and nonintact skin; to prevent transmission of pathogens on *contaminated hands* of personnel to another client; change gloves between client contacts and wash hands after gloves are removed. **Wearing gloves does not replace the need for meticulous hand hygiene.**	Same as **Standard Precautions**	Same as **Standard Precautions**	In addition to **Standard Precautions**, wear gloves when entering a room to provide direct client care, or having contact with potentially contaminated surfaces in client's environment

(continued)

TABLE 11.1 SUMMARY OF CDC GUIDELINES FOR ISOLATION PRECAUTIONS IN HEALTH CARE FACILITIES (*continued*)

	Standard Precautions	Transmission-based Precautions		
		Airborne Precautions	Droplet Precautions	Contact Precautions
Mask, eye, and face protection	Wear a mask that covers both the nose and the mouth, and goggles or a face shield during procedures and client-care activities that are likely to generate splashes or sprays of blood, body fluids, secretions, or excretions.	In addition to **Standard Precautions**, wear respiratory protection when entering the room of a client known to have or suspected of having tuberculosis.	In addition to **Standard Precautions**, wear a mask when working within 3 feet of client.	Same as **Standard Precautions**.
Gown	Wear clean, non-sterile gown to prevent contamination of clothing and protect skin from blood and body fluid exposures.	Same as **Standard Precautions**.	Same as **Standard Precautions**.	Wear clean, non-sterile gown if client is incontinent or has diarrhea, or has wound drainage; if contact with surfaces or items in client environment is expected.
Linen	Handle, transport, and launder in a manner that avoids transfer of microorganisms to clients, personnel, and environments; use hygienic and common sense storage and processing of linen.	Same as **Standard Precautions**.	Same as **Standard Precautions**.	Same as **Standard Precautions**.
Client transport		Limit movement and transport of clients only for essential purposes; use appropriate barriers (e.g., masks, impervious dressings) on the client ;notify personnel in the area to which the client is to be taken of the impending arrival of the client and of the precautions to be used; inform clients of ways they can assist in preventing the transmission of infectious microorganisms to others.	Same as **Airborne Precautions**	Same as **Airborne Precautions**

See CDC website for more information: www.cdc.gov

Summary of Key Points

1. HIV is not transmitted through casual contact but through some exposure to body fluids from a person who is infected.
2. Because of the compromised immune status, the client with AIDS is at greater risk for acquiring numerous opportunistic infections.
3. Pneumocystis carinii pneumonia is often the opportunistic infection that leads to a definitive diagnosis of AIDS.
4. Standard precautions, which include barrier guidelines and needle precautions, protect against exposure to blood-borne pathogens.
5. A health care worker is more likely to contract hepatitis; however, because AIDS is so devastating and not curable, there is greater fear; standard precautions must be followed.
6. Drug therapy does not cure AIDS but delays further destruction of the immune system.
7. Nursing care should focus on symptom management and dealing with the fears of isolation, loss, and death.

Study and Memory Aids

 ### Diet

AIDS

| ↑ Calorie | ↓ Bulk |
| Nutrient | |

Drug Review

Drug Review—AIDS

Acyclovir (*Zovirax*): 800 mg q4h
Pentamidine: 4 mg/kg/d
Ritonavir (*Norvir*): 600 mg PO bid
Trimethoprim/sulfamethoxazole (*Septra*): treatment of active disease: 15–20 mg/kg/d in 3–4 divided doses q6–8h for >2 months; prevention of *Pneumocystis carinii* pneumonia 160 mg/d
Zidovudine (*Retrovir*) (*AZT*): 200 mg q4h 5 times a day

Questions

1. A client hospitalized with AIDS who has a white blood cell count (WBC) of 1500 mm³ is scheduled for a chest x-ray. The best action on the part of the nurse would be to:
   1. Put a mask and gown on the client before transporting to the x-ray department.
   2. Arrange for an x-ray to be done with a portable machine in the client's room.
   3. Have the x-ray staff wear gowns, gloves, and masks while doing the x-ray.
   4. Have housekeeping clean the x-ray room thoroughly before the client arrives.

2. The nurse would instruct a client with AIDS who is taking zidovudine (*AZT*) to avoid taking aspirin because:
   1. This would increase the chance of gastric irritation.
   2. The risk for granulocytopenia would be increased.
   3. This will cause a further reduction in the thrombocyte count.
   4. The symptoms of infection would then be masked.

3. When caring for a client on enteric isolation, which measure would the nurse observe?
   1. Wear a gown and gloves when entering the client's room.
   2. Wear a mask when giving direct care to the client.
   3. Wear a gown and gloves if there is a chance of fecal contact.
   4. Wear a mask and gloves only when giving direct care.

4. Health care teaching about the most effective way to eliminate the transmission of infection through handwashing would include teaching all family members to:
   1. Rinse their hands with fingers pointing downward.
   2. Use friction when washing.
   3. Use friction and clean under fingernails.
   4. Rinse and dry hands well.

5. For which type of isolation should the nurse prepare a client who has a WBC of 600 mm³?
   1. Respiratory.
   2. Enteric.
   3. Reverse.
   4. General.

Answers/Rationale

1. **(2)** The client is at great risk for infection because of a severely immunosuppressed state. Obtaining the x-ray with a portable machine reduces the risk to the client. Removing the client **(1)** from protective isolation poses a risk to the client. Protecting the x-ray staff **(3)** is not as important as protecting the client. The safest environment for the client is own room; cleaning the x-ray room **(4)** may not be realistic. **IMP, APP, 1, SECE, Safety and infection control**

2. **(2)** The co-administration of aspirin or acetaminophen with *AZT* causes the metabolism of *AZT* to be inhibited, leading to granulocytopenia. The chance of gastric irritation **(1)**, although always a possible side effect of aspirin, is *not* any greater when it is taken in combination with *AZT*. The number of granulocytes, *not* thrombocytes **(3)**, would decrease. Infection may be masked **(4)** in clients taking *steroids*. **IMP, COM, 1, PhI, Pharmacological and parenteral therapies**

3. **(3)** A gown and gloves should be worn any time contact with infective material is possible. It is otherwise not necessary for a nurse to wear a gown or gloves **(1)**; in enteric isolation, a mask **(2)**, or a mask and gloves **(4)** are not necessary when giving direct care. **IMP, COM, 8, SECE, Safety and infection control**

4. **(3)** All of the techniques in the other options are appropriate, but the *most* effective one is to use friction to rub off pathogens and to clean under the fingernails where they can collect. The other options are *less* effective **(1 and 4)** or *incomplete* **(2)**. **IMP, APP, 1, SECE, Safety and infection control**

5. **(3)** The normal WBC is 5000 to 10000 mm^3; a count of 600 mm^3 is extremely low and such a client is immunosuppressed. The risk of infection is great as a result, and the client should be protected from infection by placing him/her in reverse or protective isolation. The other types of isolation **(1, 2, and 4)** are designed to protect staff and visitors from the client, *not* to protect the client. **IMP, APP, 1, SECE, Safety and infection control**

Key to Codes

Nursing process: AS, assessment; AN, analysis; PL, planning; IMP, implementation; EV, evaluation. (See **Appendix M** for explanation of nursing process steps.)

Cognitive level: RE/KN, recall/knowledge; COM, comprehension; APP, application; ANL, analysis; EVL, evaluation; SYN, synthesis. (See **Appendix M** for explanation.)

Category of human function: 1, protective; 2, sensory-perceptual; 3, comfort, rest, activity, and mobility; 4, nutrition; 5, growth and development; 6, fluid-gas transport; 7, psychosocial-cultural; 8, elimination. (See **Appendix 0** for explanation.)

Client need: SECE, safe, effective care environment; PhI, physiological integrity; PsI, psychosocial integrity; HPM, health promotion and maintenance. (See **Appendix P** for explanation.)

Client subneed: (See **Appendix P** for explanation)

Connective Tissue Disorders

Chapter Outline

- Rheumatoid Arthritis
- Systemic Lupus Erythematosus
- Lyme Disease
- Summary of Key Points

- Study and Memory Aids
  - Diet
  - Drug review
- Questions
- Answers/Rationale

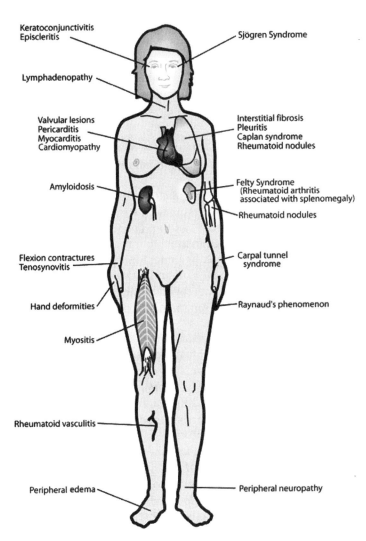

Keratoconjunctivitis
Episcleritis

Sjögren Syndrome

Lymphadenopathy

Valvular lesions
Pericarditis
Myocarditis
Cardiomyopathy

Interstitial fibrosis
Pleuritis
Caplan syndrome
Rheumatoid nodules

Amyloidosis

Felty Syndrome
(Rheumatoid arthritis
associated with splenomegaly)

Rheumatoid nodules

Flexion contractures
Tenosynovitis

Carpal tunnel
syndrome

Hand deformities

Raynaud's phenomenon

Myositis

Rheumatoid vasculitis

Peripheral edema

Peripheral neuropathy

Selected Complications Associated with Connective Tissue Disorders (especially with Rheumatoid Arthritis)

Rheumatoid Arthritis

Chronic, systemic collagen inflammatory disease; etiology unknown; may be autoimmune, viral, or genetic; affects primarily women 20–40 yr of age; present in *2%–3%* of total population; follows a course of exacerbations and remissions.

I. **Pathophysiology**: synovitis with edema → proliferation of vascular granulation tissue (formation of pannus) → destruction and fibrosis of cartilage (fibrous ankylosis); calcification of fibrous tissue (osseous ankylosis).

II. **Assessment**
   A. *Subjective data*:
      1. Joints: pain, stiffness, swelling.
      2. Easily fatigues; malaise.
      3. Anorexia; weight loss.
   B. *Objective data*:
      1. Subcutaneous nodules over bony prominences.
      2. Bilateral symmetric involvement of joints: crepitation, creaking, grating.
      3. Deformities: contractures, muscle atrophy.
      4. Lab data: blood: *decreased*—red blood cells (RBCs); *increased*—white blood cell count (WBCs) (12,000–15,000/mm^3), sedimentation rate (>20 mm/h), rheumatoid factor.

III. **Analysis/nursing diagnosis**
   A. *Pain* related to joint destruction.
   B. *Impaired physical mobility* related to joint contractures.
   C. *Risk for injury* related to the inflammatory process.
   D. *Body image disturbance* related to joint deformity.
   E. *Self-care deficit* related to musculoskeletal impairment.
   F. *Risk for activity intolerance* related to fatigue and stiffness.

G. *Altered nutrition, less than body requirements,* related to anorexia and weight loss.

H. *Self-esteem disturbance* related to chronic illness.

▶◀ IV. **Nursing care plan/implementation**

A. Goal: *prevent or correct deformities.*

1. Activity:

a. *Bed rest* during exacerbations.

☞ b. Daily range of motion (ROM) exercises—active and passive exercises *even* in acute phase for 5–10-min periods; *avoid* fatigue and persistent pain.

⬮ c. Heat and/or *pain* medication before exercise.

⬮ 2. Medications as ordered: *aspirin* (high dosages); *nonsteroidals; steroids; antacids* given for possible GI upset with ASA, steroids; *disease-modifying antirheumatic drugs* (DMARDs); *immunosuppressants;* biologic therapy.

3. *Fluids:* at least 1500 mL liquid daily to prevent renal calculi; milk for gastrointestinal (GI) upset.

▥ B. Goal: **health teaching.**

1. Side effects of medications: tarry stools (GI bleeding), tinnitus (aspirin).

2. Psychosocial aspects: possible need for early retirement, financial hardship, loss of libido, unsatisfactory sexual relations.

3. Prepare for joint repair or replacement if indicated.

▶◀ V. **Evaluation/outcome criteria**

A. Remains as active as possible, limited loss of mobility; performs self-care activities.

B. No side effects from drug therapy (e.g., GI bleeding).

C. Copes with necessary life-style changes; complies with treatment.

Systemic Lupus Erythematosus (SLE)

Chronic inflammatory disease of connective tissue; may affect or involve any organ; vague etiology, but genetic factors, viruses, hormones, or drugs are being investigated; occurs *primarily in women* aged 18–35 yr; no known cure; treatment is symptomatic.

I. **Pathophysiology**: possible toxic effects from immune complexes deposited in tissue—fibrinoid necrosis of collagen in connective tissue, small arterial walls (kidneys and heart particularly) → cellular death, obstructed blood flow.

▶◀ II. **Assessment**

A. *Subjective data:*

1. Pain: joints.

2. Anorexia, weight loss.

3. Photophobia, sensitivity to sun.

4. Weakness.

5. Nausea, vomiting.

B. *Objective data:*

1. Fever.

2. Rash: butterfly distribution across nose, cheeks.

3. Ulcerations: oral or nasopharyngeal.

〰 4. Lab data: blood: *increased* LE cells; *decreased* RBCs, WBCs, thrombocytes; *urine:* hematuria, proteinuria (nephritis).

▶◀ III. **Analysis/nursing diagnosis**

A. *Risk for injury* related to possible autoimmune disorder.

B. *Pain* related to joint inflammation.

C. *Risk for activity intolerance* related to extreme fatigue, anemia.

D. *Impaired skin integrity* related to sunlight sensitivity and rashes.

E. *Altered nutrition, less than body requirements,* related to anorexia, nausea, vomiting.

F. *Altered oral mucous membrane* related to ulcerations.

▶◀ IV. **Nursing care plan/implementation**

A. Goal: *minimize or limit immune response and complications.*

1. Activity: rest; 8–10h sleep; unhurried environment; assist with stressful activities; ☞ ROM exercises to prevent joint immobility and stiffness.

☞ ⬮ 2. Skin care: hygiene; topical *steroid* cream as ordered for inflammation, pruritus, scaling.

🍎 3. *Mouth care:* several times daily if stomatitis present; *soft, bland,* or *liquid* diet to prevent irritation.

🍎 4. *Diet: low sodium* if edematous; *low protein* with renal involvement.

5. Observe for signs of complications:

a. *Cardiac/respiratory* (tachycardia, tachypnea, dyspnea, orthopnea).

b. *GI* (diarrhea, abdominal pain, distention).

c. *Renal* (*increased* weight, oliguria, *decreased* specific gravity).

d. *Neurologic* (ptosis, ataxia).

e. *Hematologic* (malaise, weakness, chills, epistaxis); **report immediately.**

⬮ 6. Medications, as ordered:

a. *Analgesics.*

b. *Anti-inflammatory* agents (aspirin, prednisone) and *immunosuppressive* drugs (azathioprine [*Imuran*], cyclophosphamide [*Cytoxan*]) to control inflammation.

c. *Antimalarials* for skin and joint manifestations.

B. Goal: health teaching.
   1. Disease process: diagnosis, prognosis, effects of treatment.
   2. *Avoid* precipitating factors:
      a. Sun (aggravates skin lesions; thus, cover body as much as possible).
      b. Altering dosage of medications.
      c. Pregnancy (need medical clearance).
      d. Fatigue, stress.
      e. Infections.
   3. Medications: side effects of immunosuppressives and corticosteroids.
   4. Regular exercise: walking, swimming; but *avoid* fatigue.
   5. Wear MedicAlert bracelet.

V. Evaluation/outcome criteria
   A. Attains a state of remission.
   B. No organ involvement (e.g., cardiac, renal complications).
   C. Keeps active within limitations.
   D. Continues follow-up medical care—recognizes symptoms requiring immediate attention.

Lyme Disease

A spirochetal illness (syndrome) carried by infected ticks; incidence greatest during May through August when people are outdoors and wearing fewer clothes; only a small percentage of people hospitalized.

I. Classification
   A. Stages:
      I. Rash at site of tick bite; *bull's-eye* or target pattern; may appear as hives or cellulitis; common in moist areas (groin, armpit, behind knees). Flulike symptoms may occur (joint pain, chills, fever).
      II. If untreated, may progress to cardiac problems (10% of clients) or neurologic disturbances—Bell's palsy (10% of clients); occasionally meningitis, encephalitis, and eye damage may result.
      III. From 4 wk to a year after the tick bite, "arthritis" develops in half the clients. If it goes untreated, chronic neurologic problems may develop.

II. Assessment (depends on stage)
   A. *Subjective data*:
      1. Malaise (I).
      2. Headache (I).
      3. Joint, neck, or back pain (I and III).
      4. Weakness (II and III).
      5. Chest pain (II).
      6. Light-headedness (II).
      7. Numbness, pain in arms or legs (III).
   B. *Objective data*:
      1. Rash—erythema migrans (I).
      2. Dysrhythmias, heart block (II).
      3. Facial paralysis (II).
      4. Conjunctivitis, iritis, optic neuritis (II).
      5. Lab data: Lyme titer—*elevated* (II and III).
      6. *Diagnostic tests:* joint aspiration—fibrous exudate, WBCs, immune complexes; synovium biopsy—lymphocytic infiltrates.

III. Analysis/nursing diagnosis
   A. *Anxiety* related to diagnosis.
   B. *Pain* related to joint inflammation.
   C. *Fatigue* related to viral illness.
   D. *Impaired physical mobility* related to joint pain.
   E. *Altered thought processes* related to neurologic deficit.
   F. *Decreased cardiac output* related to dysrhythmias.
   G. *Knowledge deficit* related to treatment and course of disease.

IV. Nursing care plan/implementation
   A. Goal: *minimize irreversible tissue damage and complications.*
      1. Medications: *Stage* I—oral *antibiotics* for 21 d (doxycycline and penicillin V), *Stages* II *and* III—intravenous antibiotics for 14 d (penicillin or ceftriaxone).
      2. If hospitalized, monitor vital signs q4h for increased temperature, signs of heart failure; check level of consciousness and cranial nerve functioning.
      3. Note treatment response: worsening of symptoms during first 24 h; redder rash, higher fever, greater pain (*Jarisch-Herxheimer reaction*).
   B. Goal: *alleviate pain, promote comfort.*
      1. Medications: *salicylates, nonsteroidal anti-inflammatory agents*, or other *analgesic*, as ordered; observe for side effects (GI irritation).
      2. Rest: give instructions on relaxation techniques, create a quiet environment.
   C. Goal: *maintain physical and psychological well-being.*
      1. Activity: *ROM* exercises at regular intervals; medicate for pain prior to exercise; encourage proper posture to reduce joint stress, rest periods between activities and treatments.
      2. Referral: occupational and/or physical therapy as appropriate.
      3. Reassurance: give psychological support, encourage discussion of feelings.
   D. Goal: **health teaching.**
      1. Information on disease.
      2. Instructions for home IV antibiotics with heparin lock, if ordered.
      3. Side effects of antibiotics (drug specific), importance of completing therapy.
      4. Signs of disease recurrence (later stages of disease: less severe attacks).

5. Preventing subsequent infections: wear proper clothing and tick repellent on clothing; conduct "tick checks" on self, children, and pets.

V. Evaluation/outcome criteria
   A. Achieves reasonable comfort.
   B. Regains normal physiologic and psychological functioning—no irreversible complications; vital signs within normal limits.
   C. Resumes previous activity level, returns to work.
   D. Adheres to follow-up care recommendations.
   E. Knows ways to minimize risk of reinfection.

Summary of Key Points

1. Disorders of connective tissue or collagen disease characteristically involve *inflammation of multiple organs.*

2. There is *no* way to *prevent* connective tissue disorders, and there is *no cure.* Treatment is symptomatic and intended to maintain optimum functioning and self-care.

3. Rheumatoid arthritis and systemic lupus erythematosus occur more frequently in *women* aged 20–40 yr, striking during the prime of life.

4. Control of *pain* is a major nursing concern in clients with rheumatoid arthritis, as is limited *mobility* and increasing loss of *joint function.*

5. The cause of death in clients with systemic lupus erythematosus is most commonly related to *renal* failure, *cardiac* involvement, or *cerebral* infarct.

Study and Memory Aids

Diet

SLE

* Bland
* Liquid
* Soft $\quad+ \downarrow$ Protein
                    Sodium

Drug Review

Rheumatoid Arthritis

Antimalarial
Chloroquine phosphate (*Aralen* phosphate) with primaquine phosphate: 300 mg of chloroquine base once weekly with evening meal
Histamine receptor antagonist: Ranitidine (*Zantac*): 150 mg bid
Immunosuppressive agent: Methotrexate (*Mexate*): 7.5 mg/wk
Nonsteroidal anti-inflammatory
Aspirin: 325–1000 mg q4–6h, *not* to exceed 4 g/d (enteric coated to reduce gastric irritation; antacids to relieve GI upset)
Ibuprofen (*Motrin*): 300–800 mg 3–4 times a day
Naproxen (*Naprosyn*): 250—500 mg bid
Tolmetin (*Tolectin*): 400 mg tid
Steroids (should **never** be abruptly discontinued; gradually taper dose to avoid complications)
Dexamethasone (*Decadron*): 0.75—9 mg/d in single or divided doses
Methylprednisolone (*Medrol*): 4–48 mg/d
Prednisone (*Deltasone*): 5–60 mg/d.

Systemic Lupus Erythematosus

Analgesic
Aspirin: 325-1000 mg q4-6h, *not* to exceed 4 g/d (enteric coated to reduce gastric irritation; antacids to relieve GI upset)
Antimalarial
Chloroquine phosphate (*Aralen* phosphate) with primaquine phosphate: 300 mg of chloroquine base once weekly with evening meal.
Immunosuppressive agents
Azathioprine (*Imuran*): 1 mg/kg/d for 6–8 wk, increase to 2.5/kg/d
Cyclophosphamide (*Cytoxan*): 1-5 mg/kg/d
Methotrexate (*Mexate*): 7.5 mg/wk
Nonsteroidal anti-inflammatory
Ibuprofen (*Motrin*): 200-400 mg q4-6h
Naproxen (*Naprosyn*): 250-500 mg bid
Tolmetin (*Tolectin*): 400 mg tid

Lyme Disease

Ceftriaxone (*Rocephin*): 1–2 g/d
Doxycycline (*Vibramycin*): 100–200 mg in divided doses q12h
Penicillin V Potassium (*Pen Vee K*): 125–500 mg q6h
Penicillin: IV, 1–2 g/d in divided doses q4–6h

Questions

1. The nurse should encourage a client with rheumatoid arthritis who is suffering severe morning stiffness to:
   1. Use an electric blanket at night.
   2. Take a hot bath before going to bed and after arising in the morning.
   3. Drink a hot herb tea upon awakening.
   4. Take aspirin or a nonsteroidal anti-inflammatory drug (NSAID) 30 minutes before walking.
2. The nurse would conclude that the most likely cause of fever and tachycardia in a client with rheumatoid arthritis is:
   1. Dehydration and malnutrition.
   2. Drug toxicity resulting from ASA or NSAID.
   3. Joint pain and inflammation.
   4. GI tract bleeding resulting from excessive ASA use.
3. A client with acute rheumatoid arthritis is being treated with aspirin and prednisone. For what serious side effect of both drugs should the nurse monitor?
   1. Melena stool.
   2. Headaches.
   3. Diplopia.
   4. Tinnitus.
4. A client with rheumatoid arthritis is hesitant to move his acutely inflamed shoulder for fear that this may worsen his pain. The best response by the nurse would be:
   1. "Instead of exercising, let me massage your shoulder for relief."
   2. "Initially it may hurt more, but exercise can actually relieve pain."
   3. "I'll give you *aspirin* and in 30 minutes you'll be able to exercise vigorously."
   4. "Rest for your shoulder has been prescribed until the inflammation subsides."

Answers/Rationale

1. **(4)** An anti-inflammatory agent would improve mobility by easing the joint inflammation. *Aspirin* (ASA) continues to be the drug of choice for the relief of joint pain. Locally applied heat (**1** or **2**) may only work for *some* clients. Oral heat such as that provided by a hot herb tea drink (**3**) does *not* usually have any localized effect on joint stiffness. **IMP, APP, 3, PhI, Reduction of risk potential**

2. **(3)** Rheumatoid arthritis is an autoimmune, systemic inflammatory disorder of the connective tissue; the inflammation and resulting pain would cause fever and increase the heart rate. Although while dehydration (**1**) can increase temperature and heart rate, despite their ill appearance, clients with rheumatoid arthritis are *not* typically dehydrated or malnourished. Fever and tachycardia are also *not* side effects of ASA or NSAID therapy (**2**). Although GI tract bleeding is a side effect of ASA use (**4**) and tachycardia would occur if this led to severe blood loss, *fever* would *not* be expected. **AN, APP, 3, PhI, Physiological adaptation**

3. **(1)** Both drugs can cause GI tract irritation and bleeding; melena stool, or black tarry stool, signifies upper GI tract bleeding. Headaches (**2**) are a side effect of *prednisone only*. Diplopia (**3**) is *not* a side effect of either drug. Tinnitus (**4**) only occurs in clients taking high doses of *aspirin*. **EV, COM, 1, PhI, Pharmacological and parenteral therapies**

4. **(2)** Exercise is done even during an acute flare-up of rheumatoid arthritis and may help to reduce the pain. Massage (**1**) is effective but *not as much* as exercise. Pain medication should be given, but the exercise should *not* be *vigorous* (**3**). Complete rest (**4**) may increase the immobility of the limb, so *some exercise* is *needed*. **IMP, APP, 3, PhI, Basic care and comfort**

Key to Codes

Nursing process: **AS,** assessment; **AN,** analysis; **PL,** planning; **IMP,** implementation; **EV,** evaluation. (See **Appendix M** for explanation of nursing process steps.)

Cognitive level: **RE/KN,** recall/knowledge; **COM,** comprehension; **APP,** application; **ANL,** analysis; **EVL,** evaluation; **SYN,** synthesis. (See **Appendix M** for explanation.)

Category of human function: **1,** protective; **2,** sensory-perceptual; **3,** comfort, rest, activity, and mobility; **4,** nutrition; **5,** growth and development; **6,** fluid-gas transport; **7,** psychosocial-cultural; **8,** elimination. (See **Appendix 0** for explanation.)

Client need: **SECE,** safe, effective care environment; **PhI,** physiological integrity; **PsI,** psychosocial integrity; **HPM,** health promotion and maintenance. (See **Appendix P** for explanation.)

Client subneed: (See **Appendix P** for explanation)

Biliary and Pancreatic Disorders

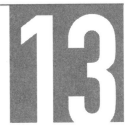

Chapter Outline

- Pancreatitis
- Diabetes
- Hyperglycemic Hyperosmolar Nonketotic Coma
- Cholecystitis/Cholelithiasis
- Summary of Key Points
- Study and Memory Aids
  - Diagnostic Studies/Procedures
    - Glucose Testing

- Ultrasound (sonagram)
- Cholecystogram
- Cholangiogram
- Diet
- Drug review
- Questions
- Answers/Rationale

Pancreatitis

Inflammatory disease of the pancreas that may result in autodigestion of the pancreas by its own enzymes.

I. **Pathophysiology:** proteolytic enzymes within the pancreas are activated by endotoxins, exotoxins, ischemia, anoxia, or trauma. Pancreatic enzymes begin process of autodigestion of pancreas and surrounding tissues; also activate other enzymes that digest cellular membranes. Autodigestion leads to: edema, hemorrhage, vascular damage, coagulation necrosis, and fat necrosis.

II. **Risk factors/causes:**
   A. Obesity.
   B. Alcoholism, alcohol consumption.
   C. Biliary tract disease.
   D. Abdominal trauma.
   E. Surgery.
   F. Drugs.
   G. Metabolic diseases.
   H. Intestinal disease.
   I. Infections.
   J. Carcinoma.
   K. Adenoma.
   L. Hypercalcemia.

III. **Assessment**
   A. *Subjective data:*
      1. Pain:
         a. Sudden onset; severe, widespread, constant, and incapacitating.
         b. Location—epigastrium, right and left upper quadrants of abdomen; radiates to back, flanks, and substernal area.
      2. Nausea.
      3. History of risk factors.
      4. Dyspnea.

   B. *Objective data:*
      1. *Elevated:* temperature, pulse, respirations, blood pressure (BP) (unless in shock).
      2. *Decreased* breath sounds related to atelectasis/pleural effusion.
      3. *Increased* crackles, cyanosis.
      4. Hemorrhage, shock.
      5. Vomiting.
      6. Fluid and electrolyte imbalances, dehydration.
      7. *Decreased* bowel sounds, abdominal tenderness with guarding.
      8. *Stools:* bulky, pale, foul smelling.
      9. *Skin:* pale, moist, cold; may be jaundiced.
      10. Muscle rigidity.
      11. Supine position leads to increased pain.
      12. Lab data:
         a. *Elevated:*
            (1) Amylase: serum and urine
            (2) Serum lipase, aspartate aminotransferase (AST) (serum glutamic-oxaloacetic transaminase [SGOT]).
            (3) Alkaline phosphatase.
            (4) Bilirubin, glucose: serum and urine.
            (5) Urine protein, white blood cell count (WBC).
            (6) Leukocytes
            (7) Blood urea nitrogen (BUN).
         b. *Decreased:*
            (1) Serum calcium.
            (2) Protein.

IV. **Analysis/nursing diagnosis**
   A. *Altered nutrition, less than body requirements,* related to nausea and vomiting.
   B. *Pain* related to inflammatory and autodigestive processes of pancreas.
   C. *Fluid volume deficit* related to inflammation, decreased intake, and vomiting.

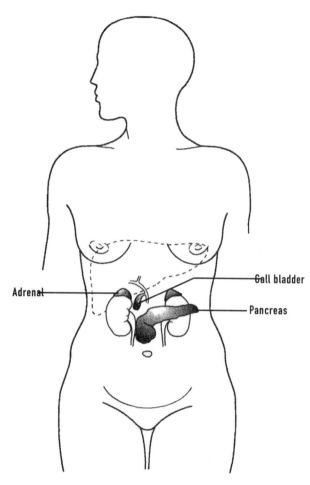

Biliary and Pancreatic Organs

D. *Ineffective breathing pattern* related to pain and pleural effusion.

E. *Knowledge deficit* related to risk factors and disease management.

V. Nursing care plan/implementation

A. Goal: *control pain.*

  1. Medications: *analgesics*—meperidine (*not* morphine or codeine due to spasmodic effect).

  2. *Position:* sitting with knees flexed.

B. Goal: *rest injured pancreas.*

  1. NPO.

  2. Nasogastric (NG) tube connected to low suction.

  3. Medications:

    a. *Antiulcer;* e.g., cimetidine (*Tagamet*); proton pump inhibitors, omeprazole (*Prilosec*).

    b. *Antiinfectives;* e.g., cephalothin (*Keflin*), cephalexin (*Keflex*).

    c. *Antiemetics;* e.g., prochlorperazine (*Compazine*).

    d. *Antispasmodics;* e.g., dicyclomine (*Bentyl*).

C. Goal: *prevent fluid and electrolyte imbalance.*

  1. Monitor: vital signs, central venous pressure.

  2. Administer IVs: fluids, blood, albumin, plasma.

D. Goal: *prevent respiratory and metabolic complications.*

  1. Cough, deep breathe, change position.

  2. Monitor: blood sugar level, as ordered.

  3. Monitor calcium levels: *Chvostek's* and *Trousseau's sign* are positive when calcium deficit exists (see **Thyroidectomy, p. 232,** for description of tests).

E. Goal: *provide adequate nutrition.*

  1. *Low fat diet.*

  2. Bland, small, frequent meals.

  3. Vitamin supplements.

  4. *Avoid* alcohol.

F. Goal: *prevent complications.*

  1. Monitor for signs of:

    a. Peritonitis.

    b. Bowel obstruction, perforation.

    c. Respiratory complications.

    d. Hypotension, shock.

    e. Disseminated intravascular coagulation.

    f. Hemorrhage from ulcers, varices.

    g. Anemia.

    h. Encephalopathy.

G. Goal: **health teaching.**

  1. Food selections for low fat, bland diet.

  2. Need for vitamin therapy.

  3. Importance of avoiding alcohol.

  4. Signs and symptoms of recurrence.

  5. Importance of rest, to prevent relapse.

  6. Desired effects and side effects of prescribed medications:

    a. *Narcotics* for pain.

    b. *Antiemetics* for nausea and vomiting.

    c. *Pancreatic hormone* and *enzymes* to replace enzymes not reaching duodenum.

VI. Evaluation/outcome criteria

A. Pain is relieved.

B. No complications (e.g., peritonitis, respiratory).

C. States dietary allowances and restrictions.

D. Takes medications as ordered; states purposes, side effects.

Diabetes

Heterogeneous group of diseases involving disruption of the metabolism of carbohydrates, fats, and protein. If it is uncontrolled, serious vascular and neurologic changes occur.

I. **Types:**
   A. *Type 1*: IDDM (insulin-dependent diabetes mellitus): formerly called *juvenile-onset diabetes*. Insulin needed to prevent ketosis; onset usually in youth but may occur in adulthood; prone to ketosis, unstable diabetes.
   B. *Type 2*: NIDDM (non–insulin-dependent diabetes mellitus): formerly called *maturity-onset* or *adult-onset diabetes*. May be controlled with diet and oral hypoglycemics or insulin; client less apt to have ketosis, except in presence of infection. May be further classified as *obese type 2 or nonobese type 2.*
   C. *Type 3*: GDM (*gestational* diabetes mellitus): glucose intolerance during pregnancy in women who were not known to have diabetes prior to pregnancy; will be reclassified after birth; may need to be treated or may return to prepregnancy state and need no treatment.
   D. *Type 4*: diabetes *secondary* to another condition, such as pancreatic disease, other hormonal imbalances, or drug therapy such as that involving glucocorticoids.

II. **Pathophysiology:**
   A. IDDM—*absolute* deficiency of insulin due to destruction of pancreatic beta cells as the result of the interaction of genetic, immunologic, hereditary, or environmental factors.
   B. NIDDM—*relative* deficiency of insulin due to:
      1. An islet cell defect resulting in a slowed or delayed response in the release of insulin to a glucose load; or
      2. Reduction in the number of insulin receptors from continuously elevated insulin levels; or
      3. A postreceptor defect; or
      4. A major peripheral resistance to insulin induced by hyperglycemia. These factors lead to the deprivation of insulin-dependent cells → a marked decrease in the cellular rate of glucose uptake, and therefore elevated blood glucose levels.

III. **Risk factors/causes:**
   A. Obesity.
   B. Family history of diabetes.
   C. Elderly.
   D. Women whose babies at birth weighed more than 9 lb.
   E. History of autoimmune disease.

IV. **Assessment**
   A. *Subjective data*:
      1. *Eyes*: blurry vision.
      2. *Skin*: pruritus vulvae.
      3. *Neuromuscular*: paresthesia, peripheral neuropathy, lethargy, weakness, fatigue, increased irritability.
      4. *Gastrointestinal (GI): polydipsia* (increased thirst).
      5. *Reproductive*: impotence.
   B. *Objective data*:
      1. *Genitourinary: polyuria*, glycosuria, nocturia (nocturnal enuresis in children).
      2. *Vital signs*:
         a. Pulse and temperature normal or elevated.
         b. BP normal or decreased, unless complications present.
         c. Respirations, increased rate and depth (*Kussmaul's* respirations).
      3. *GI*:
         a. *Polyphagia*, dehydration.
         b. Weight loss, failure to gain weight.
         c. Acetone breath.
      4. *Skin*: cuts heal slowly; frequent infections, foot ulcers, vaginitis.
      5. *Neuromuscular*: loss of strength, peripheral neuropathy.
      6. Lab data:
         a. *Elevated*:
            (1) Blood sugar > 115 mg/dL fasting or > 160 1–2 h after eating.
            (2) Glucose tolerance test.
            (3) Glycosuria (>170 mg/dL).
            (4) Potassium (>5 mEq/L) and chloride (>145 mEq/L). *[handwritten: hyperkalemia]*
            (5) Hemoglobin A_{1c} > 7%.
         b. *Decreased*: *[handwritten: metabolic acidosis]*
            (1) pH (<7.4)
            (2) PCO_2 (<32 mm Hg).
      7. *Long-term pathologic* considerations:
         a. *Cataract formation and retinopathy*: thickened capillary basement membrane, changes in vascularization and hemorrhage, due to chronic hyperglycemia.
         b. *Nephropathy*: due to glomerulosclerosis, arteriosclerosis of renal artery and pyelonephritis, progressive uremia.
         c. *Neuropathy*: due to reduced tissue perfusion; affecting motor, sensory, voluntary, and autonomic functions.
         d. *Arteriosclerosis*: due to lesions of the intimal wall.
         e. *Cardiac*: angina, coronary insufficiency, myocardial infarction.
         f. *Vascular changes*: occlusions, intermittent claudication, loss of peripheral pulses, arteriosclerosis.

V. **Analysis/nursing diagnosis**
   A. *Altered nutrition, less than body requirements*, related to inability to metabolize nutrients and weight loss.
   B. *Altered nutrition, more than body requirements*, related to excessive glucose intake.
   C. *Risk for injury* related to complications of uncontrolled diabetes.

D. *Body image disturbance* related to long-term illness.

E. *Knowledge deficit* related to management of long-term illness.

F. *Ineffective individual coping* related to inability to follow diet/medication regimen.

G. *Sexual dysfunction* related to impotence of diabetes and treatment.

VI. Nursing care plan/implementation

A. Goal: *obtain and maintain normal sugar balance.*

1. Monitor: vital signs; blood glucose before meals, at bedtime, and as symptoms demand (urine testing for glucose levels is *not* as accurate as capillary blood testing).

2. Medications: oral hypoglycemics or insulin, as ordered.

3. *Diet*, as ordered.

   a. Carbohydrates, *50%–60%*; protein, *20%*; fats, *30%* (saturated fats limited to *10%*, unsaturated fats, *90%*).

   b. Calorie reduction in adults who are obese; enough calories to promote normal growth and development for children or in adults who are not obese.

   c. Limit intake of refined sugars.

   d. Add vitamins, minerals as needed for well-balanced diet.

4. Monitor for signs of acute or chronic complications.

B. Goal: **health teaching.**

1. *Diet*: foods allowed restricted, substitutions.

2. Medications: administration *techniques*; importance of utilizing room-temperature insulin, rotating injection sites to prevent tissue damage.

3. Desired and side effects of prescribed insulin type; onset, peak, and duration of action of prescribed insulin.

4. Blood glucose testing *techniques.*

5. Signs of complications (**Table 13.1**).

6. Importance of health maintenance:

   a. Infection prevention, especially foot and nail care.

   b. Routine checkups.

   c. Maintain stable balance of glucose by carefully monitoring glucose level and making necessary adjustments in diet and activity level; seek medical attention when unable to maintain balance; engage in regular exercise program.

VII. Evaluation/outcome criteria

A. Optimal blood glucose levels achieved.

B. Ideal weight maintained.

C. Adequate hydration.

D. Carries out self-care activities: blood or urine testing, foot care, exchange diets, medication administration, exercise.

E. Recognizes and treats hyper- or hypoglycemic reactions.

F. Seeks medical assistance appropriately.

Hyperglycemic Hyperosmolar Nonketotic Syndrome (HHNS)

Profound hyperglycemia and dehydration without ketosis or ketoacidosis; occurs in clients with NIDDM. The client is *critically ill.*

I. **Pathophysiology**: hyperglycemia greater than 1000 mg/100 mL causes osmotic diuresis, depletion of extracellular fluid, and hyperosmolarity, precipitated by infection or another stressor. Client unable to replace fluid deficits with oral intake.

II. **Risk factors/causes:**

A. Old age.

B. History of NIDDM.

C. Infections: pneumonia, pyelonephritis, pancreatitis, gram-negative infections.

D. Kidney failure: uremia and peritoneal dialysis.

E. Shock:

   1. Lactic acidosis related to bicarbonate deficit.

   2. Myocardial infarction.

F. Hemorrhage:

   1. GI tract.

   2. Subdural.

   3. Arterial thrombosis.

G. Medications:

   1. *Diuretics.*

   2. *Glucocorticoids.*

III. **Assessment**

A. *Subjective data*:

   1. Confusion.

   2. Lethargy.

B. *Objective data*:

   1. Nystagmus.

   2. Dehydration.

   3. Aphasia.

   4. Nuchal rigidity.

   5. Hyperreflexia.

   6. Lab data:

      a. Blood glucose level 400 mg/dL.

      b. Serum sodium and chloride—normal to *elevated.*

      c. BUN > 60 mg/dL (higher than in ketoacidosis because of more severe gluconeogenesis and dehydration).

      d. Arterial pH—slightly depressed.

IV. **Analysis/nursing diagnosis**

A. *Risk for injury* related to hyperglycemia.

B. *Altered renal peripheral tissue perfusion* related to vascular collapse.

C. *Ineffective airway clearance* related to coma.

TABLE 13.1 COMPARISON OF DIABETIC COMPLICATIONS

	Hypoglycemia	Ketoacidosis
Pathophysiology	Major metabolic complication when too little food or too large dose of insulin or hypoglycemic agents administered; interferes with oxygen consumption of nervous tissue.	Major metabolic complication in which there is insufficient insulin for metabolism of carbohydrates, fats, and proteins; seen most frequently with clients who are insulin dependent; precipitated in the person who is known to have diabetes by stressors (such as infection, trauma, major illness) that increase insulin needs.
Risk factors/causes	Too little food. Emotional or added stress. Vomiting or diarrhea. Added exercise.	Insufficient insulin or oral hypoglycemics. Noncompliance with dietary instructions. Major illness/infections. Steroid therapy. Trauma, surgery. Elevated blood sugar: >200 mg/dL.
▶◀ Assessment	**Behavioral change:** *Subjective data*—nervous, shaky, irritable, anxious, confused, disoriented. *Objective data*—abrupt mood changes, psychosis. **Visual:** *Subjective data*—blurred vision, diplopia. *Objective data*—dilated pupils. **Skin:** *Objective data*—**diaphoresis, pale**, cool, clammy, goose bumps (piloerection), **Vitals:** *Objective data*—tachycardia; palpitations, thready. **Gastrointestinal:** *Subjective data*—hunger, nausea. *Objective data*—diarrhea, vomiting. **Neurologic:** *Subjective data*—headache; lips/tongue: tingling, numbness. *Objective data*—fainting, yawning, speech: incoherent; **convulsions**; coma. **Musculoskeletal:** *Subjective data*—weakness, fatigue. *Objective data*—trembling. Blood sugar: <80 mg/dL.	**Behavioral change:** *Subjective data*—irritable, confused. *Objective data*—drowsy. **Visual:** *Objective data*—eyeballs: soft, sunken. **Skin:** *Objective data*—loss of turgor, dry, warm, **flushed face**. **Vitals:** *Objective data*—*Kussmaul's* respiration; breath: fruity; BP: hypovolemic shock. **Gastrointestinal:** *Subjective data*—increased thirst and hunger, abdominal pain, nausea. *Objective data*—vomiting, diarrhea, dry mucous membrane; lips, tongue: red, parched. **Neurologic:** *Subjective data*—headache, irritability, confusion, lethargy, weakness. **Musculoskeletal:** *Subjective data*—fatigue, general malaise. **Renal:** *Objective data*—polyuria. Blood sugar: >130 mg/dL.
▶◀ Analysis/nursing diagnosis	*Risk for injury* related to deficit of needed glucose. *Knowledge deficit* related to proper dietary intake or proper insulin dosage. *Altered nutrition, less than body requirements,* related to glucose deficiency.	*Risk for injury* related to glucose imbalance. *Knowledge deficit* related to proper balance of diet and insulin dosage.

(continued)

TABLE 13.1 COMPARISON OF DIABETIC COMPLICATIONS (continued)

	Hypoglycemia	Ketoacidosis
▷◁ **Nursing care plan/ implementation**	Goal: *provide adequate glucose to reverse hypoglycemia*; administer simple sugar stat, PO or IV, glucose paste absorbed in mucous 〰 membrane; monitor *blood sugar levels*; identify events leading to complication.	Goal: *promote normal balance of food and insulin*: ⬭ **regular** insulin as ordered; IV saline, as ordered; bicarbonate and electrolyte replacements, as ordered; *potassium* replacements once therapy begins and urine output is adequate.
	🏠 Goal: **health teaching**: how to prevent further episodes (see **Diabetes**, Health teaching, **p. 168**); importance of careful monitoring of balance between glucose levels and insulin dosage.	🏠 Goal: **health teaching**: diet instructions; desired effects and side effects of prescribed insulin or hypoglycemic agent (onset, peak, and duration of action); importance of recognizing signs of imbalance.
▷◁ **Evaluation/ outcome criteria**	Adheres to diet and correct insulin dosage. Adjusts dosage when activity is increased.	Serious complications avoided. Accepts prescribed diet. Takes medication (correct dose and time).
	Glucose level 80-120 mg/dL	Glucose level 80-120 mg/dL

Source: ©Lagerquist SL: *Little, Brown's NCLEX-RN® Examination Review*. Boston. (out of print)

▷◁ **V. Nursing care plan/implementation**

A. Goal: *promote fluid and electrolyte balance*.

⬭ 1. Administer IVs: fluids and electrolytes, saline solution given initially to combat dehydration. Lab values will determine nature of fluid replacement.

2. Monitor intake and output (I&O) because of the high volume of fluid replaced in the critical stage of this condition.

3. Administer nursing care for problem that precipitated this serious condition.

4. Food by mouth when client is able.

B. Goal: *prevent complications*.

⬭ 1. Administer *regular* insulin (initial dose usually 5–15 U) and food, as ordered.

2. Uncontrolled condition leads to: cardiovascular disease, renal failure, blindness, diabetic gangrene.

▷◁ **VI. Evaluation/outcome criteria**

A. Blood sugar returns to normal level of 80-120 mg/dL.

B. Client is alert to time, place, and person.

C. Primary medical problem resolves.

D. Client recognizes and reports signs of imbalance.

Cholecystitis/Cholelithiasis

Inflammation of gallbladder due to bacterial infection, cholelithiasis (stones, cholesterol, calcium, or bile in the gallbladder), or choledocholithiasis (stone in the common bile duct) and/or obstruction. *Acute cholecystitis* is abrupt in onset, but the client usually has a history of several attacks of fatty-food intolerance. Client with *chronic cholecystitis* has a history of several attacks of moderate severity and has usually learned to avoid fatty foods to decrease symptoms.

I. **Pathophysiology**: calculi form as a result of the increased concentration of bile salts, pigments, or cholesterol due to metabolic or hemolytic disorders, biliary stasis → precipitation of salts into stones or inflammation causing bile constituents to become altered.

II. **Risk factors/causes**:

A. Women.

B. Obesity.

C. Pregnancy.

D. Cirrhosis of the liver.

E. Diabetes.

F. Genetic/predisposition (Native Americans).

▷◁ **III. Assessment**

A. *Subjective data*:

1. *Pain*:

a. Type—severe colic, radiating to back under the scapula and to the right shoulder.

〰 b. Positive *Murphy's sign*—a sign of gallbladder disease in which client experiences pain when taking a deep breath as pressure is placed over the location of the gallbladder.

c. Location—right upper quadrant, epigastric area, flank.

d. Duration—spasm of duct attempting to dislodge stone lasts until dislodged or relieved by medication, or sometimes by vomiting.

2. *GI*—anorexia, nausea, feeling of fullness, indigestion, intolerance of fatty foods.

B. *Objective data*:

1. *GI*—belching, vomiting, clay-colored stools.

2. *Vital signs*—increased pulse, fever.

3. *Skin*—chills, jaundice.

4. *Urine*—dark amber.

5. Lab data—*elevated*:
   a. WBC
   b. Alkaline phosphatase
   c. Serum amylase, lipase
   d. AST [SGOT]
   e. Bilirubin.

IV. Analysis/nursing diagnosis

A. *Pain* related to obstruction of bile duct due to cholelithiasis.

B. *Altered nutrition, more than body requirements,* related to consumption of fatty foods.

C. *Altered nutrition, less than body requirements,* related to hesitancy to eat due to anorexia and nausea.

D. *Risk for fluid volume deficit* related to episodes of vomiting.

E. *Knowledge deficit* related to fat free diet.

V. Nursing care plan/implementation

A. **Nonsurgical interventions:**

1. Goal: *promote comfort.*
   a. Medications as ordered: *analgesics* (meperidine), *antiinfectives, antispasmodics,* electrolytes.
   b. *Avoid* morphine due to spasmodic effect.
   c. *NG* tube connected to low suction.
   d. *Diet*: fat free when able to tolerate food.

2. Goal: **health teaching.**
   a. Signs, symptoms, and complications of disease.
   b. Fat free diet.
   c. Desired effects and side effects of prescribed medications.
   d. Prepare for possible removal of gallbladder (cholecystectomy) if conservative treatment unsuccessful.

B. **Surgical interventions:**

1. *Preoperative*—Goal: *prevent injury*: see Preoperative Preparation, **p. 127-129.**

2. *Postoperative*—Goal: *promote comfort* (see also Postoperative Experience, **p. 131-137**).
   a. Promote tube drainage.
      (1) *NG tube* connected to low suction.
      (2) *T-tube* connected to closed-gravity drainage, to preserve patency of edematous common duct and ensure bile drainage; usual amount 500–1000 mL/24h; dark brown drainage.
      (3) Provide enough tubing to allow turning without tension.
      (4) Empty and record bile drainage q8h.
   b. *Position*: low to semi-Fowler's to facilitate T-tube drainage.
   c. Dressing: dry to protect skin (because bile excoriates skin).
   d. Clamp T-tube as ordered.
      (1) Observe for: abdominal distention, pain, nausea, chills, or fever.
      (2) Unclamp tube and notify MD if symptoms appear.

3. Goal: *prevent complications.*
   a. IV fluids with vitamins.
   b. Cough, turn, and deep breathe (prone to respiratory complication because of high incision).
   c. Early ambulation to prevent vascular complications and aid in expelling flatus.
   d. Monitor for jaundice: skin, sclera, urine, stools.
   e. Monitor for signs of hemorrhage, infection.

4. Goal: **health teaching.**
   a. *Diet*: fat free for 6 wk.
   b. Signs of complications of food intolerance, pain, infection, hemorrhage.

VI. Evaluation/outcome criteria

A. No complications.

B. Able to tolerate food.

C. Plans follow-up care.

D. Possible weight reduction.

🔑 Summary of Key Points

1. The symptoms of cholecystitis are remarkably *similar* to those of many other conditions, such as angina or myocardial infarction. An accurate assessment is therefore critical.

2. *Demerol* is the preferred analgesic in cholecystitis for pain. When pain becomes intractable (unrelieved), cholecystectomy will be done.

3. The use of laser laparoscopy for removal of the gallbladder has changed the postoperative concerns from pneumonia to *injury* to the common bile duct or other organs.

4. If the common bile duct has been explored, a *T-tube* will be inserted during surgery to ensure bile drainage. When the tube is clamped, observe the client for jaundice or discomfort after eating.

5. The pain from pancreatitis is severe and intense; however, morphine sulfate is **contraindicated**.

6. The client with pancreatitis is at risk for the development of *hypovolemia* and *shock* stemming from the effects of the inflammation.

7. With diabetes mellitus the kidney excretion of excess glucose and ketones *causes* diuresis (polyuria); thirst results from the loss of water (polydipsia), and hunger (polyphagia) *results* from the impaired metabolism stemming from the deficiency of insulin.

8. Despite the glucose intolerance, most of the calories in the diabetic diet come from *complex carbohydrates*.

9. People who are diabetic are either insulin dependent (*to remember—type 1* has *none*) or non-insulin dependent (*type 2* has a *few* islet cells).

10. Although exercise may increase carbohydrate metabolism and reduce the need for insulin or increase the need for food, *stored glycogen* may be released, which increases the blood sugar level.

〰️ Diagnostic Studies/Procedures

Glucose Testing

To detect disorder of glucose metabolism, such as diabetes.

1. **Fasting blood sugar (FBS)**: Blood sample is drawn after a 12–h fast (usually overnight). H_2O is allowed. If diabetes is present, value will be >140 mg/dL.

2. **2h postprandial blood sugar (PPBS)**: blood is taken after a meal. For best results, client should be on a high *carbohydrate diet* for 2–4 d before testing. Client fasts overnight, eats a high carbohydrate breakfast; blood sample is drawn 2h after eating. Client should rest during 2h interval. Smoking and coffee may increase glucose level.

3. **Glucose tolerance test (GTT)**: done when sugar in urine or FBS or 2h PPBS results are not conclusive. A timed test, usually 2h. *High carbohydrate diet* is eaten 3d before test. Blood is drawn after overnight fast. Client drinks a very sweet glucose liquid. All of the solution must be consumed. Blood and urine sample usually taken at 30 min, 1h, 2h, and sometimes 3h after drinking solution. Blood glucose *peaks* in 30–60 min and returns to *normal*, usually *within 3h*.

Ultrasound (sonogram)

Scanning by ultrasound is *used* to diagnose disorders of the: thyroid, kidney, liver, uterus, gallbladder, fetus, and the intracranial structures in the neonate. It is not useful when visualization through air or bone is required (lung studies). In some hospitals the sonogram has taken the place of the oral cholecystogram in diagnosing gallbladder distention, bile duct distention, and calculi. *Client preparation* is minimal, i.e., NPO for at least 8h for gallbladder studies. No x-radiation. *Thirty-two ounces of water PO 30min prior* to studies of lower abdomen or uterus.

Cholecystogram

Done if gallbladder *not* seen with ultrasound—ingestion of organic iodine contrast medium: Telepaque (iopanoic acid) or Oragrafin (preparation of calcium or sodium salt of ipodate), followed in 12h by x-ray visualization; gallbladder disease is indicated if there is *poor* or no visualization of the bladder; accurate *only* if GI and liver function is intact; perform *before* barium enema or upper GI. *Client preparation*: explain purpose; administer large amount of *water* with contrast capsules; *low fat meal* evening *before* x-ray; *oral laxative or stool softener after meal; no food* allowed after contrast capsules; water, tea, or coffee, with no cream or sugar, usually allowed. *After completion of exam*: fluids, food, and rest; observe for any signs of allergy to contrast medium.

Cholangiogram

Intravenous injection of a radiopaque contrast medium, followed by fluoroscopic and x-ray examination of the bile ducts; failure of the contrast medium to pass certain points in the bile duct pinpoints *obstruction*.

Study and Memory Aids

Diabetes—Assessment: "3 P's (or "3 Poly's")

P olydipsia (↑ thirst)
P olyphagia (↑ hunger)
P olyuria (↑ urination)

Blood Glucose (rhyme)

Symptom	Implication
Wet and **clammy** (diaphoretic)	give hard **candy** (hypoglycemia).
Hot and **dry** (dehydrated) (↑ temp, ↑ resp.)	glucose is **high** (hyperglycemia)

Source: Modified from *Memory Notebook of Nursing* Dallas: Nursing Education Consultants.

Hypoglycemia: Signs and Symptoms—"DIRE"

D iaphoresis
I ncreased pulse
R estless
E xtra hungry

Diet

Pancreatitis

↓ Fat
Portions
↓ Spicy

Ⓧ Alcohol

↑ Bland foods
Frequent, small meals
↑ Vitamins

Drug Review

Pancreatitis

Analgesics
Calcium carbonate (*Titralac*): 1–2 g with water pc and hs
Magnesium and aluminum hydroxide (*Maalox* suspension): 5–30 mL pc and hs
Meperidine (*Demerol*): 50–150 mg q3–4h as needed; IV, 15–35 mg/h as a continuous infusion
No morphine, codeine
Sucralfate (*Carafate*): 1 g qid
Antiemetics
Prochlorperazine (*Compazine*): 5–30 mg qid
Promethazine (*Phenergan*): 10–25 mg q4h
Trimethobenzamide (*Tigan*): 250 mg qid
Antiinfectives—used for severe cases of pancreatitis
Cephalexin (*Keflex*): 250–500 mg q6h
Cephalothin (*Keflin*): IV 0.5–2g q4–6h
Gentamicin (*Garamycin*): 3–5 mg/kg/d in divided doses
Penicillin G: 1.2 million U IM
Antispasmodic
Propantheline (*Pro-Banthine*): 15 mg tid; 30 mg hs
Antiulcer
Aluminum hydroxide gel (*Amphojel*): 5–10 mL q2–4h or 1h pc

Replacement therapy
Exogenous pancreatic enzyme therapy includes lipase, trypsin, or histamine (H_2) receptor antagonists. Possible exogenous insulin therapy because of the destruction of islet cell tissue
Vitamin therapy
According to deficiencies

Diabetes: Antihyperglycemic

Injection
Crystalline (regular) (*Humulin R*) —rapid acting
Lente—intermediate acting
NPH—intermediate acting
Protamine zinc insulin—slow acting
Ultralente—extended acting
Oral
Acetohexamide (*Dymelor*): 200–1500 mg/d
Chlorpropamide (*Diabinese*): 100–1,000 mg/d
Tolazamide (*Tolinase*): 100–500 mg/d
Tolbutamide (*Orinase*): 500–3,000 mg/d
See **Appendix D**, Review of Pharmacology.

Cholecystitis

Antiinfectives to control infection
Cephalexin (*Keflex*): 250–500 mg q6h
Cephalothin (*Keflin*): IV, 0.5–2 g q4–6h
Erythromycin: 250–500 mg q6–12h
Gentamicin (*Garamycin*): 3–5 mg/kg/d in divided doses
Penicillin G: 1.2 million U in single IM dose
Antispasmodic
Propantheline (*Pro-Banthine*): 15 mg tid, 30 mg hs
Narcotics
Meperidine (*Demerol*): 50–150 mg q3–4h as needed; IV 15–35 mg/h as a continuous infusion
No morphine

Questions

1. When would the nurse typically expect to hear bowel sounds after exploration of the bile duct and a cholecystectomy?
   1. 4–6 hours.
   2. 6–12 hours.
   3. 12–24 hours.
   4. 24–48 hours.
2. After the ingestion of the glucose drink used in the glucose tolerance test, the nurse would know a client does not have diabetes mellitus if the blood glucose level returns to normal in:
   1. 2–3 hours.
   2. 4–6 hours.
   3. 7–8 hours.
   4. 10–12 hours.

3. Which food item would the nurse instruct a client with diabetes to exclude from the meat exchange list?
   1. Peanut butter.
   2. Dried beans.
   3. Pasta.
   4. Cottage cheese.

4. A client with diabetes tells the nurse he drinks quite a bit of nonfat milk. The nurse's response should be:
   1. "I'm glad you are watching your fat intake."
   2. "The lactose in nonfat milk is absorbed rapidly."
   3. "Have you been craving milk more lately?"
   4. "Have you decreased the amount of another exchange food?"

5. The nurse would conclude that a client was experiencing hypoglycemia if the assessment findings included:
   1. Diaphoresis and restlessness.
   2. Rapid, thready pulse.
   3. Vomiting and bradycardia.
   4. Rapid, bounding pulse.

6. The nurse is to give a client 30 units of NPH and 10 units of regular insulin subcutaneously. To administer the injection the nurse would:
   1. Take the regular insulin from the refrigerator just before giving it.
   2. Draw up the regular insulin first and then the NPH.
   3. Shake the bottle to thoroughly mix the insulin.
   4. Rub the injection site slightly after the injection.

7. Which type of insulin should the nurse prepare for a direct IV push for the treatment of ketoacidosis?
   1. Regular.
   2. Semilente.
   3. NPH.
   4. Ultralente.

8. The effectiveness of insulin given through a continuous IV infusion pump would be expected to be:
   1. More rapid because of the direct vascular access afforded.
   2. Reduced because the potency is lessened by at least 20% to 80%.
   3. The same as that of the agent given subcutaneously, because of the dilution that occurs.
   4. Variable; may be either more or less potent.

9. A client with type 1 diabetes (IDDM) asks if she will still receive insulin when she is NPO before surgery. The best response by the nurse would be:
   1. "No. Since you're not eating, there is no need."
   2. "It depends on how stressed you feel about the surgery."
   3. "Yes, because you will mostly likely receive glucose IV."
   4. "Yes, but less than your regular daily amount."

10. Which plan for a snack would be appropriate for a client receiving NPH insulin every morning at 7:00 A.M.?
    1. Coffee and half a bagel an hour after the injection.
    2. A piece of fruit about 4:00 P.M.
    3. Cheese and crackers before bed at 10:00 P.M.
    4. Hard candy every couple of hours during the day.

11. What nursing action is most important for a newly admitted client experiencing diabetic ketoacidosis?
    1. Client teaching on self-care.
    2. Insertion of a Foley catheter for urine testing.
    3. Starting a peripheral IV.
    4. Assessment of the client's level of confusion.

12. Client teaching about diabetic foot care should include the need to:
    1. Rub feet with alcohol to toughen skin.
    2. Use a heating pad to warm feet.
    3. Inspect feet daily for cracks or cuts.
    4. Disinfect scissors before removing calluses.

13. The nurse knows the client understands the teaching about diabetes when the client says:
    1. "I will need more insulin when I increase my activity."
    2. "I need to eliminate sweets from my diet."
    3. "I'll call with my questions after I read the brochure."
    4. "Managing diabetes will be a lifetime of learning."

Answers/Rationale

1. **(4)** Bowel sounds usually return between 36 and 48 hours after abdominal surgery. Bowel sounds may return the earliest by 24 hours, due to the effects of general anesthesia, but not as early as 12 hours (2 and 3). Bowel sounds would never return in 4 to 6 hours in a client receiving a general anesthetic (1). **AS, RE/KN, 8, PhI, Physiological adaptation**

2. **(1)** The blood glucose level would return to normal in 2 hours in clients under 55 years of age; this may take at least 3 hours in those over 55 years. If the blood glucose level stays above 200 mg/dL for more than 2 to 3 hours, the client is likely diabetic. The timing in all the other options (2, 3, and 4) is *longer* than that required for the blood glucose level of a client who is not diabetic to return to normal. **AN, RE/KN, 4, PhI, Reduction of risk potential**

3. **(3)** The meat exchange list contains only protein sources; pasta is a *carbohydrate*. All of the other foods (1, 2, and 4) *are* non-meat sources of *protein*. **IMP, COM, 4, PhI, Basic care and comfort**

4. **(2)** The lack of fat in the milk actually causes the absorption of lactose, or milk sugar, to increase. If a person with diabetes needs to lose weight, nonfat milk is the best type of milk to be used but the amount needs to be limited to no more than one or two 8-ounce glasses daily. Reinforcing fat reduction (1) is not wrong, but it does not address the underlying problem in a client with diabetes. If the client is not eating a balanced diet, there may be cravings (3); he/she may also not understand the limitations surrounding milk consumption. Although the diabetic diet does allow for exchanges (4), the overall percentage in each category needs to be consistent: 55% to 60% carbohydrates; 30% fats; and 12% to 20% protein. **AN, ANL, 4, PhI, Basic care and comfort**

5. **(1)** Hypoglycemia occurs when the blood glucose level drops to 60 mg/dL or lower; diaphoresis occurs because epinephrine is released when the blood glucose level declines. The client may act very restless and apprehensive, even drunk or psychotic. Although epinephrine would cause an increase in the pulse rate, there is no change in volume in hypoglycemia; a rapid, thready pulse (2) would result from *volume loss*, and a rapid, bounding pulse (4) would be a sign of *volume excess*. Other symptoms of hypoglycemia include: weakness headache, and lack of muscular coordination, but *not* vomiting or bradycardia (3). **AN, EVL, 4, PhI, Physiological adaptation**

6. **(2)** The clear insulin (regular) is drawn up first, followed by the cloudy insulin (NPH). This prevents contamination of the fast-acting (regular) insulin. The current bottle of insulin does not need to be refrigerated (1), and in fact it is *better not* to administer *cold* insulin because this fosters lipodystrophy. The bottle should be gently rolled between the palms to mix the agent, *not shaken* (3). The nurse should apply gentle direct pressure and *not rub* (4) the injection site, because absorption may be affected. **PL, COM, 1, PhI, Pharmacological and parenteral therapies**

7. **(1)** Regular insulin is the *only* insulin that may be given by direct IV administration for fast action in the treatment of diabetic ketoacidosis. The other types of insulin (2, 3, and 4) *cannot* be given IV. **IMP, COM, 4, PhI, Pharmacological and parenteral therapies**

8. **(2)** The plastic or glass container or the tubing causes the potency of the insulin to be reduced before it even reaches the venous system. The degree to which it is reduced varies, but flushing the tubing with 50 to 100 mL of IV solution minimizes the loss of potency. (Note: regular insulin is the *only* insulin that can be given IV.) Even though vascular access (1) is direct and insulin given in this way would take effect more rapidly, the *amount* received is *uncertain* and the clinical effects are less predictable. The effectiveness of insulin given by IV infusion pump is not the same as that of subcutaneously administered insulin (3), but there is a *degree of uncertainty* associated with both IV and subcutaneous administration. Insulin given by continuous IV infusion will always be *less potent*, not more (4). **EV, COM, 4, PhI, Pharmacological and parenteral therapies**

9. **(3)** Generally an IV with dextrose in the solution is started to maintain fluid and nutrition status. Insulin is given IV according to the blood glucose determinations. Insulin is still needed even though the client is not eating (1), because surgery is a stressor, which stimulates the release of glucose; the degree of stress (2) may affect the *amount* of insulin given, but *not whether* it will be given. Because of the IV glucose and the added stress, the amount administered may actually be increased, *not* decreased (4). **IMP, COM, 4, PhI, Pharmacological and parenteral therapies**

10. **(2)** NPH is an intermediate-acting insulin and the action peaks in 6 to 12 hours after administration. A reaction would therefore occur between 1:00 and 7:00 P.M. A reaction in the early morning (1) would occur in response to *regular* insulin. A reaction later in the evening or at night (3) would be more likely to occur with the *long-acting* insulins. Although people with diabetes should carry hard candy (4), hypoglycemic reactions *every few hours* are *not* common. **IMP, APP, 4, PhI, Pharmacological and parenteral therapies**

11. **(3)** A client with ketoacidosis will require the IV administration of fluids to treat the severe dehydration, insulin to manage the hyperglycemia, and possibly sodium bicarbonate to treat acidosis. Teaching (1) should be done once the client's condition is *stable* and *before* discharge. Urinalysis would be done to assess kidney function, but it is not needed for glucose testing; since blood is used for testing. Depending on the client's level of consciousness and a problem with incontinence, a catheter *may or may not* be inserted (2). Confusion (4) is *not* the change in consciousness expected in a client with ketoacidosis; the client usually becomes comatose in the presence of severe acidosis. **PL, APP, 4, PhI, Physiological adaptation**

Key to Codes

Nursing process: AS, assessment; **AN,** analysis; **PL,** planning; **IMP,** implementation; **EV,** evaluation. (See **Appendix M** for explanation of nursing process steps.)

Cognitive level: RE/KN, recall/knowledge; **COM,** comprehension; **APP,** application; **ANL,** analysis; **EVL,** evaluation; **SYN,** synthesis. (See **Appendix M** for explanation.)

Category of human function: 1, protective; **2,** sensory-perceptual; **3,** comfort, rest, activity, and mobility; **4,** nutrition; **5,** growth and development; **6,** fluid-gas transport; **7,** psychosocial-cultural; **8,** elimination. (See **Appendix O** for explanation.)

Client need: SECE, safe, effective care environment; **PhI,** physiological integrity; **PsI,** psychosocial integrity; **HPM,** health promotion and maintenance. (See **Appendix P** for explanation.)

Client subneed: (See **Appendix P** for explanation)

12. **(3)** Peripheral circulation and wound healing are poor in clients with diabetes, and they are also more susceptible to infection. Foot care is therefore very important to prevent loss of toes or the foot. Alcohol **(1)** is drying and may foster cracking. Because the circulation and sensations are decreased, going barefoot or applying extreme heat or cold to the limbs **(2)** may only cause injury. Trimming the toenails or removing calluses **(4)** should not be done by the client, but preferably by a podiatrist. **IMP, APP, 4, PhI, Basic care and comfort**

13. **(4)** Diabetes is a chronic illness; although it is manageable, it is not curable. Exercise **(1)** actually *decreases* the need for insulin. Carbohydrates constitute 55% to 60% of the diabetic diet, so "sweets" **(2)** may be included but in *limited* quantities. The statement in option **3** does *not* reflect an understanding of the teaching. **EV, EVL, 4, PhI, Pharmacological and parenteral therapies**

Hepatic Disorders

14

Chapter Outline

Hepatitis

Inflammation of the liver.

I. Pathophysiology:

  A. Infection with either hepatitis **A** (*formerly called infectious hepatitis*), hepatitis **B** (*formerly called serum hepatitis*), hepatitis **C** (caused by at least two unidentified viruses), hepatitis **D** (infection caused by a defective RNA virus that requires hepatitis **B** virus to multiply) hepatitis **E** (transmitted via fecal-oral route), or hepatitis **G** (parenterally and sexually transmitted, but is poorly characterized) → inflammation, necrosis, and regeneration of liver parenchyma. Hepatocellular injury impairs clearance of urobilinogen → elevated urinary urobilinogen; and, as injury increases → conjugated bilirubin not reaching the intestines → decreased urine and fecal urobilinogen → increased serum bilirubin → jaundice.

  B. Failure of liver to detoxify products → increased toxic products of protein metabolism → gastritis and duodenitis.

II. Risk factors/causes:

  A. Exposure to virus.

  B. Exposure to carriers of virus.

  C. Exposure to hepatotoxins, such as dry cleaning agents.

  D. Nonimmunized.

III. Assessment

  A. *Subjective data*:

  1. Anorexia, nausea.
  2. Malaise, dull ache in upper right quadrant.
  3. Repugnance to food, cigarette smoke, strong odors, alcohol.
  4. Headache.
  5. Pruritus.

  B. *Objective data*:

  1. Fever.
  2. *Liver*: enlarged (hepatomegaly), tender, smooth.
  3. *Skin*: icterus in sclera of eyes, jaundice, rash, pruritus, petechiae, bruises.
  4. *Urine*: normal, dark.
  5. *Stool*: normal, clay colored, loose.
  6. Vomiting, weight loss.
  7. *Lymph nodes*: enlarged.
  8. Lab data:
     a. Blood—leukocytosis.
     b. *Increased*: aspartate aminotransferase (AST), serum glutamic-oxaloacetic transaminase (SGOT), alanine aminotransferase (ALT), serum glutamic pyruvic transaminase (SGPT); bilirubin levels, alkaline phosphatase.
     c. Urine—*increased* urobilinogen.
  9. See **Table 14.1**, Comparison of hepatitis types.

IV. Analysis/nursing diagnosis

  A. *Pain* related to inflammation of liver.

  B. *Impaired skin integrity* related to pruritus.

  C. *Activity intolerance* related to malaise.

  D. *Risk for infection to others* related to incubation/infectious period.

  E. *Altered nutrition, less than body requirements*, related to repugnance to food.

  F. *Social isolation* related to isolation precautions.

V. Nursing care plan/implementation

  A. Goal: *promote comfort*.

  1. Bed rest to combat fatigue and reduce metabolic needs until hepatomegaly subsides; *semi-Fowler's or supine positioning*.
  2. Oral hygiene q1–2h to decrease nausea.
  3. Range of motion exercises to maintain muscle strength.

Diaphragm

Liver

Gallbladder

Cystic Duct

Common Bile Duct

Duodenum

Common Hepatic Duct

Spleen

Pancreas

Pancreatic Duct

The Liver and Biliary System

4. *Measures to reduce pruritus*:
   a. Mild, oil-based lotion to reduce itching.
   b. Nails cut short, cotton gloves, long-sleeved clothing to prevent skin injury from scratching.
   c. Environment: cool and dry
   d. Cool wet soaks to skin.
   e. Diversional activities.
   f. Medications as ordered:
      (1) *Emollients* to relieve dry skin.
      (2) *Topical corticosteroids* to reduce inflammation.
      (3) *Antihistamines* to reduce itch.
      (4) *Tranquilizers* and *sedatives* to allow rest and prevent exhaustion.

B. Goal: *prevent spread of infection to others.*
   1. Isolation according to type:
      a. *Hepatitis* A:
         (1) Enteric precautions (**Table 14.2**).
         (2) Private room preferred.
         (3) Gown/gloves for direct contact with feces.
         (4) Handwashing when in direct contact with feces.
      b. *Hepatitis* B: blood and body fluid precautions.
         (1) Needle/dressing precautions.
         (2) Private room *not* necessary.
         (3) Gown: only if enteric precautions also necessary.

         (4) Handwashing; use gloves when in direct contact with blood.
      c. *Hepatitis* C: blood and body fluid precautions—Same as precautions for hepatitis B, except when in countries with fecal-oral form; then use hepatitis A precautions also.
      d. *Hepatitis* D: Same as precautions for hepatitis B.
   2. Passive immunity for contacts:
      a. *Hepatitis* A: immune serum globulin (ISG).
      b. *Hepatitis* B: hepatitis B immune globulin (HGIB) or ISG.
      c. *Hepatitis* C: prophylaxis not as effective; immune globulin may be given.
      d. *Hepatitis* D: same as for hepatitis B.
   3. Goal: *promote healing.*
      a. *Diet* as tolerated:
         (1) NPO with parenteral infusions, when in acute stage.
         (2) *High protein, high carbohydrate, low fat*; offered in frequent, small meals.
         (3) Push fluids, if not contraindicated; intake and output (I&O).
   4. Goal: *monitor for worsening of disease process, failure to respond to treatment.*
      a. Observe urine—dark due to presence of bile and stool, clay colored.
      b. Observe sclera; monitor lab test results

TABLE 14.1 COMPARISON OF HEPATITIS A, B, C AND D: ETIOLOGY, INCIDENCE, EPIDEMIOLOGY, AND CLINICAL CHARACTERISTICS

	Hepatitis A	Hepatitis B	Hepatitis C	Hepatitis D
Incubation	2–6 wk	4 wk–6 mo	Variable: 14–160 d; average, 50 d	4 wk–6 mo
Communicable	Until 7–9 d after jaundice occurs	Several months—as long as virus present in blood	As long as virus present in blood	As long as virus present in blood
Transmission	Fecal-oral, blood, sexual	Parenteral, sexual	Percutaneous, via contaminated blood, parenteral drug abuse; some fecal-oral forms	Parenteral fecal-oral blood
Sources	Crowding; contaminated food, milk, or water	Contaminated needles, syringes, surgical instruments	Persons who have received 15 or more blood transfusions; IV drug users; persons traveling to contaminated areas	Contaminated needles, syringes
Portal of entry	GI tract; asymptomatic carriers	Integumentary: Contact with blood plasma or blood transfusion	Blood	Integumentary: blood
Hepatitis B antigen	Not present	Present	Not present	Present
Incidence	Sporadic epidemics; increased in children <15 yr	Increased in ages 15-29 yr, particularly in heroin addicts; occupational hazard for laboratory workers, nurses, physicians	All age groups; higher in adults because of exposure to risk factors	Same as for hepatitis **B**
🔋 **Immunity**	*Preexposure*: HAV vaccine. *Postexposure*: Immune globulin, 0.02 mg/kg. within 2 wk of exposure; can be used before exposure—confers passive immunity for 6–8 weeks.	*Preexposure*: hepatitis **B** vaccine *Postexposure*: immune globulin with high amounts of anti-HBs (HBIG); hepatitis **B** vaccine	None; immune globulin may be given	None
Prevention	🖐 Handwashing, use of gloves	Care when handling products contaminated by blood, use of gloves	Same as for hepatitis **B**	Same as for hepatitis **B**
Severity	Mild	Mild to moderate	Mild to moderate	Moderate to severe
Fever	Common	Uncommon	Uncommon	Uncommon
Nausea/vomiting	Common	Common	Common	Common

Source: ©Lagerquist SL; *Little, Brown's NCLEX-RN® Examination Review*. Boston: Little, Brown. (out of print)

to detect increasing jaundice.

c. Mental confusion, unusual somnolence may indicate decreased liver function.

d. Weigh daily—increase indicates fluid retention and possible ascites.

📖 5. Goal: **health teaching.**

a. Diet and fluid intake to promote liver regeneration.

b. Importance of rest and limited activity to reduce metabolic workload of liver.

TABLE 14.2 ⚠ ENTERIC PRECAUTIONS

1. Private room if the client's hygiene is poor. In general, clients with the same infection *may share* a room.

2. Masks are *not* indicated.

3. Gowns are indicated if soiling is likely.

4. Gloves are indicated for touching infective material.

5. Hands must be washed *before* and *after* touching the client or potentially contaminated articles.

6. Contaminated articles should be discarded or bagged and labeled.

Source: ©Lagerquist SL: *Little, Brown's NCLEX-RN® Examination Review.* Boston: Little, Brown. (out of print)

    c.   Personal hygiene practices to prevent contamination

    d. *Avoid*: alcohol, blood donations, and contact with communicable infections.

    e. Follow-up case referral; may take 6 mo for full recovery

    f. Teach contacts about available immunizations.

VI. Evaluation/outcome criteria

  A. Tolerates food; nausea and vomiting decreased.

  B. Signs of infection/inflammation absent.

  C. No complications, hemorrhage, liver damage, ascites.

  D. No jaundice noted.

Cirrhosis

Chronic inflammation and fibrosis of the liver in which some liver cells (hepatocytes) undergo necrosis and others undergo proliferative regeneration.

I. Pathophysiology: progressive destruction of hepatic cells → loss of normal metabolic function of the liver and formation of scar tissue. Regeneration and proliferation of fibrous tissue → obstruction of the portal vein → increased portal hypertension, ascites, liver failure, and eventual death.

II. Risk factors/causes:

  A. Alcohol abuse most common cause.

  B. Nutritional deficiency with decreased protein intake.

  C. Hepatotoxins.

  D. Virus.

  E. Severe, long-term right-sided heart failure.

III. Assessment

  A. *Subjective data*:

    1. Chronic feeling of malaise.

    2. Anorexia, nausea.

    3. Abdominal pain.

    4. Pruritus.

  B. *Objective data*:

    1. *Gastrointestinal* (GI):

      a. Malnutrition, weight loss.

      b. Vomiting.

      c. Flatulence.

      d. Ascites.

      e. Enlarged liver and spleen.

      f. Glossitis.

      g. Fetid breath (sweet, musty odor).

    2. *Blood*—coagulation defects, possible esophageal varices, portal hypertension, bleeding from gums and injection sites.

    3. *Skin and hair*—edema, jaundice, spider angioma, palmar erythema, decreased pubic and axillary hair.

    4. *Reproductive*—menstrual abnormalities, gynecomastia, testicular atrophy, impotence.

    5. *Neurologic*—memory loss, hepatic coma, decreased level of consciousness, flappy tremor, grimacing.

    6. Lab data:

      a. *Decreased*: albumin, potassium, magnesium, blood urea nitrogen;

      b. *Elevated*: prothrombin time, globulins, ammonia, AST/(SGOT), ALT/(SGPT) bromsulphalein (BSP), alkaline phosphatase, uric acid, blood sugar.

    7. *Diagnostic studies:* see **p. 182**

IV. Analysis/nursing diagnosis

  A. *Altered nutrition, less than body requirements*, related to decreased intake, nausea, and vomiting.

  B. *Risk for injury* related to decreased prothrombin production.

  C. *Activity intolerance* related to fatigue.

  D. *Fatigue* related to anorexia and nutritional deficiencies.

  E. *Self-esteem disturbance* related to physical body changes.

  F. *Risk for impaired skin integrity* related to pruritus.

V. Nursing care plan/implementation

  A. Goal: *provide for special safety needs*.

    1. Monitor vital signs (including neurologic) frequently for hemorrhage from esophageal varices (may have *Sengstaken-Blakemore* or *Linton* tube inserted).

    2. Prepare client for *LeVeen shunt* surgery for portal hypertension if needed.

    3. Assist with *paracentesis* performed for ascites; monitor vital signs to prevent shock during procedure. (See **p. 182**)

  B. Goal: *relieve discomfort caused by complications*.

    1. *Position*: semi-Fowler's or Fowler's to decrease pressure on diaphragm due to ascites.

    2. Deep breathing q2h to prevent respiratory complications.

3. Skin care: topical medications to relieve pruritus, nail care to decrease possibility of further skin injury.

4. Frequent oral hygiene necessitated by nausea, vomiting, and fetid breath.

C. Goal: *improve fluid and electrolyte balance.*

1. IV fluids and vitamins.

2. I&O, hourly urine measurements during acute attacks.

3. Daily: measure girths, weights to monitor fluid balance.

4. *Diuretics* as ordered to decrease edema.

5. May receive serum albumin to promote adequate vascular volume, prevent azotemia and encephalopathy, and promote diuresis (observe carefully, as albumin could escape quickly through cell walls and cause increase in ascites).

D. Goal: *promote optimal nutrition within dietary restrictions.*

1. NPO during acute episodes.

2. Small, frequent meals when able to eat.

3. *Low protein* (to decrease the amount of nitrogenous materials in the intestines) and *sodium* (to decrease fluid retention).

4. *Moderate carbohydrate* (to meet energy demands) and *fat* (to make diet more palatable to anorexic clients).

E. Goal: *provide emotional support.*

1. Quiet environment during acute episodes to decrease external stimuli.

2. Identify community agencies for assistance for client, e.g., Alcoholics Anonymous; for family, Alanon/Alateen.

F. Goal: **health teaching.**

1. *Avoid* alcohol, exposure to infections.

2. Dietary allowances, restrictions (see **Appendix B**, Sodium–restricted diet and Purine–restricted diet, **p. 378, 379**).

3. Drugs: names, purposes.

4. Signs, symptoms of disease and complications.

5. Stress-management techniques.

VI. **Evaluation/outcome criteria**

A. No complications.

B. Nutritional status improves; lists dietary restrictions.

C. *No* alcohol consumption.

D. Lists signs and symptoms of disease progression and complications.

E. Complies with discharge plan, becomes involved with an alcohol treatment program.

Esophageal Varices

Life-threatening hemorrhage from tortuous, dilated, thin-walled veins in submucosa of lower esophagus; may rupture when chemically or mechanically irritated or when pressure is increased because of sneezing, coughing, *Valsalva maneuver*, or excessive exercise.

I. **Pathophysiology**: portal hypertension related to cirrhosis of the liver → distended branches of the azygos vein and inferior vena cava where they join the smaller vessels of the esophagus.

II. **Risk factors for hemorrhage:**

A. Exertion that increases abdominal pressure.

B. Trauma from ingestion of coarse or poorly masticated foods.

C. Acid-pepsin erosion.

III. **Assessment**

A. *Subjective data*:

1. Fear.

2. Dysphagia.

3. History: alcohol ingestion, liver dysfunction.

B. *Objective data*:

1. Hematemesis.

2. Hemorrhage: sudden, often fatal.

3. Decreased blood pressure; increased pulse, respirations.

4. Melena (occult blood in stool).

IV. **Analysis/nursing diagnosis**

A. *Fluid volume deficit* related to blood loss.

B. *Risk for injury* related to hemorrhage.

C. *Fear* related to massive blood loss.

D. *Ineffective individual coping* related to complications of cirrhosis.

V. **Nursing care plan/implementation**

A. Goal: *provide safety measures related to hemorrhage.*

1. Recognize signs of shock; vital signs q15 min.

2. Assist with insertion of *Sengstaken-Blakemore* (or *Minnesota*) or *Linton tube* (tube is large and uncomfortable for client during insertion); explain procedure briefly to decrease fear and attempt to gain client's cooperation.

3. While tube in place, observe for respiratory distress; if occurs, *deflate the balloon by releasing pressure; do not cut the tube.*

4. Deflate the balloon as ordered to prevent necrosis.

5. NG tube connected to low gastric suction; monitor for amount of bright red blood; irrigate only as ordered using tepid, *not* iced, solutions.

6. Vitamin K as ordered to control bleeding.

B. Goal: *promote fluid balance.*

1. IV fluids, expanders, blood.

2. Fresh blood as ordered to prevent increase in ammonia; aids in coagulation.

C. Goal: *prevent complications of hepatic coma.*
1. *Saline cathartics* as ordered to remove old blood from GI tract.
2. *Anti-infectives* as ordered to prevent infection.

D. Goal: *provide emotional support.*
1. Stay with client.
2. Calm atmosphere.

E. Goal: **health teaching**.
1. Explain use of tube to client and family.
2. Bland diet instructions.
3. Recognize signs of bleeding.
4. *Avoid* straining at stool.
5. *Avoid* using aspirin because of increased bleeding tendency.

VI. **Evaluation/outcome criteria**
A. Survives acute bleeding episode.
B. Further episodes prevented by avoiding irritants, especially alcohol.
C. Nutritional status improves.
D. Recognizes symptoms of complications, e.g., bleeding.
E. Demonstrates knowledge of medications by avoiding use of aspirin.

Summary of Key Points

1. Before jaundice appears, the *symptoms* of a liver problem are rather vague and nonspecific.

2. Jaundice is a diagnostic *sign* indicating a problem, not a disease. Physically the skin itches, but changes in appearance may be most disturbing to the client.

3. Even before the visible signs of jaundice occur, the client may complain that favorite foods or drink are distasteful.

4. Check the *hard palate first* for jaundice. The sclera color is an unreliable sign in persons of color.

5. Viral hepatitis includes all of the "alphabet" types of hepatitis. They are differentiated by the *incubation* time, the *route* of transmission, and the *severity* of the clinical course.

6. Nursing interventions focus on physical and emotional rest and diet. Protein is needed for healing, but the amount consumed is adjusted according to the *blood ammonia level*. Drug therapy is used *minimally* and *cautiously* because many drugs that are normally detoxified by the liver may have toxic effects.

7. In contrast to hepatitis, which is an "itis" or inflammatory process, cirrhosis is an "osis" causing an *impaired flow* of blood, bile, or metabolites. Many of the signs and symptoms are the *result of pressure*, which "pushes," causing ascites, organ enlargement, and varices.

8. If hemorrhage occurs with cirrhosis, the prognosis is *poorer*.

Diagnostic Studies/Procedures

Celiac Angiography, Hepatoportography

Injection of a contrast medium into the portal vein or related vessel; *used* to determine patency of vessels supplying target organ or detect lesions in the organs that distort the vasculature.

Peritoneoscopy

Direct visualization of the liver and peritoneum by means of a peritoneoscope inserted through an abdominal stab wound.

Liver Biopsy

Needle aspiration of tissue for the purpose of microscopic examination; *used* to: determine tissue changes, facilitate diagnosis, and provide information regarding a disease course.

Nursing action: place client on *right side* and position pillow for pressure, to prevent bleeding.

Paracentesis

Needle aspiration of fluid from the peritoneal cavity; *used* to relieve excess fluid accumulation or for diagnostic studies.

Specific nursing actions before paracentesis

1. Have client void—to prevent possible injury to bladder during procedure.
2. *Position*—sitting up on side of bed, with feet supported by chair.
3. Check vital signs and peripheral circulation frequently throughout procedure.
4. Observe for signs of hypovolemic shock—may occur due to fluid shift from vascular compartment following removal of protein-rich ascitic fluid.

Specific nursing actions after paracentesis

1. Apply pressure to injection site and cover with sterile dressing.
2. Measure and record amount and color of ascitic fluid; send specimens to lab for diagnostic studies.

Study and Memory Aids

🍎 Diets

Hepatitis

↑ Carbohydrate   Fat
Fluids   Food by mouth
Frequent feedings   ↓ Portions
Protein

Cirrhosis

↓ Na⁺   *Moderate*:
Protein   Carbohydrate
↓ Size of meal   Fat

Esophageal Varices

NPO during and after bleeding episodes
Bland, soft diet when able to eat

💊 Drug Review

Hepatitis

Antiemetics
    Dimenhydrinate (*Dramamine*): 50–100 mg PO q4h.
    Trimethobenzamide (*Tigan*): 250 mg PO tid-qid.
Antihistamines
    Chlorpheniramine maleate (*Chlor-Trimeton*): 2–4 mg tid
    Diphenhydramine (*Benadryl*): 25–50 mg bid
Emollient
    Xipamide (*Aquaphor*) ointment
Sedative
    Diazepam (*Valium*): 2–10 mg 2–4 times a day
Topical glucocorticoid
    Hydrocortisone
Tranquilizers
    Chlordiazepoxide HCl (*Librium*): 5-25 mg 3–4 times
    daily
    Phenobarbital: 30–120 mg/d in divided doses

Cirrhosis

Corticosteroids used for postnecrotic syndrome
Diuretic
    Furosemide (*Lasix*): 20–80 mg/d
Emollient
    Xipamide (*Aquaphor*): ointment to relieve pruritus
Hydrochlorothiazide
    HydroDIURIL: 25–100 mg/d
Serum albumin for acute liver failure
Vitamins
    B; Fat-soluble vitamins (A, D, E, and K)

Esophageal Varices

Antiinfectives
Reduce portal hypertension
    Propranolol (*Inderal*)
    Vasopressin (*Pitressin*)
Saline cathartics
    Magnesium citrate: 240 mL as needed.
    Magnesium hydroxide: 5–15 mL 4 times/d.
    Magnesium sulfate: 10–15 G in water.
    Phosphate/biphosphate: 250 mg in water 4 times/d.

Esophageal Varices: Restriction

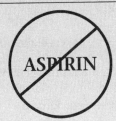

Questions

1. For which possible complication should a nurse assess a client with a LeVeen shunt, used to treat liver failure?
   1. Heart failure.
   2. Myocardial infarction.
   3. Respiratory distress syndrome.
   4. Acute renal failure.

2. Which physical assessment finding in a man would be a sign of cirrhosis?
   1. Testicular swelling.
   2. Gynecomastia.
   3. Rebound tenderness.
   4. Wheezing.

3. A client asks why he has developed cirrhosis. Which of the following in the client's history would be the most likely cause?
   1. Hepatitis A.
   2. Cholelithiasis.
   3. Acetaminophen use.
   4. Blunt abdominal trauma.

4. Which laboratory findings would the nurse expect in a client with postnecrotic cirrhosis?
   1. Decreased prothrombin time and albumin level.
   2. Increased white blood cell (WBC) and thrombocyte counts.
   3. Increased alanine aminotransferase (ALT) and aspartate aminotransferase (AST) levels.
   4. Decreased alkaline phosphatase level.

5. The nurse can anticipate that the urine of a client admitted for hepatitis will probably appear:
   1. Dark.
   2. Bloody.
   3. Clear.
   4. Diluted.

6. The nurse would use lactulose (*Cephulac*), an agent frequently used in the management of hepatic encephalopathy, in the care of a client with which chronic condition?
   1. Hypoglycemia.
   2. Constipation.
   3. Colitis.
   4. Hiatal hernia.

7. Which nursing assessment is important in a client with ascites?
   1. Hematest of all stools.
   2. Bowel sounds.
   3. Abdominal girth.
   4. Urine output.

8. A Minnesota (or Sengstaken-Blakemore) tube has been inserted in a client to manage ruptured esophageal varices. A nursing priority in this client would be to:
   1. Test for gastric hyperacidity.
   2. Test the gastric contents for blood (hematest).
   3. Ensure a means of communication.
   4. Maintain airway patency.

9. The nurse would recognize a worsening of hepatic encephalopathy if which sign were observed?
   1. Flapping tremor.
   2. Facial weakness.
   3. Drooling.
   4. Nystagmus.

Answers/Rationale

1. **(1)** The shunt is used to continuously reinfuse ascitic fluid, which accumulates as a result of liver failure, back into the venous system. One end of the catheter is implanted in the peritoneal cavity, and the other is channeled through the subcutaneous tissue to the superior vena cava. If the amount reinfused is excessive, the heart may not then be able to handle the volume. A myocardial infarction (2), respiratory distress (3) and renal failure (4) may occur *secondary* to heart failure. **AS, APP, 4, PhI, Reduction of risk potential**

2. **(2)** Men with cirrhosis suffer breast enlargement, or gynecomastia, as well as palmar erythema, because of the increased androgen production that occurs. The testicles *atrophy* rather than swell (1). Rebound tenderness (3) is indicative of *appendicitis*. Wheezing (4) would be heard in the presence of *respiratory* diseases, such as bronchitis or asthma, that cause bronchospasm. If heart failure develops in a client with cirrhosis, the client would experience crackles. **AN, COM, 4, PhI, Physiological adaptation**

3. **(1)** Hepatitis is the most significant infection of the liver, and the damage may be so extensive that cirrhosis results. The incidence of cirrhosis is *not* increased in clients with gallbladder or biliary (2) problems. The regular use of high doses of acetaminophen (3), such as *Tylenol*, has been implicated in impaired liver function, but *not consistently*. Blunt abdominal trauma (4) is more likely to result in *cholecystitis* or *pancreatitis*. **AN, COM, 4, PhI, Physiological adaptation**

4. **(3)** AST (SGOT) and ALT (SGPT) are liver enzymes, and the levels would be elevated in a client with liver disease. The *prothrombin time* (1) would be *increased*, even though the prothrombin and albumin levels are decreased. The number of thrombocytes (2), as well as red blood cells, would be *decreased*. The alkaline phosphatase (4) level is *elevated* in liver disease. **AS, APP, 4, PhI, Reduction of risk potential**

5. **(1)** The bile, which is not being broken down by the liver, is excreted in the urine, rendering the urine dark brown. Bloody urine (2), or hematuria, would occur in the presence of *bladder cancer* or *kidney disease*. Clear urine (3), if colorless, would be seen in *diuresis*; clearness in terms of turbidity would be a normal appearance. Diluted (4) urine is the same as colorless urine; it would be seen in *diuresis*. **AS, COM, 8, PhI, Basic care and comfort**

6. **(2)** Lactulose is a cathartic and may be used if other agents for constipation are ineffective. Although lactulose does not significantly affect the serum glucose level, it is a sugar and would produce *hyperglycemia*, not hypoglycemia (1), if absorbed. The client with colitis (3), or inflammation of the large bowel, suffers from frequent diarrhea, so lactulose would be *contraindicated*. A hiatal hernia (4), which is a bulging of the esophagus where it joins the stomach, causes food to "hang up." Hot liquids, *not* lactulose, would help relieve this condition. **AN, APP, 8, PhI, Pharmacological and parenteral therapies**

7. **(3)** Ascites is the accumulation of fluid in the peritoneum as a result of increased portal pressure and low serum albumin levels. Resolution of the ascites is objectively gauged by measurement of the abdominal girth. If esophageal or GI tract *bleeding* is suspected, the stools should be checked for occult blood (hematest, 1). Bowel sounds (2) may be muffled in a client with *ascites*, but the presence or absence of bowel sounds does *not* indicate the severity of the ascites. Urine output (4), if diminished, would stem from the reduced cardiac output that may occur in cirrhosis but is *unrelated* to the ascites. **AS, ANL, 6, PhI, Physiological adaptation**

8. **(4)** The Minnesota tube has inflatable balloons that are positioned in the esophagus and stomach; the tube may become dislodged and obstruct the airway. If airway obstruction is observed, the tube should not be cut; instead, the balloon, or balloons, should be deflated and the tube, or tubes, removed. An acute illness will increase gastric acidity, but *routine* testing (1) is *not done* in a client with the Minnesota tube. The client should receive an antacid or H_2

blocker to prevent hyperacidity. The tube is used to stop esophageal bleeding, so a hematest (2) result would be positive; this finding does *not* indicate a problem with the *tube*. The tube is inserted via the nose, so communication (3) would *not* be impaired. **PL, ANL, 6, PhI, Physiological adaptation**

9. **(1)** Liver flap, or asterixis, which is a flapping tremor of the hand that is seen when the arm is extended, occurs with a rising ammonia level, which is a central nervous system toxin. Facial weakness (2) and drooling (3) would be seen in a client after a *stroke* or *cranial nerve VII* (facial) damage. Nystagmus (4), or jerking eye movements, occurs with *cranial nerve damage* and *inner ear* disorders such as Meniere's disease. **AN, EVL, 2, PhI, Physiological adaptation**

Key to Codes

Nursing process: **AS**, assessment; **AN**, analysis; **PL**, planning; **IMP**, implementation; **EV**, evaluation. (See **Appendix M** for explanation of nursing process steps.)

Cognitive level: **RE/KN**, recall/knowledge; **COM**, comprehension; **APP**, application; **ANL**, analysis; **EVL**, evaluation; **SYN**, synthesis. (See **Appendix M** for explanation.)

Category of human function: **1**, protective; **2**, sensory-perceptual; **3**, comfort, rest, activity, and mobility; **4**, nutrition; **5**, growth and development; **6**, fluid-gas transport; **7**, psychosocial-cultural; **8**, elimination. (See **Appendix 0** for explanation.)

Client need: **SECE**, safe, effective care environment; **PhI**, physiological integrity; **PsI**, psychosocial integrity; **HPM**, health promotion and maintenance. (See **Appendix P** for explanation.)

Client subneed: (See **Appendix P** for explanation)

Gastric Disorders

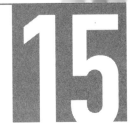

Chapter Outline

- General Nutritional Deficiencies
- Common Mineral Deficiencies
- Peptic Ulcer Disease
  - Gastric ulcers
  - Duodenal ulcers
  - Stress ulcers
- Diaphragmatic (Hiatal) Hernia
- Gastric Surgery
- Dumping Syndrome
- Summary of Key Points

- Study and Memory Aids
  - Diagnostic Studies/Procedures
    - Upper GI
    - Lower GI
    - Gastric Analysis
    - Stool Specimens
    - Esophagoscopy, Gastroscopy
  - Diets
  - Drug review
- Questions
- Answers/Rationale

General Nutritional Deficiencies

I. **Assessment**

A. *Subjective data*:
1. Mental irritability or confusion.
2. History of poor dietary intake.
3. History of lack of adequate resources to provide adequate nutrition.
4. Lack of knowledge about proper diet, food selection, or preparation.
5. History of eating disorders.
6. Paresthesia (burning and tingling): hands and feet.

B. *Objective data*:
1. *Appearance*: listless; *posture*: sagging shoulders, sunken chest, poor gait.
2. *Muscle*: weakness, fatigue, wasted appearance.
3. *Gastrointestinal (GI)*: indigestion; vomiting; enlarged liver, spleen.
4. *Cardiovascular*: tachycardia on minimal exertion, bradycardia at rest; enlarged heart; elevated blood pressure.
5. *Hair*: brittle, dry, thin, sparse; lack of natural shine; color changes; can be easily plucked out.
6. *Skin*: dryness (*xerosis*), scaly, dyspigmentation, petechiae, lack of fat under skin.
7. *Mouth*:
   a. *Teeth*: missing, abnormally placed, caries.
   b. *Gums*: bleed easily, receding.
   c. *Tongue*: swollen, sore.
   d. *Lips*: red, swollen, angular fissures at corners.

8. *Eyes*: pale conjuctiva, corneal changes
9. *Nails*: brittle, ridged.
10. *Nervous system*: abnormal reflexes.
11. Lab data: blood–*decreased* albumin, iron-binding capacity, lymphocyte, hemoglobin, and hematocrit.
12. Anthropometric measurements document nutritional deficiencies.

II. **Analysis/nursing diagnosis**

A. *Altered nutrition, less than body requirements*, related to poor dietary intake.
B. *Knowledge deficit* related to nutritional requirements.
C. *Altered health maintenance* related to inability to provide own nutritional care.
D. *Ineffective individual coping* related to eating disorders.
E. *Ineffective family coping, disabling*, related to inadequate resources or knowledge to provide appropriate family nutrition.

III. **Nursing care plan/implementation**

A. Goal: *prevent complications of specific deficiency.*
1. Identify etiology of nutritional deficiency.
2. Recognize signs of nutritional deficiencies (**Table 15.1 Common Mineral Deficiencies**).
3. Identify foods high in deficient nutrient (see **Appendix B**).
4. Evaluate economic resources to purchase appropriate foods.
5. Identify community resources for assistance.
6. Monitor progress for potential additional illnesses.

B. Goal: **health teaching.**
1. Effects of nutritional deficiencies on health.
2. Foods to include in diet to avoid deficits.

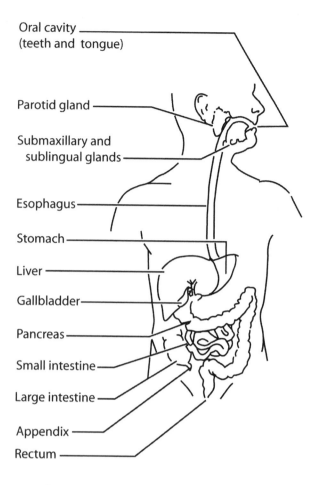

Oral cavity
(teeth and tongue)

Parotid gland

Submaxillary and
sublingual glands

Esophagus

Stomach

Liver

Gallbladder

Pancreas

Small intestine

Large intestine

Appendix

Rectum

Components of the Digestive System

IV. Evaluation/outcome criteria
    A. Complications do not occur.
    B. Client gains weight.
    C. Client selects appropriate foods to alleviate
       deficiency.

Peptic Ulcer Disease

Circumscribed loss of mucosa, submucosa, or muscle layer of the GI tract caused by decreased resistance of gastric mucosa to acid-pepsin injury. *Peptic ulcer disease* is a chronic disease and may occur in the distal esophagus, stomach, upper duodenum, or jejunum. *Gastric ulcers*, located on the lesser curvature of stomach, are larger, deeper than duodenal ulcers and tend to become *malignant. Duodenal ulcers* are located on the first part of the duodenum; they are more common than gastric ulcers. *Stress ulcers*, an acute problem, occur after a major insult to the body.

I. **Pathophysiology**: failure of the body to regenerate mucous epithelium at a sufficient rate to counterbalance the damage to tissue during the breakdown of protein; decrease in the quantity and quality of the mucus; poor local mucosal blood flow, along with individual susceptibility to ulceration.

II. **Risk factors/causes:**
    A. **Gastric ulcers:**
       1. Decreased resistance to acid-pepsin injury.
       2. Gastritis.

TABLE 15.1 COMMON MINERAL DEFICIENCIES

Mineral	Function	Deficiency Leads To:
Calcium	Aids in formation and maintenance of bones and teeth; permits healthy nerve functioning and normal blood clotting	↑ Neuromuscular irritability, impaired blood clotting
Phosphorus	Bone building	Rickets
Magnesium	Cellular metabolism of carbohydrates and protein	↓ Cellular metabolism of carbohydrates and protein; tetany
Sodium	Fluid and electrolyte balance; acid-base balance; electrochemical impulses of nerves and muscles	Fluid and electrolyte imbalance; ↓ muscle contraction
Potassium	Osmotic pressure and water balance Transmit and conduct nerve impulses; maintain: cardiac rhythm, skeletal and smooth muscle contraction, acid-base balance	Fluid and electrolyte imbalance; ↓ cardiac and skeletal muscular contractility
Chloride	Fluid and electrolyte balance, acid-base balance; digestion	Fluid imbalances; alkalosis
Iron	Hemoglobin formation; cellular oxidation	Anemia
Iodine	Synthesis of thyroid hormone; overall body metabolism	Goiter
Zinc	Constituent of cell enzyme system; CO_2 carrier in red blood cell	↓ Metabolism of protein and carbohydrates; delayed wound healing

3. Increased histamine release → inflammatory reaction.
4. Cigarette smoking, increased caffeine/alcohol use.
5. Family history.
6. Difficulty coping with high-stress environment.
7. Ulcerogenic drugs that aggravate preexisting condition.
8. Increased hydrogen ion back-diffusion.
9. Age: >50 yr.
B. Duodenal ulcers:
   1. *Elevated* gastric acid secretory rate.
   2. *Elevated* gastric acid levels postprandially (after eating).
   3. Increased rate of gastric emptying → increased amount of acid in duodenum → irritation and breakdown of duodenal mucosa.
   4. More men than women affected; possible influence of endocrine factors such as estrogen and adrenal steroids.
   5. Seasonal influence: spring and fall.
   6. Cigarette smoking; increased caffeine/alcohol use.
   7. Family history.
   8. Difficulty coping with high-stress environment (controversial).
   9. Ulcerogenic drugs that aggravate preexisting condition.
   10. Persons with type O blood.
   11. Age 25-50 yr.
C. Stress ulcers:
   1. Severe trauma or major illness.
   2. Severe burns (*Curling's ulcer*); develop in 72 h in most persons with burns over more than 35% of their body surface.
   3. Head injuries or intracranial disease (*Cushing's* ulcers).
   4. Medications in large doses: *corticosteroids*, *salicylates*, ibuprofen, indomethacin, phenylbutazone (*Butazolidin*).
   5. Shock.
   6. Sepsis.

III. **Assessment**
A. *Subjective data*:
   1. **Gastric ulcers:**
      a. *Pain*:
         (1) Type: gnawing, aching, burning.
         (2) Location: epigastric, left of midline, localized.
         (3) Occurrence: periodic pain, often 2 h after eating.
         (4) Relief: *antacids*; may be aggravated, *not relieved, by food*.
      b. Nausea.
      c. History of risk factors, as above.
   2. **Duodenal ulcers:**
      a. *Pain*:
         (1) Type: gnawing, aching, burning, hungerlike, boring.
         (2) Location: right epigastric, localized; steady pain near midline of back may indicate perforation.
         (3) Occurrence: 1–3h after eating, worse at end of day or during the night; initial attack occurs in spring or fall; history of remissions and exacerbations.
         (4) Relief: food and/or *antacids*.
      b. Nausea.
      c. History of risk factors (see **p. 188-189**).
   3. **Stress ulcers:**
      a. *Pain*: often painless until serious complication (hemorrhage, perforation) occurs.
      b. History of risk factors (see **p. 188-189**).
B. *Objective data*:
   1. **Gastric ulcers:**
      a. Vomiting.
      b. Melena (tarry stools).
      c. Weight loss.
      d. X-ray (*upper GI series*) confirms "crater" (punched-out appearance, clean base).
      e. *Endoscopy* confirms presence of ulcer; biopsy for cytologic data.
      f. Lab data—positive for H. *pylori*
      g. Monitor for blood loss: complete blood count, stool for occult blood.
   2. **Duodenal ulcers:**
      a. Eructation.
      b. Vomiting.
      c. Regurgitation of sour liquid into back of mouth.
      d. Constipation.
      e. X-ray (*upper GI series*) confirms ulcer craters and niches as well as outlet deformities: round or oval funnel-like lesion extending into musculature.
      f. Lab data—positive for H. *pylori*
      g. Common complications: hemorrhage or perforation.
   3. **Stress ulcers:**
      a. GI tract bleeding.
      b. Multiple, superficial erosions affecting large area of gastric mucosa (as documented by GI series or endoscopy).

IV. **Analysis/nursing diagnosis (all types)**
A. *Pain* related to erosion of gastric lining.
B. *Ineffective individual coping* related to inability to change life-style.
C. *Altered nutrition, less than body requirements*, related to inadequate intake.
D. *Knowledge deficit* regarding preventive measures.
E. *Risk for injury* related to possible hemorrhage or perforation.

V. Nursing care plan/implementation (all types)
  A. Goal: *promote comfort.*
    1. Medications as ordered to decrease pain (see Goal: **health teaching**, below.
    2. Prepare for diagnostic tests.
      a. X-rays: *upper GI series* (barium swallow), *lower GI* (barium enema).
      b. *Endoscopy.*
      c. *Gastric analysis*, to determine amount of hydrochloric acid in GI tract.
  B. Goal: *prevent/recognize signs of complications.*
    1. Monitor vital signs for shock.
    2. Check stool for occult blood/hemorrhage.
    3. Palpate abdomen for perforation (rigid, board-like), arterial bleeding.
  C. Goal: *provide emotional support.*
    1. Stress-management techniques.
    2. Restful environment.
    3. Prepare for surgery, if necessary.
  D. Goal: **health teaching.**
    1. Medications:
      a. *Antiulceratives: give 1–3h after meals and at bedtime* to decrease pain by lowering acidity; monitor for:
        (1) Diarrhea (seen most often with magnesium carbonate and magnesium oxide).
        (2) Constipation (seen most often with calcium carbonate or aluminum hydroxide).
        (3) Electrolyte imbalance (seen with systemic antacid, soda bicarbonate).
        (4) Best 1–3h *after meals.*
        (5) Liquids more effective than tablets; if taking tablets, chew slowly.
      b. *Histamine antagonists: taken with meals and at bedtime* to block the action of histamine-stimulated gastric secretions (basal and stimulated); inhibits pepsin secretion and reduces the volume of gastric secretion.
        (1) Cimetidine (*Tagamet*) inhibits gastrin release, can be given PO, IV, or IM; *cannot* be given within 1h of antacid therapy.
        (2) Ranitidine (*Zantac*) causes greater reduction of acid secretion, has longer duration, requires less frequent administration (bid vs qid), and has fewer side effects than cimetidine.
      c. *Proton pump inhibitors*: block ATPase enzyme necessary for secretion of hydrochloric acid; more effective than H_2 receptor blockers.
        (1) Omeprazole (*Prilosec*) should be taken before eating; do **not** break, crush, or chew; give PO qd.
        (2) Esomeprazole (*Nexium*) is similar to omeprazole; taken once a day.
      d. *Protectant*: Sucralfate (*Carafate*): *given 1h before meals and at bedtime.*
        (1) Locally active topical agent that forms a protective coat on mucosa, prevents further digestive action of both acid and pepsin.
        (2) Must *not* be given within ½ h of antacids.
      e. *Antiinfectives*: take as directed in combination with *antiulcerative* or H_2 *antagonists*. Optimal treatment regimen is under investigation.
      f. *Anticholinergic, when used, given before meals* to decrease gastric acid secretion and delay gastric emptying.
      g. Important: *avoid* aspirin use (could increase bleeding possibility).
    2. Diet:
      a. *Avoid*:
        (1) Stress at mealtimes.
        (2) Milk (increases gastric acid production).
        (3) Substances that provoke pain.
        (4) Coffee with or without caffeine.
        (5) Foods or liquids containing caffeine.
        (6) Alcohol.
        (7) Tobacco.
      b. *Plan*:
        (1) Small, frequent meals (to prevent exacerbation of symptoms related to an empty stomach).
        (2) Weight control.
    3. Complications: signs and symptoms:
      a. Gastric ulcers may be premalignant.
      b. Perforation.
      c. Hemorrhage.
      d. Obstruction.
    4. Lifestyle changes:
      a. *Decrease*:
        (1) Smoking.
        (2) Noise.
        (3) Rush.
        (4) Confusion.
      b. *Increase*:
        (1) Communication; verbalize concerns.
        (2) Mental/physical rest.
        (3) Compliance with medical regimen.

VI. Evaluation/outcome criteria
  A. Remains on specified diet.
  B. Takes prescribed medications.
  C. Pain decreases.

D. No complications.

E. States signs and symptoms of complications.

F. Participates in stress-reduction activities.

G. No further ulcers.

Diaphragmatic (Hiatal) Hernia

Protrusion of part of stomach through diaphragm and into thoracic cavity. *Types*: sliding (most common), paraesophageal "rolling."

I. **Pathophysiology:** weakening of the musculature of the diaphragm, aggravated by increased intraabdominal pressure → protrusion of the abdominal organs through the esophageal hiatus → reflux of gastric contents → esophagitis.

II. **Risk factors/causes:**

A. Congenital abnormality.

B. Penetrating wound.

C. Age (middle-aged or elderly).

D. Women more affected than men.

E. Obesity.

F. Ascites.

G. Pregnancy.

H. History of constipation.

III. **Assessment**

A. *Subjective data*:

1. Pressure: substernal.

2. Pain: epigastric, burning.

3. Eructation, heartburn after eating.

4. Dysphagia.

5. Symptoms aggravated when recumbent.

B. *Objective data*:

1. Cough, dyspnea.

2. Tachycardia, palpitations.

3. Bleeding: hematemesis, melena, signs of anemia due to gastroesophageal irritation, ulceration, and bleeding.

4. *Diagnostic tests*:

a. Chest x-rays showing protrusion of abdominal organs into thoracic cavity.

b. *Barium swallow* (upper GI series) to show presence of hernia.

IV. **Analysis/nursing diagnosis**

A. *Pain* related to irritation of lining of GI tract.

B. *Altered nutrition, less than body requirements,* related to dysphagia.

C. *Sleep pattern disturbance* related to increase in symptoms when recumbent.

D. *Risk for aspiration* related to reflux of gastric contents.

E. *Activity intolerance* related to dyspnea.

F. *Anxiety* related to palpitations.

V. **Nursing care plan/implementation**

A. **Preoperative care:**

1. Goal: *promote relief of symptoms.*

a. *Diet*:

(1) Small, frequent feedings of soft, bland foods, to reduce abdominal pressure and reflux.

(2) *Fluid* when swallowing solids; may push food into stomach; hot fluid may work best.

(3) *Avoid* eating 2h before bedtime.

(4) *High protein, low fat* foods to decrease heartburn.

b. *Positioning: head elevated* to increase movement of food into stomach. Symptoms may decrease if head of bed at home is elevated on 8-in. blocks.

c. Weight reduction to decrease abdominal pressure.

d. Medications as ordered:

(1) 30 mL of *antacid* 1h after meals and at bedtime.

(2) *Avoid* anticholinergic drugs, which decrease gastric emptying.

B. **Postoperative care:**

1. Goal: *provide for postoperative safety needs.*

a. Respiratory: deep breathing, coughing; splint incision area.

b. *Nasogastric (NG) tube*: check patency

(1) Drainage: should be small amount.

(2) Color: dark brown 6–12h after surgery, changing to greenish yellow.

(3) Do *not* disturb tube placement to *avoid* traction on suture line.

c. *Position*: initially head of bed elevated slightly, then semi-Fowler's; turn side to side frequently to prevent pressure on diaphragm.

d. Maintain *closed-chest drainage* if indicated (see **Chap. 6 p. 86**, **Tubes** box).

e. Check for return of bowel sounds.

2. Goal: *promote comfort and maintain nutrition.*

a. IVs for hydration and electrolytes.

b. Initiate feeding through *gastrostomy* tube, if present.

(1) Usually attached to intermittent, low *suction* after surgery.

(2) *Aspirate* gastric contents before feeding—delay if 75 mL or more is present; report these findings to physician.

(3) Feed in *high-Fowler's* or *sitting position*; keep head elevated for 30 min *after* eating.

(4) *Warm* feeding to room temperature; *dilute* with water if too thick.

(5) Give 50 mL of water *before* feeding; 200–500 mL feeding by gravity over 10–15 min; *follow* with 50 mL of water.

(6) Give frequent mouth care.

3. Goal: **health teaching.**

  a. *Avoid* constricting clothing and activities that increase intraabdominal pressure, e.g., lifting, bending, straining at stool.

  b. Weight reduction.

  c. Dietary needs: small, frequent, soft, bland meals; chew thoroughly; *upright* position for at least 1h *after* meals.

VI. Evaluation/outcome criteria

  A. Relief from symptoms, comfortable.

  B. Receiving adequate, balanced nutrition.

  C. Describes dietary changes, recommended positioning, and activity limitations to prevent recurrence.

Gastric Surgery

Performed when: medical treatment for ulcer is unsuccessful, ulcer is determined to be precancerous, or complications are present.

I. Types:

  A. *Subtotal gastrectomy*: removal of a portion of the stomach.

  B. *Total gastrectomy*: removal of the entire stomach.

  C. *Antrectomy*: removal of entire antrum (lower) portion of the stomach.

  D. *Pyloroplasty*: repair of the pyloric opening of the stomach.

  E. *Vagotomy*: interruption of the impulses carried by the vagus nerve, which results in reduction of gastric secretions and decreased physical activity of the stomach (this procedure is now being done less often).

  F. Combination of vagotomy and gastrectomy.

II. Analysis/nursing diagnosis

  A. *Pain* related to surgical incision.

  B. *Ineffective breathing pattern* related to high surgical incision.

  C. *Risk for trauma* related to possible complications after gastrectomy.

  D. *Knowledge deficit* related to inability to manage ulcer disease on medical regimen.

  E. *Fear* related to possible precancerous lesion.

  F. *Ineffective individual coping* related to risk factors for peptic ulcer disease.

III. Nursing care plan/implementation

  A. Goal: *promote comfort in the postoperative period.*

  1. *Analgesics*: to relieve pain and allow client to cough, deep breathe to prevent pulmonary complications.

  2. *Position*: semi-Fowler's to aid in breathing.

  B. Goal: *promote wound healing.*

  1. Keep dressing dry.

2. *NG tube* connected to low intermittent (*Levin*) or low continuous (*Salem sump*) suction.

  a. Check drainage from NG tube; normally bloody first 2–3h after surgery, then brown to dark green.

  b. Excessive bright red blood drainage: take vital signs; report: vital signs, color, and volume of drainage to MD **immediately**.

  c. Irrigate *gently* with saline in amount ordered; do **not** irrigate against resistance; may not be done in early postoperative period.

  d. Tape securely to face, but prevent obstructed vision.

  e. Frequent mouth and nostril care.

  C. Goal: *promote adequate nutrition and hydration.*

  1. Administer parenteral fluids as ordered.

  2. Accurate intake and output.

  3. Check bowel sounds, at least q4h; NPO 1–3 days; bowel sounds normally return after 24–36h; *oral fluids* as ordered when bowel sounds present—usually 30 mL, then *small* feedings, then *bland* liquids to *soft* diet.

  4. Observe for nausea and vomiting due to suture line edema, food intake (too much, too fast).

  D. Goal: *prevent complications.*

  1. Check dressing q4h for bleeding.

  2. Vitamin B_{12} and *iron* replacement as ordered to prevent pernicious or iron deficiency anemia.

  3. Prevent dumping syndrome (see below).

IV. Evaluation/outcome criteria

  A. Hemorrhage, dumping syndrome prevented.

  B. Healing begins.

  C. Adjusts life-style to prevent recurrence/marginal ulcer.

Dumping Syndrome

Hypoglycemic-type episode; occurs postoperatively after gastric resection (may also occur after vagotomy, antrectomy, or gastroenterostomy), when food and fluids that are more hyperosmolar than the jejunal secretions pass *quickly* into jejunum, producing fluid shifts from bloodstream to jejunum. This is a mild problem for about 20% of clients and disappears in a few months to a year. Symptoms are serious in about 7% of the clients. This discomfort may occur during a meal or up to 30 min after the meal and last from 20–60 min. The reaction is greatest after the ingestion of sugar.

I. Assessment

  A. *Subjective data*:

  1. Feeling of fullness, weakness, faintness.

2. Palpitations.
3. Nausea.
4. Discomfort during or after eating.

B. *Objective data*:
1. Diaphoresis.
2. Diarrhea.
3. Fainting.
4. Symptoms of hypoglycemia.

▶◀ **II. Analysis/nursing diagnosis**

A. *Altered nutrition, more than body requirements*, related to body's inability to properly digest high carbohydrate, high sodium foods.

B. *Diarrhea* related to food passing into jejunum too quickly.

C. *Risk for injury* related to hypoglycemia.

D. *Knowledge deficit* related to dietary restrictions.

▶◀ **III. Nursing care plan/implementation**

A. Goal: *slow gastric emptying.*
🍎 1. *Increase fat, protein* in diet to delay emptying; fiber.
2. Rest after meals.
3. Eat small, frequent meals.
4. Drink fluids *between* meals.
▭ 5. Medications: *anticholinergics* (ephedrine).

📖 B. Goal: **health teaching.**
🍎 1. *Avoid* foods high in *refined carbohydrate.*
2. Practice portion control.
3. Stress management, particularly at mealtime.
4. Symptom management.

▶◀ **IV. Evaluation/outcome criteria**

A. No complications.
B. Client heals.
C. Incorporates health teaching into life-style and prevents syndrome.

〰️ Diagnostic Studies/Procedures

Common Fluoroscopic Examinations

Upper GI—ingestion of barium sulfate or meglumine diatrizoate (Gastrografin, a white, chalky, radiopaque substance), followed by fluoroscopic and x-ray examination; *used* to determine:

1. Patency and caliber of *esophagus*; may also detect esophageal varices.
2. Mobility and thickness of *gastric* walls, presence of ulcer craters, filling defects due to tumors, pressures from outside the stomach, and patency of pyloric valve.
3. Rate of passage in *small bowel* and presence of structural abnormalities.

Lower GI—rectal instillation of barium sulfate followed by fluoroscopic and x-ray examination; *used* to determine contour and mobility of colon and presence of any space-occupying tumors; perform *before* upper GI. **Client preparation:** explain purpose; *no food after evening meal* the evening before test; *stool softeners, laxatives, enemas, and suppositories* to cleanse the bowel before the test; NPO *after midnight* prior to test; oral medications *not* permitted day of test.

After completion of exam: food, *increased liquid* intake, and rest; *laxatives for at least 2 d* or until stools are normal in color and consistency.

Examination of Gastric Contents

Gastric analysis—aspiration of the contents of the fasting stomach for analysis of free and total acid.

1. Gastric acidity is generally *increased* in presence of duodenal ulcer.
2. Gastric acidity is usually *decreased* in pernicious anemia, cancer of the stomach.

Stool specimens—*examined for*: amount, consistency, color, character, and melena; *used to* determine presence of: urobilinogen, fat, nitrogen, parasites, and other substances.

Esophagoscopy and gastroscopy—visualization of the esophagus, the stomach, and sometimes the duodenum by means of a lighted tube inserted through the mouth.

🔑 Summary of Key Points

1. Gastric disorders may include problems with *ingestion* (getting the food to the stomach) *digestion* (the process of secreting gastric juices and breaking down protein), or absorption (transfer of food porticles into circulation).

2. Regardless of the disorder, the client often complains of pain (erosion or stretching), loss of appetite (impaired gastric emptying), nausea (gastric tension), bleeding (erosion or trauma), diarrhea (increased peristalsis), belching or flatus, dyspepsia (heartburn), or a combination of these.

3. Enteral (NG or gastric tube) or parenteral (TPN) feedings may be *supplemental or replacement*. If they are replacing oral feedings, mouth care and satisfying oral needs are important.

4. Though similar in many ways, the differences

between a duodenal and gastric ulcer are distinctive. A *duodenal* ulcer is more common, the characteristic gnawing pain occurs hours *after* a meal or at night, and food *relieves* the pain.

5. Treatment is medical (rest, drugs, diet, decreased stress), unless the ulcer: becomes chronic, recurs, perforates, causes obstruction, or bleeds—then surgery is indicated.

▭ 6. Drug therapy *inhibits* acid secretion and *neutralizes* or *protects* the gastric mucosa. Client teaching must include whether a drug is taken *before, with,* or how long *after* meals.

🍎 7. The dumping syndrome is controlled by regulating the *volume* and type of food—*decrease carbohydrates* and *fluids, increase protein* and *fat* to delay gastric emptying.

Study and Memory Aids

🍎 Diets

Diaphragmatic Hernia

↑ Feedings	↓ Fat
Protein	Size of portions
Soft, bland	

Dumping Syndrome

↑ Fat	↓ Carbohydrate
Fiber	Fluids at mealtime
Frequency	↓ Portion size
Protein	

💊 Drug Review

Peptic Ulcer Disease

Anticholinergic
Propantheline bromide (*ProBanthine*): 15 mg tid, 30 mg hs

Antiinfectives
Amoxicillin: 250–500 mg q8h
Clarithromycin: (*Biaxin*) 250–500 mg q 12h
Metronidazole: (*Flagyl*) 250 mg tid
Tetracycline: 500 mg qid

Antiulceratives
Aluminum hydroxide gel (*Amphojel*): 5–10 mL q2–4h or 1h pc
Calcium carbonate (*Titralac*): 1–2 g with water after meals and hs
Magnesium and aluminum hydroxides (*Maalox* suspension): 5–30 mL pc and hs
Omeprazole (*Prilosec*): 20 mg qd for 4–8 wk

Histamine antagonists
Cimetidine (*Tagamet*): 300–600 mg q6h
Ranitidine (*Zantac*): 150 mg bid

Proton pump inhibitors
Lansoprazole (*Prevacid*): 15 mg PO qd.
Omeprazole (*Prilosec*): 20 mg PO qd for 4–8 wk.

Protectant
Sucralfate (*Carafate*): 1 g ac and hs

Diaphragmatic Hernia

Antacid therapy
Magnesium and aluminum hydroxide
(*Mylanta*): 500–1000 mg 3–6 times/day
(*Maalox* suspension): 5–30 mL pc and hs
(*Gaviscon*): 30–60 mL pc and hs

Histamine receptor antagonists
Ranitidine (*Zantac*): 150 mg bid.
Avoid anticholinergic drugs because they decrease lower esophageal sphincter function

Proton pump inhibitors
Lansoprazole (*Prevacid*): 15 mg PO qd
Omeprazole (*Prilosec*): 20 mg PO qd for 4–8 wk

Dumping Syndrome

Anticholinergic
(e.g., propantheline): to decrease gastric activity
Vasopressor
(e.g., ephedrine): to relieve vasomotor symptoms

Questions

1. After esophagoscopy is done to diagnose gastroesophageal reflux, the most important nursing action would be to:
   1. Check the client's vital signs frequently, as ordered.
   2. Assess for cervical crepitus in the neck.
   3. Place the client in a side-lying position to prevent aspiration.
   4. Give the client an anesthetic lozenge for sore throat.

2. Which instruction should be included in health care counseling for a client with a hiatal hernia?
   1. Restrict intake of high carbohydrate foods, which speed emptying.
   2. Increase fluid intake with meals to facilitate food passage.
   3. Increase fat intake to delay gastric emptying.
   4. Eat three regular meals daily at least 5 hours apart.

3. When giving morphine sulfate (5 mg) in an IV push to a 65-year-old client after a gastrectomy, the best technique would be to:
   1. Dilute it in 5 mL of normal saline and give it over 4 to 5 minutes.
   2. Dilute it in 10 mL of 5% dextrose in water and give it over 30 minutes.
   3. Give it undiluted at the injection site closest to the client.
   4. Give it undiluted at the injection site farthest from the client.

4. An important nursing action for a client with a nasogastric feeding tube is to:
    1. Measure the residual contents in the stomach every morning.
    2. Clean and lubricate the external nares.
    3. Administer the feeding over 1 to 2 hours.
    4. Check the client's blood glucose level before each feeding.

5. A client is receiving *Carafate* (sucralfate) qid and *Mylanta* tid. The nurse explains to the client that the best schedule for these drugs is to take:
    1. *Carafate* AC and HS and *Mylanta* PC.
    2. *Carafate* PC and HS and *Mylanta* AC.
    3. *Carafate* PC and HS and *Mylanta* PC.
    4. *Carafate* AC and *Mylanta* AC and HS.

    Mylanta 2-3 hours after eating

6. A client accidentally receives a bolus of *Tagamet* as the result of a faulty IV administration set. The nurse's first action would be to:
    1. Ask another nurse what problems are caused by getting an overdose of *Tagamet*.
    2. Consult a nursing textbook to find out the potential complications.
    3. Assess the client for signs of adverse drug effects.
    4. Consult the drug formulary to find out the implications of this.

    Carafate: before meals, hour of sleep

7. Which pair of drugs should the nurse plan to give at different times?
    1. *Diuril* (chlorothiazide) and *Questran* (cholestyramine) PO. — *always take alone*
    2. *Atarax* (hydroxyzine) and *Demerol* (meperidine) IM.
    3. *Tylenol* (acetaminophen) and *Coumadin* (warfarin sodium) PO.
    4. *Decadron* (dexamethasone) and *mannitol* IV.

8. While being assisted to the bathroom, the client complains of a "giving" sensation in the abdominal incision. The first nursing action would be to:
    1. Return the client to bed and place in a supine position.
    2. Call the physician immediately.
    3. Sit the client in a chair and check the vital signs.
    4. Culture the wound and reinforce the dressing.

9. The nurse irrigates a client's nasogastric tube with iced saline until it is cleared of blood. What would the nurse record on the intake and output record?
    1. The amount of irrigant aspirated as output.
    2. The amount of irrigant instilled as input.
    3. The difference between the amount of the irrigant and the amount of the aspirate.
    4. Nothing about the irrigation procedure.

10. Which finding is a complication of ulcer disease and should be reported immediately?
    1. A fine rash on body.
    2. Black stool.
    3. Constipation or diarrhea.
    4. Dizziness or headache.

11. Only a small amount of fluid is draining from a client's nasogastric tube. What is the first action the nurse should take?
    1. Irrigate the nasogastric tube.
    2. Position the client on the right side.
    3. Determine the placement of the tube.
    4. Record the amount of drainage.

12. Which sign of bleeding would the nurse expect in a client with a duodenal ulcer?
    1. Bright red blood in the stool.
    2. Bright red emesis.
    3. Coffee-ground emesis.
    4. Black, tarry stool.

13. Assessment of a client with a perforated ulcer would reveal:
    1. A boardlike abdomen, tachycardia, and hypotension.
    2. A distended abdomen and hyperactive bowel sounds.
    3. A distended abdomen and belching.
    4. A boardlike abdomen, restlessness, and bradycardia.

    hypovolemic shock

Answers/Rationale

1. **(3)** All of the nursing actions are correct, but the *first* priority is to position the client to prevent aspiration because a local anesthetic is sprayed on the posterior pharynx to ease the discomfort and prevent gagging when the tube is inserted, which may impair the swallowing reflex for a while. The client should be NPO for 2 to 4 hours afterward. Checking the vital signs (1) is *less important* than maintaining a clear airway. The finding of cervical crepitus (2) would indicate perforation, a *rare* complication. A sore throat (4) may result from the tube insertion, but it is a *less serious* concern; lozenges or a saline gargle may soothe the irritation. **IMP, ANL, 3, PhI, Reduction of risk potential**

2. **(2)** The main problem in a hiatal hernia is the food "hanging up" in the dilated area above the

Key to Codes

Nursing process: **AS**, assessment; **AN**, analysis; **PL**, planning; **IMP**, implementation; **EV**, evaluation. (See **Appendix M** for explanation of nursing process steps.)

Cognitive level: **RE/KN**, recall/knowledge; **COM**, comprehension; **APP**, application; **ANL**, analysis; **EVL**, evaluation; **SYN**, synthesis. (See **Appendix M** for explanation.)

Category of human function: 1, protective; 2, sensory-perceptual; 3, comfort, rest, activity, and mobility; 4, nutrition; 5, growth and development; 6, fluid-gas transport; 7, psychosocial-cultural; 8, elimination. (See **Appendix O** for explanation.)

Client need: **SECE**, safe, effective care environment; **PhI**, physiological integrity; **PsI**, psychosocial integrity; **HPM**, health promotion and maintenance. (See **Appendix P** for explanation.)

Client subneed: (See **Appendix P** for explanation)

sphincter of the stomach. Hot fluids are often most effective in relaxing the sphincter. Restricting carbohydrate intake (1) and increasing fat intake (3) are appropriate measures for clients with the *dumping syndrome*. Eating three regular meals a day (4) is incorrect; the clients should instead eat *smaller* and *more frequent* meals. **PL, APP, 4, HPM, Health promotion and maintenance**

3. **(1)** Morphine sulfate should be diluted when being given to an older adult to lessen potential adverse effects of IV push administration. For direct IV administration the drug should be diluted in at least 5 mL of sterile water or normal saline; 2.5 to 15 mg may be given over 4 to 5 minutes. Thirty minutes for the administration of' an IV push (2) is *too long*, and 5% dextrose in water is used for a continuous IV, *not* an IV push. Morphine sulfate *should be* diluted to lessen the side effects **(3 and 4)**. **IMP, APP, 1, PhI, Pharmacological and parenteral therapies**

4. **(2)** The nose may become very irritated, dried, and cracked because of the irritating effects of the tube. The residual gastric contents (1) should be measured *before every feeding*. The feeding should be given as prescribed (3); such intermittent feedings are usually administered in *less* than 1 hour. The blood glucose level (4) is *not* routinely tested before tube feedings. **IMP, COM, 4, PhI, Reduction of risk potential**

5. **(1)** *Carafate* is an agent used for the short-term treatment of an ulcer; it works by coating the ulcered area and should be taken 1 hour before eating and at bedtime. It does not decrease acidity or reduce H_2 (histamine) production. To effectively coat the ulcer the stomach needs to be empty, *not* full **(2 and 3)**. *Mylanta*, an antacid, should be taken 2 to 3 hours *after* meals when acid production is greatest, *not* before meals **(2 and 4)**. **PL, ANL, 4, PhI, Pharmacological and parenteral therapies**

6. **(3)** The first priority is assessing the client, noting any immediate effects from the excessive fluid or the large dose of the drug received. Side effects could include diarrhea, vomiting, headache, and dizziness. A colleague (1) and a nursing textbook (2) could provide inaccurate or dated data, or these actions could take time away from observation of the client. Consulting the formulary (4) would be the *next* appropriate action after the client's status has been assessed. **IMP, ANL, 1, SECE, Management of care**

7. **(1)** *Questran* is an antilipemic that is taken alone; administration with any other oral medication would cause the absorption of the *Questran* to be decreased. *Atarax* (2) or *Vistaril*, and *Demerol* are a common preoperative combination. *Tylenol* (3) is an analgesic that *can* be taken safely with *Coumadin*, an anticoagulant. *Decadron* and *mannitol* (4) *are* frequently administered together to clients with head injuries and cerebral edema. **PL, APP, 4, PhI, Pharmacological and parenteral therapies**

8. **(1)** The priority is to place the client supine to keep the intestines in the abdomen if evisceration

has occurred. The nurse should return the client to bed if it is nearby; lying the client on a gurney or a couch would also be appropriate. The MD should be called (2), but *not first*. Sitting (3) would *not* involve the use of gravity to keep the bowel in the abdomen. Wound culture (4) is *not* indicated in dehiscence or evisceration. **IMP, ANL, 1, PhI, Physiological adaptation**

9. **(4)** The fluid used in the irrigation of a nasogastric tube in a client suffering from gastrointestinal tract bleeding does not count as either intake or output fluid because the fluid instilled is withdrawn immediately, so there is no effect on the intake or output. The other options (1, 2, and 3) are wrong because there *should be no entry* on the intake and output record for the reasons just given. **IMP, COM, 1, SECE, Management of care**

10. **(2)** Black stool, or melena, is a sign of gastrointestinal tract bleeding. Other complications are perforation, hemorrhage, shock, and peritonitis. A rash (1), constipation or diarrhea (3), and dizziness or headache (4) are possible side effects of one of the drugs used in the treatment of ulcers (cimetidine [*Tagamet*]), but they are *not potentially life-threatening* and do *not* need to be *reported immediately*. These side effects usually resolve as the body adjusts to the effects of the drug. **AS, ANL, 4, PhI, Physiological adaptation**

11. **(3)** The small amount of drainage could be the result of either displacement or occlusion, but to prevent possible instillation of irrigant into the lungs, tube placement must be determined before the tube is irrigated. Irrigation (1) would therefore *not* be the *first* action. Positioning the client on the right side (2) could be tried *after* tube placement in the stomach is confirmed. This would promote gastric emptying and might cause the end of the tube to move if it is up against the stomach wall. Recording the output (4) is not wrong but it does *not improve* tube functioning. **IMP, ANL, 4, PhI, Reduction of risk potential**

12. **(4)** The digestion of blood in the duodenum results in black, tarry stools. Bright red blood in the stool (1) would be seen in a client with *colitis* or *hemorrhoids*. Bright red emesis (2) or hemorrhage, is more common in clients with *gastric* ulcers. Acid digestion in the stomach (*gastric* ulcers) results in dark, granular emesis (3). **AS, COM, 6, PhI, Physiological adaptation**

13. **(1)** The abdomen becomes rigid as a consequence of the resulting chemical peritonitis, and the vital signs indicate the occurrence of hypovolemic shock. The abdomen does *not* distend **(2 and 3)** with a perforated ulcer but is tender, hard, and rigid. Peristalsis would diminish and paralytic ileus develop, so bowel sounds would be *absent* (2). Gas (3) is not a problem. There would be tachycardia, *not* bradycardia (4), with perforation. **AS, COM, 4, PhI, Physiological adaptation**

Intestinal Disorders

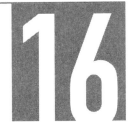

Chapter Outline

- Celiac Disease (Nontropical Sprue)
- Appendicitis
- Hernia
- Diverticulosis
- Ulcerative Colitis
- Crohn's Disease
- Intestinal Obstruction
- Fecal Diversion
- Hemorrhoids

- Summary of Key Points
- Study and Memory Aids
    - Diagnostic Studies/Procedures
        - Proctoscopy
        - Small Bowel Biopsy
    - Diets
    - Drug review
- Questions
- Answers/Rationale

Celiac Disease (Nontropical Sprue)

Gluten-induced intestinal disease affecting adults and children, characterized by inability to digest and utilize sugars, starches, and fats.

I. **Pathophysiology:** intolerance to the gliadin fraction of grains, causing degeneration of the epithelial surface of the intestine, atrophy of the intestinal villi, and impaired absorption of essential nutrients.

II. **Risk factors/causes:**
   A. Possible genetic or familial factors.
   B. Hypersensitivity response.
   C. History of childhood celiac disease.

III. **Assessment**
   A. *Subjective data*: family history.
   B. *Objective data*:
      1. Loss: weight, fat deposits, musculature.
      2. Anemia.
      3. Vitamin deficiencies.
      4. Abdomen: distended with flatus.
      5. Stools: diarrhea, foul smelling, bulky, fatty, float in commode.
      6. History of acute attacks of fluid/electrolyte imbalances.
      7. *Diagnostic tests: small bowel biopsy, stool for fat.*
      8. *Gluten-free diet* leads to remission of symptoms.

IV. **Analysis/nursing diagnosis**
   A. *Altered nutrition, less than body requirements,* related to inability to digest and utilize sugars, starches, and fats.
   B. *Diarrhea* related to intestinal response to gluten in diet.
   C. *Fluid volume deficit* related to loss through excessive diarrhea.

   D. *Knowledge deficit* related to dietary restrictions to control symptoms.

V. **Nursing care plan/implementation**
   A. Goal: *prevent weight loss.*
      1. *Diet*: high in calories, protein, vitamins, and minerals; gluten free.
         a. *Avoid* wheat, rye, oats, barley.
         b. All other foods permitted.
      2. Daily weights to monitor changes.
   B. Goal: **health teaching.**
      1. Nature of disease.
      2. Dietary restrictions and allowances.
      3. Complications of noncompliance.
      4. Medications: *antidiarrhea* and *anticholinergic.*

VI. **Evaluation/outcome criteria**
   A. No further weight loss.
   B. Normal stools.
   C. Fluid/electrolyte balance obtained and maintained.

Appendicitis

Obstruction of appendiceal lumen and subsequent bacterial invasion of appendiceal wall; **acute emergency.**

I. **Pathophysiology:** when obstruction is partial or mild, inflammation begins in mucosa with slight appendiceal swelling, accompanied by periumbilical pain. As the inflammatory process escalates and/or obstruction becomes more complete, appendix becomes more swollen, lumen fills with pus, and mucosal ulceration begins. When inflammation extends to peritoneal surface, pain is referred to right lower abdominal quadrant. *Danger*: rigidity over the entire abdomen is usually indicative of ruptured appendix; client is then prone to peritonitis.

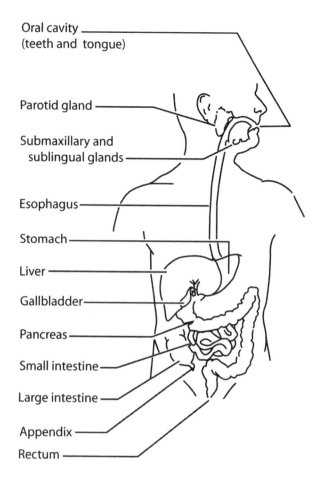

Oral cavity
(teeth and tongue)

Parotid gland

Submaxillary and
sublingual glands

Esophagus

Stomach

Liver

Gallbladder

Pancreas

Small intestine

Large intestine

Appendix

Rectum

Components of the Digestive System

II. Risk factors/causes:
   A. Men affected more often than women.
   B. Most frequently seen in 10-30 yr old.

III. Assessment
   A. *Subjective data*:
      1. Pain: generalized, then right lower quadrant at McBurney's point, with rebound tenderness.
      2. Anorexia, nausea.
   B. *Objective data*:
      1. Vital signs: elevated temperature, shallow respirations.
      2. Either diarrhea or constipation.
      3. Vomiting, fetid breath odor.
      4. Splitting of abdominal muscles, flexion of knees onto abdomen.
      5. Lab data: *elevated*—white blood cell count (>10,000/mm³), neutrophil count (>75%).

IV. Analysis/nursing diagnosis
   A. *Pain* related to inflammation of appendix.
   B. *Risk for infection* related to ruptured appendix.
   C. *Knowledge deficit* related to possible surgery.

V. Nursing care plan/implementation
   A. Goal: *promote comfort preoperatively and postoperatively.*

1. Explain procedures; pain medications often withheld pending diagnosis.
2. Assist with diagnostic workup.
3. Medications as ordered: *analgesics.*
   B. Goal: *prevent complications.*
      1. Prevent infection: wound care, dressing technique, *antiinfectives.*
      2. Prevent dehydration: IVs, intake and output (I&O), fluids to solids by mouth as tolerated.
      3. Promote ambulation to prevent postoperative complications.

VI. Evaluation/outcome criteria
   A. No infection.
   B. Tolerates fluid, bowel sounds return.
   C. Heals with no complications.

Hernia

Protrusion of the intestine through a weak portion of the abdominal wall.

I. Types:
   A. *Reducible*: visceral contents return to their normal position, either spontaneously or by manipulation.
   B. *Irreducible, or incarcerated*: contents cannot be returned to normal position.
   C. *Strangulated*: blood supply to the structure within the hernia sac becomes occluded (usually a loop of bowel).
   D. *Most common hernias*: umbilical, femoral, inguinal, incisional, and hiatal (see **Chap. 15** for **hiatal hernia**).

II. Pathophysiology: weakness in the wall may be either congenital or acquired. Herniation occurs when there is an increase in intraabdominal pressure from: coughing, lifting, crying, straining, obesity, or pregnancy.

III. Assessment
   A. *Subjective data*:
      1. Pain, discomfort.
      2. History of feeling a lump.
   B. *Objective data*:
      1. Soft lump, especially when straining or coughing.
      2. Sometimes alteration in normal bowel pattern.
      3. Swelling.

IV. Analysis/nursing diagnosis
   A. *Activity intolerance* related to pain and discomfort.
   B. *Risk for trauma* related to lack of circulation to affected area of bowel.
   C. *Pain* related to protrusion of intestine into hernia sac.

V. Nursing care plan/implementation

A. Goal: *prevent postoperative complications.*

1. Monitor bowel sounds.
2. Prevent postoperative scrotal swelling with inguinal hernia by applying ice and support to scrotum.

B. Goal: **health teaching.**

1. Prevent recurrence with correct body mechanics.
2. Gradual increase in exercise.

VI. Evaluation/outcome criteria: healing occurs with no hernia recurrence.

Diverticulosis

A *diverticulum* is a small *pouch* or sac composed of mucous membrane that has protruded through the muscular wall of the intestine. *Diverticulosis* is the name for the condition in which several of these are present. *Inflammation* of the diverticula is called *diverticulitis.*

I. **Pathophysiology:** weakening in a localized area of muscular wall of the colon (especially the sigmoid colon), accompanied by increased intraluminal pressure.

II. **Risk factors/causes:**

A. Diverticulosis.

1. Age: seldom before 35 yr; 60% incidence in older adults.
2. History of constipation.
3. Diet history: low in vegetable fiber, high in carbohydrate.

B. Diverticulitis: highest incidence between ages 50 and 60 yr.

III. **Assessment**

A. *Subjective data:* pain: cramplike left lower quadrant of abdomen.

B. *Objective data:*

1. Constipation or diarrhea, flatulence.
2. Fever.
3. Rectal bleeding.
4. *Diagnostic procedures:*
   a. Palpation reveals tender colonic mass.
   b. *Barium enema* (done only in absence of inflammation) reveals presence of diverticula.
   c. *Sigmoidoscopy.*

IV. **Analysis/nursing diagnosis**

A. *Constipation* related to dietary intake.

B. *Pain* related to inflammatory process in intestines.

C. *Risk for fluid volume deficit* related to episodes of diarrhea or bleeding.

D. *Risk for injury* related to bleeding.

E. *Knowledge deficit* related to prevention of constipation.

V. Nursing care plan/implementation

A. Goal: *bowel rest during acute episodes.*

1. *Diet:* soft, liquid.
2. Fluids, IVs if oral intake not adequate.
3. *Pain* medications, as ordered.
4. Monitor stools for signs of bleeding.

B. Goal: *promote normal bowel elimination.*

1. *Diet:* bland, high in vegetable fiber if no inflammation.
   a. *Include:* fruits, vegetables, whole-grain cereal, unprocessed bran.
   b. *Avoid:* foods difficult to digest (corn, nuts).
2. *Bulk-forming agents* as ordered: methylcellulose, psyllium.
3. Monitor: abdominal distention, acute bowel symptoms.

C. Goal: **health teaching.**

1. Methods to prevent constipation.
2. Foods to include/avoid in diet.
3. Relaxation techniques.
4. Signs and symptoms of complications of chronic inflammation: abscess, obstruction, fistulas, perforation, or hemorrhage.

VI. Evaluation/outcome criteria

A. Inflammation decreases.

B. Bowel movements return to normal.

C. Pain decreases.

D. No perforation, fistulas, abscesses, obstruction, or hemorrhage noted.

Ulcerative Colitis

Inflammation of mucosa and submucosa of the distal colorectal area; inflammation leads to ulceration with bleeding; involved areas are continuous; disease is characterized by remissions and exacerbations.

I. **Pathophysiology:** etiology is poorly understood. Edema and hyperemia of colonic mucous membrane → superficial bleeding with increased peristalsis, shallow ulcerations, abscesses; bowel wall thins and shortens and becomes vulnerable to perforation. Increased rate of flow of liquid ileal contents → decreased water absorption and diarrhea.

II. **Risk factors/causes:**

A. Highest occurrence in young adults (20–40 yr).

B. Genetic predisposition: greater in whites, Jews.

C. Autoimmune response.

D. Infections.

E. More common in urban areas (upper–middle incomes and higher educational levels).

F. May be influenced by smoking.

G. Exacerbations often related to stressful event.

III. Assessment

A. *Subjective data*:
1. Urgency to defecate, particularly when standing; tenesmus.
2. Loss of appetite, nausea.
3. Coliclike stomach pain.
4. History of intolerance to dairy products.
5. Depression, frustration, anxiety.

B. *Objective data*:
1. *Diarrhea*: 10–20 stools/d; can be chronic or intermittent, episodic or continual; stools contain blood, mucus, and pus.
2. Weight loss and malnutrition, dehydration.
3. Fever.
4. Lab data: *decreased*: red blood cells, potassium, sodium, calcium bicarbonate, related to excessive diarrhea.
5. Lymphadenitis.
6. *Diagnostic* procedures:
   a. *Sigmoidoscopy* for visualization of lesions.
   b. *Barium* enema.

IV. Analysis/nursing diagnosis

A. *Diarrhea* related to increased flow rate of ileal contents.
B. *Self-esteem disturbance* related to progression of disease and increased number and odor of stools.
C. *Pain* related to inflammatory process.
D. *Fluid volume deficit* related to frequent episodes of diarrhea.
E. *Knowledge deficit* related to methods to control symptoms.
F. *Social isolation* related to continual diarrhea episodes.

V. Nursing care plan/implementation

A. Goal: *reduce psychological stress*.
1. Provide quiet environment.
2. Encourage verbalization of concerns.
3. Psychotherapy as indicated.

B. Goal: *relieve discomfort*.
1. Administer medications as ordered.
   a. *Sedatives* and *tranquilizers* to promote rest and comfort.
   b. *Absorbents*, kaolin-pectin (*Kaopectate*).
   c. *Anticholinergics* and *antispasmodics* to relieve cramping and diarrhea e.g., phenobarbital, atropine sulfate—diphenoxylate HCl (*Lomotil*).
   d. *Antiinfectives* to relieve bacterial overgrowth in bowel and limit secondary infection.
   e. *Steroids* to relieve inflammation and produce remission.
   f. *Potassium supplements* to relieve deficiencies.

C. Goal: **health teaching**—*Diet*:
1. *Avoid*: coarse-residue, high fiber foods (e.g., raw fruits and vegetables, whole milk, cold beverages) because of inflammation.
2. *Include*: bland, *high* protein, *high* vitamin, *high* mineral, *high* calorie foods.
3. Parenteral hyperalimentation for severely ill.
4. *Force fluids* by mouth.

D. Goal: *prepare for surgery if medical regimen unsuccessful*—possible surgical procedures:
1. Permanent ileostomy.
2. Continent ileostomy (*Koch pouch*).
3. Total colectomy, anastomosis with rectum.
4. Total colectomy, anastomosis with anal sphincter.

VI. Evaluation/outcome criteria

A. Fluid balance is obtained and maintained.
B. Alterations in life-style managed.
C. Stress-management techniques successful.
D. Complications such as fistulas, obstruction, perforation, and peritonitis are prevented.
E. Client is prepared for surgery if medical regimen is unsuccessful or complications develop.

Crohn's Disease

A chronic, progressive inflammatory disease usually affecting the terminal ileum.

I. **Pathophysiology:** *one of two conditions called "inflammatory bowel disease"* (ulcerative colitis is the other) that affect all layers of the ileum and/or the colon, causing patchy, shallow, longitudinal mucosal ulcers; possible correlation with autoimmune disease and adenocarcinoma of the bowel.

II. **Risk factors:**
A. Age: 15–20, 55–60 yr.
B. White, especially Jewish.
C. Familial predisposition.
D. Possible virus involvement.
E. Possible hormonal or dietary influences.

III. **Assessment**
A. *Subjective data*:
1. Abdominal pain.
2. Anorexia.
3. Nausea.
4. Malaise.
5. History of isolated, intermittent, or recurrent attacks.

B. *Objective data*:
1. Diarrhea.
2. Weight loss, vomiting.
3. Fever, signs of infection.
4. Fluid/electrolyte imbalances.
5. Malnutrition, malabsorption.
6. Occult blood in feces.

▶ **IV.** (See **Ulcerative Colitis, p. 199-200,** for analysis/nursing diagnosis, nursing care plan/implementation, and evaluation/outcome criteria)

Intestinal Obstruction

Blockage of movement of intestinal contents through small or large intestine. **Medical emergency** because of potential for shock.

I. **Pathophysiology:**

　　A. *Mechanical causes*—physical impediments to passage of intestinal contents, e.g., adhesions, hernias, neoplasms, inflammatory bowel diseases, foreign bodies, fecal impactions, congenital or radiational strictures, intussusception, or volvulus.

　　B. *Paralytic causes*—passageway remains open, but peristalsis ceases, e.g., after abdominal surgery, abdominal trauma, hypokalemia, myocardial infarction, pneumonia, spinal injuries, peritonitis, or vascular insufficiency.

▶ **II.** **Assessment**

　　A. *Subjective data*: pain related to:

　　☞ **1.** *Proximal loop obstruction*: upper abdominal, sharp, cramping, intermittent pain.

　　　2. *Distal loop obstruction*: poorly localized, cramping pain.

　　B. *Objective data*:

　　☞ **1.** Bowel sounds: initially loud, high pitched; then when smooth muscle atony occurs, bowel sounds absent.

　　　2. Increased peristalsis above level of obstruction in attempt to move intestinal contents through the obstructed area.

　　　3. Obstipation (no passage of gas or stool through obstructed portion of bowel; no reabsorption of fluids).

　　　4. Distention.

　　　5. Vomiting:

　　　　a. *Proximal loop obstruction*: profuse nonfecal vomiting.

　　　　b. *Distal loop obstruction*: less frequent fecal-type vomiting.

　　〰 **6.** Urinary output: decreased.

　　　7. Elevated temperature, tachycardia, hypotension → shock if untreated.

　　〰 **8.** Dehydration, hemoconcentration, hypovolemia.

　　　9. Lab data:

　　　　a. Leukocytosis.

　　　　b. *Decreased*: sodium (<138 mEq/L), potassium (<3.5 mEq/L).

　　　　c. *Increased*: pH (>7.45); bicarbonates (>26 mEq/L); blood urea nitrogen (BUN) (>18 mg/dL).

▶ **III.** **Analysis/nursing diagnosis**

　　A. *Fluid volume deficit* related to vomiting.

　　B. *Pain* related to increased peristalsis above the level of obstruction.

　　C. *Altered nutrition, less than body requirements,* related to vomiting.

　　D. *Risk for trauma* related to potential perforation.

▶ **IV.** **Nursing care plan/implementation**

　　A. Goal: *obtain and maintain fluid balance.*

　　☞ **1.** Nursing care of client with nasogastric (NG) tube (see **Tubes** box in **Chap. 9**).

　　　　a. *Miller-Abbott tube*: dual lumen, balloon inflated with air or mercury after insertion.

　　　　b. *Cantor tube*: has mercury in distal sac, which helps move tube to point of obstruction.

　　　　c. *Caution*: do *not* tape either tube to face until tube reaches point of obstruction.

　　▭ **2.** Nothing by mouth, IV therapy, strict I&O.

　　☞ **3.** Take daily weights (early morning), monitor central venous pressure (CVP) for hydration status.

　　☞ **4.** Monitor abdominal girth for signs of distention and urinary output for signs of retention or shock.

　　B. Goal: *relieve pain and nausea.*

　　▭ **1.** Medications, as ordered:

　　　　a. *Analgesics, antiemetics.*

　　　　b. If problem is paralytic: medical treatment includes neostigmine to *stimulate peristalsis.*

　　　2. Observe for bowel sounds, flatus (tape intestinal tube to face once peristalsis begins).

　　　3. Skin and frequent mouth care.

　　C. Goal: *prevent respiratory complications.*

　　　1. Encourage coughing and deep breathing.

　　　2. *Semi-Fowler's* or position of comfort.

　　D. Goal: *postoperative nursing care* (if treated surgically): see **Postoperative Experience, p. 131-137.**

▶ **V.** **Evaluation/outcome criteria**

　　A. Fluid balance obtained and maintained.

　　B. Shock is prevented.

　　C. Obstruction resolves.

　　D. Pain decreases.

　　E. Fluids tolerated by mouth.

　　F. Complications such as perforation and peritonitis prevented.

Fecal Diversion

Stomas: created because of disease or trauma; may be temporary or permanent.

I. **Types (Table 16.1):**

　　A. *Temporary*—fecal stream rerouted to allow distal GI tract to heal or to provide outlet for stool when obstructed.

TABLE 16.1 COMPARISON OF ILEOSTOMY AND COLOSTOMY

	Ileostomy	Colostomy
Procedure	Surgical formation of a fistula, or stoma, between the abdominal wall and *ileum*; continent ileostomy (*Koch pouch*) may be constructed.	Surgical formation of an artificial opening between the surface of the abdominal wall and *colon*. *Single barrel*—only one loop of bowel is opened to the abdominal surface. *Double barrel*—two loops of bowel, a proximal and distal portion, are open to the abdominal wall; feces are expelled from the proximal loop, mucus is expelled from the distal loop; client may expel some excreta from rectum as well.
Reasons Performed	Unresponsive ulcerative colitis: complications of ulcerative colitis, e.g., hemorrhage, carcinoma (suspected).	*Single barrel*: colon or rectal cancer. *Double barrel*: relieve obstruction.
Results	Permanent stoma.	*Single barrel*: permanent stoma. *Double barrel*: temporary stoma.
Discharge	Green liquid, nonodorous.	Consistency of feces dependent on diet and portion of the bowel used as the stoma; from brown odorous liquid to normal stool consistency.
Nursing Care	See **Fecal Diversion**, p. 202.	See **Tables 16.2 to 16.4** and **Fecal Diversion**, p. 203-204.

Source: ©Lagerquist SL: *Little, Brown's NCLEX-RN® Examination Review*. Boston: Little, Brown. (out of print).

B. *Permanent*—intestine cannot be reconnected. Rectum and anal sphincter removed (abdominal perineal resection). Often performed for cancer of the colon and/or rectum.

II. Analysis/nursing diagnosis
  A. *Bowel incontinence* related to lack of sphincter in newly formed stoma.
  B. *Altered health maintenance* related to knowledge of ostomy care.
  C. *Body image disturbance* related to stoma.
  D. *Fluid volume deficit* related to increased output through stoma.

III. Nursing care plan/implementation
  A. **Preoperative care:**
    1. Goal: *prepare bowel for surgery.*
      a. Administer neomycin as ordered to reduce colonic bacteria.
      b. Administer cathartics, *enemas* as ordered to cleanse the bowel of feces.
      c. Administer *low residue or liquid diet* as ordered.
    2. Goal: *relieve anxiety and assist in adjustment to surgery.*
      a. Provide accurate, brief, and reassuring explanations of procedures; allow time for questions.
      b. Have enterostomal nurse visit to discuss ostomy management and placement of stoma appliance.
      c. Offer opportunity for a visit with an Ostomy Association Visitor.
    3. Goal: **health teaching.**
      a. Determine knowledge of surgery and potential impact.
      b. Begin teaching regarding ostomy.

  B. **Postoperative care:**
    1. Goal: *maintain fluid balance.*
      a. Monitor I&O, as large volume of fluid is lost through stoma.
      b. Administer IV fluids as ordered.
      c. Monitor losses through *NG tube*.
    2. Goal: *prevent other postoperative complications.*
      a. Monitor for signs of intestinal obstruction.
      b. Maintain sterility when changing dressings; *avoid* fecal contamination of incision.
      c. Observe appearance of stoma: rosy pink, raised.
    3. Goal: *initiate ostomy care.*

    > a. Protect skin around stoma: use commercial preparation to toughen skin and use protective barrier wafer (*Stomahesive*) or paste (karaya or substitute) to keep drainage (which can cause excoriation) off the skin.
    > b. Keep skin around stoma clean and dry; empty appliance frequently. Check for drainage in appliance at least twice during each shift. If drainage (diarrhea-type stool) is present, empty colostomy appliance (**Table 16.2**).
    > c. Change appliance when drainage leaks around seal, or approximately every 2–3 d. Initially, stoma will be large due to edema. Pouch opening should be slightly larger than stoma, so it will not constrict. Stoma will need to be measured for each change until swelling subsides to ensure appropriate fit. (**See Table 16.3**). (*continued on next page*)

TABLE 16.2 ☞ EMPTYING COLOSTOMY APPLIANCE

Check for drainage in appliance at least twice during each shift. If drainage present (diarrhea-type stool):

Do	Do Not
1. Unclip the bottom of bag.	1. Remove appliance each time it needs emptying.
2. Drain into bedpan.	2. Use any materials that could irritate bowel.
3. Use a squeeze-type bottle filled with warm water to rinse inside of appliance.	3. Ignore client's needs.
4. Clean off clamp if soiled.	
5. Put a few drops of deodorant in appliance if not odorproof.	
6. Fasten bottom of appliance securely (fold bag over clamp 2–3 times before closing).	
7. Check for leakage under appliance every 2–4 h.	
8. Communicate with client while attending to appliance.	

Source: ©Lagerquist SL: *Little, Brown's NCLEX-RN® Examination Review*. Boston: Little, Brown (out of print).

d. Use deodorizing drops in appliance and provide adequate room ventilation to decrease odors. *Caution*: deodorizing drops must be safe for mucous membranes. *No* pinholes in pouch.

e. If a continent ileostomy, a *Koch pouch*, has been constructed, the client does not have to wear an external pouch. The stool is stored intraabdominally. The client drains the pouch several times daily, when there is a feeling of fullness, using a catheter. The stoma is flat and on the right side of the abdomen.

4. Goal: *promote psychological comfort.*

a. Support client and family—accept feelings and behavior.

b. Recognize that such a procedure may initiate the grieving process.

5. Goal: **health teaching.**

a. Self-care management skills related to ostomy appliance, skin care, and irrigation, if indicated (**Table 16.4**).

b. *Diet*: adjustments to control character of feces; *avoid* foods that increase flatulence.

c. Signs of complications of infection, obstruction, or electrolyte imbalance.

d. Community referral for follow-up care.

IV. **Evaluation/outcome criteria**

A. Demonstrates self-care skill for independent living.

B. Makes dietary adjustments.

C. Ostomy functions well.

D. Adjusts to alteration in bowel elimination pattern.

Hemorrhoids

Enlarged vein in mucous membrane of rectum.

I. **Pathophysiology**: venous congestion and interference with venous return from hemorrhoidal veins → increase in pelvic pressure, swelling, and distortion.

II. **Risk factors/causes:**

A. Straining to expel constipated stool.

B. Pregnancy.

C. Intraabdominal or pelvic masses.

D. Interference with portal circulation.

E. Prolonged standing or sitting.

F. History of low fiber, high carbohydrate diet, which contributes to constipation.

G. Family history of hemorrhoids.

H. Enlarged prostate.

III. **Assessment**

A. *Subjective data*: discomfort, anal pruritus, pain.

B. *Objective data*:

1. Bleeding, especially on defecation.

2. Narrowing of stool.

3. Grapelike clusters around anus (pink, red, or blue).

4. *Diagnostic* procedures:

a. Visualization for *external* hemorrhoids.

b. *Digital exam* or *proctoscopy* for *internal* hemorrhoids.

IV. **Analysis/nursing diagnosis**

A. *Pain* related to defecation.

B. *Constipation* related to dietary habits and pain at time of defecation.

C. *Knowledge deficit* related to foods to prevent constipation.

V. **Nursing care plan/implementation**

A. Goal: *reduce anal discomfort.*

1. Sitz baths, as ordered; perineal care to prevent infection.

2. Hot or cold compresses, as ordered, to reduce inflammation and pruritus.

3. Topical medications as ordered.

a. *Anti–inflammatory*: hydrocortisone cream.

b. *Astringents*: witch hazel–impregnated pads.

c. *Topical anesthetics*: dibucaine (*Nupercaine*).

TABLE 16.3 ☞ CHANGING COLOSTOMY APPLIANCE

Gather equipment: gloves, skin prep packet, colostomy appliance measured to fit stoma properly (if new surgical stoma, it will continue to shrink with healing; use stoma measuring guide), skin barrier, warm water and soap, face cloth/towel, plastic bag for disposal of old equipment. Remember that bowel is very fragile; also, working near bowel increases peristalsis, and feces and flatulence may be expelled.

Do	Do Not
1. Remove old appliance carefully, pulling from area with least drainage to area with most drainage.	1. Tear appliance quickly from skin.
2. Wash skin area with soap and water.	2. Wash stoma with soap; put anything dry onto stoma.
3. Observe skin area for potential breakdown.	3. Irritate skin or stoma.
4. Use packet of skin prep on the skin around the stoma; allow skin prep solution to dry on skin before applying colostomy appliance.	4. Put skin prep solution onto stoma; it will cause irritation.
5. Apply skin barrier you have measured and cut to size.	5. Make opening too large (increases risk of leakage) or too small (impinges on stoma).
6. Put appliance on so that the bottom of the appliance is easily accessible for emptying (e.g., if client is *out* of bed most of the time, put the bottom facing the feet; if client is *in* bed most of the time, have bottom face the side); picture-frame the adhesive portion of the appliance with 1-in. (2.5-cm) tape.	6. Have appliance attached so client can't be involved in own care.
7. Put a few drops of deodorant in appliance if not odor-proof.	7. Use any materials that would irritate bowel.
8. Use clamp to fasten bottom of appliance.	8. Avoid conversation/eye contact.
9. Talk to client (or communicate in best way possible for client) during and after procedure. This is a very difficult alteration in body image.	9. Contaminate other incisions.
10. Use good handwashing technique.	

Source: ©Lagerquist SL: *Little, Brown's NCLEX-RN® Examination Review.* Boston: Little, Brown. (out of print).

B. Goal: *prevent complications related to surgery.*
1. Encourage postoperative ambulation.
2. Pain relief until packing removed.
3. Monitor for: bleeding, infection, pulmonary emboli, phlebitis.
4. Facilitate bowel evacuation: *stool softeners, laxatives, suppositories, oil enemas,* as ordered.
5. Monitor for syncope/vertigo during first postoperative bowel movement.
6. *Diet*:
   a. *Low* residue (postoperative)—*until* healing has begun.
   b. *High* fiber to prevent constipation *after* healing.
7. *Increase* fluid intake.
C. Goal: **health teaching**—methods to avoid constipation.

VI. **Evaluation/outcome criteria**
A. No complications.
B. Client has bowel movement.
C. Incorporates knowledge of correct foods into lifestyle.

TABLE 16.4 ☞ COLOSTOMY IRRIGATION

1. Assemble all equipment for irrigation and appliance change.
2. Remove and discard old pouch.
3. Clean the peristomal skin.
4. Apply the irrigating sleeve; place in toilet or bedpan.
5. Fill container with 500–1000 mL of warm water, never more than 1000 mL. Clear air from tubing. Insert lubricated cone 2–4 in. (5–10 cm) into stoma. Do *not* force. Hold container about 18 in. (45 cm) above stoma. Infuse gently over 7–10 min.
6. Allow stool to empty into toilet. Evacuation usually occurs in 20–25 min.
7. If no return after irrigation, ambulate, gently massage abdomen, or give client a warm drink.
8. Once complete, remove the sleeve and follow guidelines for applying appliance.

Source: ©Lagerquist SL: *Little, Brown's NCLEX-RN® Examination Review.* Boston: Little, Brown. (out of print).

Summary of Key Points

1. *Auscultation* of bowel sounds is done *after* inspection because palpation or percussion done before auscultation will change the bowel sounds.

2. Only an intestinal obstruction is more of an emergency than appendicitis. The chance of a ruptured appendix places the client at risk for *peritonitis* leading to sepsis.

3. Instruct a client with a hernia to seek assistance if the hernia cannot be reduced or pain occurs that could be indicative of *strangulation*.

4. If the client has an inflammatory bowel condition (an "itis"), the diet should be *low fiber or low residue*.

5. Clients with ulcerative colitis may have more than 20 diarrhea stools per day. Assess for *fluid* and *electrolyte* imbalance.

6. Surgical removal of the entire inflamed colon is the common treatment for ulcerative colitis, but only sections of the diseased bowel are removed in clients with Crohn's disease. Surgical options include *a permanent ileostomy* with a stoma and an external appliance; a *Koch's pouch*, a *continent* ileostomy (a stoma but no appliance), or a *restorative* procedure (anastomosis or *J pouch* reservoir), which allows for rectal evacuation.

7. A colostomy is indicated after *removal* of the rectum or part of the colon (*permanent*) or when the colon is being allowed to rest (*temporary*).

8. For all types of fecal diversion, a sufficient oral intake of fluid is essential; high fiber foods may cause obstruction of an ileostomy but are needed to manage constipation in a client with a colostomy.

9. An intestinal obstruction is an **emergency** situation because fluid and electrolyte absorption is seriously impaired and mortality is high if it goes untreated.

10. With a *mechanical* obstruction, bowel sounds (peristalsis) will be increased initially in an attempt to move the obstruction. Bowel sounds are *absent* from the beginning of a paralytic ileus (*functional* obstruction).

Study and Memory Aids

Diagnostic Studies/Procedures

Proctoscopy
Visualization of rectum and colon by means of a lighted tube inserted through the anus.

Small Bowel Biopsy
A specimen is obtained by passing a tube through the oral cavity and is microscopically examined for changes in cellular morphology.

☞ *Nursing responsibilities*: *no* food or fluids 8 h before procedure. Obtain written consent. Remove dentures if present. Monitor vital signs before, during, and after procedure for indications of hemorrhage. Procedure takes about an hour.

Diets

Celiac Disease

↑ Calories
　Minerals
　Protein
　Vitamins

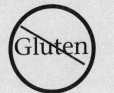

Diverticulosis

Bowel rest (dietary progression):
　NPO initially
　　↓
　Liquid to soft food to high fiber (after ↓ inflammation); Increase fluids
Bowel cleansing:
　Bland food
　High fiber food (fruits, vegetables, whole-grain cereal, unprocessed bran)
Avoid foods that are difficult to digest (corn, nuts)

Hemorrhoids

Postoperative: ↓ Residue　　　After healing: ↑ Fiber
　　　　　　　　　　　　　　　　　　　　　　 Fluids

Ulcerative Colitis

↑ Bland
　Calories
　Minerals
　Protein
AVOID:
- Coarse residue, high fiber foods
- Cold beverages
- Raw fruits and vegetables
- Whole milk

⊂ **Drug Review**

Appendicitis

Analgesics
  Meperidine HCl (*Demerol*): IM or IV, 50–150 mg
  Morphine sulfate: IM or IV, 5–20 mg
Other drugs used according to client's medical history and
  postoperative health status
Antibiotic
  Ampicillin: 1–2 g/day q6–12h

Celiac Disorders

Anticholinergic
  Belladonna alkaloid: PO or sublingual, 0.25–0.5 mg 3
    times/d to inhibit gastric motility
Antidiarrheals
  Diphenoxylate HCl with atropine sulfate (*Lomotil*):
    2.5–5 mg 4 times/d
  Kaolin with pectin (*Kaopectate*): 60–120 mL after each
    loose bowel movement

Crohn's Disease

Anticholinergic
  Propantheline (*Pro-Banthine*): 15 mg tid, 30 mg hs
Antidiarrheal
  Loperamide hydrochloride (*Imodium*): 4 mg initially,
    then 2 mg after each loose stool
  No opiate preparations
Antiinfective/anti-inflammatory
  Sulfasalazine (*Azulfidine*): 500 mg 4/d
Antispasmodics (to reduce postprandial pain)
  Belladonna Alkaloid: 0.25–0.5 mg 3 times/d
  Glycopyrrolate (*Robinol*):1 mg tid
  Propantheline bromide (*Pro-Banthine*): 15 mg tid,
    30 mg hs
Antiulceratives
  Aluminum hydroxide gel (*Amphojel*): 5–10 mL q2–4h
    or 1 h pc
  Calcium carbonate (*Titralac*): 1–2 g with *water pc* and
    hs
  Magnesium and aluminum hydroxide (*Maalox*
    suspension): 5–30 mL pc and hs
  Sucralfate (*Carafate*): 1 g qid
Histamine antagonists
  Cimetidine (*Tagamet*): 300–600 mg q6h
  Ranitidine (*Zantac*): 150 mg bid
Hydrophilic mucilloids
  Methylcellulose (*Citrucel*): 15 mL in water 1–3 times/d
    (for stool consistency)
  Psyllium (*Metamucil*): 1 rounded tsp in water 1–3
    times/d
Immunosuppressive agent
  6-Mercaptopurine

Proton pump inhibitors
  Lansoprazole (*Prevacid*): PO 15 mg daily
  Omeprazole (*Prilosec*): PO 20 mg daily
Steroids (should **never** be abruptly discontinued; gradually
  taper dose to prevent complications)
  Dexamethasone (*Decadron*): 0.5–9 mg/d in single or
    divided doses
  Methylprednisolone (*Medrol*): 4–48 mg/d
  Prednisone: 5–60 mg/d

Diverticulosis

Analgesics
  Morphine sulfate: IM or IV, 5–20 mg
  Oxycodone (*Roxicodone*) with acetaminophen
    (*Percocet*): 5 mg q6h as needed
Antiinfective
  Cephalothin sodium (*Keflin*): IV 0.5–1 g q6h

Fecal Diversion

Antiinfective
  Neomycin: 1 g/h for 4 h, then 1 g q4h for 24 h
    preoperatively

Hemorrhoids

Anti–inflammatory: hydrocortisone cream
Astringent: witch hazel–impregnated pads
Topical anesthetic: dibucaine (*Nupercaine*)

Hernia

Analgesics
  Meperidine HCl (*Demerol*): 50–150 mg
  Morphine sulfate: IM or IV, 5–20 mg (may use client
    controlled analgesia—PCA)
  Oxycodone (*Roxicodone*) with acetaminophen
    (*Percocet*): 5 mg q6h as needed

Intestinal Obstruction

Analgesics
  Meperidine HCI (*Demerol*): IM or IV, 50–150 mg
  Morphine sulfate: IM or IV, 5–20 mg
Antiemetics
  Prochlorperazine (*Compazine*): IM 5–10 mg; repeat
    once as needed
  Promethazine (*Phenergan*): 12.5–25 mg q4–6h as
    needed
  Trimethobenzamide (*Tigan*): IM 200 mg; 3–4 times/d
Cholinergic
  Neostigmine (*Prostigmin*): used for paralytic ileus, SC
    or IM, 0.5–1 mg

Ulcerative Colitis

Anticholinergics/antispasmodics
    Atropine: 0.3–1.2 mg q 4–6h
    Phenobarbital: 30–120 mg/d in divided doses
Antidiarrheals
    Diphenoxylate HCl and atropine sulfate (*Lomotil*):2.5–
       5 mg 4 times/d
    Kaolin with pectin (*Kaopectate*): 60–120 mL after each
       loose bowel movement
    Loperamide hydrochloride (*Imodium*): 4 mg initially,
       then 2 mg after each loose bowel movement
Antiinfectives
    Ampicillin: 1–2 g/d q6–12h
    Cephalexin (*Keflex*): 250–500 mg q6h
    Cephalothin (*Keflin*): IV 0.5–2 g q4–6h
    Erythromycin: 250–500 mg q6–12h
    Gentamicin (*Garamycin*): 3–5 mg/kg/d in divided
       doses
    Penicillin G: IM 1.2 million U in single dose
    Tetracycline: 1–2 g/d q6–12h
Potassium supplement
    Potassium chloride: 16–24 mEq/d in divided doses,
       or in IV maintenance fluid. Titrate according to
       client's serum K+.
Sedatives/tranquilizers
    Chlordiazepoxide HCl (*Librium*): 5–25 mg 3–4 times/d
    Diazepam (*Valium*): 2–10 mg 2–4 times/d
Steroids (should **never** be discontinued abruptly; gradually
    taper dose to prevent complications)
    Dexamethasone (*Decadron*): 0.5–9 mg/d in single or
       divided doses
    Methylprednisolone (*Medrol*): 4–48 mg/d
    Prednisone: 5–60 mg/d

Questions

1. The dietary instructions the nurse gives a client with ulcerative colitis would include a recommendation to eat foods that are low in:
   1. Residue.
   2. Carbohydrate.
   3. Fat.
   4. Calories.

2. The nursing priority in a client who 2 days before has undergone an uncomplicated abdominoperineal resection and a colostomy would be to:
   1. Give instructions regarding colostomy irrigation.
   2. Record the client's vital signs and intake and output.
   3. Check stomal drainage and the condition of the incision.
   4. Institute dietary restrictions and plan menus because client is ready to start eating.

3. Which client complaint should the nurse recognize as a symptom or sign of colorectal cancer?
   1. Nausea and vomiting.
   2. Left lower quadrant pain.
   3. Increased flatulence.
   4. Change in stool color.

4. Which statement that a client makes about a scheduled colonoscopy would indicate to the nurse a need for further teaching?
   1. "A flexible tube will be inserted into my rectum."
   2. "I will be conscious, but sedated."
   3. "A scope will be inserted through my belly button."
   4. "I will need to have several enemas before the test."

5. Before the surgical removal of a rectal mass and a sigmoid colostomy, a client will be receiving neomycin PO. The nurse knows that the purpose of this medication is to:
   1. Sterilize the bowel before surgery.
   2. Treat the infection caused by the tumor.
   3. Provide prophylactic anti-infective therapy.
   4. Decrease intestinal motility.

6. Which food should the nurse remove from the tray of a client on a low residue diet?
   1. Cottage cheese.
   2. Chicken breast.
   3. Mashed potatoes.
   4. Green beans.

7. The nurse explains to a colleague that the purpose of keeping a Foley catheter in place for several days after an abdominal perineal resection with a colostomy is to:
   1. Prevent a urinary tract infection.
   2. Prevent urine retention and resulting perineal wound pressure.
   3. Minimize the chance of wound contamination from urine.
   4. Determine whether the surgery caused bladder trauma.

8. Which nursing diagnosis would be a priority during the first 72 hours after surgery in a client who has undergone a sigmoid colostomy?
   1. Knowledge deficit.
   2. Risk for infection.
   3. Body image disturbance.
   4. Self-care deficit.

9. The most important nursing action in a client experiencing an acute episode of ulcerative colitis would be to:
   1. Replace the fluid and sodium lost as a result of the diarrhea.
   2. Monitor regularly for an increased serum glucose level from steroid therapy.
   3. Restrict dietary intake of high potassium foods.
   4. Note change in color and consistency of stool.

10. About which side effects of propantheline (*Pro-Banthine*), given for the control of gastrointestinal tract spasms, would the nurse educate a client?
    1. Pupillary constriction and photophobia.
    2. Urinary frequency and urgency. *tachycardia*
    3. Bradycardia and dizziness.
    4. Dry mouth and constipation.

anticholinergic

11. The greatest concern in a 74-year-old client who has been given midazolam (*Versed*) and fentanyl (*Sublimaze*) to produce conscious sedation during colonoscopy would be:
    1. An increased risk of postural hypotension.
    2. Management of abdominal discomfort resulting from constipation.
    3. Decreased bowel function stemming from reduced peristalsis.
    4. Assessment for return of motor function.

12. After self-irrigation of a sigmoid colostomy, there is no return. What should the nurse tell the client to do?
    1. Massage the abdomen gently.
    2. Instill another 150 mL of water.
    3. Lie down, supine, until there is a return.
    4. Wait 45 minutes for initial emptying to occur.

13. When performing a physical assessment in a client complaining of abdominal pain, the nurse would first:
    1. Auscultate to determine whether there are changes in bowel sounds.
    2. Observe the contour of the abdomen.
    3. Palpate the abdomen for a mass.
    4. Percuss the abdomen to determine whether fluid is present.

14. To assess the function of a colostomy 3 days after the procedure, the nurse would assess for:
    1. An appliance filled with flatus (gas).
    2. Semiformed stool. *— 4-5 days postop*
    3. Continuous liquid drainage.
    4. A flat, pale-pink stoma.

Answers/Rationale

1. **(1)** It is important for a client with *colitis*, an inflammation, to consume a low residue, low fiber diet. (A high fiber diet is called for in clients with *diverticulosis*.) The carbohydrate (2), fat (3), and calorie (4) content of foods is *not* a concern in inflammatory bowel disease. **IMP, COM, 4, PhI, Basic care and comfort**

2. **(3)** Around 36 hours the wound should be assessed for signs of infection, and the character of any drainage should be noted. Instruction on irrigation (1) should be done *before discharge*. Vital signs and I&O (2) would be the priority during the *first 24 hours* after surgery. Dietary planning (4) would also be an emphasis around this time, but this is a priority question and diet would be a *lesser* concern. **IMP, ANL, 8, PhI, Reduction of risk potential**

3. **(1)** Nausea and vomiting, as well as rectal bleeding, a change in bowel habits, abdominal pain, weight loss, and anorexia, may occur in colorectal cancer. Tumors of the small bowel and ascending (right) colon are usually associated with nausea and vomiting. Rectal bleeding is the usual finding that alerts a client to a problem. Left lower quadrant pain (2) is more consistent with *ulcerative colitis*. Flatulence (3) is seen with *gallbladder* problems and *dietary* intolerance. A change in stool color (4) would more likely be due to a problem in the *biliary* system, such as gallstones. **AS, ANL, 8, PhI, Physiological adaptation**

4. **(3)** In a colonoscopy the lining of the large intestine is visualized by means of a flexible endoscope that is inserted rectally. (A *laparoscope* is inserted through the navel.) The statement in option **1** is therefore accurate, and requires *no* further teaching. Conscious sedation (2) *is* used, often a combination of midazolam (*Versed*) and fentanyl (*Sublimaze*). Bowel preparation *does* include enemas (4) to clean the bowel and ensure visualization. **EV, EVL, 8, PhI, Reduction of risk potential**

5. **(1)** It is important to minimize the bacterial growth in the bowel, because otherwise, when the bowel is incised, bacteria from the bowel could contaminate the peritoneum. Sterilizing the bowel before surgery minimizes the chance of postoperative infection. Infection (2) is *not* a common characteristic of colorectal cancer. General antiinfective therapy (3) is a plausible choice, but bowel sterilization is a *more specific* answer. Antiinfectives frequently cause diarrhea, which stems from an increase, *not* decrease (4), in motility. **PL, APP, 8, PhI, Pharmacological and parenteral therapies**

6. **(4)** Green beans are high in fiber, or residue, and such foods are usually eliminated from the diet of a client with a bowel inflammation to reduce fecal bulk and mechanical irritation. The other foods (1, 2, and 3) *are* low in residue and would be easily tolerated. **IMP, COM, 4, PhI, Basic care and comfort**

7. **(2)** Because general anesthesia and abdominal pain may make voiding difficult, the Foley catheter would be placed to prevent urine retention and the resultant bladder distention, which would then exert pressure on the surgical area. Catheters actually *increase* the risk of a urinary tract infection; they *do not prevent* such infections (1). There has been no intentional surgical incision into the urinary tract, so urine should *not* be leaking into the surgical wound (3). Bladder trauma (4) is always a possibility, and the appearance of the urine draining from the catheter would alert the nurse to blood in the urine or inadequate output; however, this is *not* the *initial* purpose of the catheter. **PL, APP, 8, SECE, Management of care**

8. **(2)** All of the diagnoses could apply in a client who has undergone a sigmoid colostomy, but the diagnosis of postoperative complications is a *priority* during the first few days after surgery. The bowel sterilization procedure carried out preoperatively should minimize the risk for infection however. Other complications to observe for include:

hemorrhage, wound disruption, thrombophlebitis, and abnormal stomal function. Knowledge about stoma care (1) would need to be *assessed before discharge. Once* the risk of postoperative complications is reduced, body image (3) becomes a major concern. The client's ability to care for the stoma (4) would also need to be determined *before discharge.* **AN, ANL, 8, SECE, Management of care**

9. (1) If a client is suffering an acute episode of ulcerative colitis, there will be a minimum of 20 diarrhea stools per day, with a resultant fluid loss of as much as 17,000 mL in 24 hours. Steroid therapy will be ordered and will reduce the inflammation, but it is not curative. Steroids will increase the serum glucose level over a long term, but hyperglycemia (2) is *not* a priority concern during treatment for an acute episode. Steroids cause a loss of potassium; if the client were eating, the dietary intake of potassium would therefore be increased, *not* restricted (3). The frequency of the stools, *not* the color (4), is important. **IMP, ANL, 8, PhI, Physiological adaptation**

10. (4) Propantheline is an anticholinergic drug that causes dry mouth and constipation. It also causes pupillary dilatation, *not* constriction, and photophobia (1); urinary retention, *not* frequency and urgency (2); and tachycardia, *not* bradycardia, and dizziness (3). **IMP, COM, 8, PhI, Pharmacological and parenteral therapies**

11. (1) Both drugs cause hypotension, and this risk is greater in the elderly. Position changes should therefore be made slowly and with assistance to prevent fainting and falls. The drugs do *not* cause constipation. Air is used during the colonoscopy to increase visualization, thus cramping may occur during the procedure, but there is little subsequent discomfort resulting from the gas distention or the drugs (2). These drugs have *no* effect on peristalsis (3). The drugs do *not* have an effect on motor function (4) (e.g. no paralysis) per se. Any problems with ambulation would be related to fainting. **PL, ANL, 1, PhI, Pharmacological and parenteral therapies**

12. (1) Usually 300 to 500 mL of fluid, and up to 1000 mL, is instilled over 3 to 5 minutes. If there is no return, the nurse should tell the client to massage the abdomen gently. Additional fluid (2) would *only* be indicated if the fluid was returning as it was being instilled. If unable to sit up, the client should lie on the left side to facilitate drainage, *not* on the back (3). The whole procedure may take an hour, but the bowel is usually stimulated soon after the fluid is instilled; it should *not* take 45 minutes for initial emptying to occur (4). **IMP, APP, 8, HPM, Health promotion and maintenance**

13. (2) The nurse should always observe or inspect before proceeding with the next step in the physical assessment. Auscultation (1) should be done after inspection and before palpation (3) and percussion (4). **AS, RE/KN, 8, HPM, Health promotion and maintenance**

14. (1) Initially there would be gas or mucus in the appliance. Stool is *not* present until 4 to 5 days postoperatively, and the expected *consistency cannot be determined* in this question because the location of the colostomy is not specified. Semiformed stool (2) would be expected with a *transverse* colostomy; continuous liquid (3) would be expected with an *ascending* (right) colostomy. Option 4 describes the stoma and is *unrelated to functioning.* **AS, COM, 8, PhI, Basic care and comfort**

Key to Codes

Nursing process: AS, assessment; AN, analysis; PL, planning; IMP, implementation; EV, evaluation. (See **Appendix M** for explanation of nursing process steps.)

Cognitive level: RE/KN, recall/knowledge; COM, comprehension; APP, application; ANL, analysis; EVL, evaluation; SYN, synthesis. (See **Appendix M** for explanation.)

Category of human function: 1, protective; 2, sensory-perceptual; 3, comfort, rest, activity, and mobility; 4, nutrition; 5, growth and development; 6, fluid-gas transport; 7, psychosocial-cultural; 8, elimination. (See **Appendix 0** for explanation.)

Client need: SECE, safe, effective care environment; PhI, physiological integrity; PsI, psychosocial integrity; HPM, health promotion and maintenance. (See **Appendix P** for explanation.)

Client subneed: (See **Appendix P** for explanation)

Renal Disorders

Chapter Outline

Pyelonephritis

Acute or chronic inflammation due to bacterial infection of the parenchyma and pelvis of the kidney; 95% of cases caused by gram-negative enteric bacilli (*Escherichia coli*); occurs more frequently in young women and older men

I. **Pathophysiology**: inflammation of renal medulla or lining of the renal pelvis → nephron destruction; hypertrophy of nephrons needed to maintain urine output → impaired sodium reabsorption (salt wasting); inability to concentrate urine; progressive renal failure; hypertension (two-thirds of all cases).

II. **Risk factors/causes**:
   A. Obstruction.
   B. Hypertension.
   C. Hypokalemia.
   D. Diabetes mellitus.
   E. Pregnancy.
   F. Catheterization.

III. **Assessment**
   A. *Subjective data*:
       1. *Pain*: flank—one or both sides, back, dysuria; headache.
       2. *Loss of appetite*, weight loss.
       3. *Night sweats*, chills.
       4. *Urination*: frequency, urgency, pain.
   B. *Objective data*:
       1. Fever.
       2. Lab data:
           a. *Blood*—polymorphonuclear leukocytosis > 11,000/mm^3.

   b. *Urine*—leukocytosis, hematuria, white blood cell casts; proteinuria (<3 g in 24 h); *positive* cultures; specific gravity—normal or *increased* with acute pyelonephritis; *decreased* with chronic pyelonephritis; cloudy, foul smelling.

   3. *Intravenous pyelogram (IVP)*—may show structural changes; see **p. 224**.

IV. **Analysis/nursing diagnosis**
   A. *Altered urinary elimination* related to kidney disease.
   B. *Pain* related to dysuria and kidney damage.
   C. *Altered nutrition, less than body requirements*, related to impaired sodium reabsorption and protein loss.
   D. *Risk for fluid volume excess* related to renal failure.

V. **Nursing care plan/implementation**
   A. Goal: *combat infection, prevent recurrence, alleviate symptoms*.
       1. Medications:
           a. *Antiinfectives, urinary antiseptics*, and/or *sulfonamides* appropriate for causative organism; also reduces pain.
           b. *Analgesics* for pain—phenazopyridine (*Pyridium*); stronger if calculi present.
           c. *Antipyretics* for fever—acetaminophen (*Tylenol*).
       2. *Fluids*: 1500–2000 mL/d to: flush kidneys, relieve dysuria, reduce fever, prevent dehydration.
       3. Observe hydration status: intake and output (I&O) (output minimum, 1500 mL/24 h);

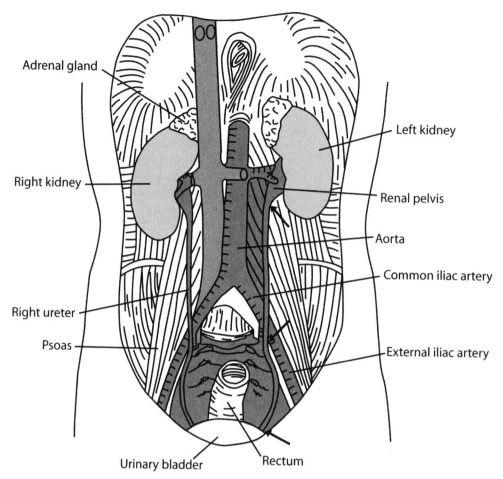

Posterior Abdominal Wall, showing kidneys and ureters in situ. **Arrows indicate three sites where ureter is narrowed.**

daily weight; urine—check each voiding for *protein, blood, specific gravity*; vital signs q4h to monitor for hypertension, tachycardia; skin turgor.

4. Hygiene: meticulous *perineal* care, cleanse with soap and water, *antiinfective* ointment may be used around urinary meatus with retention catheter.

5. Cooling measures: tepid sponging.

6. *Diet*: sufficient calories and protein to prevent malnutrition; sodium supplement as ordered.

B. Goal: *promote physical and emotional rest.*

  1. Activity: bed rest or as tolerated—depends on whether anemia or fever is present; encourage activities of daily living as tolerated.

  2. Emotional support: encourage expression of fears (possible renal failure, dialysis); provide diversional activities; include family in care; answer questions.

C. Goal: **health teaching.**

  1. Medications: take regularly to maintain blood level; side effects.

  2. Personal care: perineal hygiene, *avoid* urethral contamination, *avoid* tub baths.

3. Possible recurrence with pregnancy.

4. Monitor daily weight.

VI. Evaluation/outcome criteria

A. Normal renal function (minimum 1500 mL of urine/24 h).

B. Blood pressure (BP) within normal range.

C. No recurrence of symptoms.

Acute Glomerulonephritis

Acute glomerulonephritis (AGN) is a bilateral inflammation of the glomeruli of the kidneys. It is twice as common in men as in women. Like rheumatic fever, AGN is thought to result from an antigen-antibody reaction to a *Streptococcus* infection; however, unlike rheumatic fever, it does *not* tend to recur, because specific immunity is conferred after the first episode of AGN. Postinfectious AGN is primarily a disease of children occurring about 21 d after infection. AGN from other bacterial, viral, or parasitic infections occurs within a few days after illness.

I. **Pathophysiology**: immunologic disorder often associated with an infection; circulating antigen–antibody complexes are trapped within glomerulus

→ inflammation → ↓ glomerular function, ↑ glomerular porosity → proteinuria and hematuria.

II. Risk factors/causes:

A. Beta-hemolytic streptococcal infection of skin or upper respiratory system

B. Systemic lupus erythematosus

C. Vascular injury (e.g., hypertension)

D. Diabetes

E. Disseminated intravascular coagulation

III. Assessment

A. Typical concerns from family about urine: change in color/appearance of urine (thick, reddish brown; decreased amounts).

B. **Acute edematous phase**—usually lasts 4–10 d.

  1. Lab examination of urine:
    a. Severe **hematuria**.
    b. Mild proteinuria
    c. *Increased* specific gravity.

  2. **Hypertension**
    a. Headache.
    b. Potential hypertensive encephalopathy → seizures, increased intracranial pressure.

  3. Mild–moderate edema, chiefly periorbital; increased weight due to fluid retention.

  4. Vomiting.

  5. Fever.

  6. General (*subjective data*):
    a. Abdominal pain.
    b. Malaise.
    c. Anorexia.
    d. Pallor.
    e. Irritability.
    f. Lethargy

C. **Diuresis phase** (*objective data*):

  1. Copious diuresis.

  2. Decreased body weight.

  3. Marked clinical improvement.

  4. Decrease in gross hematuria, but microscopic hematuria may persist for weeks/months.

IV. Analysis/nursing diagnosis

A. *Fluid volume excess* related to decreased urine output.

B. *Pain* related to fluid retention.

C. *Altered nutrition, less than body requirements*, related to anorexia and vomiting.

D. *Impaired skin integrity* related to immobility.

E. *Activity intolerance* related to fatigue.

F. *Knowledge deficit* related to disease process, treatment, and follow-up care.

V. Nursing care plan/implementation

A. Goal: *monitor fluid balance, observing carefully for complications.*

  1. Check and record BP at least every 4 h to monitor hypertension.

  2. Monitor daily weights.

  3. Urine: strict I&O; specific gravity and dipstick for blood every void.

  4. Note edema: extent, location, progression.

  5. Adhere to fluid restrictions if ordered.

  6. Bed rest, chiefly necessitated by hypertension: monitor for possible development of hypertensive encephalopathy (seizures, increased intracranial pressure); report any changes **stat** to physician.

  7. Administer medications as ordered:
    a. *Antiinfectives*—eradicate any lingering *Streptococcus* infection.
    b. *Antihypertensives*, e.g., hydralazine HCl (*Apresoline*).
    c. Rarely use diuretics—limited value.
    d. *If heart failure develops—may use digoxin.*
    e. Refer to **Appendix D** for additional information on medications.

B. Goal: *provide adequate nutrition.*

  1. *Diet: low sodium, low potassium*—to prevent fluid retention and hyperkalemia; Protein depends on BUN and level of protein in urine. Refer to **Appendix B** for additional information on diets.

  2. Stimulate appetite: offer small portions, attractively prepared; meals with family or others; offer preferred foods, if possible; encourage family to bring in special foods, e.g., culturally related preferences.

C. Goal: *provide reasonable measure of comfort.*

  1. Encourage visiting by family.

  2. Provide for positional changes, give good skin care.

  3. Provide appropriate diversion, as tolerated.

D. Goal: *prevent further infection.*

  1. Use good handwashing technique.

  2. Screen staff, other clients, visitors to limit contact with people who are infectious.

  3. Administer *antiinfectives* if ordered (usually only for clients with positive cultures).

  4. Keep warm and dry, stress good hygiene.

  5. Note possible sites of infection: increased skin breakdown secondary to edema.

E. Goal: **health teaching**.

  1. Teach how to check urine at home: dipstick for protein and blood. (*Note*: occult hematuria may persist for months.)

  2. Teach activity restriction: *no strenuous activity until hematuria is completely resolved.*

  3. Teach family how to prepare *low* sodium, *low* potassium diet.

  4. Arrange for follow-up care: physician, home health nurse.

  5. *Stress*: subsequent recurrences are *rare* because specific immunity is conferred.

⋈ **VI. Evaluation/outcome criteria**
   A. No permanent renal damage occurs.
   B. Normal fluid balance is maintained/restored.
   C. Adequate nutrition is maintained.
   D. No secondary infections occur.
   E. Verbalizes understanding of the disease, its treatment, and its prognosis.

Acute Renal Failure

< 400 mL/24h

Broadly defined as the rapid onset of oliguria accompanied by a rising blood urea nitrogen (BUN) and serum creatinine; usually reversible.

I. **Pathophysiology**: acute renal ischemia → tubular necrosis → decreased urine output. *Oliguric phase* (<400 mL/24 h)—waste products are retained → metabolic acidosis → water and electrolyte imbalances → anemia. *Recovery phase*—diuresis → dilute urine → rapid depletion of sodium, chloride, and water → dehydration.

II. **Types and risk factors:**
   A. *Prenal*—due to factors outside of kidney; usually *circulatory* collapse—hemorrhage, severe dehydration, myocardial infarction, shock, vascular obstruction.
   B. *Intrinsic renal*—parenchymal disease resulting from ischemia or *nephrotoxic* damage; nephrotoxic agents—poisons, (such as carbon tetrachloride); heavy metals (arsenic, mercury); anti-infectives (kanamycin sulfate, neomycin sulfate); incompatible blood transfusion; alcohol myopathies; acute renal disease—AGN, acute pyelonephritis.
   C. *Postrenal*—*obstruction* in collecting system: renal or bladder calculi; tumors of bladder, prostate, or renal pelvis; gynecologic or urologic surgery in which ureters are accidentally ligated.

⋈ **III. Assessment**
   A. *Subjective data*:
      1. Sudden *decrease* or cessation of urine output (<400 mL/24 h).
      2. Anorexia, nausea, vomiting resulting from azotemia.
      3. Headache.
   B. *Objective data*:
      1. Sudden weight gain resulting from fluid accumulation.
      2. Vital signs (vary according to cause and severity):
         a. *BP*—usually *elevated*.
         b. *Pulse*—tachycardia, irregularities.
         c. *Respirations*—*increased* rate, depth, crackles.
      3. *Neurologic*: decreasing mentation, unresponsive to verbal or painful stimuli, psychoses, convulsions.

4. Mouth/oral: halitosis, cracked mucous membranes.
5. *Skin*: dry, rashes, purpura, itchy, pale.
6. Lab data:
   a. Blood: *increased*—potassium, BUN; creatinine, white blood cell count (WBC); *decreased*—pH, bicarbonate, hematocrit, hemoglobin.
   b. Urine: *decreased*—volume, specific gravity (↓ 1,010); *increased*—protein, casts, red and white blood cells, sodium.

⋈ **IV. Analysis/nursing diagnosis**
   A. *Altered urinary elimination* related to kidney malfunction.
   B. *Fluid volume excess* related to decreased urine output.
   C. *Altered nutrition, less than body requirements,* related to anorexia.
   D. *Altered oral mucous membrane* related to stomatitis.
   E. *Altered thought processes* related to uremia.

⋈ **V. Nursing care plan/implementation**
   A. Goal: *maintain fluid and electrolyte balance and nutrition.*
      1. Monitor: daily weight (should not vary more than ± 1 lb); vital signs—include central venous pressure (CVP).
      2. Blood chemistries: BUN 6–20 mg/dL; creatinine 0.6–1.5 mg/dL.
      3. *Fluids*: IV as ordered; blood: plasma, packed cells; electrolyte solutions to replace losses; restricted to 400 mL/24 h if hypertension present or during oliguric phase to prevent fluid overload.
      4. *Diet*: as tolerated: *high* carbohydrate, *low* protein, may be *low* potassium and *low* sodium; hypertonic glucose (total parenteral nutrition) if oral feedings not tolerated; intravenous L-amino acids and glucose.
      5. Control hyperkalemia: infusions of hypertonic glucose and insulin to force potassium into cells; calcium gluconate (IV) to reduce myocardial irritability from potassium; sodium bicarbonate (IV) to correct acidosis; sodium polystyrene sulfonate (*Kayexalate*) or other exchange resins, orally or rectally (*enema*), to remove excess potassium (K^+); *peritoneal dialysis or hemodialysis.*
      6. Medications—*diuretics* (mannitol, furosemide [*Lasix*]).
   B. Goal: *use assessment and comfort measures to reduce occurrence of complications.*
      1. Respiratory: monitor rate, depth, breath sounds, *arterial blood gases*; encourage deep breathing, coughing, turning; use *incentive spirometer* or *nebulizer* as indicated.
      2. Frequent oral care to prevent stomatitis.

3. Observe for signs of:
   a. *Infection*—elevated temperature, localized redness, swelling, heat, or drainage.
   b. *Bleeding*—stools, gums, venipuncture sites.

C. Goal: *maintain continual emotional support.*
  1. Same caregivers, consistency in procedures.
  2. Give opportunities to express concerns, fears.
  3. Allow family interactions.

D. Goal: **health teaching.**
  1. Preparation for dialysis (indications: uremia, uncontrolled hyperkalemia, or acidosis).
  2. *Dietary restrictions*: low sodium, fluid restriction.
  3. Disease process; treatment.

VI. Evaluation/outcome criteria
A. Return of kidney *function*—normal creatinine level (<1.5 mg/dL), urine output.
B. Resumes normal life pattern (about 3 mo after onset).

Chronic Renal Failure

Because of progressive destruction of kidney tissue, the kidneys are no longer able to maintain their homeostatic functions; considered irreversible.

I. **Pathophysiology**: destruction of glomeruli → reduced glomerular filtration rate → retention of metabolic waste products; decreased urine output; severe fluid, electrolyte, acid-base imbalances → uremia. Clinical picture includes:
  A. Ammonia in skin and alimentary tract resulting from bacterial interaction with urea → inflammation of mucous membranes.
  B. Retention of phosphate → decreased serum calcium → muscle spasms, tetany, and increased parathormone release → demineralization of bone.
  C. Failure of tubular mechanisms to regulate blood bicarbonate → metabolic acidosis → hyperventilation.
  D. Urea osmotic diuresis → flushing effect on tubules → decreased reabsorption of sodium → sodium depletion.
  E. Waste product retention → depressed bone marrow function → decreased circulating red blood cells (RBCs) → renal tissue hypoxia → decreased erythropoietin production → further depression of bone marrow functioning → anemia.

II. **Risk factors/causes:**
  A. Polycystic kidney disease.
  B. Chronic glomerulonephritis.
  C. Chronic urinary obstruction, ureteral stricture, calculi, neoplasms.

  D. Chronic pyelonephritis.
  E. Severe hypertension.
  F. Congenital or acquired renal artery stenosis.
  G. Systemic lupus erythematosus.

III. **Assessment**
  A. *Subjective data*: excessive fatigue, weakness.
  B. *Objective data:*
   1. Skin: bronze-colored, uremic frost.
   2. Ammonia breath.
   3. See also **Acute Renal Failure**, p. 214; symptoms gradual in onset.

IV. **Analysis/nursing diagnosis**
  A. In addition to the following, see **Acute Renal Failure**, p. 214.
  B. *Fatigue* related to severe anemia.
  C. *Risk for impaired skin integrity* related to pruritus.
  D. *Ineffective individual coping* related to chronic illness.
  E. *Body image disturbance* related to need for dialysis.
  F. *Noncompliance* related to denial of illness.

V. **Nursing care plan/implementation**
  A. Goal: *maintain fluid/electrolyte balance and nutrition.* (See also Acute Renal Failure, **p. 214.**)
   1. *Diet: low:* sodium, protein, phosphorus; foods *high* in: calcium, vitamin B complex, vitamins C and D, and iron (to reduce edema, replace deficits, and promote absorption of nutrients).
   2. Administer medications: calcium carbonate; supplemental vitamins if deficient; electrolyte modifier (aluminum hydroxide [*Alu-Cap, Amphojel*]).
   3. I&O; intake should be *limited* to no more than 600–800 mL more than previous day's output to prevent fluid retention.
  B. Goal: *employ comfort measures that reduce distress and support physical function.*
   1. Activity: bed rest; facilitate ventilation; turn, cough, deep breathe q2h; range of motion exercises—active and passive, to prevent thrombi.
   2. Hygiene: *mouth care* to prevent stomatitis and reduce discomfort from mouth ulcers; *perineal care.*
   3. Skin care: soothing lotions to reduce pruritus.
   4. Encourage communication of concerns.
  C. Goal: **health teaching.**
   1. Dietary restrictions: *no* added salt when cooking; change cooking water in vegetables during process to decrease potassium; read food labels to *avoid* sodium and potassium intake; *restrict protein* to 0.6–1.3 mg/kg IBW; *restrict phosphorus* to 800–1000 mg.
   2. Importance of daily weight: same scale, time, clothing.
   3. Prepare for dialysis, transplantation.

[handwritten margin notes: diet: ↓ 3 Ps: Protein Phosphorus Potassium; ↓ sodium; ↑ Ca⁺ ↑ iron; ↑ K acidosis]

⋈ VI. Evaluation/outcome criteria

    A. Acceptance of chronic illness (no indication of indiscretions, destructive behavior, suicidal tendency).

    B. Compliance with dietary restriction—no signs of protein excess (e.g., nausea, vomiting) or fluid/sodium excess (e.g., edema, weight gain).

Dialysis

Diffusion of solute through a semipermeable membrane that separates two solutions; direction of diffusion depends on concentration of solute in each solution; rate and efficiency depend on concentration gradient, temperature of solution, pore size of membrane, and molecular size; (**Table 17.1**).

I. *Indications*: acute poisonings, acute or chronic renal failure, hepatic coma, metabolic acidosis, extensive burns with azotemia.

II. *Goals*:

    A. *Reduce level of nitrogenous waste.*

    B. *Correct acidosis, reverse electrolyte imbalances, remove excess fluid.*

III. Hemodialysis: circulation of client's blood through a compartment formed of a semipermeable membrane (cellophane or cuprophane) surrounded by dialysate fluid.

    A. Types of dialyzers:

        1. Coil type.

        2. Parallel plate.

        3. Capillary.

    B. Types of venous access for hemodialysis:

        1. *Temporary venous access.*

            a. Flexible double lumen catheter is inserted into the internal jugular or femoral vein when *immediate* dialysis is needed. Subclavian vein can be used, but is usually *last* choice due to central stenosis that tends to occur.

            b. Internal jugular and subclavian catheters can remain in place 1–3 weeks.

            c. Femoral vein catheter can be used up to 1 week. Additional disadvantages are that the location is awkward, and groin area presents increased risk for infection.

        2. *External shunt* (**Figure 17.1**).

            a. Cannula is placed in a large vein and a large artery that are approximate.

            b. External shunts, which provide easy and painless access to bloodstream, are prone to infection and clotting and cause erosion of the skin around the insertion area.

              ☞ (1) Daily cleansing and application of a sterile dressing.

                 (2) Prevention of physical trauma and *avoidance* of some activities, such as swimming.

        2. *Arteriovenous fistulas* (**Figure 17.2**).

            a. Large artery and vein are sewn together (anastomosed) below the surface of the skin.

            b. Purpose is to create one blood vessel for withdrawing and returning blood.

            c. *Advantages*: greater activity range than arteriovenous shunt and no protective asepsis.

            d. *Disadvantage*: need for two venipunctures with each dialysis.

    C. **Complications** during hemodialysis:

        1. *Dysequilibrium syndrome*—rapid removal of urea from blood → reverse osmosis, with water moving into brain cells → cerebral edema → possible headache, nausea, vomiting, confusion, and convulsions; usually occurs with initial dialysis treatments; shorter dialysis time and slower rate minimizes.

        2. *Hypotension*—results from excessive ultrafiltration or excessive antihypertensive medications.

        3. *Hypertension*—results from volume overload (water and/or sodium), causing *dysequilibrium syndrome* or anxiety.

        4. *Transfusion reactions* (see **Chap. 5**).

        5. *Arrhythmias*—due to hypotension, fluid overload, or rapid removal of potassium.

        6. *Psychological problems*:

            a. Clients react in varying ways to dependence on hemodialysis.

            b. Nurse needs to identify client reactions and defense mechanisms and to employ supportive behaviors, i.e., include client in care; continual repetition and reinforcement; do *not* interpret client's behavior—for example, do not say, "You're being hostile" or "You're acting like a child"; answer questions honestly regarding quality and length of life with dialysis and/or transplantation; encourage independence as much as possible.

IV. Intermittent peritoneal dialysis: involves introduction of a dialysate solution into the abdomen, where the peritoneum acts as the semipermeable membrane between the solution and blood in abdominal vessels. *Procedures*:

    A. Area around umbilicus is prepared, anesthetized with local anesthetic, and a catheter is inserted into the peritoneal cavity through a trocar; the catheter is then sutured into place to prevent displacement.

    B. Warmed dialysate is then allowed to flow into the peritoneal cavity. Inflow time: 5–10 min; 2 liters of solution are used in each cycle in the adult; solutions contain glucose, Na^+, Ca^{2+}, Mg^{2+}, K^+, Cl^-, and lactate or acetate.

TABLE 17.1 COMPARISON OF HEMODIALYSIS AND PERITONEAL DIALYSIS

	Hemodialysis	Peritoneal Dialysis
Process	*Rapid*—uses temporary central venous access, external AV shunt (acute renal failure) or internal AV fistula (chronic renal failure); typical treatment is 3–4 h, 3 d/wk; also used for barbiturate overdoses to remove toxic agent quickly.	*Intermittent*—up to 24–72 h for hospitalized clients; ambulatory care: 10–14 h 3–4 times a week; *dwell time*: 30–45 min for manual dialysis, or 10–20 min for automatic cycler; either rigid stylet catheter or surgically inserted soft catheter; advantage for clients who cannot tolerate rapid fluid and electrolyte changes. *Continuous*—four cycles in 24 h; *dwell time* is 4–5 h during the day and 8 h overnight; no need for machinery, electricity, or water source; surgically inserted soft catheter; closely resembles normal renal function.
Vascular access	Required.	Not necessary; therefore suitable for clients with vascular problems.
Heparinization	Required; systemic or regional.	Little or no heparin necessary; therefore suitable for clients with bleeding problems.
Complications (other than fluid and electrolyte imbalances, which are common to all)	Dialysis dysequilibrium syndrome (preventable) Mechanical dysfunctions of dialyzer	Peritonitis Hypoalbuminemia Bowel or bladder perforation Plugged or dislodged catheter.

AV = arteriovenous.

Source: ©Lagerquist SL: *Little, Brown's NCLEX-RN® Examination Review*. Boston: Little, Brown. (out of print).

C. When solution bottle is empty, dwell time (exchange time) begins. *Dwell time*: 10–20 min, up to 8 hours depending on method of peritoneal dialysis. Processes of diffusion, osmosis, and filtration begin to move waste products from bloodstream into peritoneal cavity.

D. Draining of the dialysate begins with the unclamping of the outflow clamp. *Outflow time*: usually 20 min; return of <2 liters usually results from incomplete peritoneal emptying; turn side to side to increase return; 30 cycles in 24 h is ideal.

V. **Continuous ambulatory peritoneal dialysis (CAPD)**: functions on the same principles as peritoneal dialysis, yet allows greater freedom and independence for client. *Procedure*:

A. Dialysis solution is infused into peritoneum three times daily and once before bedtime.

B. Dwell time—5 h for each daily exchange, overnight for the fourth (8 h).

C. Indwelling peritoneal catheter is connected to solution bag at all times—serves to fill and drain peritoneum; concealed in cloth pouch, strapped to the body during dwell time; client can move about doing usual activities.

Kidney Transplantation

Placement of a donor kidney (from sibling, parent, cadaver) into the iliac fossa of a recipient and the anastomosis of its ureter to the bladder of the recipient; indicated in end-stage renal disease.

I. *Criteria for recipient*: irreversible kidney function; under 70 yr of age; patent and functional lower urinary tract; and good surgical risk, free of serious cardiovascular complications. *Contraindicated* in metastatic carcinoma and oxalosis (excessive oxalate in urine).

II. *Donor selection*:
A. Sibling or parent—survival rate of kidney is greater; preferred for transplantation.
B. Cadaver—greater rate of rejection after transplantation, although cadaver kidneys are used for most transplantations.

III. *Bilateral nephrectomy*: necessary for clients with rapidly progressive glomerulonephritis, malignant hypertension, or chronic kidney infections; prevents complications in transplanted kidney (see **Nephrectomy** for nursing care, p. 219).

IV. Analysis/nursing diagnosis
A. *Altered urinary elimination* related to kidney failure.
B. *Fear* related to potential transplant rejection.
C. *Risk for infection* related to immunosuppression.
D. *Body image disturbance* related to immunosuppression.

FIGURE 17.1 ARTERIOVENOUS SHUNT (CANNULAS).

(Adapted from an illustration provided by Ann Holmes, RN.)

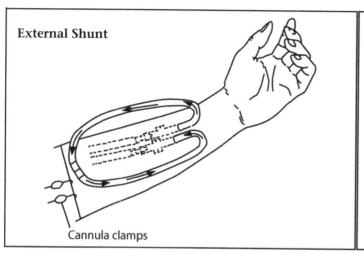

FIGURE 17.2 ARTERIOVENOUS FISTULA.

(Adapted from an illustration provided by Ann Holmes, RN..)

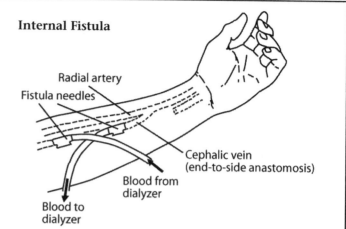

▶◀ V. **Nursing care plan/implementation**
   A. **Preoperative care:**
      1. Goal: *promote physical and emotional adjustment.*
         a. Informed consent.
         b. Lab work completed—histocompatibility, complete blood count, urinalysis, blood type and cross-match.
         c. Skin preparation.
      2. Goal: *encourage expression of feelings:* origin of donor, fear of complications, rejection.
      3. Goal: *minimize risk of organ rejection:* give medications: begin *immunosuppression (azathioprine, corticosteroids, cyclosporine); antiinfectives* if ordered.
      4. Goal: **health teaching.**
         a. Nature of surgery, placement of kidney.
         b. Postoperative expectations: deep breathing, coughing, turning, early ⚠ ambulation; *reverse isolation.*
         c. Medications: immunosuppressive therapy: purpose, effect.
   B. **Postoperative care:**
      1. Goal: *promote uncomplicated recovery of recipient.*
         a. *Vital signs;* CVP; I&O—may see large amounts urine (3–20 L) in early postoperative period from sodium diuresis; or kidney may not work for a week or more and dialysis will be needed within 24–48 h.
         ⚠ b. *Isolation:* strict *reverse isolation* with immunosuppression; client should wear face mask when out of room.
         c. *Position:* back to nonoperated sides; semi-Fowler's to promote gas exchange.
         ☞ d. *Indwelling catheter care:* characteristics of urine (see **p. 223**)—report gross

hematuria, heavy sediment; clots; perineal care.
         e. *Activity:* ambulate 24 h after surgery, *avoid* prolonged sitting.
         f. *Weigh daily.*
         g. *Medications: immunosuppressives, analgesics* as ordered.
         ☞ h. *Drains:* irrigate *only* on physician's order; *meticulous* catheter care.
         🍎 i. *Diet:* regular; liberal amounts of protein; *restrict* fluids, sodium, potassium *only if* oliguric.
      2. Goal: *observe for signs of rejection—most dangerous complication. Three classifications:*
         a. *Hyperacute*—occurs within 5–10 min up to 48 h after transplantation (RARE).
         b. *Acute*—signs and symptoms are evident at approximately 6 weeks after transplantation. Rejection is most common at 3 mos. after transplantation.
         c. *Chronic*—occurs several months to years after transplantation.
         ▶◀ d. **Assessment**
            (1) *Subjective data:*
               (a) Lethargy, anorexia.
               (b) Tenderness over graft site.
            (2) *Objective data:*
               (a) Lab data: urine: *decreased*—output, creatinine clearance, sodium; *increased*—protein; blood; *increased*—BUN, creatinine.
               (b) Rapid weight gain.
               (c) Vital signs: BP, temperature—*elevated.*
      3. Goal: *maintain immunosuppressive therapy.*
         a. Azathioprine (*Imuran*)—an anti-

metabolite that interferes with cellular division. *Side effects*:
- (1) Gastrointestinal (GI) bleeding (give PO form *with food*).
- (2) Bone marrow depression, *leukopenia, anemia.*
- (3) Development of malignant neoplasms.
- (4) Infection.
- (5) Liver damage.

b. Prednisone—believed to affect lymphocyte production by inhibiting nucleic acid synthesis; antiinflammatory action helps prevent tissue damage if rejection occurs. *Side effects*:
- (1) Stress ulcer with bleeding (give with food).
- (2) *Decreased* glucose tolerance (hyperglycemia).
- (3) Muscle weakness.
- (4) Osteoporosis.
- (5) Moon facies.
- (6) Acne and striae.
- (7) Depression and hallucinations.

c. Cyclosporine (*Cyclosporin* A)—a polypeptide antibiotic used to prevent rejection of kidney, liver, or heart allografts; PO dose given *with* room temperature chocolate milk or orange juice in a glass dispenser. *Side effects*:
- (1) Nephrotoxicity (*increased* BUN, creatinine).
- (2) Hypertension.
- (3) Tremor.
- (4) Hirsutism, gingival hyperplasia.
- (5) GI—nausea, vomiting, anorexia, diarrhea, abdominal pain.
- (6) *Infections*—pneumonia, septicemia, abscesses, wound.

d. Additional drugs may include cyclophosphamide (*Cytoxan*), methylprednisolone, antithymocyte (ATGAM), antilymphocyte globulin, and anti-T-lymphocyte monoclonal antibody.

4. Goal: **health teaching.**
a. Signs of rejection (see **Goal 2**).
b. Drugs: side effects of immunosuppression (see **Goal 3**).
c. Self-care activities: temperature, BP, I&O, urine specimen collection.
d. Prevention of infection.
e. See also goals of care, **Postoperative Experience, p. 132.**

VI. Evaluation/outcome criteria
A. No signs of rejection (e.g., weight gain, oliguria).
B. No depression.
C. Resumes role responsibilities.

Nephrectomy

Removal of kidney through flank, retroperitoneal, abdominal, thoracic, or thoracic-abdominal approach; indicated with malignant tumors, severe trauma, or under certain conditions before renal transplantation (see **Kidney Transplantation, p. 217-219**).

I. Analysis /nursing diagnosis
A. *Pain* related to surgical incision.
B. *Risk for infection* related to wound contamination.
C. *Risk for aspiration* related to vomiting.
D. *Constipation* related to paralytic ileus.
E. *Anxiety* related to possible loss of function in remaining kidney.
F. *Dysfunctional grieving* related to perceived loss.

II. Nursing care plan/implementation
A. **Preoperative care**: Goal: *optimize physical and psychological functioning* (see **Preoperative Preparation, p. 127-129**).
B. **Postoperative care**: Goal: *promote comfort and prevent complications.*
1. Observe for signs of:
a. *Paralytic ileus*—abdominal distention, absent bowel sounds, vomiting (common complication following renal surgery).
b. *Hemorrhage.*
2. Fluid balance: daily weight—maintain within 2% of preoperative level.

III. Evaluation/outcome criteria
A. No complications (e.g., hemorrhage, paralytic ileus, wound infection).
B. Acceptance of loss of kidney.

Renal Calculi (Urolithiasis)

Formation of calculi (stones) in renal calyces or pelvis that pass to lower regions of urinary tract—ureters, bladder, or urethra; occurs after age 30 yr, with greatest incidence in *men*, particularly over age 50 yr.

I. **Pathophysiology**: organic crystals form (75% of stones contain calcium) → obstruction, infection; increased backward pressure in kidney → hydronephrosis → atrophy, fibrosis of renal tubules.

II. **Risk factors/causes:**
A. Changes in urine pH and concentration from readily precipitable, crystalline materials—sulfonamides, uric acid, calcium salts, oxalate.
B. Urinary tract infection.
C. Indwelling Foley catheter.
D. Vitamin A deficiency.

III. **Assessment** (depends on size, shape, location of stone)

A. *Subjective data*:
1. Pain: occasional, dull, in loin or back when stones are in calyces or renal pelvis; *excruciating* in flank area (renal colic), radiating to groin when stones are ureteral.
2. Nausea associated with pain.
B. *Objective data*:
1. Pallor, sweating, syncope, shock, and vomiting due to pain.
2. Palpable kidney mass with hydronephrosis.
3. Fever and pyuria with infection.
4. Lab data:
   a. Urinalysis: abnormal—pH (acidic or alkaline), RBCs (injury), WBCs (infection); *increased*—specific gravity, casts, crystals, other organic substances, depending on type of stone (i.e., uric acid, calcium); positive culture.
   b. Blood: *increased*—calcium phosphorus, total protein, alkaline phosphatase, creatinine, uric acid, BUN.
5. *Diagnostic tests*:
   a. IVP: reveals nonopaque stones, degree of obstruction. See **p. 224**.
   b. X-ray: radiopaque stones seen.
   c. Ultrasound may also be used.

IV. Analysis/nursing diagnosis
A. *Pain* related to passage of stone.
B. *Altered urinary elimination* related to potential obstruction.
C. *Urinary retention* related to obstruction of urethra.

V. Nursing care plan/implementation
A. Goal: *reduce pain and prevent complications.*
1. Medication: *narcotics, antiemetics, antiinfectives.*
2. *Fluids*: 3–4 L/d; IVs if nauseated, vomiting.
3. Activity: ambulate to promote passage of stone, except bed rest during acute attack (colic).
4. Reduce spasms: warm soaks to affected flank.
5. Observe for signs of:
   a. *Obstruction—decreased* urinary output, *increased* flank pain.
   b. *Passage of stone*—cessation of pain; filter urine with gauze.
6. Monitor: hydration status—I&O, daily weight; vital signs—particularly temperature for sign of infection; urine—color, odor.
B. Goal: **health teaching.**
1. Importance of *fluids*: minimum 3000 mL/d; 2 glasses during night.
2. *Diet*: modify according to stone type and amount of urinary excretion of organic substance (i.e., calcium).
   a. *Uric acid stones—low* purine.
   b. *Calcium oxalate and calcium phosphate stones—low* calcium, phosphorus, and oxalate (e.g., *avoid* tea, cocoa, cola, beans, strawberries, nuts, salt, spinach, acidic fruits). Low calcium diet may be **contraindicated**, as it may cause bone demineralization, particularly in postmenopausal women. Vitamins C and D supplements may also increase the risk of stone formation.
   c. *Cystine stones—low* protein.
3. *Acid-ash diet* with: calcium oxalate and calcium phosphate stones, magnesium and ammonium phosphate stones.
4. *Alkaline-ash diet* with: uric acid, and cystine stones (see Review of Nutrition in **Appendix B**).
5. Signs of urinary tract infection: dysuria, frequency, hematuria; seek immediate treatment.
6. Prepare for removal if indicated; 60%–80% of clients will have lithotripsy done (see below); cystoscopy (see **p. 224**) or ureterolithotomy may also be ordered; nephrectomy in *extreme cases*.

VI. Evaluation/outcome criteria
A. Relief from pain.
B. No signs of urinary obstruction (e.g., increased flank pain, decreased urine output).
C. No recurrence of lithiasis (adheres to diet and fluid regimen).

Extracorporeal Lithotripsy

A noninvasive mechanical procedure used to break up renal calculi so they can pass spontaneously, in most cases. The trunk of the client is submerged in water. In addition to being strapped to a frame, the client may also be sedated, as the procedure takes 30–45 min and remaining still is important. An underwater electrode generates shock waves that fragment the stone, so it can be excreted in the urine a few days after the procedure. A degree of renal colic may occur, necessitating treatment with *antispasmodics.*

Nursing measures: encourage ambulation and promote diuresis through *forcing fluids.*

Urinary Diversion (Ileal Conduit)

Implantation of ureters into a portion of the terminal ileum, with formation of a stoma; common method for urinary diversion; also known as *Bricker's procedure.*

I. *Indications*:
A. Congenital anomalies of bladder.
B. Neurogenic bladder.
C. Mechanical obstruction to urine flow (e.g., bladder cancer).
D. Severe cystitis.

E. Trauma to lower urinary tract.

II. Analysis /nursing diagnosis

A. *Altered urinary elimination* related to surgical diversion.

B. *Risk for impaired skin integrity* related to leakage of urine.

C. *Risk for infection* related to contamination of stoma.

D. *Constipation* related to absence of peristalsis.

E. *Body image disturbance* related to stoma.

III. Nursing care plan/implementation

A. **Preoperative care**: optimal bowel and stoma site preparation.

    1. *Diet*: nonresidue several days before surgery.

    2. Medications:

       a. Neomycin.

    3. Bowel cleansing activities

       a. Cathartics

       b. Enemas

    4. Site selection: appliance faceplate must bond securely; *avoid* areas where there would be pressure from clothing (waistline); usual site is right or left lower abdominal quadrant.

    5. See also Preoperative Preparation, **p. 127-128.**

B. **Postoperative care:**

    1. Goal: *prevent complications and promote comfort.*

       a. Observe for signs of:

         (1) *Paralytic ileus* (common complication)—keep *nasogastric tube* patent.

         (2) *Stoma necrosis*—dusky or cyanotic color (**emergency** situation).

       b. Skin care: check for leakage around ostomy bag.

       c. See Postoperative Experience, **p. 132.**

    2. Goal: **health teaching.**

       a. Self-care activities:

         (1) *Peristomal skin care*—prevent irritation, breakdown; proper cleansing—soap and water; adhesive remover, if needed.

         (2) *Appliance application and emptying*—do *not* remove each day; change appliance every 4–5 d or when leaking.

         (3) *Odor control*—dilute urine; *acid ash diet*; hygiene; *avoid* asparagus, tomatoes; an increase in mucus is normal.

         (4) *Use of night drainage system* if necessary for uninterrupted sleep.

       b. Signs of *complications*: change in urine: color, clarity, quantity, smell; stomal color change.

IV. Evaluation/outcome criteria

A. Acceptance of new body image.

B. Regains independence.

C. Demonstrates confidence in management of self-care activities.

Prostatic Hyperplasia (Prostatism)

Malfunction of the urinary tract resulting from a lesion (benign or malignant) of the prostate gland.

I. **Pathophysiology**: prostate enlarges, bulges upward, blocks flow of urine from bladder into urethra → obstruction → hydroureter, hydronephrosis.

II. **Risk factors/causes:**

A. *Benign*:

    1. Changes in estrogen and androgen levels.

    2. Men >50 yr.

B. *Malignant*:

    1. Genetic tendency.

    2. Hormonal factors (e.g., late puberty, greater sperm count).

    3. Diet (high fat).

    4. Exposure to chemical carcinogens (fertilizer, rubber, cadmium batteries).

III. **Assessment**

A. *Subjective data—urination*:

    1. Difficulty starting stream.

    2. Smaller, less forceful.

    3. Dribbling.

    4. Frequency.

    5. Urgency.

    6. Nocturia.

    7. Retention (incomplete emptying).

    8. Inability to void after ingestion of alcohol or exposure to cold.

B. *Objective data*:

    1. Catheterization for residual urine: 25-50 mL after voiding.

    2. Enlarged prostate on digital rectal exam (DRE).

    3. Lab data:

       a. Urine—*increased* RBC, WBC.

       b. Blood—*increased* creatinine. Prostate Specific Antigen (PSA)—*elevated* with cancer.

IV. **Analysis/nursing diagnosis**

A. *Urinary retention* related to incomplete emptying.

B. *Altered urinary elimination* related to obstruction.

C. *Urinary incontinence* related to urgency, pressure.

D. *Anxiety* related to potential surgery.

E. *Body image disturbance* related to threat to masculine identity.

V. **Nursing care plan/implementation**

A. Goal: *relieve urinary retention.*

☞ 1. Catheterization: release maximum of 1000 mL initially; *avoid* bladder decompression, which results in hypotension, bladder spasms, ruptured blood vessels in bladder; empty 200 mL every 5 min.

☞ 2. Patency: irrigate intermittently or continually, as ordered.

3. *Fluids*: minimum of 2000 mL/24 h.

🏠 B. Goal: **health teaching.**

1. Preparation for surgery (cystostomy, prostatectomy):

    a. Expectations—indwelling catheter (will feel urge to void).

    b. *Avoid* pulling on catheter (this increases bleeding and clots).

    c. Bladder spasms common 24–48 h after surgery, particularly with transurethral resection (TUR) and suprapubic approaches.

    d. Threatening nature of procedure (possibility of impotence and/or incontinence).

2. See also **Preoperative Preparation, p. 127-129.**

Prostatectomy

Surgical procedure to relieve urinary retention and frequency caused by benign prostatic hypertrophy or cancer of the prostate.

I. **Types**

A. *Transurethral resection (TUR)*—removal of obstructive prostatic tissue surrounding urethra by an electric wire (resectoscope) introduced through the urethra; hypertrophy may recur, and TUR may need to be repeated.

B. *Suprapubic*—low midline incision is made directly over the bladder; bladder is opened and large mass of prostatic tissue is removed through incision in urethral mucosa.

C. *Retropubic*—removal of hypertrophied prostatic tissue high in pelvic area through a low abdominal incision; bladder is not opened.

D. *Perineal*—removal of prostatic tissue low in pelvic area is accomplished through an incision made between the scrotum and the rectum; usually results in impotency because procedure involves nerve transection.

◄ II. **Nursing care plan/implementation**

A. **Preoperative care:** see **Prostatic Hyperplasia, p. 221.**

B. **Postoperative care:**

1. Goal: *promote optimal bladder function and comfort.*

    ☞ a. *Urinary drainage*: sterile closed-gravity system—maintain external traction as ordered.

    b. Reinforce: purposes, sensations to expect.

    ☞ c. *Bladder irrigation* to control bleeding, keep clots from forming (see Three-way Foley, p. 223).

    d. *Suprapubic catheter* care (suprapubic prostatectomy)—closed-gravity drainage system; observe character, amount, flow of drainage see **p. 223.**

    e. *After removal*:

        (1) Observe for urinary drainage q4h for 24 h.

        (2) Skin care.

        (3) Report excessive drainage to physician.

    ☞ f. *Dressings*: keep dry, clean; reinforce if necessary (may need to change suprapubic dressing if urinary drainage); notify physician of *excessive bleeding*.

    g. Observe for signs of:

        (1) *Bladder distention*—distinct mound over pubis, slow drop in collecting bottle; irrigate catheter as ordered.

        (2) *Increased bleeding*—bright red drainage and clots; cool, clammy, pale skin; increased pulse rate.

2. Goal: *assist in rehabilitation.* Emotional support: *fears* of incontinence, loss of masculine identity, impotence.

🏠 3. Goal: **health teaching.**

    a. Expectations: mild incontinence, dribbling for a while (several months) after surgery; need to void as soon as urge is felt; *push fluids*.

    b. Exercises: perineal 1–2 d after surgery—buttocks are tightened for a count of ten, 20–50 times daily.

    c. *Avoid*:

        (1) Long auto trips, vigorous exercise, heavy lifting, and sexual intercourse until medical permission given, as this may increase tendency to bleed.

        (2) Alcoholic beverages for 1 mo, as this may cause burning on urination.

        (3) Tub baths, as this increases chance of infection.

    ⬤ d. Medications: *stool softeners* or mild *cathartics* to decrease straining.

◄ III. **Evaluation/outcome criteria**

A. Relief of symptoms.

B. No complications (e.g., hemorrhage impotence).

REVIEW OF THE USE OF COMMON TUBES

Tube or Apparatus	Purpose	Examples of Use	☞ Key Points
Three-way Foley	To provide avenues for *constant irrigation and constant drainage* of the urinary bladder.	1. Transurethral resection. 2. *Bladder* infections.	1. Watch for blocking by clots—causes bladder spasms 2. Irrigant solution often has anti-infective added to normal saline or sterile water 3. Sterile water rather than normal saline may be used for lysis of clots
Suprapubic catheter	To *drain bladder* via an opening through the abdominal wall above the pubic bone.	*Suprapubic* prostatectomy.	May have orders to irrigate prn or continuously
Ureteral catheter	To *drain urine* from the pelvis of one kidney, or for *splinting* ureter.	1. *Cystoscopy* for diagnostic workups. 2. *Ureteral surgery*. 3. *Pyelotomy*	1. **Never** clamp the tube—pelvis of kidney only holds 4–8 mL. 2. Use *only* 5 mL of sterile normal saline if ordered to irrigate.

Note: This review focuses on care of the tubes, not on total client care.

Source: Jane Vincent Corbett, RN, MS, EdD, Professor Emerita, School of Nursing, University of San Francisco. Used with permission.

🔑 Summary of Key Points

1. Kidney infections such as pyelonephritis and glomerular nephritis, may result in kidney failure. It is therefore important to recognize clients at high risk, such as those with an untreated streptococcal infection, bowel incontinence, or history of urinary reflux.

2. A classic symptom of a kidney infection is *flank pain.*

3. *Acute* renal failure is considered *reversible. Chronic* renal failure is *irreversible.*

4. Frequently the *specific gravity* of the scanty urine output in renal failure is *low* because the kidney is unable to concentrate water. Reduced urine output resulting from dehydration will lead to an elevated specific gravity, indicating concentration of particles from water loss.

5. The best indicator of the status of glomerular function is the serum *creatinine* level. BUN is *increased* in renal failure, dehydration, and malnutrition.

6. Dialysis may be: permanent *or* temporary; stationary *or* ambulatory; fast *or* slow; intermittent *or* continuous; and the access external *or* internal. Client needs will be varied.

7. The effectiveness of dialysis is measured by both a *decrease* in serum creatinine and BUN, but also the *reduction in fluid retention* (1 kg = 1000 mL).

8. After a kidney transplantation the greatest concern is *rejection*, which may be immediate or take months or a year or more to develop.

9. *Pain* is usually greater after a nephrectomy than after a kidney transplantation. The pain from renal colic (renal calculi) is excruciating, requiring pain management and rest until the pain is relieved.

10. Expect *mucus* in the urine after the construction of an ileal conduit.

11. *Impotence* is expected after a perineal prostatectomy because the procedure involves nerve transection. If present after the other approaches, the cause may be psychological.

💡 Study and Memory Aids

〰️ Diagnostic Studies/Procedures

Kidney, Ureter, and Bladder X-ray

Used to: determine size, shape, and position of kidneys, ureters, and bladder.

Cystogram

Installation of radiopaque medium through a catheter into the bladder; *used to:* visualize bladder wall and evaluate ureterovesical valves for reflux.

Cystoscopy

Visualization of bladder, urethra, and prostatic urethra by insertion of a tubular, lighted, telescopic lens (cystoscope) through the urinary meatus.

1. *Used to:* directly inspect the bladder, collect urine from the renal pelvis, obtain biopsy specimens from bladder and urethra, remove calculi, and treat lesions in the bladder, urethra, and prostate.
☞ 2. *Nursing actions following* procedure:
    a. Observe for urinary retention.
    b. Warm sitz baths to relieve discomfort.

Intravenous Urography (IVU) or Pyelography (IVP)

Injection of a radiopaque contrast substance, followed by fluoroscopic and x-ray films of kidneys and urinary tract; *used to:* identify lesions in kidneys and ureters and provide a rough estimate of kidney function.

Renal Angiogram

Small catheter is inserted into the femoral artery and passed into the aorta or renal artery, radiopaque fluid is instilled, and serial films are taken.

1. *Used to:* diagnose renal hypertension and pheochromocytoma and differentiate renal cysts from renal tumors.
☞ 2. *Postangiogram nursing actions:* check pedal pulse for signs of decreased circulation.

Renal biopsy

Needle aspiration of tissue from the kidney for the purpose of microscopic examination.

24-h Urine Collection

A true and accurate evaluation of kidney function, primarily glomerular filtration. Substances excreted by the kidney are excreted at different rates, amounts, and times of day or night. Timed urine collection is done for *protein, creatinine, electrolytes, urinary steroids,* etc. A large container is used, with or without preservative. Label with client name, type of test, and exact time test starts and ends. Not usually necessary to measure urine. Have client void, discard urine; test starts at this time. Have client void as close to the end of the 24-h period as possible. If refrigeration is required, urine may be stored in iced container.

🍎 Diets

Acute Glomerulonephritis

↓ Potassium	↑ Protein
↓ Sodium	

Acute Renal Failure

↓ Potassium	↑ Carbohydrate
Protein	
Sodium	
Fluid restriction	

Chronic Renal Failure

↑ Calcium	↓ Sodium
Iron	
Vitamins: B, C, D	

Kidney Transplantation

If oliguric: ↓ sodium, potassium, fluids

💊 Drug Review

Pyelonephritis

Analgesic
  Phenazopyridine (*Pyridium*): 200 mg tid
Antiinfectives
  Cephalexin (*Keflex*): 250–500 mg q6h
  Cephalothin (*Keflin*): IV 0.5–2 g q4–6h
  Erythromycin: 250–500 mg q6–12h
  Gentamicin (*Garamycin*): 3–5 mg/kg/d in divided doses q 8h
  Penicillin G: IM 1.2 million U in single dose
  Sulfamethoxazole (*Gantanol* DS): 1 g q8–12h; with trimethoprim (*Septra*)
Antipyretics
  Acetaminophen (*Tylenol*): 325–1000 mg q6h
  Aspirin: 325–1000 mg q4–6h, *not to exceed* 4 g/d

Acute Renal Failure

Diuretics
  Furosemide (*Lasix*): 20–80 mg/d
  Mannitol (*Osmitrol*): IV 50–100 g as 5–10% solution
Electrolyte modifier
  Sodium polystyrene sulfonate (*Kayexalate*): 15 g qid

Chronic Renal Failure

Electrolyte modifiers
  Aluminum hydroxide (*Amphojel*): 1.9–4.8 g 3–4 times/d
  Calcium carbonate (dose varies with symptoms)
Vitamin supplements: water soluble: folic acid 0.4–1 mg/day; pyridoxine 2.5–10 mg/day; ascorbic acid 45–60 mg/day; vitamin D supplements 0.25 mcg/day (if deficient)

Kidney Transplantation

Analgesics

Meperidine (*Demerol*): 50–150 mg q3–4h as needed; IV 15–35 mg/h as a continuous infusion

Morphine: IV 2.5–15 mg q4h or loading dose of 15 mg with 0.8–10 mg/h rate increased as needed; SC 5–20 mg q4h as needed

Corticosteroids

Dexamethasone (*Decadrom*): 0.5-9 mg daily in single on divided doses

Methylprednisolone (*Medrol*): 4-48 mg/d

Prednisone (*Deltasone*): 5-60 mg/d

Immunosuppresive therapy

Antithymocyte (*ATGAM*) (antilymphocyte globulin): 10–30 mg/kg for 14 days, then alternate days for total of 21 doses in 4 weeks

Anti-T-lymphocyte monoclonal antibody (*OKT₃*): 5 mg/d for 14 days

Azathioprine (*Imuran*): 3–5 mg/kg/d

Cyclophosphamide (*Cytoxan*): 1–5 mg/kg/d

Cyclosporine (*Sandimmune*): 15 mg/kg/d

Renal Calculi

Antiemetics

Prochlorperazine (*Compazine*): IM 5–10 mg—repeat once as needed

Promethazine (*Phenergan*): IM 12.5–25 mg q4–6h as needed

Trimethobenzamide (*Tigan*): IM 200 mg 3–4 times/d

Antiinfectives

Cephalexin (*Keflex*): 250–500 mg q6h

Cephalothin (*Keflin*): IV 0.5–2 g q4–6h

Erythromycin: 250–500 mg q6–12h

Gentamicin (*Garamycin*): 3–5 mg/kg/d in divided doses

Penicillin G: IM 1.2 million U in single dose

Narcotics

Meperidine (*Demerol*): 50–150 mg q3–4h as needed; IV, 15–35 mg/h as a continuous infusion

Urinary Diversion

Neomycin (*Mycifradin*): 1 g/h for 4h, then 1 gm q4h for 24h preoperatively to decrease incidence of infection

Questions

1. During the immediate postoperative period after a transurethral resection of the prostate (TURP), for what common physical problem should the nurse observe?
   1. Sexual impotence.
   2. Thrombophlebitis.
   3. Venous bleeding.
   4. Atelectasis.

2. Three days after renal transplantation, a client's urine output decreases to 720 mL in 24 hours. The nurse would respond to this by:
   1. Calling the client's physician.
   2. Increasing the intravenous infusion rate.
   3. Checking the urine specific gravity.
   4. Checking the output hourly for 8 hours.

3. To minimize bleeding after a TURP, the most important nursing action would be to maintain:
   1. Traction on the indwelling catheter.
   2. Continuous irrigation of the bladder.
   3. The client on bedrest until bleeding diminishes.
   4. The patency of the catheter drainage system.

4. The nurse would recognize which of the following as a complication of peritoneal dialysis?
   1. Oliguria.
   2. Pink-tinged urine.
   3. Cloudy dialysate return.
   4. Yellow dialysate drainage.

5. What characteristic urinalysis findings would the nurse note in a client with glomerulonephritis?
   1. Decreased specific gravity and hematuria.
   2. Decreased specific gravity and proteinuria.
   3. Increased specific gravity and glycosuria.
   4. Increased specific gravity and proteinuria.

6. After a cystectomy and construction of an ileal conduit, against which complication should the nurse advise the client to take special precautions?
   1. Paralytic ileus.
   2. Urinary calculi.
   3. Pyelonephritis.
   4. Mucus in the urine.

7. When the amount of peritoneal dialysate returned is less than that infused, the nurse should:
   1. Turn the client from side to side gently.
   2. Apply suction to the abdominal catheter.
   3. Reduce the amount of dialysate infused during the next exchange.
   4. Apply gentle pressure to the abdomen to move the catheter tip.

8. The nurse should advise a middle-aged man that it is recommended that the prostate be examined:
   1. Once a month, when showering, after age 40.
   2. Every 3 months after age 50.
   3. During an annual physical examination after age 40.
   4. Every other year after age 50.

9. Which nursing diagnosis is a priority concern in a client in acute renal failure?
   1. Risk for impaired skin integrity.
   2. Altered nutrition: less than body requirements.
   3. Fluid volume excess.
   4. Anxiety.

10. The nursing care plan for a client suffering from acute renal failure should include a diet that is:
    1. High in protein and calories.
    2. Low in protein and high in calories.
    3. High in protein and low in calories.
    4. Low in protein and calories.

low potassium low Nat

11. Which fruit should the nurse suggest as a snack for a client in acute renal failure?
    1. Apricots.
    2. Apples. → *low in K⁺*
    3. Nectarines.
    4. Oranges.

12. Client teaching on the way in which continuous ambulatory peritoneal dialysis works would include the fact that:
    1. The dialysate is absorbed intravascularly, and waste products are excreted by the kidneys.
    2. Urine is drawn into the dialysate and eliminated with each exchange.
    3. Waste products move out of the blood into the dialysate and are drained out.
    4. The instillation of fluid into the abdomen stimulates the kidneys to concentrate waste products.

13. The nurse tells a client undergoing continuous ambulatory peritoneal dialysis that a common side effect of the treatment is:
    1. Diarrhea.
    2. Bloody effluent.
    3. Back pain.
    4. Nausea.

14. The nurse should anticipate, during an attack of ureteral colic stemming from a kidney stone, what change in the urine would a client most likely show?
    1. Ketonuria.
    2. Glycosuria.
    3. Hematuria.
    4. Proteinuria.

15. Intravenous pyelography has been ordered to search for kidney stones. In preparation, the nurse must first:
    1. Weigh the client.
    2. Determine whether the client has any allergy to iodine.
    3. Note the last bowel movement.
    4. Record the baseline vital signs.

16. Which nursing measure is a priority for a client with renal calculi?
    1. Monitoring for extreme variations in blood pressure.
    2. Straining the urine to obtain sediment or stone particles.
    3. Encouraging the client to drink 3 to 4 liters of fluids daily.
    4. Recording the urine output to assess kidney function.

17. Which assessment finding would be an early indication of a postoperative complication that frequently occurs after the construction of an ileal conduit?
    1. Mucus in the urinary drainage.
    2. Absent bowel sounds.
    3. Boardlike abdomen.
    4. Diminished breath sounds.

18. Which discharge teaching should the nurse question in a client with calcium renal calculi?
    1. Limit amount of protein in the diet.
    2. Drink 3 to 4 liters of fluid daily.
    3. Void every 2 to 3 hours.
    4. Take vitamin C daily.

19. The nurse should anticipate that an infection in the kidney would most likely produce which complaint?
    1. Burning on urination. — *bladder*
    2. Flank or abdominal pain.
    3. Blood in the stool.
    4. Difficulty starting urinary stream.

20. Which statement regarding the usual postoperative urinary elimination would guide the nursing actions?
    1. A well-hydrated client usually voids within 6 to 8 hours after surgery.
    2. The amount of fluids administered IV after abdominal surgery is restricted to prevent diuresis.
    3. The amount of the first voiding after surgery is usually 800 to 1000 mL.
    4. The total urinary output the day of surgery usually exceeds 3000 mL.

Answers/Rationale

1. **(3)** Venous bleeding is common for several days after a TURP. The blood is dark red, and it is also less viscous than arterial blood. Sexual dysfunction (**1**) is not an expected complication of the transurethral approach, because there would be *no physiologic* cause for impotence. The client ambulates early after a TURP to prevent problems stemming from immobility (**2**). Atelectasis (**4**) would be more likely in a client who receives a general anesthetic, *not* spinal anesthesia, which is used for a TURP. **AS, COM, 8, PhI, Physiological adaptation**

2. **(3)** The 24-hour volume equals 30 mL/h, the minimum hourly output, so additional data are needed to determine whether this change is due to dehydration or rejection. Calling the physician (**1**) turns the decision-making process over to the MD. Increasing the infusion rate (**2**) is *not* an *independent nursing action*. Waiting another 8 hours (**4**) would not be in the client's best interests, because intervention may be needed in the meantime. **EV, ANL, 8, PhI, Reduction of risk potential**

3. **(1)** Venous bleeding is often controlled by the pressure exerted by the fluid-filled balloon of the urethral catheter. Irrigation (**2**) would prevent clogging of the drainage system with clots but would *not stop* the bleeding. Lengthy bedrest (**3**) would lead to problems stemming from immobility. Keeping the

catheter drainage system patent (4) would also *not stop* the bleeding. **IMP, ANL, 8, PhI, Reduction of risk potential**

4. (3) Cloudy dialysate would indicate the presence of peritonitis caused by organisms that have entered the peritoneum after insertion of the dialysis catheter. Small urine volume, or oliguria (1), would indicate that renal function is compromised and is *not* a complication of the treatment. Blood in the urine (2) would indicate the existence of bladder or kidney problems. If blood were in the dialysate, this would indicate that trauma occurred during insertion of the trocar. Protein would color the dialysate yellow (4), but this is *not* a complication of peritoneal dialysis. **AS, ANL, 8, PhI, Physiological adaptation**

5. (4) The urinalysis findings would reflect damage to the glomeruli with the resultant leaking of protein and red blood cells into the urine, but the kidney would still have the ability to concentrate wastes, so specific gravity would be increased. Hematuria (1) and proteinuria (2) would be found, but the specific gravity is *increased* in glomerulonephritis. Sugar in the urine, or glycosuria (3), would *not* occur in glomerulonephritis. **EV, ANL, 8, PhI, Reduction of risk potential**

6. (3) This urinary diversion procedure increases the risk of infection because the bladder has been removed which normally reduces the chance of organisms reaching the kidneys. There is *nothing* the client can do to *prevent* ileus (1), which is a complication of surgery. The likelihood of kidney stones (2) forming is not greater in clients who undergo this procedure, and this is *not necessarily preventable*. The mucus in the urine (4) is *normal* and expected after the surgery. **IMP, APP, 8, PhI, Reduction of risk potential**

7. (1) The tip of the catheter may lodge up against the bowel. By turning the client, the tip of the catheter may shift and the dialysate return increase. Suction is *not* applied (2); return of the dialysate is achieved by gravity. Reducing the amount of the next exchange (3) is *not an independent nursing decision*. The use of even gentle pressure (4) may cause trauma to the bowel if the trocar is rigid. **IMP, APP, 8, PhI, Pharmacological and parenteral therapies**

8. (3) The prostate is examined annually during a rectal examination performed by a physician. The prostate is not examined while showering (1), and self-examination *is not possible*. Examination every 3 months (2) is *more often* than necessary. Examination every other year (4) after age 50 is *not often enough*. **IMP, COM, 8, HPM, Health promotion and maintenance**

9. (3) Acute renal failure is a reversible dysfunction of the kidneys; if the kidneys are not working, elimination of water, electrolytes and waste products is impaired and there would be a fluid excess. Skin problems (1) occur in *chronic* renal failure. As electrolytes (K^+, Na^+) accumulate, there would be more, *not* less, nutrition to meet body requirements (2). Anxiety (4) is *not* specific to acute renal failure but may be due to many other client circumstances. Changes in the client's psychological status are seen in *chronic* renal failure as the level of metabolic wastes increases in the serum. **AN, ANL, 8, SECE, Management of care**

10. (2) During the acute phase of renal failure the kidney cannot eliminate the nitrogenous waste products given off during protein metabolism, so protein intake is restricted to those proteins consisting of essential amino acids. A high calorie intake is necessary to prevent catabolism, and the source is carbohydrates, not protein. Options 1 and 3 are incorrect because the diet should be *low* in protein. Option 4 is incorrect because the diet should be *high* in calories. The diet may also be low in sodium and potassium. **PL, APP, 4, PhI, Basic care and comfort**

11. (2) Apples are acceptable as a snack for clients in acute renal failure because they are low in potassium, which is restricted in renal failure. All of the other fruits (1, 3, and 4) are high in potassium and therefore not acceptable. **IMP, COM, 4, PhI, Basic care and comfort**

12. (3) The peritoneal membrane acts as a semipermeable membrane. When the dialysate comes in contact with the peritoneal blood vessels, the waste substances in the blood are exchanged for the bicarbonate and acetate in the dialysate. In continuous ambulatory dialysis there is continuous exchange and better clearance of certain elements during the prolonged 4 to 8-hour dwell time. The concentration gradient between the serum and dialysate causes wastes to move *out of the serum, not* into the vascular space (1). In renal failure, the kidneys are *not* producing sufficient amounts of urine to eliminate waste (2) and to concentrate waste products. (4). **IMP, RE/KN, 8, PhI, Physiological adaptation**

13. (3) Low back pain may develop because of the added abdominal weight from the fluid which affects posture. Appropriate exercises may help relieve

Key to Codes

Nursing process: **AS**, assessment; **AN**, analysis; **PL**, planning; **IMP**, implementation; **EV**, evaluation. (See **Appendix M** for explanation of nursing process steps.)

Cognitive level: **RE/KN**, recall/knowledge; **COM**, comprehension; **APP**, application; **ANL**, analysis; **EVL**, evaluation; **SYN**, synthesis. (See **Appendix M** for explanation.)

Category of human function: 1, protective; 2, sensory-perceptual; 3, comfort, rest, activity, and mobility; 4, nutrition; 5, growth and development; 6, fluid-gas transport; 7, psychosocial-cultural; 8, elimination. (See **Appendix O** for explanation.)

Client need: **SECE**, safe, effective care environment; **PhI**, physiological integrity; **PsI**, psychosocial integrity; **HPM**, health promotion and maintenance. (See **Appendix P** for explanation.)

Client subneed: (See **Appendix P** for explanation)

the discomfort. Diarrhea (**1**) is a symptom of *bowel perforation*. Bloody effluent (**2**), although usually insignificant initially, may also be an indication of *bowel perforation*. Nausea (**4**) is a symptom of *peritonitis*. **IMP, COM, 8, PhI, Pharmacological and parenteral therapies**

14. (**3**) As the stone moves through the ureter, there is trauma to the ureter, with the result that the ureter becomes infected and blood appears in the urine. Ketonuria (**1**) and glycosuria (**2**) would occur in *diabetes*. Proteinuria (**4**) is a sign of *renal disease*. **AN, RE/KN, 8, PhI, Physiological adaptation**

15. (**2**) The contrast dye used for pyelography is an iodine-based agent, and severe, even fatal, allergic reactions can occur in a client allergic to iodine or seafood. Weight (**1**) is the best indicator of *fluid status*; it would be important to determine this *if* the client had hydronephrosis stemming from obstruction. It is important to know the status of the bowel (**3**), but the presence of stool would *not* be *life-threatening*; if the bowel were full of fecal matter, visualization of the kidneys would be partially or totally obscured. Cathartics, enemas, or suppositories are used to clear the bowel and ensure good visualization. Vital signs (**4**) are important, but the first action is to determine whether the client is at any risk for anaphylaxis. **IMP, ANL, 8, PhI, Reduction of risk potential**

16. (**2**) It is important to collect the stone so that its composition can be determined. Dietary changes can be made on the basis of the stone's composition to minimize the formation of more stones. Blood pressure changes (**1**) are *not* expected in clients with calculi unless the obstruction leads to renal failure. Fluid intake (**3**) is very important, and 3 to 4 liters per day may be needed to produce sufficient urine to flush out the stone; however, knowing the composition of the stone is *more* important clinically. Keeping track of the urine output (**4**) is also important, but collecting the stone is *more* important from the standpoint of long-term treatment. **IMP, ANL, 8, PhI, Physiological adaptation**

17. (**2**) Paralytic ileus is a frequent complication of ileal conduit construction. Resection of the bowel segment and general anesthesia inhibit peristalsis, causing bowel sounds to be absent. Mucus in the urine (**1**) is *normal*, because the urine irritates the bowel mucosa of the ileal pouch. A boardlike abdomen (**3**) would *not* be expected unless there was gastrointestinal tract bleeding. Diminished breath sounds (**4**) are a possible complication of general anesthesia and hypoventilation but are *not* directly related to the surgical procedure. **AS, ANL, 8, PhI, Physiological adaptation**

18. (**4**) Vitamin C supplements increase oxalate, not calcium, excretion. If calcium phosphate stones are present, protein intake *should* be restricted (**1**); otherwise a high protein diet promotes calcium excretion and stone formation. Fluid intake *should be* increased regardless of the type of stone (**2**). The client *should*, and will need to, void every 2 to 3 hours (**3**). An acid-ash diet is also indicated for clients with calcium stones. Such food includes meat, fish, poultry, grains, corn, cranberries, prunes, and plums. **EV, ANL, 8, SECE, Management of care**

19. (**2**) Infection in the kidney causes edema and swelling, and the symptom of this is flank pain. The pain often radiates down the ureter or toward the epigastric area, causing the abdominal pain. Burning (**1**) is a symptom of a *bladder* infection. Blood in the stool (**3**) would be seen in *hemorrhoids* or *colorectal* problems; a kidney infection would most likely cause blood to be excreted in the *urine*. Difficulty starting urine flow (**4**) is a characteristic problem associated with an enlarged *prostate*. **AS, COM, 6, PhI, Physiological adaptation**

20. (**1**) Before surgery a client is NPO; however, IV solutions administered during surgery should maintain hydration unless the client hemorrhages during surgery. If a catheter is not inserted during the surgery, the client should need to void within 6 to 8 hours. It is important to check for bladder distention. In addition, abdominal pain may affect the client's ability to relax the sphincter muscles. The amount of fluids administered IV is increased, *not* decreased (**2**), after surgery because PO intake is generally restricted. The bladder is palpable when it contains 250 mL of urine; if the client voids 800 to 1000 mL (**3**) initially there would have been bladder distention, which should be avoided. Retention of sodium and water is common, but, diuresis does not occur until 5 to 7 days after surgery, *not* the *day* of surgery (**4**). **AN, ANL, 1, SECE, Management of care**

Endocrine Disorders

Chapter Outline

- Syndrome of Inappropriate Antidiuretic Hormone
- Thyroid and Parathyroid Disorders
  - Hyperthyroidism (Thyrotoxicosis or Graves' disease)
  - Thyroid storm (crisis)
  - Thyroidectomy
  - Hypothyroidism (myxedema)
- Adrenal Disorders
  - Cushing's disease
  - Adrenalectomy
  - Addison's disease
- Diabetes—see Chap. 13

- Pheochromocytoma
- Summary of Key Points
- Study and Memory Aids
  - Diagnostic Studies/Procedures
    - [131] I Uptake
    - ACTH Test (8 h IV)
  - Diets
  - Drug review
- Questions
- Answers/Rationale

Syndrome of Inappropriate Antidiuretic Hormone (SIADH)

A condition characterized by overproduction or over-secretion of antidiuretic hormone (ADH).

I. **Pathophysiology:** abnormal production or sustained secretion of ADH resulting in fluid retention, serum hypoosmolality, hyponatremia, hypochloremia, concentrated urine with normal intravascular volume, normal renal function. Thought to be the most common cause of hyponatremia in older adults.

II. **Risk factors/causes:**
   A. Small cell carcinoma of the lung (most common cause).
   B. Pancreatic cancer.
   C. Lymphoid cancers.
   D. Head injury.
   E. Brain tumors.
   F. Infection (encephalitis, meningitis).
   G. Drug therapy with carbamazepine, chlorpropamide, opioids, oxytocin, thiazide diuretics, general anesthesia agents, tricyclic antidepressants, antineoplastic agents.
   H. Hypothyroidism.
   I. Lung infection (pneumonia, tuberculosis, lung abscess).
   J. COPD.
   K. Positive pressure mechanical ventilation.

III. **Assessment**
   A. *Subjective data:*
      1. Thirst.
      2. Dyspnea on exertion.
      3. Fatigue.
      4. Dull sensorium.
      5. As hyponatremia *worsens:*
         a. Abdominal cramps.
         b. Nausea & vomiting.
         c. Muscle cramping.
   B. *Objective data:*
      1. Decreased urinary output.
      2. Increased body weight.
      3. Lab data:
         a. Serum Na^+ < 134 mEq/L; serum osmolality < 280 mOsm/kg; urine specific gravity > 1.05; *decreased:* BUN, creatinine clearance, Hct, Hgb.
      4. As hyponatremia *worsens:*
         a. Decreased neurological function.
         b. Seizures.

IV. **Analysis/nursing diagnosis**
   A. *Fluid volume excess* related to abnormal production and secretion of ADH.
   B. *Thirst* related to fluid restriction.
   C. *Risk for injury* related to possible altered mental status secondary to hyponatremia.

V. **Nursing care plan/implementation**
   A. Goal: *restore fluid balance.*
      1. Restrict fluids to 800–1000 mL/day.
      2. *Position:* supine, with head of bed elevated no more than 10° (this increases venous return to the right side of the heart, increases left atrial filling pressure, which reduces release of ADH).
      3. Administer furosemide as ordered, if serum Na^+ is greater than 125 mEq/L.

B. Goal: *protect from injury*.
1. Put side-rails up.
2. Assist with ambulation.
3. Position close to nurse's station and visit room frequently.
4. Institute seizure precautions.
5. Frequent turning and repositioning.
C. Goal: **health teaching**.
1. For chronic SIADH, teach client to self-manage by restricting fluids to 800–1000 mL/day.
2. Suck on hard candy to relieve dry mouth and thirst.
3. Supplement diet with sodium and potassium.
4. Teach client signs and symptoms of Na⁺ and K⁺ imbalance.
5. Stress need for close follow-up care.

VI. **Evaluation/outcome criteria**
A. Fluid and electrolyte balance restored to normal range.
B. Client will manage therapeutic regimen to maintain fluid and electrolyte balance.

Thyroid and Parathyroid Disorders

Hyperthyroidism

Spectrum of symptoms of accelerated metabolism caused by excessive amounts of circulating thyroid hormone. (also called *thyrotoxicosis, Graves' disease*)

I. **Pathophysiology**: diffuse hyperplasia of thyroid gland → overproduction of thyroid hormone and increased blood serum levels. Hormone stimulates mitochondria to increase energy for cellular activities and heat production. As metabolic rate increases, fat reserves are utilized, despite increased appetite and food intake. Cardiac output is increased to meet increased tissue metabolic needs, and peripheral vasodilation occurs in response to increased heat production. Neuromuscular hyperactivity → accentuation of reflexes, anxiety, and increased alimentary tract mobility. *Graves' disease* is caused by stimulation of the gland by immunoglobulins of the G class.

II. **Risk factors/causes**:
A. Possible autoimmune response resulting in increase of a gamma globulin called *long-acting thyroid stimulator* (LATS).
B. Occurs in third and fourth decades.
C. Affects women more than men.
D. Emotional trauma, infection, increased stress.
E. Overdose of medications used to treat hypothyroidism.
F. Use of certain weight-loss products.

III. **Assessment**
A. *Subjective data*:
1. Nervousness, mood swings.
2. Palpitations.
3. Heat intolerance.
4. Dyspnea.
5. Weakness.
B. *Objective data*:
1. *Eyes*: exophthalmos, characteristic stare, lid lag.
2. *Skin*:
    a. Warm, moist, velvety.
    b. Increased sweating, melanin pigmentation.
    c. Pretibial edema with thickened skin and hyperpigmentation.
3. *Weight*: loss *despite* increased appetite.
4. *Muscle*: weakness, tremors, hyperkinesia.
5. *Vital signs*: blood pressure (BP)—*increased* systolic pressure, widened pulse pressure; tachycardia.
6. Goiter: thyroid gland noticeable and palpable.
7. GYN: abnormal menstruation.
8. GI: frequent bowel movements.
9. *Activity* pattern: overactivity leads to fatigue, which leads to depression, which stimulates client to overactivity, and pattern continues. *Danger*: total exhaustion.
10. Lab data:
    a. *Elevated*: serum thyroxine (T_4) (>11 mcg/dL); free T_4 or free T_4 index; triiodothyronine (T_3) level (>35%) and free T_3 level.
    b. *Elevated*: thyroid uptake of radioiodine (see **Diagnostic Studies** box).
    c. *Elevated*: basal metabolic rate (BMR).
    d. *Decreased*: white blood cell count (WBC) caused by *decreased* granulocytosis (<4500 mm³).

IV. **Analysis/nursing diagnosis**
A. *Altered nutrition, less than body requirements*, related to elevated BMR.
B. *Risk for injury* related to exophthalmos and tremors.
C. *Activity intolerance* related to fatigue from over-activity.
D. *Fatigue* related to overactivity.
E. *Anxiety* related to tachycardia.
F. *Sleep pattern disturbance* related to excessive amounts of circulating thyroid hormone.

V. **Nursing care plan/implementation**
A. Goal: *protect from stress*: private room, restrict visitors, quiet environment.
B. Goal: *promote physical and emotional equilibrium*.
1. Environment: quiet, cool, well ventilated.
2. Eye care:

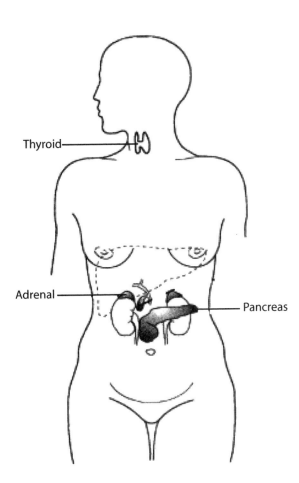

Endocrine Organs

a. Sunglasses to protect from photophobia, dust, wind.

b. Protective drops (methylcellulose) to soothe exposed cornea.

3. *Diet*:

a. *High*: calorie, protein, vitamin B.

b. 6 meals/d, as needed.

c. Weigh daily.

d. *Avoid* stimulants (coffee, tea, colas, tobacco).

C. Goal: *prevent complications.*

1. Medications as ordered:

a. Propylthiouracil to *block thyroid synthesis*; hyperthyroidism returns when therapy is stopped.

b. Methimazole (*Tapazole*) to inhibit synthesis of thyroid hormone.

c. Iodine preparations: used in combination with above medications when hyperthyroidism not well controlled; saturated solution of potassium iodide (*SSKI*) or *Lugol's* solution; more palatable if *diluted* with water, milk, or juice; give through a *straw* to prevent staining teeth. Takes 2–4 wk before results are evident.

d. Propranolol to *relieve tachycardia, tremors, and anxiety.*

2. Monitor for **thyroid storm** (*crisis*)—**medical emergency**: acute episode of thyroid overactivity caused when increased amounts of thyroid hormone are released into the bloodstream and metabolism is markedly increased.

a. **Risk factors/causes—*thyroid storm***: client with uncontrolled hyperthyroidism (usually *Graves' disease*) subjected to severe, sudden stress, such as:

(1) Infection.

(2) Surgery.

(3) Beginning of labor.

(4) Taking inadequate antithyroid medications before thyroidectomy.

b. **Assessment**

(1) *Subjective data*:

(a) Apprehension.

(b) Restlessness.

(2) *Objective data*:

(a) Vital signs: elevated temperature (106° F), hypotension, extreme tachycardia.

(b) Marked respiratory distress, pulmonary edema.

(c) Weakness and delirium.

(d) **If untreated, client could die of heart failure.**

c. Medications—*thyroid storm*:

(1) Propylthiouracil or methimazole (*Tapazole*) to decrease synthesis of thyroid hormone.

(2) Sodium iodide IV, *Lugol's* solution orally to *facilitate thyroid hormone synthesis.*

(3) Propranolol (*Inderal*) to *slow heart rate.*

(4) Aspirin to *decrease temperature.*

(5) *Steroids* to *combat crisis.*

(6) *Diuretics*, digitalis to *treat heart failure.*

D. Goal: **health teaching.**

1. Stress-reduction techniques.

2. Importance of medications, their desired and side effects.

3. Methods to protect eyes from environmental damage.

4. Signs and symptoms of thyroid storm (see above p. 231).

E. Goal: *prepare for additional treatment as needed.*

1. *Radioactive iodine therapy:* [131]I, a radioactive isotope of iodine to decrease thyroid activity.

a. [131]I dissolved in water and given by mouth.

b. Hospitalization necessary only when large dose is administered.

c. Minimal precautions needed for usual dose:

(1) Sleep alone for several nights.

(2) Flush toilet several times after use.

d. Effectiveness of therapy seen in 2–3 wk; single dose controls 90% of clients.

e. Monitor for signs of hypothyroidism.

2. Surgery: see **Thyroidectomy**, below.

VI. Evaluation/outcome criteria

A. Complications avoided.

B. Compliance with medical regimen.

C. No further weight loss.

D. Able to obtain adequate sleep.

Thyroidectomy

Partial removal of thyroid gland (for hyperthyroidism) or total removal (for malignancy of thyroid).

I. **Risk factor/causes**: unsuccessful medical treatment of hyperthyroidism.

II. **Analysis/nursing diagnosis**

A. *Risk for injury* related to possible trauma to parathyroid gland during surgery.

B. *Ineffective breathing pattern* related to neck incision.

C. *Pain* related to surgical incision.

D. *Altered nutrition, less than body requirements,* related to difficulty in swallowing because of neck incision.

E. *Impaired verbal communication* related to possible trauma to nerve during surgery.

F. *Risk for altered body temperature* related to thyroid storm.

III. **Nursing care plan/implementation:** *prepare for surgery* (see **Preoperative Preparation, p. 132-137**). *Postoperative Care:*

A. Goal: *promote physical and emotional equilibrium.*

1. *Position:* semi-Fowler's to reduce edema.

2. Immobilize head with pillows/sandbags.

3. Support head during position changes to prevent stress on sutures, flexion or hyperextension of neck.

B. Goal: *prevent complications of hypocalcemia and tetany*, due to accidental trauma to parathyroid gland during surgery; signs of tetany indicate need for *calcium gluconate IV*.

1. Check *Chvostek's sign*—tapping face in front of ear produces spasm of facial muscles.

2. Check *Trousseau's sign*—compression of upper arm (usually with BP cuff) elicits carpal (wrist) spasm.

3. Monitor for *respiratory distress* (due to laryngeal nerve injury, edema, bleeding); keep tracheostomy set/suction equipment at bedside.

4. Monitor for elevated temperature, indicative of *thyroid storm* (see objective assessment data for **thyroid storm, p. 231**).

5. Monitor vital signs, check dressing and beneath head, shoulders for bleeding q1h and prn for 24 h; *hemorrhage* is possible complication; if swallowing is difficult, loosen dressing. If client still complains of tightness when dressing is loosened, look for further signs of hemorrhage.

6. Check voice postoperatively as soon as client is responsive after anesthesia and every hour (assessing for possible *laryngeal nerve damage*); crowing voice sound indicates laryngeal nerves on both sides have been injured, making *respiratory distress possible due to swelling*.

a. *Avoid* unnecessary talking to lessen hoarseness.

b. Provide alternative means of communication.

C. Goal: *promote comfort measures.*

1. *Narcotics*, as ordered.

2. Offer *iced fluids*.

3. Ambulation and *soft diet*, as tolerated.

D. Goal: **health teaching.**

1. How to support neck to prevent pressure on suture line: place both hands behind neck when moving head or coughing.

2. Signs of hypothyroidism; needs supplemental thyroid hormone if total thyroidectomy.

3. Signs and symptoms of hemorrhage and respiratory distress.

4. Importance of adequate rest and nutritious diet.

5. Importance of voice rest in early recuperative period.

IV. **Evaluation/outcome criteria**

A. No respiratory distress, hemorrhage, laryngeal damage, tetany.

B. Preoperative symptoms relieved.

C. Normal range of neck motion obtained.

D. States signs and symptoms of possible complications.

Hypothyroidism (Myxedema)

Deficiency of circulating thyroid hormone; often a final consequence of *Hashimoto's thyroiditis* and *Graves' disease.*

I. **Pathophysiology:** atrophy, destruction of gland by endogenous antibodies or inadequate pituitary thyrotropin production → insidious slowing of body processes, personality changes, and generalized, interstitial non-pitting (mucinous) edema—myxedema; pronounced involvement in systems with high protein turnover (e.g., cardiac, gastrointestinal [GI], reproductive, hematopoietic).

II. **Risk factors/causes:**
   A. Total thyroidectomy, inadequate replacement therapy.
   B. Inheritance of autosomal recessive genes coding for disorder.
   C. Hypophyseal failure.
   D. Dietary iodine deficiencies.
   E. Irradiation of thyroid gland.
   F. Overtreatment of hyperthyroidism.

III. **Assessment**
   A. *Subjective data*:
      1. Weakness, fatigue, lethargy.
      2. Headache.
      3. Slowed memory, psychotic behavior.
      4. Loss of interest in sexual activity.
      5. Menstrual disturbances.
      6. Depression
   B. *Objective data*:
      1. Depressed BMR.
      2. Cardiomegaly, bradycardia, hypotension, anemia.
      3. Menorrhagia, amenorrhea, infertility.
      4. Dry skin, brittle nails, coarse hair, hair loss.
      5. Slowed speech, hoarseness, thickened tongue.
      6. Weight gain: edema, generalized interstitial; peripheral nonpitting; periorbital puffiness.
      7. Intolerance to cold.
      8. Hypersensitivity to narcotics and barbiturates.
      9. Radioactive iodine uptake test: *low* uptake (see **Diagnostic Studies** at end of chapter).
      10. Lab data:
         a. *Elevated*: thyroid releasing hormone (TRH), thyroid stimulating hormone (TSH), cholesterol (>200 mg/dL), lipids (>850 mg/dL), protein (>8 g/dL).
         b. Normal-low: serum thyroxine (T_4), serum triiodothyronine (T_3).
         c. *Decreased*: radioactive iodine uptake (RAIU) (see **Diagnostic Studies** box p. 237).

IV. **Analysis/nursing diagnosis**
   A. *Risk for injury* related to hypersensitivity to drugs.
   B. *Altered nutrition, more than body requirements*, related to decreased BMR.
   C. *Activity intolerance* related to fatigue.
   D. *Constipation* related to decreased peristalsis.
   E. *Decreased cardiac output* related to hypotension and bradycardia.
   F. *Risk for impaired skin integrity* related to dry skin and edema.
   G. *Social isolation* related to lethargy.
   H. *Hypothermia* related to cold intolerance.

V. **Nursing care plan/implementation**
   A. Goal: *provide for comfort and safety*.
      1. Monitor for infection or trauma; may precipitate **myxedema coma**, which is manifested by: unresponsiveness, bradycardia, hypoventilation, hypothermia, hypotension.
      2. Provide warmth, prevent heat loss and vascular collapse.
      3. Administer thyroid medications as ordered: levothyroxine (*Synthroid*)—most common drug used; liothyronine sodium (*Cytomel*); dosage adjusted according to symptoms.
   B. Goal: **health teaching.**
      1. *Diet*: *low* calorie, *high* protein.
      2. Signs and symptoms of hypothyroidism and hyperthyroidism.
      3. Life-long medications, dosage, desired and side effects.
      4. Medication dosage adjustment: take $^1/_3$-$^1/_2$ usual dose of narcotics and barbiturates.
      5. Stress-management techniques.
      6. Exercise program.

VI. **Evaluation/outcome criteria**
   A. No complications noted. Most common complications: atherosclerotic coronary heart disease, acute organic psychosis, and myxedema coma.
   B. Dietary instructions followed.
   C. Medication regimen followed.
   D. Thyroid hormone balance obtained and maintained.

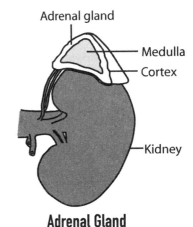

Adrenal Gland

Adrenal Disorders

Cushing's Disease

Overactivity of adrenal gland, leading to prolonged elevated plasma concentration of adrenal steroids.

I. **Pathophysiology**: excess glucocorticoid production, leading to:
   A. *Increased* gluconeogenesis → raised serum glucose levels → glucose in urine, increased fat deposits in face and trunk.

B. *Decreased* amino acids → protein deficiencies, muscle wasting, poor antibody response, lack of collagen.

II. Risk factors/causes:
   A. Adrenal hyperplasia.
   B. Excessive hypothalamic stimulation.
   C. Tumors: adrenal, hypophyseal, pituitary, bronchogenic, gallbladder.
   D. Excessive steroid therapy.

III. Assessment
   A. *Subjective data*:
      1. Headache, backache.
      2. Weakness, decreased work capacity.
      3. Mood swings.
   B. *Objective data*:
      1. Hypertension, weight gain, pitting edema.
      2. Characteristic supraclavicular fat deposits (*buffalo hump*).
      3. Pendulous abdomen, purple striae, easy bruising.
      4. Moon face, acne.
      5. Hirsutism: face, arms, legs.
      6. Hyperpigmentation.
      7. Menstrual changes.
      8. Impotence.
      9. Lab data:
         a. Urine: *elevated* 17-ketosteroids (>12 mg/24 h), glucose (>120 mg/dL).
         b. Plasma: *elevated* 17-hydroxycortico-steroids, cortisol (>10 mg/dL). Cortisol level does *not* decrease during the day as it *should*.
         c. Serum: *elevated*—glucose; red blood cells, WBC; *diminished*—potassium, chloride, eosinophils, lymphocytes.
      10. X-rays and scans to determine tumors/metastasis (see also 8 h IV ACTH test in **Diagnostic Studies** box).

IV. Analysis/nursing diagnosis
   A. *Body image disturbance* related to changes in physical appearance.
   B. *Activity intolerance* related to backache and weakness.
   C. *Risk for injury* related to infection and bleeding.
   D. *Knowledge deficit* related to management of disease.
   E. *Pain* related to headache.

V. Nursing care plan/implementation
   A. Goal: *promote comfort.*
      1. Assist with preparation for diagnostic workup.
      2. Explain procedures.
      3. Protect from trauma.
   B. Goal: *prevent complications*; monitor for:
      1. Fluid balance—intake and output (I&O), daily weights.

   2. Glucose metabolism—blood, urine for sugar and acetone.
   3. Hypertension—vital signs.
   4. Infection—skin, urinary tract; check temperature.
   5. Mood swings—observe behavior.
   C. Goal: **health teaching.**
      1. *Diet: increased* protein, potassium; *decreased* calories, sodium.
      2. Medications:
         a. *Cytotoxic* agents: aminoglutethimide (*Cytadren*), trilostane (*Modrastane*), mitotane (*Lysodren*)—decrease cortisol production.
         b. *Replacement hormones* as needed.
      3. Signs and symptoms of increased disease as noted in assessment.
      4. Preparation for adrenalectomy if medical regimen unsuccessful.

VI. Evaluation/outcome criteria
   A. Symptoms controlled by medication.
   B. No complications—adrenal steroids within normal limits.
   C. If adrenalectomy necessary, see following section.

Adrenalectomy

Surgical removal of adrenal glands due to tumors or uncontrolled overactivity; also, bilateral adrenalectomy may be performed to control metastatic breast or prostate cancer.

I. Risk factors/causes:
   A. Pheochromocytoma.
   B. Adrenal hyperplasia.
   C. Cushing's syndrome.
   D. Metastasis of prostate or breast cancer.
   E. Adrenal cortex or medulla tumors.

II. Assessment
   A. *Objective data*: validated evidence of:
      1. Benign lesion (unilateral adrenalectomy) or malignant tumor (bilateral adrenalectomy).
      2. Adrenal hyperfunction that cannot be managed medically.
      3. Metastasis of breast cancer.
      4. Metastasis of prostate carcinoma.

III. Analysis/nursing diagnosis
   A. *Knowledge deficit* related to planned surgery.
   B. *Risk for physical injury* related to hormone imbalance.
   C. *Risk for decreased cardiac output* related to possible hypotensive state resulting from surgery.
   D. *Risk for infection* related to decreased normal resistance.
   E. *Altered health maintenance* related to need for self-administration of steroid medications, orally or by injection.

IV. Nursing care plan/implementation

A. Goal: **preoperative**: *reduce risk of postoperative complications.*

1. Prescribed *steroid* therapy, given 1 wk before surgery, is gradually decreased; will be given again postoperatively.

2. *Antihypertensive* drugs are discontinued, as surgery may result in severe hypotension.

3. *Sedation* as ordered.

4. General preoperative measures (see **p. 127-128**).

B. Goal: **postoperative**: *promote hormonal balance.*

1. Administer hydrocortisone parenteral therapy, as ordered; rate determined by fluid and electrolyte balance, blood sugar level, and blood pressure.

2. Monitor for signs of adrenal crisis (see **p. 235-236**).

C. Goal: *prevent postoperative complications.*

1. Monitor vital signs until stability is regained; if on *vasopressor* drugs such as metaraminol (*Aramine*):

   a. Maintain flow rate as ordered.

   b. Monitor BP q5–15min; notify physician of significant elevations in BP (dose needs to be *decreased*) or drop in BP (dose needs to be *increased*). Note: readings that are normotensive for some may be hypotensive for clients who have been hypertensive.

2. NPO—attach nasogastric (*NG*) tube to intermittent suction; abdominal distention is common side effect of this surgery.

3. Respiratory care:

   a. Turn, cough, deep breathe.

   b. Splint flank incision when coughing.

   c. Administer *narcotics* to reduce pain and allow client to cough; flank incision is close to diaphragm, making coughing very painful.

   d. Auscultate breath sounds q2h; decreased or absent sounds could indicate *pneumothorax.*

   e. Sudden chest pain and dyspnea should be reported **immediately**, as spontaneous pneumothorax can occur.

4. *Position*: flat or semi-Fowler's.

5. Mouth care.

6. Monitor dressings for bleeding; reinforce prn.

7. Ambulation, as ordered.

   a. Check BP q15min when ambulation is first attempted.

   b. Place elastic stockings on lower extremities to enhance stability of vascular system.

8. Diet—as tolerated, once NG tube removed.

D. Goal: **health teaching.**

1. *Signs and symptoms of* **adrenal crisis**:
   a. Pulse: rapid, weak, or thready.
   b. Temperature: elevated.
   c. Severe weakness and hypotension.
   d. Headache.
   e. Convulsions, coma.

2. Importance of adhering to *steroid* therapy schedule to ensure therapeutic serum level.

3. Weigh daily.

4. Monitor blood glucose levels daily.

5. Report undesirable side effects of steroid therapy or adrenal crisis to physician.

6. *Avoid* persons with infections, due to decreased resistance.

7. Daily schedule: include adequate rest, moderate exercise, good nutrition.

V. Evaluation/outcome criteria

A. Adrenal crisis avoided.
1. Vital signs within normal limits.
2. No neurologic deficits noted.

B. Healing progresses: no signs of infection or wound complications.

C. Adjusts to alterations in physical status.
1. Complies with medication regimen.
2. Avoids infections.
3. Incorporates good nutrition, periods of rest and activity into daily schedule.

Addison's Disease

Chronic primary adrenocorticotropic hormone (ACTH) insufficiency.

I. Pathophysiology:

A. Atrophy of adrenal gland is most common cause of adrenal insufficiency; manifested by *decreased* adrenocortical secretions.

1. Deficiency in mineralocorticoid secretion (*aldosterone*) → increased sodium excretion → dehydration → hypotension → decreased cardiac output and resulting decrease in heart size.

2. Deficiency in glucocorticoid secretion (*cortisol*) → decrease in gluconeogenesis → hypoglycemia and liver glycogen deficiency, emotional disturbances, diminished resistance to stress. Cortisol deficiency → failure to inhibit anterior pituitary secretion of ACTH and melanocyte-stimulating hormone → increased levels of ACTH and hyperpigmentation.

3. Deficiency in androgen hormone → less axillary and pubic hair in women (testes supply adequate sex hormone in men, so no symptoms are produced).

II. Risk factors/causes:

A. Autoimmune processes.

B. Infection.

C. Malignancy.
D. Vascular obstruction.
E. Bleeding.
F. Environmental hazards.
G. Congenital defects.
H. Bilateral adrenalectomy.

III. Assessment

A. *Subjective data*:
1. Muscle weakness, fatigue, lethargy.
2. Dizziness, fainting.
3. Nausea, food idiosyncrasies, anorexia.
4. Abdominal pain, cramps.

B. *Objective data*:
1. *Vital signs*: decreased BP, orthostatic hypotension, widened pulse pressure.
2. *Pulse*: increased, collapsing, irregular.
3. *Temperature*: subnormal.
4. *GI*: vomiting, diarrhea.
5. Tremors.
6. *Skin*: poor turgor, excessive pigmentation (bronze tone).
7. Lab data:
   a. Blood
      (1) *Decreased*: sodium (<135 mEq/L); glucose (<60 mg/dL); chloride (<98 mEq/ L), bicarbonate (<23 mEq/L).
      (2) *Increased*: hematocrit, potassium (>5 mEq/L).
   b. Urine: *decreased* (or absent) 17-ketosteroids (<5 mg/24 h), 17-hydroxycorticosteroids (<2 mg/24 h).
8. See also **Diagnostic Studies** box, **p. 237.**

IV. Analysis/nursing diagnosis

A. *Fluid volume deficit* related to decreased sodium level.
B. *Altered renal tissue perfusion* related to hypotension.
C. *Decreased cardiac output* related to aldosterone deficiency.
D. *Risk for infection* related to cortisol deficiency.
E. *Activity intolerance* related to muscle weakness and fatigue.
F. *Altered nutrition, less than body requirements,* related to nausea, anorexia, and vomiting.

V. Nursing care plan/implementation

A. Goal: *decrease stress.*
1. Environment: quiet, nondemanding schedule.
2. Anticipate events where extra resources will be necessary.
B. Goal: *promote adequate nutrition.*
1. *Diet: acute phase—high* sodium, *low* potassium; *nonacute phase—increased* carbohydrates and protein.
2. *Fluids*: force, to balance fluid losses; monitor I&O, daily weights.

3. Administer life-long exogenous replacement therapy as ordered.
   a. *Glucocorticoids—*prednisone, hydrocortisone.
   b. *Mineralocorticoids—*fludrocortisone (*Florinef*).
C. Goal: *prevent serious complications if Addisonian crisis evident.*
1. Complete bed rest, *avoid* stimuli.
2. High dose of *hydrocortisone IV* or *cortisone* IM.
3. Treat shock—IV saline.
4. I&O, vital signs q15min to 1 h or prn until crisis passes.
D. Goal: **health teaching.**
1. Take medications *with* food or milk.
2. May need *antacid* therapy to prevent GI disturbances.
3. Side effects of steroid therapy.
4. *Avoid* stress; may need adjustment in medication dosage when stress is increased.
5. Signs and symptoms of *adrenal (Addisonian) crisis*: very serious condition characterized by: severe hypotension, shock, coma, and vasomotor collapse related to strenuous activity, infection, stress, omission of prescribed medications. **If untreated, could quickly lead to death.**

VI. Evaluation/outcome criteria

A. No complications occur.
B. Medication regimen followed, is adequate for client's needs.
C. Adequate nutrition and fluid balance obtained.

Pheochromocytoma

Rare tumor of the adrenal medulla.

I. **Pathophysiology**:
A. Tumor of adrenal medulla stimulates excessive production of catecholamines (epinephrine, norepinephrine), which causes severe hypertension.
1. Tumor usually benign and encapsulated.
2. Can be fatal if not diagnosed and treated.

II. **Risk factor/causes:** pheochromocytoma is a rare condition found most often in young to middle-aged adults of either gender.

III. **Assessment**
A. *Subjective data*:
1. Complaint of severe, pounding headache.
2. Anxiety and palpitations.
B. *Objective data*:
1. Episodic, severe hypertension.
2. Tachycardia.
3. Profuse sweating.

IV. **Analysis/nursing diagnosis**
  A. *Anxiety* related to effects of tumor, lack of knowledge about condition, and/or impending surgery.
  B. *Knowledge deficit* related to condition and surgical intervention.
  C. *Ineffective tissue perfusion* related to effects of hypertension.

V. **Nursing care plan/implementation**
  A. Goal: *control hypertension preoperatively.*
    1. Monitor vital signs closely.
    2. Administer *antihypertensive* meds as ordered.
  B. Goal: *reduce stress.*
    1. Provide quiet, calm environment.
  C. Goal: **health teaching.**
    1. Expectations before, during, and after surgery.
    2. See **Chapter 9**: Perioperative Nursing, for general care of the surgical client.

VI. **Evaluation/outcome criteria**
  A. Maintain blood pressure within normal range. Client will take antihypertensive medications if necessary.
  B. No complications from surgery.

Diagnostic Studies/Procedures

Radioactive Iodine Uptake Test (^{131}I Uptake)—ingestion of a tracer dose of ^{131}I, followed in 24 h by a scan of the thyroid for amount of radioactivity emitted.

1. *High* uptake indicates hyperthyroidism.
2. *Low* uptake indicates hypothyroidism.

Eight-hour Intravenous ACTH Test—administration of 25 U of ACTH in 500 mL of saline over an 8h period.

1. *Used to* determine function of adrenal cortex.
2. 24-h urine specimens are collected, before and after administration, for measurement of 17-ketosteroids and 17-hydroxycorticosteroids.
3. In *Addison's disease*, urinary output of steroids does *not increase* after administration of ACTH; *normally* steroid excretion *increases three-to five-fold* after ACTH stimulation.
4. In *Cushing's syndrome*, hyperactivity of the adrenal cortex *increases* the urine output of steroids tenfold in the second urine specimen.

Summary of Key Points

1. In hyperthyroidism the body responses and systems are *accelerated*, resulting in: tachycardia, agitation, muscle tremors, diarrhea, and fever. In hypothyroidism the same responses and systems are *depressed*, resulting in: bradycardia, sluggishness, and sensitivity to cold.
2. Drug doses may need to be *increased* in hyperthyroidism and *reduced* in hypothyroidism.
3. After complete or partial removal of the thyroid gland, observing for *airway obstruction* is a priority.
4. Note signs of *tetany* (*carpopedal spasm*), indicating injury to or accidental removal of the parathyroid glands.
5. Cushing's disease involves an *excess* of sugar (increased glucose), salt (increased sodium), and sex hormones (increased androgens). These changes adversely affect body image, with weight gain and abnormal hair distribution as a result.
6. The signs and symptoms of Cushing's disease are the *same* regardless of whether it is caused by *hyperadrenalism* or *steroid therapy*.
7. The greatest concern in a client with Addison's disease is the occurrence of a *crisis*, causing severe *hypovolemic shock* and *vascular collapse*.

Study and Memory Aids

Cushing's Syndrome: Signs—"3 S's"

Salt (hypernatremia)
Sex (excess androgens)
Sugar (hyperglycemia)

Diets

Addison's Disease

Acute: ↓ Potassium
       ↑ Sodium
Non acute: ↑ Carbohydrate
           ↑ Protein

Cushing's Syndrome

| ↑ Potassium | Calories |
| ↑ Protein | ↓ Sodium |

Hyperthyroidism

↑ Calorie
Protein
Vitamin B

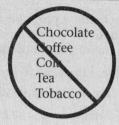

Chocolate
Coffee
Cola
Tea
Tobacco

⊂▬ Drug Review

Hyperthyroidism

Methimazole (*Tapazole*): 15–60 mg/d for 6–8 wk; maintenance dose, 15–30 mg/d in single or divided doses

Potassium iodide (SSKI): 250 mg (5 drops) tid. **Mix with fruit juice.** Used for 10 d before thyroidectomy.

Propylthiouracil: 50–600 mg/d in single or divided doses

Strong iodine solution (*Lugol's* solution): 0.1–0.3 mL tid. Used for 10 d before thyroidectomy.

Thyroid Storm Crisis

Antiarrhythmics
   Digoxin (*Lanoxin*): IV 0.6–1 mg in divided doses over 24 h; maintenance dose; rapid loading dose, 150 mcg/d.
   Propranolol (*Inderal*): IV 1–3 mg; repeat in 2 min if needed
Antipyretic
   Aspirin: 325–1000 mg q4–6h, *not* to exceed 4 g/d
Antithyroids
   Methimazole (*Tapazole*): 15–60 mg/d for 6–8 wk; maintenance dose, 15–30 mg/d in single or divided doses
   Propylthiouracil: 50–600 mg/d in single or divided doses
   Strong iodine solution (*Lugol's* solution): 0.1–0.3 mL tid. Used for 10 d before thyroidectomy
Diuretics
   Furosemide (*Lasix*): 20–80 mg/d
   Mannitol (*Osmitrol*): IV 50–100 g as 5%–25% solution
Steroids (should **never** be abruptly discontinued; gradually taper dose to prevent complications)
   Dexamethasone (*Decadron*): 0.5–9 mg/d in single or divided doses
   Methylprednisolone (*Medrol*): 4–48 mg/d
   Prednisone: 5–60 mg/d

Thyroidectomy

Potassium iodide (SSKI): 250 mg (5 drops) tid. **Mix with fruit juice.** Used for 10 d before thyroidectomy.

Strong iodine solution (*Lugol's* solution): 0.1–0.3 mL tid. Used for 10 d before thyroidectomy

Hypothyroidism

Levothyroxine (*Synthroid*): 0.05 mg/d; increase by 0.025 mg q 2–3 weeks; maintenance dose, 0.1–0.2 mg/d

Liothyronine (*Cytomel*): 25 mcg/d; increase by 12.5–25 mcg/d at 1 to 2-wk intervals; usual maintenance dose, 25–50 mcg/d

Cushing's Disease

Aminoglutethimide (*Cytadren*): 250 mg q6h increased by 250 mg/d at 1- to 2-wk intervals up to daily total of 2 g

Mitotane (o, p'-DDD, *Lysodren*): 3–6 g/d in 3–4 divided doses, decreased to maintenance dose of 500 mg twice/wk (half-life, 18–159 d)

Adrenalectomy

Steroids (should **never** be abruptly discontinued; gradually taper dose to prevent complications)
   Dexamethasone (*Decadron*): 0.5–9 mg/d in single or divided doses
   Hydrocortisone (*Solu-Cortef*): 10–320 mg/d in divided doses; succinate—IM or IV, 100–500 mg q2–6 h
   Methylprednisolone (*Medrol*): 4–48 mg/d
   Prednisone: 5–60 mg/d
Tranquilizers
   Chlordiazepoxide HCl (*Librium*): 5–25 mg 3–4 times/d
   Diazepam (*Valium*): 2–10 mg 2–4 times/d
   Phenobarbital: 30–120 mg/d in divided doses

Addison's Disease

Antiulcers
   Aluminum hydroxide gel (*Amphojel*): 5–10 mL q2–4h or 1 h pc
   Calcium carbonate (*Titralac*): 1–2 g with water pc and hs
   Magnesium and aluminum hydroxides (*Maalox* suspension): 5–30 mL pc and hs
   Sucralfate (*Carafate*): 1 g qid
Glucocorticoids
Short acting
   Cortisone (*Cortone*): 20–300 mg/d
   Hydrocortisone (*Solu-Cortef*): 10–320 mg/d in divided doses; succinate—IM or IV, 100–500 mg q2–6h
Intermediate acting
   Methylprednisolone (*Medrol*): 4–48 mg/d in single or divided doses
   Prednisolone (*Deltasone*): 5–60 mg in single or divided doses
Long acting
   Betamethasone (*Valisone*): 0.6–7.2 mg/d
   Dexamethasone (*Decadron*): 0.5–9 mg/d in single or divided doses
Mineralocorticoids: Fludrocortisone (*Florinef*): 100 mcg/d (range, 100 mcg 3 times/wk to 200 mcg/d)
Note: **Steroids** should **never** be abruptly discontinued; gradually taper dose to prevent complications.

Questions

1. The nurse would counsel a client taking cortisone to observe a diet:
   1. High in protein, calcium, and potassium. *low carbs*
   2. High in carbohydrates and low in sodium. *low sodium*
   3. Low in sodium, calcium, and carbohydrates.
   4. Low in protein, potassium, and sodium.

2. What are signs and symptoms of hyperthyroidism?
   1. Nervousness and weight loss.
   2. Lethargy and slow pulse.
   3. Weight gain and diaphoresis.
   4. Slow pulse and increased appetite.

3. The nurse tells a client that the most appropriate diet to follow the week before surgery to remove a suspected thyroid tumor is one that is:
   1. Increased in carbohydrates and protein.
   2. Decreased in carbohydrates and increased in protein.
   3. Decreased in fat and protein.
   4. Increased in fat and decreased in protein.

4. To assess for laryngeal nerve damage after a thyroidectomy, the nurse would observe the client for:
   1. Dyspnea, intercostal muscle retraction, and stridor.
   2. Difficulty swallowing, deviated uvula, and hoarseness.
   3. Stridor, difficulty swallowing, and cough.
   4. Dysphagia, weakened voice, and wheezing.

Answers/Rationale

1. **(1)** Corticosteroids, such as cortisone, have a catabolic effect on protein, resulting in a negative nitrogen balance, so protein is needed to compensate for this loss. Aldosterone secretion is also stimulated, leading to sodium retention and potassium loss, and thus making added potassium intake important. Cortisone also decreases the intestinal transport of calcium and promotes calcium loss through the kidneys, and so extra calcium is needed in the diet to make up for the loss. The diet should be *low* in carbohydrates (2). As already noted, calcium (3) as well as protein and potassium (4) intake should be *increased*. The sodium intake, however, should be *decreased* to compensate for the sodium retained. **PL, APP, 4, PhI, Basic care and comfort**

2. **(1)** Hyperthyroidism, or Graves' disease, results from an overproduction of thyroid-stimulating hormone. This causes the metabolic rate of the client to be accelerated, leading to: agitation, weight loss, heat intolerance, tachycardia, exophthalmos, goiter, diaphoresis, increased appetite, and diarrhea. Lethargy (2) and slow pulse (2 and 4) would be seen in *hypothyroidism*. Weight gain (3) is also a symptom of *hypothyroidism*. **AS, RE/KN, 3, PhI, Physiological adaptation**

3. **(1)** Because of the increased metabolism in such a client, the caloric and protein intake would need to be high to prevent catabolism (a negative nitrogen balance) before surgery. The carbohydrate (2) and protein (3 and 4) intake should both be *increased*. **PL, APP, 4, PhI, Basic care and comfort**

4. **(4)** Thyroidectomy is the most common cause of laryngeal nerve damage because of the proximity of the gland and the nerve. The primary symptom is hoarseness or a weakened voice. There may also be temporary dysphagia, or difficulty swallowing, and if both vocal cords are involved, there would be airway compromise (wheezing). The problems listed in option 1 may occur if the person is active but would *not* be seen in the *early* postoperative period. A deviated uvula (2) would be seen in a client with *glossopharyngeal* nerve damage. A cough (3) is *not* characteristic. **AS, COM, 3, PhI, Reduction of risk potential**

Key to Codes

Nursing process: AS, assessment; AN, analysis; PL, planning; IMP, implementation; EV, evaluation. (See **Appendix M** for explanation of nursing process steps.)

Cognitive level: RE/KN, recall/knowledge; COM, comprehension; APP, application; ANL, analysis; EVL, evaluation; SYN, synthesis. (See **Appendix M** for explanation.)

Category of human function: 1, protective; 2, sensory-perceptual; 3, comfort, rest, activity, and mobility; 4, nutrition; 5, growth and development; 6, fluid-gas transport; 7, psychosocial-cultural; 8, elimination. (See **Appendix 0** for explanation.)

Client need: SECE, safe, effective care environment; PhI, physiological integrity; PsI, psychosocial integrity; HPM, health promotion and maintenance. (See **Appendix P** for explanation.)

Client subneed: (See **Appendix P** for explanation)

Sensory Disorders

19

Chapter Outline

Ear Disorders

Meniere's Disease

Chronic, recurrent disorder of inner ear; attacks of vertigo, tinnitus, and vestibular dysfunction; lasts 30 min to full day; usually no pain or loss of consciousness.

I. **Pathophysiology**: associated with excessive dilatation of cochlear duct (unilateral) resulting from overproduction or decreased absorption of endolymph → progressive sensorineural hearing loss.

II. **Risk factors/causes:**
   A. Emotional or endocrine disturbance (diabetes mellitus).
   B. Spasms of internal auditory artery.
   C. Head trauma.
   D. Allergic reaction.
   E. High salt intake.
   F. Smoking.
   G. Ear infections.

III. **Assessment**
   A. *Subjective data*:
      1. Tinnitus.
      2. Headache.
      3. True vertigo: sudden attacks, room appears to spin.
      4. Depression, irritability, withdrawal.
      5. Nausea with sudden head motion.
   B. *Objective data*:
      1. Impaired hearing, especially *low* tones.
      2. Change in gait, lack of coordination.
      3. Vomiting with sudden head motion.
      4. Nystagmus—during attacks.

   5. *Diagnostic test*: *caloric* (cold water in ear canal)—may precipitate attack; audiometry—loss of hearing (See **Diagnostic Studies** box).

IV. **Analysis/nursing diagnosis**
   A. *Risk for injury* related to vertigo, lack of coordination.
   B. *Auditory sensory/perceptual alteration* related to progressive hearing loss.
   C. *Anxiety* related to uncertainty about treatment.
   D. *Risk for activity intolerance* related to sudden onset of vertigo.
   E. *Sleep pattern disturbance* related to tinnitus.
   F. *Ineffective individual coping* related to chronic disorder.

V. **Nursing care plan/implementation**
   A. Goal: *provide safety and comfort during attacks.*
      1. Activity: *bed rest* during attack, siderails up; lower to chair or floor if attack occurs while standing; assist with ambulation (sudden dizziness common).
      2. *Position*: recumbent, affected ear uppermost usually.
      3. Identify prodromal symptoms (aura, ear pressure, increased tinnitus).
      4. Call bell within reach.
   B. Goal: *minimize occurrence of attacks.*
      1. Give medications as ordered:
         a. *Diuretics* (chlorothiazide [*Diuril*], acetazolamide [*Diamox*]) to decrease endolymphatic fluids.
         b. *Antihistamines* (dimenhydrinate [*Dramamine*], diphenhydramine HCl [*Benadryl*]) to inhibit tissue edema.
         c. *Vasodilators* (nicotinic acid) to control vasospasms.

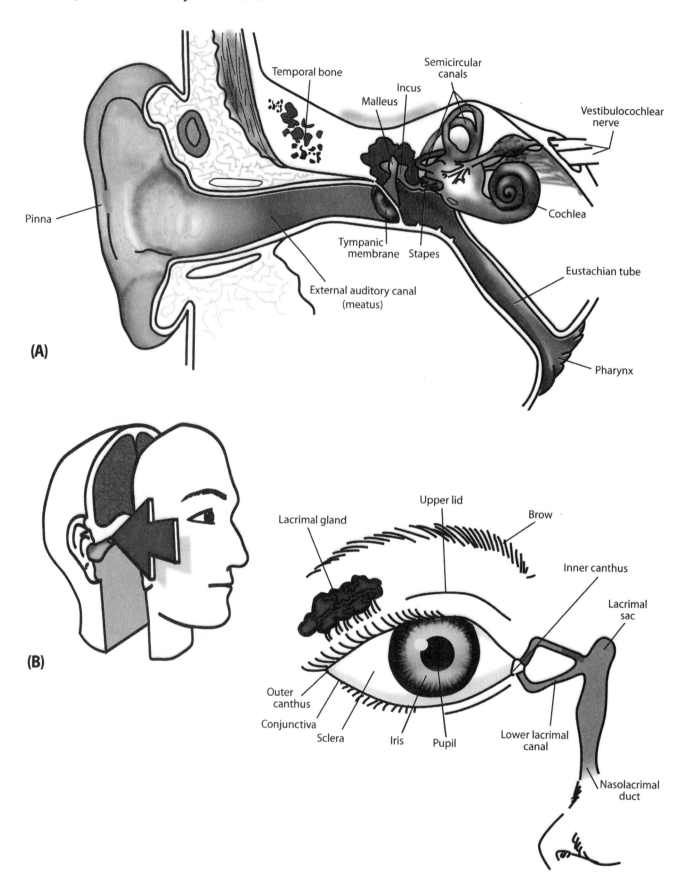

(A) THE EAR, SHOWING THE EXTERNAL, MIDDLE, AND INTERNAL SUBDIVISIONS.

(B) STRUCTURES OF THE EXTERNAL EYE AND POSITION OF THE INTERNAL LACRIMAL STRUCTURES.

d. *Antiemetics and antivertigo agents*
(diazepam [*Valium*], meclizine HCl
[*Antivert*]).

2. *Diet*: *low* sodium; *limited* fluids to reduce
endolymphatic pressure.

3. *Avoid* precipitating stimuli: bright, glaring
lights; noise; sudden jarring; turning head
or eyes (stand in front of client when
talking).

C. Goal: **health teaching.**

1. No smoking (causes vasospasm) or alcoholic
beverages (fluid retention, contraindicated
with medications).

2. Management of symptoms: play radio to
mask tinnitus, particularly at night.

3. Keep medication available at all times.

4. Prepare for surgery if indicated
(*labyrinthectomy* if hearing is gone or
endolymphatic sac decompression to preserve
hearing).

VI. **Evaluation/outcome criteria**

A. Decreased frequency of attacks.

B. Complies with treatment regimen and
restrictions (e.g., low sodium diet, no smoking).

C. Hearing preserved.

Otosclerosis

Insidious, progressive deafness; most common cause of
conductive deafness; cause unknown.

I. **Pathophysiology**: formation of new spongy bone
in labyrinth → fixation of stapes → prevention of
sound transmission through ossicles to inner ear
fluids.

II. **Risk factors:**

A. Heredity.

B. Women, puberty to 45 yr.

III. **Assessment**

A. *Subjective data*:

1. Tinnitus.

2. Difficulty hearing—gradual loss in both
ears.

B. *Objective data*: *diagnostic tests*.

1. *Rinne* (tuning fork placed over mastoid
bone)—reduced sound conduction by air
and intensified by bone.

2. *Weber* (tuning fork placed on top of head)—
increased sound conduction to affected ear.

3. *Audiometry*—diminished hearing.

IV. **Analysis/nursing diagnosis**

A. *Auditory sensory/perceptual alteration* related to
hearing loss.

B. *Body image disturbance* related to hearing aid.

C. *Ineffective individual coping* related to grief
reaction to loss.

D. *Impaired social interaction* related to hearing loss.

V. **Nursing care plan/implementation, evaluation/
outcome criteria**: see **Stapedectomy**, following.

Stapedectomy

Removal of the stapes and replacement with a prosthesis
(steel wire, Teflon piston, or polyethylene); treatment
for deafness due to otosclerosis, which fixes the stapes,
preventing it from oscillating and transmitting vibrations
to the fluids in the inner ear.

I. **Analysis /nursing diagnosis**

A. *Sensory/perceptual alteration* related to edema and
ear packing.

B. See **Perioperative Experience, p. 127**, for
diagnoses relating to surgery.

II. **Nursing care plan/implementation**

A. **Preoperative care: health teaching.**

1. Important postoperatively to keep head in
position ordered by physician.

2. *Avoid*: sneezing, blowing nose, vomiting,
coughing—all of which increase pressure in
eustachian tubes.

3. Breathing exercises.

B. **Postoperative care:**

1. Goal: *promote physical and psychological
equilibrium.*

a. *Position*: as ordered by physician—varies
according to preference; side-rails up, as
vertigo is common.

b. Activity: assist with ambulation; *avoid*
rapid turning, which might increase
vertigo.

c. Dressings: check frequently; may
change cotton pledget in outer ear.

d. Give medications as ordered:

(1) *Antiemetics*.

(2) *Analgesics*.

(3) *Antibiotics*.

e. Reassurance: reduction in hearing is
normal, hearing may *not* immediately
improve after surgery.

2. Goal: **health teaching.**

a. Ear care: keep covered outdoors; keep
outer ear plug clean, dry, and changed.

b. *Avoid*:

(1) Washing hair for 2 wk.

(2) Swimming for 6 wk.

(3) Air travel for 6 mo.

(4) People with upper respiratory tract
infections.

(5) Heavy lifting or straining.

III. **Evaluation/outcome criteria**

A. Hearing improves—evaluate 1 mo
postoperatively (may require hearing aid).

B. Returns to work (usually 2 wk after surgery).

C. Continues medical supervision.

Deafness

Hard of hearing—slight or moderate hearing loss that is serviceable for performing activities of daily living. *Deaf*—hearing is nonfunctional for carrying out activities of daily living.

I. **Risk factors/causes:**

    A. *Conductive* hearing losses (transmission deafness):

        1. Impacted cerumen (wax).

        2. Foreign body in external auditory canal.

        3. Defects (thickening, scarring) of eardrum.

        4. Otosclerosis of ossicles.

    B. *Sensorineural* hearing losses (perceptive or nerve deafness):

        1. Arteriosclerosis.

        2. Infectious diseases (mumps, measles, meningitis).

        3. Drug toxicities (quinine, streptomycin, neomycin sulfate).

        4. Tumors.

        5. Head trauma.

        6. High-intensity noises.

II. **Assessment**—*objective data:*

    A. Inattentive or strained facial expression.

    B. Excessive loudness or softness of speech.

    C. Frequent need to clarify content of conversation or inappropriate responses.

    D. Tilting of head while listening.

    E. Lack of response when others speak.

III. **Analysis/nursing diagnosis**

    A. *Auditory sensory/perceptual alteration* related to loss of hearing.

    B. *Impaired social interaction* related to deafness.

IV. **Nursing care plan/implementation**

    A. Goal: *maximize hearing ability and provide emotional support.*

        1. Gain person's attention before speaking, *avoid* startling.

        2. Provide adequate lighting so person can see you when you are speaking.

        3. Look at the person when speaking.

        4. Use nonverbal cues to enhance communication, e.g., writing, hand gestures, pointing.

        5. Speak slowly, distinctly; do *not* shout (excessive loudness distorts voice).

        6. If person does not understand, use different words; write it down.

        7. Use alternative communication system:

           a. Speech (lip) reading.

           b. Sign language.

           c. Hearing aid.

           d. Paper and pencil.

           e. Flash cards.

         8. Supportive, nonstressful environment.

    B. Goal: **health teaching.**

TABLE 19.1 ☞ CARE OF HEARING AID

Clean earmold as often as needed. Warm water and mild soap may be used, or wipe nightly with alcohol. Use a pipe cleaner to remove wax. Dry earmold completely before connecting to hearing aid.

Keep the hearing aid dry. Do *not* wear in the shower or at the hairdresser. Aid may not work as well in hot, humid climate because of moisture in ear or hearing aid.

Turn hearing aid off at night or when not in use. Keep spare batteries. Batteries may be removed completely at night.

Store away from pets. Dogs and cats like the smell of ear wax and will chew or roll on hearing aid.

Leave the aid in the same place every night.

If the aid does not work: check on-off switch, inspect for wax, examine battery for correct insertion, replace batteries (may only last a few days or a few weeks), check for correct placement of earmold.

        1. Prepare for evaluative studies—audiogram.

        2. Appropriate community resources: National Association of Hearing and Speech Agencies for *counseling* services; National Association for the Deaf to assist with *employment, education, legislation*; Alexander Graham Bell Association for the Deaf, Inc., serves as *information* center for those working with the deaf; American Hearing Society provides educational information, employment services, *social clubs.*

        3. Use of hearing aid: care, testing, carry spare battery at all times. (See **Table 19.1** for care of hearing aid.)

        4. Safety precautions: when crossing street, driving.

V. **Evaluation/outcome criteria**

    A. Method of communication established.

    B. Achieves independence (use of Dogs for Deaf, special telephones, visual signals).

    C. Copes with life-style changes (minimal depression, anger, hostility).

Eye Disorders

Glaucoma (Acute and Chronic)

Increased intraocular pressure; affects 2% of population >40 yr.

I. **Pathophysiology:**

    A. *Acute (closed-angle)*—impaired passage of aqueous humor into the circular canal of Schlemm due to closure of the angle between the cornea and the iris. **Medical emergency;** *requires surgery.*

    B. *Chronic (open-angle)*—local obstruction of aqueous humor between the anterior chamber and the canal. *Most common; treated with* medication (miotics, carbonic anhydrase inhibitors).

C. Untreated: imbalance between rate of secretion of intraocular fluids and rate of absorption of aqueous humor → increased intraocular pressures → decreased peripheral vision → corneal edema → halos and blurring of vision → blindness.

II. **Risk factors/causes**—unknown, but associated with:
   A. Emotional disturbances.
   B. Hereditary factors.
   C. Allergies.
   D. Vasomotor disturbances.
   E. Age.

III. **Assessment**
   A. *Subjective data*:
      1. *Acute* (closed-angle):
         a. Pain: severe, in and around eyes.
         b. Headache.
         c. Rainbow halos around lights.
         d. Blurring of vision.
         e. Nausea, vomiting.
      2. *Chronic* (open-angle):
         a. Eyes tire easily.
         b. Loss of peripheral vision.
   B. *Objective data*:
      1. Corneal edema.
      2. Decreased peripheral vision.
      3. Increased cupping of optic disc.
      4. Tonometry—pressures >22 mm Hg.
      5. Pupils: dilated.
      6. Redness of eye.

IV. **Analysis/nursing diagnosis**
   A. *Visual sensory/perceptual alterations* related to increased intraocular pressure.
   B. *Pain* related to sudden increase in intraocular pressure.
   C. *Risk for injury* related to blindness.
   D. *Impaired physical mobility* related to impaired vision.

V. **Nursing care plan/implementation**
   A. Goal: *reduce intraocular pressure.*
      1. Activity: bed rest.
      2. *Position*: semi-Fowler's.
      3. Medications as ordered:
         a. *Miotics* (pilocarpine, carbachol).
         b. *Carbonic anhydrase inhibitors* (acetazolamide [*Diamox*]).
         c. *Anticholinesterase* (demecarium bromide [*Humorsol*]) to facilitate outflow of aqueous humor.
         d. *Ophthalmic* (*Timolol*) to decrease intraocular pressure.
   B. Goal: *provide emotional support.*
      1. Place personal objects within field of vision.
      2. Assist with activities.

3. Encourage verbalization of concerns, fears of blindness, loss of independence.

C. Goal: **health teaching.**
   1. *Prevent* increased intraocular pressure by avoiding:
      a. Anger, excitement, worry.
      b. Constrictive clothing.
      c. Heavy lifting.
      d. Excessive *fluid* intake.
      e. Atropine or other mydriatics, which cause dilation.
      f. Straining at stool.
      g. Eye strain.
   2. Relaxation techniques; stress-management techniques, if indicated.
   3. Prepare for surgical intervention, if ordered: *laser trabeculoplasty, trabeculectomy* (filtering).
   4. Medications: purpose, dosage, frequency; eyedrop installation; have extra bottle in case of breakage or loss.
   5. Activity: moderate exercise—walking.
   6. Safety measures: eye protection (shield or glasses); MedicAlert band or tag; *avoid* driving 1–2 h after instilling miotics.
   7. Community resources as necessary.

VI. **Evaluation/outcome criteria**
   A. Eyesight preserved if possible.
   B. Intraocular pressure lowered (<22 mm Hg).
   C. Continues medical supervision for life—reports reappearance of symptoms immediately.

Cataract

Developmental or degenerative opacification of the crystalline lens.

I. **General**
   A. **Risk factors/causes:**
      1. Aging (most common).
      2. Trauma.
      3. Toxins.
      4. Congenital defect.
   B. **Assessment**
      1. *Subjective data*—vision: blurring, loss of acuity (see best in low-lit conditions); distortion; diplopia; photophobia.
      2. *Objective data*:
         a. Blindness: unilateral or bilateral (particularly in congenital cataracts).
         b. Loss of red reflex, gray opacity of lens.
   C. **Analysis/nursing diagnosis**
      1. *Visual sensory/perceptual alterations* related to opacity of lens.
      2. *Risk for injury* related to accidents.
      3. *Social isolation* related to impaired vision.

II. **Cataract removal**: removal of opacified lens because of loss of vision; extracapsular cataract extraction followed by intraocular lens (IOL) insertion is procedure of choice.

mydriatic — dilation
myotic — constriction

A. Nursing care plan/implementation
1. **Preoperative care:**
   a. Goal: *prepare for surgery.* Antibiotic drops or ointment, *mydriatic* eyedrops as ordered; note dilatation of pupils; *avoid* glaring lights; usually done under local anesthesia with sedation.
   b. Goal: **health teaching.** Postoperative expectations: do *not* rub, touch, or squeeze eyes shut after surgery; eye patches will be on; assistance will be given for needs; overnight hospitalization not required unless complications occur; mild iritis usually occurs.
2. **Postoperative care:**
   a. Goal: *reduce stress on the sutures and prevent hemorrhage.*
      (1) Activity: ambulate as ordered, usually soon after surgery; generally discharged 5–6 h after surgery.
      (2) *Position:* flat or low Fowler's; on back or turn to *nonoperative* side, as turning to operative side increases pressure.
      (3) *Avoid* activities that increase intraocular pressure: straining at stool, vomiting, coughing, brushing teeth, brushing hair, shaving, lifting objects over 20 lb, *bending,* or *stooping;* wear glasses or shaded lens during day, eyeshield at night.
      (4) Provide: mouthwash, hair care, personal items within easy reach, "step-in" slippers.
   b. Goal: *promote psychological well-being.* With elderly, frequent contacts to prevent sensory deprivation.
   c. Goal: **health teaching.**
      (1) If prescriptive glasses are used (*aphakic* glasses), explain about magnification, perceptual distortion, blind areas in peripheral vision; guide through activities with glasses; need to look through central portion of lens and turn head to side when looking to the side to decrease distortion.
      (2) Eye care: *instillation of eyedrops* (mydriatics and carbonic anhydrase inhibitors to prevent glaucoma and adhesions if intraocular lens [IOL] not inserted; with intraocular lens, steroid-antibiotic used); eye shield at night to prevent injury for 1 mo.
      (3) Signs/symptoms of: *infection* (redness, pain, edema, drainage); *iris prolapse* (bulging or pear-shaped pupil); *hemorrhage* (sharp eye pain, half-moon of blood).
      (4) *Avoid:* heavy lifting, potential eye trauma.

B. Evaluation/outcome criteria
1. Vision restored.
2. No complications (e.g., severe eye pain, hemorrhage).
3. Performs self-care activities (e.g., instills eyedrops).
4. Returns for follow-up ophthalmology care—recognizes symptoms requiring immediate attention.

Retinal Detachment

Separation of retina from choroid.

I. **Risk factors/causes:**
   A. Trauma.
   B. Degeneration.
II. **Assessment**
   A. *Subjective data:*
      1. Flashes of light before eyes.
      2. Vision: blurred, sooty (*sudden onset*); sensation of floating particles; blank areas of vision.
   B. *Objective data*—ophthalmic exam: retina is grayish in area of tear; bright red, horseshoe-shaped tear.
III. **Analysis/nursing diagnosis**
   A. *Visual sensory/perceptual alteration* related to blurred vision.
   B. *Anxiety* related to potential loss of vision.
   C. *Risk for injury* related to blindness.
IV. **Nursing care plan/implementation**
   A. **Preoperative care:**
      1. Goal: *reduce anxiety and prevent further detachment.*
         a. Encourage verbalization of feelings, answer all questions, reinforce physician's explanation of surgical procedures.
         b. Activity: *bed rest,* eyes usually covered to promote rest and maintain normal position of retina, siderails up.
         c. *Position:* according to location of retinal tear: involved area of eye should be in a *dependent* position.
         d. Give medications as ordered: *cycloplegic* or *mydriatics* to dilate pupils widely and decrease intraocular movement.
         e. Relaxing diversion: conversation, music.
      2. Goal: **health teaching.** Prepare for surgical intervention:
         a. *Cryotherapy*—supercooled probe is applied to the sclera, causing a scar, which pulls the choroid and retina together.

  b. *Laser photocoagulation*—a beam of intense light from a carbon arc is directed through the dilated pupil onto the retina; seals hole if retina not detached.

  c. *Scleral buckling*—the sclera is resected or shortened to enhance the contact between the choroid and retina.

  d. *Banding or encirclement*—silicone band or strap is placed under the extraocular muscles around the globe.

B. **Postoperative care:**

1. Goal: *reduce intraocular stress and prevent hemorrhage.*

   a. *Position*: flat or low-Fowler's; sandbags may be used to position head; turn to *nonoperative side* if allowed, retinal tear dependent. Special positions: prone, side-lying, or sitting with face down on table.

   b. Activity: *bed rest*; decrease intraocular pressure by *not* stooping, bending, or assuming prone position.

   c. Give medications as ordered:
      (1) *Mydriatics.*
      (2) *Antiinfectives.*
      (3) *Corticosteroids* to reduce eye movements, inflammation, and prevent infection.

   d. Range of motion exercises—isometric, passive; elastic stockings to prevent thrombus related to immobility.

2. Goal: *support coping mechanisms.*

   a. Plan all care with client.
   b. Encourage verbalization of feelings, fears.
   c. Encourage family interaction.
   d. Diversional activities.

3. Goal: **health teaching.**

   a. Eye care: eye patch or shield at night to prevent touching of the eye while asleep; dark glasses; *avoid* rubbing, squeezing eyes.
   b. Limitations: *no* reading for 3 wk, no physical exertion for 6 wk.
   c. Medications: dosage, frequency, purpose, side effects; *avoid* nonprescription medications.
   d. *Signs of redetachment*: flashes of light, increase in "floaters," blurred vision.

V. **Evaluation/outcome criteria**

A. Vision restored.
B. No further detachment—recognizes signs and symptoms.
C. No injury occurs—accepts limitations.

Blindness

Legally defined as vision less than 20/200 with the use of corrective lenses, or a visual field of no greater than 20 degrees; greatest incidence after 65 yr.

I. **Risk factors/causes:**

A. Glaucoma.
B. Cataracts.
C. Diabetic retinopathy.
D. Atherosclerosis.
E. Trauma.

II. **Analysis/nursing diagnosis**

A. *Visual sensory/perceptual alteration* related to blindness.
B. *Impaired social interaction* related to loss of sight.
C. *Risk for injury* related to visual impairment.
D. *Self-care deficit* related to visual loss.

III. **Nursing care plan/implementation**

A. Goal: *promote independence and provide emotional support.*

1. Familiarize with surroundings, encourage use of touch.
2. Establish communication lines, answer questions.
3. Deal with feelings of loss, overprotectiveness by family members.
4. Provide diversional activities: radio, records, talking books, tapes.
5. Encourage self-care activities; allow voicing of frustrations when activity is not done to satisfaction (spilling or misplacing something), to decrease anger and discouragement.

B. Goal: *facilitate activities of daily living.*

1. *Eating*:
   a. Establish routine placement for tableware, (e.g., plate, glass).
   b. Help person mentally visualize the plate as a clock or compass (e.g., "3 o'clock" or "east").
   c. Take person's hand and guide the fingertips to establish spatial relationship.

2. *Walking*:
   a. Have person hold your *forearm*; walk a half step in front.
   b. Tell the person when approaching stairs, curb, incline.

3. *Talking*:
   a. Speak when approaching person; tell them *before* you touch them.
   b. Tell them who you are and what you will be doing.
   c. Do *not avoid* using words such as "see" or discussing the appearance of things.

C. Goal: **health teaching.**

1. Accident prevention in the home.

2. Community resources:
   a. Voluntary agencies:
      (1) American Foundation for the Blind—provides catalogs of devices for visually handicapped.
      (2) National Society for the Prevention of Blindness—comprehensive educational programs and research.
      (3) Recording for the Blind, Inc.— provides recorded educational books on free loan.
      (4) Lion's Club.
      (5) Catholic Charities.
      (6) Salvation Army.
   b. Government agencies;
      (1) Social and Rehabilitation Service— counseling and placement services.
      (2) Veterans Administration—screening and pensions.
      (3) State Welfare Department, Division for the Blind—vocational.
3. Care of artificial eye—see **Table 19.2.**

IV. Evaluation/outcome criteria
   A. Acceptance of disability—participates in self-care activities, remains socially involved.
   B. Regains independence with rehabilitation.

TABLE 19.2 ☞ CARING FOR AN ARTIFICIAL EYE

With gloved hand pull lower eyelid down over the infraorbital bone and exert pressure below the eyelid.
Pressure will make the eye pop out.
Handle eye prosthesis carefully.
Using aseptic techniques, cleanse socket with saline-moistened gauze, stroking from the inner to outer canthus.
Wash the prosthesis in warm normal saline.
To reinsert, gently pull the client's lower lid down, raise the upper lid if necessary, slip the saline-moistened eye prosthesis gently into the socket, and release the lids.

Source: ©Lagerquist SL: *Little, Brown's NCLEX-RN® Examination Review.* Boston: Little, Brown. (out of print)

⌇⌇⌇ Diagnostic Study/Procedure

Caloric Stimulation Test
Used to: evaluate the vestibular portion of the eighth cranial nerve, identify the impairment or loss of thermally induced nystagmus. Reflex eye movements (nystagmus) result in response to cold or warm irrigations of the external auditory canal if the nerve is intact. A *diminished or absent* response occurs in Meniere's disease or acoustic neuroma. Nausea, vomiting, or dizziness can be precipitated by the test.

🔑 Summary of Key Points

1. Regardless of the type of sensory disorder, concern for client safety is a priority because of the accompanying *dizziness* (vertigo), impaired vision, or *altered depth perception.*

2. Meniere's disease is a relatively common disorder of *balance.* Medical treatment is instituted first; hospitalization is necessary only if surgery is needed to preserve hearing or manage symptoms.

3. Ringing in the ears (tinnitus) is *not* normal and usually indicates a problem.

4. The client should be told that hearing will not immediately improve after surgery for otosclerosis.

5. Hearing losses are either *conductive or sensorineural.* A conductive loss involves the *external, middle,* or *inner* ear. Sensorineural loss means there is *nerve damage.*

6. When talking to a client with an inner ear problem, stand *in front* of the client to avoid causing head movement and prevent dizziness.

7. Talking *louder* does *not* improve communication with a person who is blind.

8. The client with glaucoma must *avoid* using drugs that dilate the pupil and impair the outflow of aqueous humor. *Miotics* are used to constrict the pupil.

9. A rule of thumb—unless otherwise stated, the client should *not lie* on the *operative* side after eye surgery.

10. The most common cause of cataract is *aging.* An intraocular *lens* will most likely be inserted after cataract removal. Postoperative complications are less with such a lens implant, and depth perception is not altered; therefore accidents are less likely. Contact lenses are less desirable for older adults with decreased manual dexterity.

11. If a gas or air bubble is injected to seal a retinal tear, postoperative *positioning is key* to maximizing the gravitational force. The client may need to assume a *head-down* position while sitting and lie *prone* while sleeping.

Study and Memory Aids

Eye Medications

Mydriatic = dilated (big) pupils
Miotic = tiny (constricted) pupils

Source: Modified from Zerwekh J, et al. *Memory Notebook of Nursing.* Dallas: Nursing Education Consultants.

🍎 Diet

Meniere's Disease

↓ Sodium

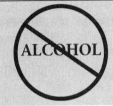

Drug Review

Meniere's Disease

Antiemetics
Prochlorperazine (*Compazine*): 5–10 mg qid
Promethazine (*Phenergan*): 10–25 mg q4h
Trimethobenzamide (*Tigan*): 250 mg qid
Antihistamines
Dimenhydrinate (*Dramamine*): 5–200 mg q4–6h, *not* to exceed 400 mg/d
Diphenhydramine HCl (*Benadryl*): 25–50 mg q4–6h
Antivertigos
Diazepam (*Valium*): 2–10 mg 3–4 times daily
Meclizine (*Antivert*): 25–100 mg/d in divided doses
Diuretics
Acetazolamide (*Diamox*): 250 mg 2–4 times/d
Hydrochlorothiazide (*Diuril, HydroDIURIL*): 25–100 mg/d in 1–2 doses
Vasodilator
Niacin (nicotinic acid): 500 mg/d in divided doses

Stapedectomy

Analgesics
Acetaminophen/codeine (*Tylenol #1, #2, #3*): 1–2 tablets q3–4h, as needed
Meperidine HCl (*Demerol*): IM or SC, 50–150 mg
Morphine sulfate: IM or SC, 5–20 mg
Oxycodone/acetaminophen (*Tylox, Percocet*): 5 mg q3–6h, as needed
Antiemetics
Prochlorperazine (*Compazine*): 5–10 mg qid
Promethazine (*Phenergan*): 10–25 mg q4h
Trimethobenzamide (*Tigan*): 250 mg qid
Antiinfectives
Cephalexin (*Keflex*): 250–500 mg q6h
Cephalothin (*Keflin*): IV 0.5–2 g q4–6h
Erythromycin: 250–500 mg q6–12h
Gentamicin (*Garamycin*): 3–5 mg/kg/d in divided doses
Penicillin G: IM 1.2 million U in single dose

Glaucoma

Anticholinesterase
Demecarium bromide (*Humorsol*): 1–2 drops twice/wk, up to 1–2 drops bid
Carbonic anhydrase inhibitor
Acetazolamide (*Diamox*): 250 mg 2–4 times/d
Miotics (pupil will *constrict*)
Carbachol (*Miostat Intraocular*): 1–2 drops qid
Pilocarpine (*Ocusert*): 1–2 drops up to 6 times/d
Ophthalmic
Timolol (*Timoptic*) 1 drop 1–2 times/d

Cataract Removal: Restriction

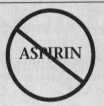

Cataract

Mydriatics (pupil will *dilate*)
Cyclopentolate (*Cyclogyl*): 1 drop/d
Homatropine (*Homatrine*): 1–2 drops/d

Questions

1. The nurse would question a client's understanding of the discharge instructions after removal of a cataract if he says:
    1. "I'll protect my eye with glasses or a shield."
    2. "I'll remember to drink plenty of fluids."
    3. "I'll wash around my eye with warm water."
    4. "I'll take a laxative every night."

2. Client teaching about what to expect after cataract surgery would include the fact that:
    1. Nausea and vomiting may result from general anesthesia.
    2. Narcotics will be available to manage surgical pain.
    3. The client will be tested for increased intraocular pressure.
    4. The client will need to significantly restrict activities after surgery.

3. The nurse would know that a client understands the possible precipitating causes of Meniere's disease if she states that she:
    1. Will increase her fluid intake.
    2. Plans to quit smoking.
    3. Must begin to do vigorous exercises regularly.
    4. Likes wine with her dinner.

4. The nurse knows that the vertigo in Meniere's disease may be relieved if the client lies:
    1. On the side with the affected ear uppermost.
    2. On the side with the unaffected ear uppermost.

3. Supine with the head of the bed elevated 30 degrees.
4. Supine with the head of the bed flat.

5. The best technique the nurse can use to improve communication with a client with hearing impairment is to:
   1. Speak loudly and accentuate the words.
   2. Tap the client's shoulder before talking.
   3. Stand with a light on his/her face while talking.
   4. Give one-word answers to the client's questions.

6. Besides frontal headaches, the nurse would expect a client with open-angle glaucoma to:
   1. Experience a decrease in peripheral vision.
   2. See colored halos around lights.
   3. Have dilated pupils, even in light.
   4. Have cloudy corneas.

7. Routine discharge teaching in a client who has undergone removal of a cataract from the right eye would include the need to:
   1. Avoid sexual activity for a month.
   2. Report immediately any eye aching.
   3. Sleep supine or lying on the nonoperated side.
   4. Remove the eye patch at night only.

8. Which aspect of a physical assessment of the eyes would be unaffected in a client with a cataract?
   1. Red reflex testing.
   2. Funduscopy.
   3. Visual acuity.
   4. Pupillary reaction.

9. Which nursing action would be inappropriate in a client with Meniere's disease suffering an attack of vertigo?
   1. Supporting each side of the client's head with a pillow.
   2. Speaking into the client's unaffected ear to facilitate hearing.
   3. Keeping the client on bed rest with siderails up.
   4. Having the client ask for assistance when turning.

10. A client is preparing to go home after surgery for glaucoma. Which instruction would not be included in the discharge teaching?
    1. Washing hands well before instilling eye drops.
    2. Refraining from smoking for 1 week postoperatively.
    3. Avoiding driving at night for 6 weeks.
    4. Wearing a protective eyeshield during sleep for several weeks.

11. Which instruction is part of the proper care of a hearing aid?
    1. Cleaning off the ear mold weekly. *daily*
    2. Storing the hearing aid in a warm, dry place.
    3. Removing accumulated lint from the casing monthly.
    4. Replacing the batteries every month.

12. Which action to determine the cause of hearing aid failure should the nurse take first?
    1. Replacing the existing batteries.
    2. Checking for proper fit in the ear.
    3. Examining the ear for cerumen.
    4. Checking to see if the hearing aid is "on."

Answers/Rationale

1. (2) The intake of plenty of fluids, although an important measure in most clients, is *not* going to promote recovery after cataract surgery. Protecting the eye (1), careful cleaning (3), and preventing straining at stool (4) *are* all important and *appropriate* measures. EV, EVL, 2, HPM, **Health promotion and maintenance**

2. (3) Secondary glaucoma is one of the major complications of cataract extraction. Usually this resolves within 24 to 72 hours, however. *Local* anesthesia, *not* general anesthesia, is used for the procedure, so nausea and vomiting (1) are *not* expected. Acetaminophen (*Tylenol*) is usually effective enough to relieve the postoperative discomfort (2). Restrictions are *minimal* (4). Normally, clients should avoid lifting and straining but they may resume other usual activities within 24 hours. IMP, RE/KN, 2, PhI, **Reduction of risk potential**

3. (2) Quitting smoking eliminates one source of vasospasm and vasoconstriction, which may inhibit the absorption of endolymph and cause ear pressure to increase. If fluid intake is increased (1), fluid retention may result and the symptoms will be aggravated. Vigorous, sudden movement (3) may precipitate an attack, so vigorous exercise should be *avoided*. Alcohol (4), like smoking, may cause vasoconstriction and hence increased endolymph accumulation. EV, EVL, 2, PhI, **Physiological adaptation**

4. (1) Some clients have experienced relief if they lie on their side with the affected ear uppermost. This may reduce inner ear pressure. Lying with the unaffected ear up (2), with the head elevated (3), or supine (4) has *not* been found to produce *any relief.* IMP, COM, 2, PhI, **Basic care and comfort**

5. (3) Standing with a light on the nurse's face helps the client to speech-read. It is best to speak slowly in a *normal* tone and *not* to overaccentuate (1). To get the client's attention, the nurse should raise an arm or hand; tapping the client on the shoulder (2) may startle the client. It is also best *not* to use one-word answers (4), but to use phrases, which convey more meaning. In general, the nurse should not avoid conversation with a client who is hearing-impaired. IMP, APP, 2, PsI, **Psychosocial integrity**

6. (1) A client with open-angle glaucoma suffers a gradual loss of peripheral vision, but central vision

remains good. A client with *closed*-angle glaucoma sees colored halos around lights (2). *Cranial nerve III* (oculomotor) damage or drugs cause pupillary dilatation (3). Clients with *cataracts* have cloudy corneas (4). **AS, RE/KN, 2, PhI, Physiological adaptation**

7. (3) Discharge teaching should emphasize the need to avoid activities that place strain on the eye. Unless otherwise stated, sleeping on the back or the nonoperated side is recommended. Sexual activity (1) is *not* routinely restricted, but this varies with each client and MD. *Mild* pain and aching (2) are *expected* and relieved with mild analgesia. Sudden, sharp pain should be reported. A patch *is* worn at night (4) to protect the eye from rubbing against the bedclothes and keep the client from rubbing the eye during sleep. **IMP, RE/KN, 2, SECE, Management of care**

8. (4) The pupillary response, which is controlled by cranial nerve III, would still be intact, because this is elicited by light, which can still penetrate the cornea. Cataract *would interfere* with the red reflex (1), which is the bright red-orange glow seen through the pupil. The opacity of the lens caused by a cataract *would* make it difficult for the examiner to see through the lens into the posterior portion of the eye (2) and the central vision acuity (3) of the client *would be impaired.* **AS, RE/KN, 2, HPM, Health promotion and maintenance**

9. (2) It is inappropriate to make the client turn the head or move the eyes to look at the nurse, because this may worsen dizziness. Head support (1) and assistance in turning (4) *can* minimize sudden movements or jerking, which could increase discomfort and aggravate the symptoms. The side rails (3) *would* be up to prevent falls during dizzy spells. **IMP, ANL, 2, SECE, Management of care**

10. (3) There are usually no driving restrictions unless visual impairment has resulted. The instructions in

options 1, 2, and 4 *are* appropriate for clients who have undergone glaucoma surgery. **IMP, RE/KN, 2, SECE, Management of care**

11. (4) Replacing the batteries every month will prevent battery failure as a source of a client's inability to hear. The instructions in options 1 and 3 specify exact times for cleaning, whereas cleaning is actually done *only as needed* when wax or lint buildup warrant. The ear mold is cleaned off daily with soap and warm water, and with a pipe cleaner if necessary. The hearing aid is usually *not stored* (2) when not in use; when it is not in the ear, it is kept on the client's bedside stand. **IMP, RE/KN, 2, SECE, Management of care**

12. (4) The nurse should start with the obvious: checking to see if the hearing aid is on. Next check to see if the ear mold is clean. After this, the battery should be checked to make sure it is correctly inserted. The other actions would *follow* these steps: replacing the battery if necessary (1), then checking the position of the hearing aid in the ear (2), and finally checking to see if there has been a buildup of cerumen (3). **IMP, ANL, 2, PhI, Reduction of risk potential**

Key to Codes

Nursing process: AS, assessment; AN, analysis; PL, planning; IMP, implementation; EV, evaluation. (See **Appendix M** for explanation of nursing process steps.)

Cognitive level: RE/KN, recall/knowledge; COM, comprehension; APP, application; ANL, analysis; EVL, evaluation; SYN, synthesis. (See **Appendix M** for explanation.)

Category of human function: 1, protective; 2, sensory-perceptual; 3, comfort, rest, activity, and mobility; 4, nutrition; 5, growth and development; 6, fluid-gas transport; 7, psychosocial-cultural; 8, elimination. (See **Appendix 0** for explanation.)

Client need: SECE, safe, effective care environment; PhI, physiological integrity; PsI, psychosocial integrity; HPM, health promotion and maintenance. (See **Appendix P** for explanation.)

Client subneed: (See **Appendix P** for explanation)

Musculoskeletal Disorders

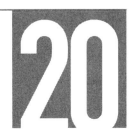

Chapter Outline

Fractures

Disruptions in the continuity of bone as the result of trauma or various disease processes, such as Cushing's syndrome, that weaken the bone structure.

I. **Types:**
- A. *Open or compound*—fractured bone extends *through skin* and mucous membranes; increased potential for infection.
- B. *Closed or simple*—fractured bone *does not* protrude through skin.
- C. *Complete*—fracture extends through *entire bone*, disrupting the periosteum on both sides of the bone, producing two or more fragments.
- D. *Incomplete*—fracture extends *only part way* through bone; bone continuity is not totally interrupted.
- E. *Greenstick or willow-hickory stick*—fracture of *one* side of bone; *other side merely bends*; usually seen only in children.
- F. *Impacted or telescoped*—fracture in which bone fragments are *forcibly driven into* other or adjacent bone structures.
- G. *Comminuted*—fracture having *more than one* fracture line and with bone fragment broken into *several pieces*.
- H. *Depressed*—fracture in which bone or bone fragments are driven *inward*, as in skull or facial fractures.
- I. *Pathologic*–spontaneous fracture at site of bone disease.
- J. *Displaced* (overriding)–fracture that involves a displaced fracture fragment that is overriding the other bone fragment.
- K. *Spiral*–line of fracture extends in a spiral direction along the shaft of the bone.

II. **Methods used to reduce/immobilize fractures:** reduction or setting of the bone—restores bone alignment as nearly as possible.

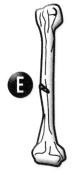 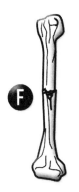 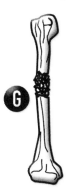 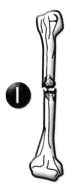 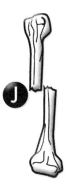 

Greenstick   Impacted   Comminuted   Pathologic   Displaced   Spiral

FIGURE 20.1   SELECTED EXAMPLES OF FRACTURES

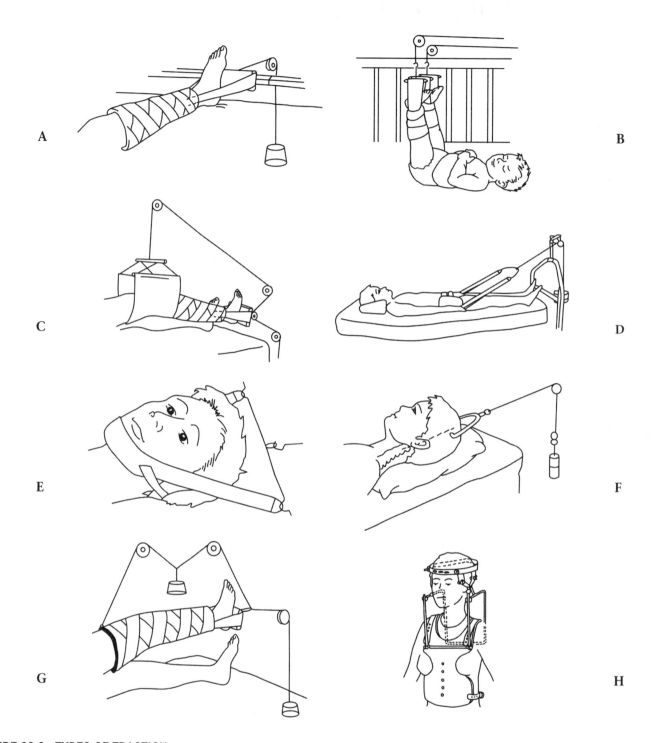

FIGURE 20.2 TYPES OF TRACTION.

A. **Buck's extension.** Skin traction applied to the medial and lateral aspects of an extremity with adhesive foam, moleskin, or use of "Buck's boot."

B. **Bryant's traction.** Vertical suspension skin traction in which pelvis is elevated from the bed.

C. **Russell's traction.** Skin traction composed of **Buck's** extension on the foreleg, three pulleys at the bottom, and a sling under the knee. Affords more freedom of movement than **Buck's**.

D. **Pelvic traction.** Skin traction applied to the lumbosacral region by means of a pelvic belt.

E. **Head halter.** Cervical traction applied to the head by means of a halter under the chin.

F. **Crutchfield tongs.** Cervical traction using tongs into the skull.

G. **Thomas' splint.** Full-leg splint that keeps the leg fully extended and the long bones in alignment. Pressure is on the ischium and perineal area. May be used with skin or skeletal traction.

H. **Halo vest assembly.** Applied in operating room. Client will usually be ambulatory 24 hours after application.

Adapted from: Saxton DF. The Addison-Wesley Manual of Nursing Practice. Menlo Park, CA. Addison-Wesley, (out of print)

A. *Closed reduction*—manual traction or manipulation. Usually done under local or general anesthesia to reduce pain and muscle spasm. Maintenance of reduction and immobilization is accomplished by casting (fiberglass or plaster of Paris).

B. *Open reduction*—operative procedure utilized to achieve bone alignment; pins, wire, nails, or rods may be used to secure bone fragments in position; prosthetic implants may also be used.

C. *Traction reduction*—force is applied in two directions, to obtain alignment and to reduce or eliminate muscle spasm. Used for fractures of long bones. May be:

1. *Continuous*—used with fractures or dislocations of bones or joints.

2. *Intermittent*—used to reduce flexion contractures or lessen pain and muscle spasm.

3. Applied as follows:

   a. *Skin*—traction applied to skin using a commercial foam-rubber *Buck's* traction splint or an adhesive, plastic, or moleskin strip bound to the extremity by elastic bandage; exerts indirect traction on bone or muscles (e.g., *Buck's* extension, Bryant's, *Russell's,* pelvic*)*. (**Figure 20.2A** to **20.2D**.)

   b. *Skeletal*—direct traction applied to bone using pins (*Steinman*), wires (*Kirschner*). Pin is inserted through the bone in or close to the involved area and usually protrudes through skin on both sides of the extremity. Skeletal traction for fractured vertebrae accomplished with tongs (*Crutchfield tongs, Gardner-Wells tongs*).

4. **Specific types of traction:**

   a. *Cervical*

      (1) *Cervical skeletal traction*—direct traction applied to cervical vertebrae using *Crutchfield, Gardner-Wells*, or *Vinke* tongs that are inserted into the skull (see **Figure 20.2E** and **20.2F**). Traction is increased with weights until vertebrae move into position and alignment is regained. After reduction is obtained, weights are decreased to the amount needed to maintain reduction. *Weight amount is prescribed by physician.*

      (2) *Cervical skin traction*—applied via head halter; used to treat soft tissue disorders and cervical disc disease; often used to treat the client at home; *not* used for vertebral fracture reduction.

   b. *Balanced suspension*—countertraction produced by a force other than client's body weight; additional weights supply countertraction. Extremity is suspended in a traction apparatus that maintains the line of traction despite changes in the client's position (e.g., *Russell's* leg traction, *Thomas'* splint with *Pearson's* attachment). (See **Figure 20.2C** and **20.2G**.) Client has more freedom to move about than in straight or running traction.

   c. *Running*—traction that exerts a pull in one plane; countertraction is supplied by the weight of the client's body (this must not be less than the pull of the traction) or can be increased through use of weights and pulleys in the opposite direction (e.g., *Buck's* extension, *Russell's* traction; see **Figure 20.2A** and **20.2C**). Check specific orders to determine how much the head may be elevated.

   d. *Halo*—an apparatus that employs both a plastic and metal frame; molded frame extends from the axilla to iliac crest and houses a metal frame. The struts of the frame extend to skull and attach to round metal (halo) device. The halo is attached to skull by four pins—two located anterolaterally and two located posterolaterally. They are inserted into external cortex of the cranium. (See **Figure 20.2H**.) Used to immobilize the cervical spine after spinal fusion, somewhat corrects scoliosis before spinal fusion, immobilizes nondisplaced fracture of spine.

D. *Immobilization*—maintains reduction and promotes healing of bone fragments. Achieved by:

1. *External fixation*:

   a. *Casts*—types:

      (1) *Spica*—applied to immobilize hip or shoulder joints.

      (2) *Body cast*—applied to trunk.

      (3) Arm or leg cast—joints above and below site included in cast.

   b. *Splints*—continuous traction.

   c. *External fixation devices*—multiple pins/rods through limb above and below fracture site, attached to external metal supports; client able to become ambulatory.

2. *Internal fixation*—pins, wires, nails, rods. See **Total Hip Replacement, p. 271-273**, and Total **Knee Replacement, p. 273**.

▶ **III. Assessment**

A. *Subjective data*:

1. Pain, tenderness.

2. Tingling, numbness.

(continued on p.259)

TABLE 20.1 COMPLICATIONS OF FRACTURES

⧗ Complication	⧗ Assessment	⧗ Analysis/Nursing Diagnosis	⧗ Nursing Care Plan/Implementation	⧗ Evaluation/Outcome Criteria
Shock (see Chap. 8). **Compartment Syndrome** (see p. 262). **Thrombophlebitis** (see p. 20). **Fat emboli:** serious, potentially life-threatening complication in which pressure changes in interior of fracture force molecules of fat from marrow into systemic circulation; may cause problems in respiratory or nervous system; seen most frequently on *third day* after multiple fractures, fractures of long bones, or comminuted fracture.	*Subjective data:* dyspnea, severe chest pain; confusion, agitation; decrease in level of consciousness; numbness; feeling faint; history of diabetes, obesity. *Objective data:* cyanosis; papillary changes, muscle twitching; *petechiae*—chest, buccal cavity, axilla, conjunctiva, soft palate; *extremities*—pallor, cold; shock, vomiting.	*Risk for injury* related to fat emboli. *Altered tissue perfusion* related to fat emboli.	1. *Position:* high-Fowler's to relieve respiratory symptoms. 2. Administer *oxygen STAT*, to relieve anoxia and reduce surface tension of fat globules. 3. Institute respiratory support measures, as ordered—intermittent positive-pressure breathing, respiratory assistive devices; **be prepared for cardiopulmonary resuscitation** in event of respiratory failure. 4. Monitor vital signs, cardiac monitor, q15min during acute episode and prn (shock/cardiac failure possible). 5. Obtain baseline data and monitor *level of consciousness, neurologic* signs q15min during acute episode and prn (neurologic involvement possible). 6. Administer *parenteral fluids*, as ordered; IV alcohol, blood and fluid replacements. 7. Administer medications as ordered; corticosteroids, digitalis, aminophylline, heparin sodium. 8. DO NOT RUB ANY LEG CRAMPS, BUT REPORT IMMEDIATELY.	Alert, oriented. Pain relieved. Respiratory, cardiac, and neurologic problems cause no permanent damage.

(Continued)

TABLE 20.1 COMPLICATIONS OF FRACTURES *(continued)*

Complication	⧗ Assessment	⧗ Analysis/Nursing Diagnosis	⧗ Nursing Care Plan/Implementation	⧗ Evaluation/Outcome Criteria
Nerve compression: pressure on nerve in affected area from edema, dislocation of bone, or immobilization apparatus; if pressure not relieved, permanent paralysis can result.	*Subjective data:* discomfort, pain, referred pain, burning, tingling, "stinging sensation," numbness, altered sensation, inability to distinguish touch. *Objective data:* limited movement; muscle weakness; paralysis; *reflexes*—diminished, irritable, or absent; color changes related to impaired circulation.	*Pain* related to pressure on nerve. *Risk for physical injury* related to pressure on nerve. *Impaired tissue perfusion* related to impaired circulation. *Impaired physical mobility* related to joint contracture, numbness.	1. Monitor for potential signs q1h for first 48 h; neurovascular assessment q12h and prn as condition indicates *(CSM [circulation, sensation, motion]).* 2. *Position: elevate* affected limb; flex hand or foot of affected extremity; passive and active ROM exercises. 3. **Be prepared to cut cast or remove constrictions if signs of impairment present.** 4. Begin active ROM exercises to unaffected extremities. 5. Use footboard to prevent footdrop. 6. Encourage use of trapeze if applicable. 7. Isometric exercises, as ordered. 8. Ambulation, weight bearing as ordered; support casts.	Sensation, motor function are normal. No complications noted.
Avascular necrosis/ circulatory impairment: interference with normal circulation to affected area due to interruption of blood vessel, pressure on the vessel from dislocation, edema, or immobilization devices; impaired circulation leads to discomfort and, if not eliminated, to necrosis of tissue and bone due to lack of oxygen supply.	*Subjective data:* tenderness; pain, especially on passive motion. *Objective data:* edema, swelling in affected area; *decreased:* color, temperature, mobility; bleeding from wound.	*Risk for altered peripheral tissue perfusion,* related to vessel damage.	1. Monitor for potential signs q1h for first 48 h: blanching, coolness, edema; palpate pulse above and below injury; report absent or major discrepancies **stat.** 2. *Position: elevate* affected limb to decrease edema. 3. Report to physician if signs persist. 4. **Be prepared to assist with bivalving of casts, or cut cast to relieve pressure.** 5. Monitor size of drainage stains on casts; measure accurately and report if they enlarge.	Circulation adequate to limb, to prevent tissue damage.

(Continued)

TABLE 20.1 COMPLICATIONS OF FRACTURES (continued)

Complication	⌛ Assessment	⌛ Analysis/Nursing Diagnosis	⌛ Nursing Care Plan/Implementation	⌛ Evaluation/Outcome Criteria
Infection	*Subjective data:* pain. *Objective data: elevated* temperature and pulse; *erythema*—discoloration of surrounding skin; *edema*—sudden, local, induration; *drainage*—thin, watery, foul-smelling exudate; *crepitation* (may be indicative of gas gangrene); with cast—warm area, foul smell.	*Risk for injury* related to tissue destruction. *Altered peripheral tissue perfusion* related to swelling.	1. Monitor vital signs, drainage. 2. Ensure client has had prophylactic tetanus toxoid. 3. May have prophylactic *anti-infectives* ordered if wound was contaminated at time of injury. 4. Instruct client *not* to touch open wound, pin sites or put anything inside cast (could interrupt skin integrity and become potential source of infection).	No infection or heals with no serious complications.
Delayed union/ nonunion: failure of bone to heal within normal time related to lack of use, inadequate circulation, other complicating medical conditions such as diabetes or poor nutrition.	*Subjective data:* pain. *Objective data:* lack of callus formation on x-ray, poor alignment.	*Risk for injury* related to poor healing of bone fracture. *Impaired physical mobility* related to lower limb fractures. *Dressing/grooming, bathing/hygiene, self-care deficit* related to upper limb fracture.	1. Maintain immobilization and alignment of affected limb. 2. Maintain adequate nutrition. 3. *Avoid* trauma to affected limb. 4. Monitor for circulatory or infective complication. 5. Dietary instructions regarding foods containing *calcium* and *protein* necessary for bone healing.	Bone heals. No complications noted. Pain decreases. Ambulation and self-care return to preinjury state.
Skin breakdown (related to cast).	*Subjective data:* pain. *Objective data:* temperature and pulse elevated; *erythema; edema*—cast edges, exposed distal portion of limb, limb area within cast; *drainage* and *foul odor* from break in skin, may be under cast and stain through or exit at ends of cast; *crepitus* (crackling sound could indicate gas gangrene); hyperactive reflexes.	*Impaired skin integrity* related to cast trauma.	1. If open wound: verify tetanus administration; monitor site through cast window, change *dressing* daily and prn. 2. Apply lotion or cornstarch to exposed skin (*no* powder). 3. Petal tape edges of cast to reduce irritation. 4. Inspect skin for: irritation, edema, odor, drainage—q2h initially, then q3h. 5. Instruct client *not* to place any object under cast as skin abrasions may lead to decubitus ulcers. 6. Promote drying of cast by leaving it uncovered and exposed to air for 48 h; use *no* plastic. 7. Prevent indenting casts with fingertips or hard surface; place on pillows, use palms of hands when positioning affected limb. 8. *Avoid* excessive padding of Thomas splint in groin area—padding traps moisture, leading to skin breakdown.	No skin breakdown.

(Continued)

TABLE 20.1 COMPLICATIONS OF FRACTURES (continued)

Complication	Assessment	Analysis/Nursing Diagnosis	Nursing Care Plan/Implementation	Evaluation/Outcome Criteria
Duodenal distress (with spica cast): spica cast incorporates the trunk and affected limb and can cause respiratory or abdominal distress when edema is present under the cast; or cast is too tight to allow for normal body functions.	*Subjective data:* anorexia, nausea, abdominal pain. *Objective data:* duodenal distress, vomiting, distention, cast too tight.	*Ineffective breathing pattern* related to pressure from cast. *Pain* related to abdominal distress from pressure. *Fear* related to cast constriction.	1. Place on firm mattress; use bed boards if necessary to reduce muscle spasm. 2. Maintain warmth by covering uncasted areas. 3. *Avoid* turning for first 8 h; *when turning:* use enough personnel to *log-roll; do not use* bar between legs while turning; support chest with pillows. 4. Monitor for signs of respiratory distress: increased respirations, apprehension. 5. Monitor for signs of duodenal distress: vomiting, distention; *if these signs occur: place in prone position;* have cast bivalved; may need NG tube; monitor for fluid imbalance. 6. Protect cast with nonabsorbent material during elimination.	Complications prevented or detected early enough to prevent serious damage.

Source: ©Lagerquist SL: *Little, Brown's NCLEX-RN® Examination Review.* Boston: Little, Brown (out of print).

TABLE 20.2 ASSESSING NEUROVASCULAR STATUS IN THE EXTREMITIES

■ Assessing *circulation* to the extremity:
1. Warmth and color.
2. Peripheral pulses (radial for upper extermities, dorsalis pedis and posterior tibial for lower extermities).
3. Capillary refill.
4. Presence of edema.

■ Assessing *neurologic function* of the limb
1. Upper extremities:
   a. *Sensory:* numbness or tingling over fingertips, dorsum of hand.
   b. *Motor:* dorsiflexion and palmar flexion of wrist and fingers.
2. Lower extremities:
   a. *Sensory:* numbness or tingling over heel and dorsum of foot.
   b. *Motor:* dorsiflexion and plantar flexion of foot.

Note: The affected extremity should always be compared to the unaffected extremity.

3. Nausea.
4. History of trauma.
5. Muscle spasm.

B. *Objective data:*
1. Function: abnormal or lost.
2. Deformities, shortening of limb
3. Ecchymosis, increased heat over injured part.
4. Localized edema.
5. Crepitation (grating sensations heard or felt as bone fragments rub against each other).
6. Signs of shock.
7. Indicators of anxiety.
8. X-ray: *fracture*—positive interruption of bone; *dislocation*—abnormal position of bone.

IV. Analysis/nursing diagnosis
A. *Pain* related to interruption in bone.
B. *Impaired physical mobility* related to fracture/treatment.
C. *Risk for injury* related to complications of fractures.
D. *Knowledge deficit* regarding cast care, crutch walking, traction.
E. *Constipation* related to immobilization.
F. *Risk for impaired skin integrity* related to immobility or friction from materials used to immobilize the fracture during healing.

V. Nursing care plan/implementation
A. Goal: *promote healing and prevent complications of fractures* (Table 20.1).
   1. *Diet: high* protein, iron, vitamins, *to improve tissue repair; moderate* carbohydrates, to

prevent weight gain; *no* increase in calcium, to *prevent kidney stones* (decalcification and demineralization occur when client is immobilized).

2. Encourage *increased fluid intake,* to *prevent kidney stones.*

🍎 3. *Prevent* or alleviate *constipation* by *increasing bulk foods, fruits, and fruit juices* or by 💊 administering prescribed *stool softeners, laxatives,* or *cathartics,* as necessary.

4. Provide activities to reduce perceptual deprivation—reading, handicrafts, music, special interests/hobbies that can be done while maintaining correct position for healing.

B. Goal: *prevent injury or trauma in relation to:*

☞ 1. *Fracture care:*

  a. Maintain affected part in optimal alignment.

  b. Maintain skin integrity; check all bony prominences for evidence of pressure q4h and prn, depending on amount of pressure.

  c. Monitor: *circulation* in, *sensation* of, and *motion* (CSM) of affected part q15min for first 4 h; q1h until 24 h; then q4h and prn, depending on amount of edema (**Table 20.2**).

  d. Maintain mobility in unaffected limb and unaffected joints of affected limb by active and passive range of motion (ROM) exercises, prevent footdrop by using ankle-top sneakers.

☞ 2. *Skin traction:*

  a. Maintain correct alignment:

    (1) If tape or moleskin is used, shave 💊 extremity and apply benzoin to improve adherence of strip and reduce itching.

    (2) Check apparatus for slippage, bunching; replace prn.

  b. Prevent tissue injury:

    (1) Check all bony prominences for evidence of pressure: q15min for first 4 h; q1h until 24 h; then q4h and prn, depending on amount of edema.

    (2) Nonadhesive traction may be removed q8h to check skin (e.g., *Bryant's*).

☞ 3. *Skeletal traction:*

  a. Maintain affected part in optimal alignment:

    (1) Ropes on pulleys.

    (2) Weights hang free.

    (3) *Position: elevate* head of bed as prescribed.

    (4) Check knots routinely.

  b. Maintain skin integrity:

    (1) Frequent skin care.

    (2) Keep bed linens free of crumbs and wrinkles.

  c. Prevent *infection:* special skin care to pin insertion site tid. Keep area around pins clean and dry. Utilize prescribed solution for cleansing.

  d. Monitor: *circulation, sensation, motion* of affected part (see *Fracture care*, p. 260).

  e. Maintain mobility in unaffected limb and unaffected joints; prevent footdrop of affected limb.

☞ 4. *Running traction:*

  a. Keep well centered in bed.

  b. *Position: elevate head of bed only* to point of countertraction.

  c. *No* turning from side to side—will cause rubbing of bony fragments.

  d. Check distal circulation frequently.

  e. Frequent back care to prevent skin breakdown.

  f. Fracture bedpan for toileting.

  g. *Avoid* excessive padding of splints in groin area to prevent tissue trauma.

☞ 5. *Balanced suspension traction:*

  a. Maintain alignment and countertraction:

    (1) Ropes on pulleys.

    (2) Weights hang free.

    (3) *Position: elevate* head of bed as prescribed.

    (4) Check knots routinely.

  b. May move client, but turn only slightly (*no more* than 30 degrees to *unaffected* side).

  c. Heel of affected leg *must* remain free of the bed.

  d. *20-degree angle* between thigh and bed.

  e. Check for pressure to popliteal area exerted by sling.

  f. Provide foot support to prevent footdrop.

  g. Maintain *abduction* of extremity.

  h. Check for signs of infection at pin insertion sites; cleanse tid as ordered.

  i. If tape or moleskin is used, shave 💊 extremity and apply *benzoin* to improve adherence of strip and reduce itching.

☞ 6. *Cervical traction:*

  a. May be placed on specialized bed (e.g., *Stryker frame*).

  b. *Position:* maintain body alignment.

  c. Keep tongs free from bed, keep weights hanging freely to allow traction to function properly.

☞ 7. *Halo traction:*

  a. Several times a day: check screws to the head and screws that hold the upper portion of the frame, to determine correct position.

b. Pin sites cleansed tid with *bacteriostatic* solution to prevent infection.

c. Monitor for signs of infection.

d. *Position* as any other client in body cast, except *no pressure* on halo—pillows may be placed under abdomen and chest when client is prone.

e. Institute ROM exercises to prevent contractures.

f. Turn frequently to prevent development of pressure areas.

g. Allow client to verbalize about having screws placed in skull.

h. Postapplication, nursing care same as that for pin insertion for other forms of traction.

☞ 8. *External fixation devices*:

a. Pin care same as that for skeletal traction.

b. Teach clothing adjustment.

c. Teach to adjust for size of apparatus.

☞ 9. *Internal fixation devices*:

a. Monitor for signs of infection/ allergic reaction to materials used for maintenance of reduction (drainage, pain, increased temperature).

b. *Position*: as ordered to prevent dislocation.

☞ 10. *Casts*:

a. Support drying cast on firm pillow, prevent finger imprints on cast.

b. *Position: elevate* limb to reduce edema.

c. Prevent complications of fractures, as listed.

d. Closely monitor: *circulation* (blanching, swelling, decreased temperature), *sensation* (absence of feeling, pain, burning), *motion* (inability to move digits of affected limb).

e. **Be prepared to notify MD or cut cast if circulatory impairment occurs.**

f. Protect skin integrity: *avoid* pressure from edges of cast, petal tape edges of cast as needed.

g. Monitor for signs of infection if skin integrity impaired.

☞ C. Goal: *provide care related to ambulation with crutches.*

1. Measure crutches correctly (also see **Table 20.4**).

a. Subtract 16 in. from total height, top of crutch should be 2 in. below the axilla.

b. Complete extension of the elbows should be possible without axilla bar exerting pressure into the axilla.

c. Handgrip should be adjusted so that complete wrist extension is possible.

d. Instruct in correct body alignment:

(1) Head erect.

TABLE 20.3 ☞ TEACHING CRUTCH WALKING

A. When only *one* leg can bear weight:

1. *Swing-to gait*: crutches forward; swing body to crutches:

a. Move both crutches forward.

b. Move both legs to meet the crutches.

c. Continue pattern.

2. *Swing-through gait*: crutches forward; swing body through crutches:

a. Move both crutches forward.

b. Move both legs farther ahead than crutches.

c. Continue pattern.

3. *Three-point gait*: crutches and *affected* extremity forward; swing forward, placing *nonaffected* foot ahead or between crutches:

a. Both crutches and affected limb move at same time.

b. Move both crutches and *affected* leg (e.g., left) ahead 6 in.

c. Move *unaffected* leg (e.g., right) to same places as left and crutches.

d. Continue pattern.

B. When *both* legs can move separately and bear some weight:

1. *Four-point gait*: right crutch forward, left foot forward; swing weight to right side while bringing left crutch forward, then right foot forward; gait simulates normal walking:

a. Move right crutch forward 4–6 in.

b. Move left foot forward same distance as right crutch.

c. Move left crutch forward ahead of left foot.

d. Move right foot forward to meet right crutch.

e. Continue pattern.

2. *Two-point gait*: same as four-point gait but faster; one crutch and opposite leg moving forward at same time:

a. Opposite crutch and limb move together.

b. Move right crutch and left leg ahead 6 in.

c. Move left crutch and right leg ahead.

d. Continue pattern.

C. When client is *unable* to walk: *tripod gait*: crutches forward at a wide distance; drag legs to point just behind crutches, balance, and repeat.

Source: ©Lagerquist SL: *Little, Brown's NCLEX-RN® Examination Review*. Boston: Little, Brown (out of print).

(2) Back straight.

(3) Chest forward.

(4) Feet 6–8 in. apart, wide base for support.

2. See **Table 20.3**.

D. Goal: *provide safety measures related to possible complications following fracture* (see **Table 20.1**).

⌂ E. Goal: **health teaching**.

1. Explain and show apparatus before application, if possible.

TABLE 20.4 ☞ MEASURING CRUTCHES CORRECTLY

1. Have client lie on a flat surface. Measure from anterior fold of axilla to 4 in. lateral to heel.
2. Have client stand. Measure from 1–2 in. below axilla to 2 in. in front of and 6 in. to the side of the foot.
3. Hand placement on bar of crutch: have client stand upright, support body weight with hand on bar (*not* putting weight on axilla). Elbow flexion should be *30 degrees*.
4. Slightly pad the shoulder rests of the crutches for general comfort.
5. Make sure there are nonskid rubber tips on the crutches.

Source: ©Lagerquist SL: *Little, Brown's NCLEX-RN® Examination Review.* Boston: Little, Brown (out of print).

2. Pin care at least once daily to prevent granulation and cellulitis.
3. Correct position for rest/sleep and prevention of injury with halo traction—*no* pressure on halo.
4. Purpose of cast: to immobilize, to support body tissues, to prevent or correct deformities.
5. Teach signs and symptoms of complications to report related to cast care (i.e., numbness; odor; crack/break in cast; extremity cold, bluish).
6. Isometric exercises for use with affected joint.
7. *Safety measures with crutches*:
   a. Weight bearing on hands, *not* axilla.
   b. *Position* crutches 4 in. to side and 4 in. to front.
   c. Use short strides, looking ahead, *not* at feet.
   d. *Prevent* injury: if client begins to fall, throw crutches to side to prevent falling on them; body should be relaxed.
   e. Check for environmental hazards: rugs, water spills

◄ VI. **Evaluation/outcome criteria**
   A. No injury or complications related to apparatus or immobilization (e.g., infection, tissue injury, altered circulation/sensation, dislocation).
   B. Bone remains in correct alignment and begins to heal.
   C. Demonstrates elevated limb position to relieve edema with casted extremity.
   D. Lists complications related to circulation and/or neurologic impairment and infection.
   E. Begins to use affected part.
   F. Demonstrates correct technique for ambulation with crutches—no pressure on axilla, utilizes strength of arms and wrists.
   G. No falls while using crutches.

Compartment Syndrome

An accumulation of fluid in the muscle compartment, resulting in an increase in pressure that reduces blood flow to the tissues; can lead to neuromuscular deficit, amputation, death.

I. **Risk factors/causes:**
   A. Fractures.
   B. Burns.
   C. Crushing injuries.
   D. Restrictive bandages.
   E. Cast.
   F. Prolonged lithotomy positioning.

II. **Pathophysiology:** inability of the fascia surrounding the muscle group to expand to accommodate the increased volume of fluid → increased compartment pressure → impaired venous flow → continued arterial flow, increasing capillary pressure → pushing of fluid into the extravascular space → further increased intracompartment pressure → prolonged or severe ischemia → destruction of muscle and nerve cells; contracture; loss of function; necrotic tissue; infection; release of potassium, hydrogen, and myoglobin into bloodstream.

◄ III. **Assessment**
   A. *Subjective data*:
      1. Severe, unrelenting *pain*, unrelieved by narcotics and associated with passive stretching of muscle.
      2. *Paresthesias*.
   B. *Objective data*:
      1. Edema; tense skin over limb.
      2. *Paralysis*.
      3. Decreased or absent peripheral *pulses*.
      4. Poor capillary refill.
      5. Limb temperature change (colder).
      6. Ankle-arm pressure index *decreased*: 0.4 indicates ischemia (see **Chap. 3, Doppler ultrasonography, p. 33**).
      7. Urine: *decreased* output (developing acute tubular necrosis), reddish brown.

◄ IV. **Analysis/nursing diagnosis**
   A. *Pain* related to tissue swelling and ischemia.
   B. *Risk for injury* related to neuromuscular deficits.
   C. *Impaired physical mobility* related to contracture and loss of function.
   D. *Risk for infection* related to tissue necrosis.
   E. *Altered urinary elimination* related to acute tubular necrosis resulting from myoglobin accumulation.
   F. *Body image disturbance* related to limb disfigurement.

◄ V. **Nursing care plan/implementation**
   A. Goal: *recognize early indications of ischemia*
      ☞ 1. Assess neurovascular status frequently (q1h): skin temperature, capillary refill, peripheral pulses, mobility, and sensation.

2. Listen to client complaints; report suspected complications.
3. Report nonrelief of pain with narcotics.
4. Recognize unrelenting pain with passive muscle stretching (*positive Homans's* sign in lower extremities).

B. Goal: *prevent complications.*
   1. *Position*: if compartment syndrome suspected, keep extremity at heart level to prevent compensatory increase in blood flow; *do not* elevate.
   2. *Do not* apply ice, which would further hinder already-impaired arterial flow.
   3. *Avoid tight* bandages, splints, or casts.
   ☞ 4. Monitor intravenous infusion for signs of infiltration.
   5. Prepare to remove dressings or cast.
   6. Prepare client for *fasciotomy* (incision of skin and fascia to release tight compartment).

VI. Evaluation/outcome criteria
   A. Relief from pain; normal perfusion restored.
   B. Neurovascular status within normal limits.
   C. Retains function of limb; no contractures or infection.
   D. Compartment pressure returns to normal (<20 mm Hg).
   E. No systemic complications (e.g., normal cardiac and renal function, acid-base balance within normal limits).

Immobility

Impaired physical mobility or limitation of physical movement resulting from various causes that may be accompanied by many complications that can involve any or all of the major systems of the body. The complications are summarized in **Table 20.5.**

I. **Types of immobility:**
   A. *Physical*—caused by limitation in physical movement or physiologic processes (e.g., breathing).
   B. *Intellectual*—caused by lack of knowledge (e.g., mental retardation, brain damage).
   C. *Emotional*—caused by highly stressed situations (e.g., after loss of loved person, diagnosis of terminal illness).
   D. *Social*—occurring when social interaction decreased due to separation from family when hospitalized or alone, as in old age.

II. **Risk factors/causes:**
   A. Pain, trauma, injury.
   B. Loss of body function or body part.
   C. Chronic disease.
   D. Emotional, mental illness; neglect.
   E. Malnutrition.
   F. Bed rest, traction, surgery, medications.

III. Assessment
   A. *Subjective data: psychological/social effects* of immobility:
      1. Decreased motivation to learn, retention.
      2. Decreased problem-solving abilities.
      3. Diminished drives, hunger (anorexia).
      4. Changes in body image, self-concept.
      5. Exaggerated emotional reactions, inappropriate to situation or person; aggression, apathy, withdrawal.
      6. Deterioration of time perception.
      7. Fear, anxiety, worthlessness related to change in role activities (e.g., when no longer employed).
   B. *Objective data: physical effects* of immobility:
      1. *Cardiovascular*:
         a. Orthostatic hypotension.
         b. Increased cardiac load.
         c. Thrombus formation.
      2. *Gastrointestinal*:
         a. Diarrhea.
         b. Constipation.
      3. *Metabolic*:
         a. Tissue atrophy and protein catabolism.
         b. Basal metabolic rate *reduced.*
         c. Fluid/electrolyte imbalances.
      4. *Musculoskeletal*:
         a. Demineralization (osteoporosis).
         b. Contractures and atrophy.
         c. Skin breakdown.
      5. *Respiratory*:
         a. Decreased respiratory movement.
         b. Accumulation of secretions in respiratory tract.
         c. Oxygen/carbon dioxide level imbalance.
      6. *Urinary*:
         a. Calculi.
         b. Bladder distention, stasis.
         c. Infection.
         d. Frequency.

IV. Analysis/nursing diagnosis
   A. *Impaired physical mobility* related to specific client condition.
   B. *Impaired skin integrity* related to physical immobilization.
   C. *Urinary retention* related to incomplete emptying of bladder.
   D. *Constipation* related to inactivity.
   E. *Risk for disuse syndrome* related to lack of ROM.
   F. *Bathing/hygiene self-care deficit* related to musculoskeletal impairment.
   G. *Sensory/perceptual alteration* related to complications of immobility.
   H. *Body image disturbance* related to physical limitations.

⋈ V. **Nursing care plan/implementation**

A. Goal: *prevent physical, psychological hazards.*

1. Apply nursing measures to promote venous flow, muscle strength, endurance, joint mobility, skin integrity.

2. Assess and counteract *psychological* effect of immobility (e.g., feelings of helplessness, hopelessness, powerlessness).

3. Help maintain accurate sensory processing to prevent or lessen *sensory disturbances.*

4. Help adapt to *altered body image* due to increased dependency, sensory deprivation, changes in status and power that accompany immobility.

5. Offer counseling when sexual expression is impaired.

B. Goal: **health teaching**: ways to prevent physical problems related to immobility (e.g. UTI, *anticonstipation* diet, ROM exercises, skin care); teach activities that encourage independence and provide sensory stimulation while immobile.

⋈ VI. **Evaluation/outcome criteria**

A. Minimal contractures, skin breakdown, muscle atrophy or loss of strength.

B. Interest in self and environment; positive self-image.

C. Returns to optimal level of physical activity.

Osteoarthritis

Joint disorder characterized by degeneration of articular cartilage and formation of bony outgrowths at edges of weight-bearing joints.

I. **Pathophysiology**: excessive friction combined with risk factors → thinning of articular cartilage, narrowing of joint space, and loss of joint stability; erosion of cartilage → formation of shallow pits on articular surface, exposure of bone in joint space. Bone responds by becoming denser and harder.

II. **Risk factors/causes:**

A. Aging (>50 yr).

B. Rheumatoid arthritis.

C. Arteriosclerosis.

D. Obesity.

E. Trauma.

F. Family history.

⋈ III. **Assessment**

A. *Subjective data*:

1. Pain; tender joints.

2. Fatigability, malaise.

3. Anorexia.

4. Cold intolerance.

5. Extremities: numb, tingling.

B. *Objective data*:

1. *Joints*:

a. Enlarged.

b. Stiff, limited movement.

c. Swelling, redness, heat around affected joint.

d. Shiny stretched skin over and around joint.

e. Subcutaneous nodules.

2. Weight loss.

3. Fever.

4. Crepitation (creaking or grating of joints).

5. Deformities, contractures.

6. Cold, clammy extremities.

7. Lab data: *decreased* hemoglobin; *elevated* white blood cell count (WBC).

〰 8. *Diagnostic tests*: x-ray studies, thermography, arthroscopy (see **Diagnostic Studies** box at end of chapter).

⋈ IV. **Analysis/nursing diagnosis**

A. *Pain* related to friction of bones in joints.

B. *Bathing/hygiene self-care deficit* related to decreased mobility of involved joints.

C. *Risk for injury* related to fatigue.

D. *Impaired physical mobility* related to stiff, limited movement.

E. *Impaired home maintenance management* related to contractures.

⋈ V. **Nursing care plan/implementation**

A. Goal: *promote comfort: reduce pain, spasms, inflammation, swelling.*

1. Medications as prescribed:

a. *Anti-inflammatory* agents: aspirin (*Ecotrin*), ibuprofen (*Motrin*), indomethacin (*Indocin*).

b. Prepare client for intraarticular injections of *corticosteroids* or *hyaluronic acid*, as prescribed.

☞ 2. Heat to reduce muscle spasm.

☞ 3. Cold to reduce swelling and pain.

4. Prevent contractures:

a. Exercise.

b. Bed rest on firm mattress during attacks.

☞ c. Splints to maintain proper alignment.

5. *Position: elevate* extremity to reduce swelling.

6. Rest.

7. Assistive devices to decrease weight bearing on affected joints (canes, walkers.)

B. Goal: **health teaching** *to promote independence.*

1. Encourage self-care with assistive devices for activities of daily living.

2. Activity, as tolerated, with ambulation-assistive devices.

3. Scheduled rest periods.

4. Correct body posture and body mechanics.

C. Goal: *provide for emotional needs.*

1. Accept feelings of frustration regarding long-term debilitating disorder.

2. Provide diversional activities appropriate for age and physical condition to promote comfort and satisfaction.

(continued on p. 271)

TABLE 20.5 COMPLICATIONS OF IMMOBILIZATION

Disorder	Pathophysiology	▶ Assessment	▶ Analysis/Nursing Diagnosis	▶ Nursing Care Plan/Implementation	▶ Evaluation/Outcome Criteria
ORTHOSTATIC HYPOTENSION	A decrease in BP >30/15 mm Hg caused by failure of vasomotor responses to compensate for change from a recumbent to an upright position.	*Subjective data:* weakness; dizziness with position change. *Objective data:* decreased BP >30/15 mm Hg measured 2 min after moving from a supine to a sitting or standing position; loss of muscle tone and strength; client may faint.	*Decreased cardiac output related* to orthostatic hypotension. *Risk for injury* related to vertigo. *Activity intolerance,* related to dizziness.	*Prevent trauma due to sudden decrease in BP:* 1. Change position gradually. 2. Elastic stockings. 3. Leg exercises. 4. Dangle before getting up. 5. Tilt table. 6. Sitting and lying BP. 7. Monitor side effects of drugs. **☞ Health teaching:** 1. Explain signs and symptoms to client. 2. Encourage client to dangle before standing. 3. Encourage slow movement from sitting to standing. 4. Exercises to maintain muscle tone.	Client tolerates increased activity. No trauma occurs. BP remains within normal limits.
CARDIAC OVERLOAD	When the body is recumbent, some of the total blood volume that would be in the legs due to gravity is redistributed to other parts of the body, thereby increasing the circulating volume and increasing the workload of the heart; heart rate, which is decreased because blood is prevented from entering the thoracic vessels by pressure from the *Valsalva maneuver,* increases when normal breathing resumes.	*Subjective data:* fear, apprehension. *Objective data:* *Valsalva maneuver* (pressure against the closed glottis when breath is held) 10–20 times/h, when trying to move in bed; tachycardia; decreased exercise tolerance.	*Risk for injury* related to increased workload of heart. *Activity intolerance* related to increased workload of heart. *Fear* related to tachycardia.	*Prevent injury and further ischemic damage to cardiac tissue* by decreasing workload of heart: 1. Out of bed in chair when possible. 2. *Semirecumbent position* when in bed; pillows between legs when side-lying. 3. Exercises: passive and active ROM, isometric. 4. Encourage participation in self-care. 5. Turn every 2 h, dangle. 6. *Avoid* Valsalva maneuver, fatigue. 7. Minimize constipation. 8. Encourage slow, deep breathing when moving in bed. **☞ Health teaching:** 1. Exhale while turning, don't hold breath. 2. Measures to conserve energy.	No complications noted. Client tolerates increased activity. Heart rate within normal limits.

(Continued)

TABLE 20.5 COMPLICATIONS OF IMMOBILIZATION *(continued)*

Disorder	Pathophysiology	⊠ Assessment	⊠ Analysis/Nursing Diagnosis	⊠ Nursing Care Plan/Implementation	⊠ Evaluation/Outcome Criteria
THROMBUS FORMATION	Mass of blood constituents formed in the heart or blood vessels due to pooling of blood from lack of activity; increased viscosity related to dehydration or possible external pressure.	*Subjective data:* discomfort over involved vessel. *Objective data:* increased: RBC, venous stasis, hypercoagulability.	*Altered peripheral tissue perfusion* related to obstructed vessel. *Risk for injury* related to emboli.	*Prevent injury* by reducing risk factors and venous stasis: 1. *Position:* change q1–2h 2. *Do not gatch* bed (causes pressure against leg vessels). 3. *Increase fluid* intake. 4. Monitor coagulation lab values. 5. *Medications: anticoagulation* therapy, as prescribed for clients at risk (immobilized, trauma, low pelvic surgery). 6. Ambulate as soon as possible. ☞ **Health teaching:** 1. How to recognize signs of thrombophlebitis/thromboemboli. 2. Leg exercise program to strengthen muscles for improved tone, to prevent pooling of blood in vessels. 3. Precautions necessary when on anticoagulation therapy. 4. Side effects of anticoagulation therapy (bleeding from gums, body fluids, obvious bleeding).	
RESPIRATORY CONGESTION— *decreased respiratory movements.*	Decreased thoracic movement due to restriction against bed or chair, lack of position change, restrictive clothing or binders/bandages, or abdominal distention.	*Subjective data:* dyspnea; pain. *Objective data:* trauma; immobilization of thorax or abdomen, due to position in bed; inability to cough or deep breathe; abdominal distention.	*Ineffective breathing pattern* related to splinting to reduce pain. *Ineffective airway clearance* related to retained secretions. *Impaired physical mobility* related to trauma.	*Prevent complications related to respiratory status:* 1. Maintain a clear airway, assist with *ventilation prn.* 2. Remove or minimize causes of dyspnea. 3. Conserve client's energy (periods of rest and activity—client able to cough more effectively when rested). 4. Incentive spirometry. *Promote comfort:* 1. Maintain hydration and nutrition 2. *Position:* change q2h; out of bed in chair when possible (chest expansion greater when sitting in chair). ☞ **Health teaching:** 1. Methods to allay anxieties precipitated by dyspnea. 2. Effective breathing and coughing exercises.	No respiratory complications or excess secretions noted.

(Continued)

TABLE 20.5 COMPLICATIONS OF IMMOBILIZATION (*continued*)

Disorder	Pathophysiology	Assessment	Analysis/Nursing Diagnosis	Nursing Care Plan/Implementation	Evaluation/Outcome Criteria
RESPIRATORY CONGESTION—*pooled secretions*	Inability of cilia to move normal secretions out of bronchial tree due to: ineffective coughing, lack of thoracic expansion, or effects of medications.	*Subjective data:* dyspnea, pain. *Objective data:* dehydration; drugs—anticholinergic, CNS depressants, anesthesia; inadequate coughing; stationary position.	*Ineffective airway clearance* related to pooled secretions. *Impaired gas exchange* related to ineffective coughing.	*Prevent atelectasis, infection, stasis of air and secretions in lungs:* 1. Maintain patent airway; cough; suction; change position 2. See nursing care plan for Respiratory congestion related to *decreased respiratory movements*, **p. 266**. **Health teaching:** 1. Effective coughing techniques. 2. Importance of adequate hydration	No respiratory complications. Client coughs and removes secretions
OXYGEN-CARBON DIOXIDE IMBALANCE	Imbalance in oxygen and carbon dioxide levels related to pulmonary congestion, ineffective breathing patterns, trauma, or effects of medications.	*Subjective data:* confusion, irritable, restless, dyspnea. *Objective data:* hypoxia, hypercapnia, cyanosis.	*Impaired gas exchange* related to immobilization.	*Promote improved respirations:* 1. Change position frequently 2. Increase *humidification.* 3. Monitor side effects of administered medication, especially *narcotics, barbiturates.* 4. See nursing care plan for Respiratory congestion related to *decreased respiratory movements*, **p. 266**.	No respiratory complications. Respiratory rate and depth are adequate for maintaining balance of oxygen and carbon dioxide.

(*Continued*)

TABLE 20.5 COMPLICATIONS OF IMMOBILIZATION (continued)

Disorder	Pathophysiology	⋈ Assessment	⋈ Analysis/Nursing Diagnosis	⋈ Nursing Care Plan/Implementation	⋈ Evaluation/Outcome Criteria
MALNUTRITION of immobilized adult	Lack of adequate diet intake to maintain healthy tissue related to lack of food; lack of knowledge about food; problems with ingestion, digestion, or absorption; psychosocial factors that influence client's motivation to eat.	*Subjective data:* anorexia, nausea; diet history validating lack of adequate nutritional intake; mental irritability. *Objective data:* 1. Recent weight loss of >10%. 2. *Decreased:* healing ability, GI motility, absorption, secretion of digestive enzymes. 3. *Appearance:* listlessness, muscle weakness; posture—sagging shoulders, sunken chest. 4. Anthropometric data (measurement of size, weight, and body proportions) <85% of standard. 5. *Cardiovascular:* tachycardia (>100 beats/min) on minimal exertion; bradycardia at rest. 6. *Hair:* brittle, dry, thin. 7. *Skin:* dry, scaly. 8. Lack of financial resources: sociocultural influences. 9. *Decreased* blood values: serum albumin, iron-binding capacity, lymphocyte levels, hematocrit, and hemoglobin.	*Altered nutrition, less than body requirements,* related to decreased appetite. *Knowledge deficit* related to nutrition requirements.	*Improved nutritional intake* to maintain basal metabolism requirements and replace losses from catabolism: 1. Provide balanced or prescribed diet, *soft or ground food* if cannot chew or is edentulous. 2. *Increase fluid* intake. 3. Attain/maintain normal weight. 4. Feed, assist with feeding, or place foods within client's reach. *Promote comfort:* 1. Mouth care: to facilitate mastication of food → improved digestion and absorption. 2. Relieve constipation (see nursing care plan for **Constipation, p. 269**). 3. Observe for stomatitis; bleeding; color changes in skin texture, color. 4. Medications: monitor nausea and vomiting side effects of prescribed medications; administer *antiemetics* as ordered to control nausea and vomiting. 5. Ambulate to alleviate flatulence and distention. 6. Alleviate pain and discomfort by providing distractions, increased social interactions, pleasant environment, back-rubs; administering *pain* medications prn, as ordered. **Health teaching:** 1. Diet and elimination 2. See **Appendix B** for foods high in *protein and carbohydrate.*	No complications. Client obtains/ maintains normal weight. No tissue breakdown.

(Continued)

TABLE 20.5 COMPLICATIONS OF IMMOBILIZATION (continued)

Disorder	⧗ Pathophysiology	⧗ Assessment	⧗ Analysis/Nursing Diagnosis	⧗ Nursing Care Plan/Implementation	⧗ Evaluation/Outcome Criteria
CONSTIPATION	Waste material in the bowel is too hard to pass easily; or bowel movements are so infrequent that client has discomfort.	*Subjective data:* discomfort, pain, distress, pressure in the rectum; reported decrease in normal elimination pattern. *Objective data:* immobilization; hard-formed stool, possible palpable impaction; decreased bowel sounds; bowel elimination less frequent than usual.	*Constipation* related to decreased water and fiber intake. *Knowledge deficit* related to dietary and exercise requirements to prevent constipation.	*Promote normal pattern of bowel elimination:* 1. Administer: *stool softeners* or bulk *cathartics* as ordered; oil retention, soap suds *enemas* as ordered. 2. Encourage change of position and activity as tolerated. 3. Provide *high bulk diet.* 4. *Increase* fluid intake. 5. Provide for privacy. 6. Encourage regular time for evacuation. **Health teaching:** 1. Dietary instructions regarding increased fiber 2. Exercise program as tolerated. 3. Increase fluids.	Client has normal bowel elimination pattern. No impactions. Increases fluid and fiber in diet.
OSTEOPOROSIS	Metabolic bone disorder in which there is a generalized loss of bone density due to an imbalance between formation and bone resorption; immobilization can cause calcium losses of 200–300 mg/d.	*Subjective data:* backache. *Objective data:* demineralization of bone seen on x-ray; kyphosis; spontaneous fracture of bone.	*Pain* related to bone fractures or body structural changes.	*Prevent injury related to decreased bone strength:* 1. *Position:* correct body alignment, firm mattress. 2. Encourage self-care activities plan maximal activity allowed by physical condition; muscle exercises against resistance as tolerated. 3. Rest/activity pattern: encourage ROM exercise; *avoid* fatigue. 4. Weight-bearing positions, tilt table. 5. *Diet: high* protein, vitamin C and B complex. 6. *Increase fluids* to prevent renal calculi (calcium from bones could cause kidney stones). 7. Calcium supplement if client is mobile and has normal Ca⁺. **Health teaching:** 1. Dietary instructions, foods to include for *high* protein, *high* vitamin C. 2. Exercise programs. 3. Signs and symptoms of renal calculi.	No fractures. No renal calculi. Incorporates dietary improvements in daily menu selection. Participates in exercise program on a regular basis.

(Continued)

TABLE 20.5   COMPLICATIONS OF IMMOBILIZATION   (continued)

Disorder	Pathophysiology	⌛ Assessment	⌛ Analysis/Nursing Diagnosis	⌛ Nursing Care Plan/Implementation	⌛ Evaluation/Outcome Criteria
CONTRACTURES	Abnormal shortening of muscle tissue, rendering the muscle highly resistant to stretching; related to lack of active or passive ROM, or improper support and positioning of joints affected by arthritis or injury.	*Subjective data:* pain. *Objective data:* muscles—fixed, shortened, decreased tone; resistance of muscles to stretch; decreased ROM in affected limb.	*Impaired physical mobility* related to muscle weakness and contractures. *Pain* related to injury. *Self-care deficit* related to immobility.	*Prevent deformities:* 👉 1. Active and/or passive ROM exercises. 2. *Position:* functional, correct alignment. 3. Footboard to prevent footdrop. 4. *Avoid* foot gatch. 📖 **Health teaching:** 1. Importance of ROM exercises. 2. Correct anatomic positions.	ROM maintained. No deformities noted.
SKIN BREAKDOWN	Presence of risk factors that could lead to skin breakdown, (e.g., immobility, inadequate nutrition, lack of position changes).	*Subjective data:* fatigue, pain, inability to turn on own. *Objective data:* interruption of skin integrity, especially over: ears, occiput, heels, sacrum, scrotum, elbows, trochanter, ischium, scapula; immobilization; malnutrition.	*Impaired skin integrity* related to lack of frequent position change.	*Prevent skin breakdown:* 🖐 1. Change *position* q1–2h and prn, out of bed when possible. 2. Protect from infection. 3. *Increase* dietary intake: *protein, carbohydrates.* 4. *Increase fluids.* *Assess for/reduce contributing factors known to cause decubitus ulcers:* incontinence, stationary position, malnutrition, obesity, sensory deficits, emotional disturbances, paralysis. *Promote healing:* 1. Wash gently, pat dry—to prevent skin abrasion. 2. Clean dry, wrinkle-free bed linens and pads. 3. Massage skin with lotion that does *not* contain alcohol (alcohol dries skin). 👉 4. Protect with *"wafer barrier,"* alternating mattress, sheepskin pads, protectors, flotation devices. 5. *No "doughnuts"* or rubber rings (interfere with circulation of tissue within center of ring).	*No skin breakdown.*

(Continued)

TABLE 20.5 COMPLICATIONS OF IMMOBILIZATION (*continued*)

Disorder	Pathophysiology	⋈ Assessment	⋈ Analysis/Nursing Diagnosis	⋈ Nursing Care Plan/Implementation	⋈ Evaluation/Outcome Criteria
URINARY STASIS	Immobility leads to inability to completely empty the bladder, which increases risk for urinary tract infection and renal calculi.	*Subjective data:* pain, due to infection or renal calculi. *Objective data:* difficulty in urinating due to position or lack of privacy; infection related to catheter insertion or stasis of urine; hematuria.	*Altered urinary elimination* related to inability to empty bladder.	*Prevent urinary infections, stasis, or renal calculi:* 1. Increase activity as allowed. 2. Check for distended bladder. 3. *Increase fluids,* I&O. 4. *Diet: acid-ash* to increase acidity, thereby preventing infection. 5. *Avoid catheterization; use intermittent catheterization instead of Foley whenever possible or Credé maneuver to empty bladder* (manual exertion of pressure on the bladder to force urine out). 6. Bladder training.	No urinary tract infections or evidence of renal calculi. Bladder emptied, no urinary stasis.

P = blood pressure; ROM = range of motion; RBC = red blood cell count; CNS = central nervous system; GI = gastrointestinal; I&O = intake and output.
Source: ©Lagerquist SL: *Little, Brown's NCLEX-RN® Examination Review.* Boston: Little, Brown (out of print).

⋈ **VI. Evaluation/outcome criteria**
   A. Remains independent as long as possible.
   B. No contractures.
   C. States comfort has improved.
   D. Uses adjunctive methods to successfully control pain.

Total Hip Replacement

Femoral head and acetabulum are replaced by a prosthesis, which is cemented into the bone with plastic cement. Performed to replace a joint with limited and painful function due to bony alkalosis and deformity, caused by degenerative joint disease. Goal of the surgery: restore or improve mobilization of hip joint, prevent complications of extended immobilization.

I. **Risk factors/causes:**
   A. Rheumatoid arthritis.
   B. Osteoarthritis.
   C. Complications of femoral neck fractures (**Table 20.6**).
   D. Congenital hip disease.

⋈ II. **Analysis/nursing diagnosis**
   A. *Risk for injury* related to implant surgery.
   B. *Knowledge deficit* regarding joint replacement surgery.
   C. *Impaired physical mobility* related to major hip surgery.
   D. *Pain* related to surgical incision.
   E. *Risk for impaired skin integrity* related to immobility.

⋈ III. **Nursing care plan/implementation**
   A. **Preoperative care:**
      1. Goal: *prevent thrombophlebitis and pulmonary emboli.*
         a. Antiembolic stockings.
         b. *Increase fluid intake.*
      2. Goal: *prevent infection.*
         a. *Antiinfectives* as ordered, given prophylactically.
         b. Assist client with skin scrubs using *antibacterial* soap.
      3. Goal: **health teaching.**
         a. *Isometric exercises*—gluteal, abdominal, and quadriceps-setting; dorsiflexion and plantar flexion of the feet.
         b. Use of trapeze.
         c. Explain position of operative leg and hip postoperatively to prevent *adduction* and flexion.
         d. *Transfer techniques*—bed to chair and chair to crutches; dangle at bedside first time out of bed.
   B. **Postoperative care:**
      1. Goal: *prevent respiratory complications.*

TABLE 20.6 TYPES OF HIP FRACTURES

Type	▶◀ Assessment	Treatment	Complications
Femoral neck (intrascapular)	History of slight trauma Pain in groin and hip Pain with hip movement Usually occurs in women >60 yr Lateral rotation and shortening of leg with minimal deformity	Femoral head replacement with prosthesis, threaded pins Occasionally, primary total hip replacement	Avascular necrosis of femoral head Nonunion Pin complications Dislocation of prosthesis
Intertrochanteric (extracapsular)	History of direct trauma over trochanter Severe pain Tenderness over trochanter Usually women 60–85 yr or younger women with osteoporosis External rotation and shortening of leg with obvious deformity Loss of hip motion	Open reduction: internal fixation with nail, pin, compression plate with screw	Shortening of the leg Traumatic arthritis Pin migration; bending or breaking of pin Fracture impaction Loss of reduction Delayed union or nonunion of bone
Subtrochanteric (extracapsular)	History of direct trauma of great force Proximal leg pain Usually women >60 yr External rotation and shortening of leg with some deformity Large hematoma	Open reduction: internal fixation with intramedullary nail, sliding nail plates, and other fixed plates Closed reduction with nail insertion Closed intramedullary device (nail)	Shortening of the leg Lateral displacement of proximal fragment Metal fatigue

a. Turn, cough, deep breathe.

☞ b. Incentive spirometry.

2. Goal: *prevent complications of shock or infection.*

☞ a. Check dressings for drainage q1h for first 4 h, then q4h and prn; may have Hemovac or other drainage tubes inserted in wound to keep dressing dry.

b. Monitor intake and output, vital signs hourly for 4 h, then q4h and prn.

3. Goal: *prevent contractures, muscle atrophy:*

☞ initiate exercises as soon as allowed: isometric quadriceps, dorsiflexion and plantar flexion of foot, flexion and extension of the ankle.

4. Goal: *promote early ambulation and movement.*

a. Use trapeze.

☞ b. Transfer technique (pivot on unaffected leg), crutches/walker.

c. Initiate progressive ambulation as ordered, ensure maximum extension of leg when walking.

▭ d. Administer *anticoagulants* as ordered to prevent thromboemboli.

e. Recognize early side effects of medications and report appropriately.

5. Goal: *prevent constipation.*

a. *Increase fluid* intake.

b. Use fracture bedpan.

☞ 6. Goal: *prevent dislocation of prosthesis.*

a. Maintain *abduction* of the affected joint (prevent external rotation); *elevate head of bed* (but *not* >90 degrees), turn according to physician's order. When turning to unaffected side, turn with abduction pillow *between* legs to maintain abduction.

b. *Buck's* extension or *Russell's* traction may be applied (temporary skin traction).

c. *Plaster booties* with an abduction bar may be used.

d. Use wedge-shaped *Charnley pillow* to *maintain abduction* between knees and lower legs.

e. Provide periods throughout day when client lies flat in bed to *prevent hip flexion* and strengthen hip muscles.

f. Report signs of dislocation: *anteriorly*—knee flexes, leg turns outward, leg looks longer than other, femur head may be felt in groin area; *posteriorly*—leg turns inward, appears shorter than other, greater trochanter elevated.

7. Goal: *promote comfort.*
   a. Initiate skin care, monitor pressure points for redness; back care q2h.
   b. Alternating pressure mattress, sheepskin when sitting in chair.
8. Goal: **health teaching**.
   a. Exercise program with written list of activity restrictions.
   b. Methods to prevent hip adduction.
   c. *Avoid* sitting for more than 1 h; stand, stretch, and walk frequently to prevent hip flexion contractures.
   d. Advise *not to exceed 90 degrees of hip flexion* (dislocation can occur, particularly with posterior incisions); *avoid* sitting in low chairs.
   e. Teach alternative methods of usual self-care activities to prevent hip dislocation—e.g., *avoid*: bending from waist to tie shoes, sitting up straight in a low chair, using a low toilet seat.
   f. *Avoid*: crossing legs, driving a car for 6 wk.
   g. Wear support hose for 6 wk to enhance venous return and prevent thrombus formation.

IV. **Evaluation/outcome criteria**
   A. Participates in postoperative nursing care plan to prevent complications.
   B. Reports pain has decreased.
   C. Ambulates with assistive devices.
   D. Complications of immobility prevented.
   E. Able to resume self-care activities.

Total Knee Replacement

Both sides of the joint are replaced by metal or plastic implants.

I. **Analysis: see Total Hip Replacement, p. 271.**

II. **Nursing plan/implementation**
   A. See **Total Hip Replacement, p. 271.**
   B. Goal: *to achieve active flexion beyond 70 degrees.*
      1. *Immediately postoperatively*: may have continuous passive motion (CPM) device for flexion/extension of affected knee. Maximum flexion: 110 degrees.
      2. Monitor drainage in *Hemovac*: q15min for first 4 h, q1h until 24 h, then q4h and prn.
      3. *Analgesics*, as ordered.
      4. While dressings are still on: *quadriceps-setting exercises* for approximately 5 d (consult with physical therapist for specific instructions).
      5. After dressings removed: *active flexion exercises*.
      6. *Avoid* pressure on heel.

III. **Evaluation/outcome criteria**
   A. No complications of infection, hemorrhage noted.
   B. ROM of knee increases with exercises.

Amputation

Surgical removal of a limb due to trauma or circulatory impairment (gangrene). The amount of tissue amputated is determined by the severity of disease or trauma and the ability of the remaining tissue to heal.

I. **Risk factors/causes:**
   A. Atherosclerosis obliterans.
   B. Uncontrolled diabetes mellitus.
   C. Malignancy.
   D. Extensive and intractable infection.
   E. Severe trauma.

II. **Assessment**—*preoperative*:
   A. *Subjective data*: pain in affected part.
   B. *Objective data*:
      1. Soft-tissue damage.
      2. Partial or complete severance of a body part.
      3. Lack of peripheral pulses.
      4. Skin color changes, pallor → cyanosis → gangrene.
      5. Infection, hemorrhage, or shock.

III. **Analysis/nursing diagnosis**
   A. *Impaired physical mobility* related to lower limb amputation.
   B. *Body image disturbance* related to loss of body part.
   C. *Pain* related to interruption of nerve pathways.
   D. *Anxiety* related to potential change in lifestyle.
   E. *Knowledge deficit* related to rehabilitation goals.

IV. **Nursing care plan/implementation**
   A. Goal: *prepare for surgery, physically and emotionally.*
      1. Validate that client and family are aware that amputation of body part is planned.
      2. Validate that informed consent is signed.
      3. Allow time for grieving.
      4. If time allows, prepare client for postoperative phase (e.g., teach arm-strengthening exercises if lower limb is to be amputated; teach alternate methods of ambulation).
      5. Provide time to discuss feelings.
      6. Prepare surgical site to decrease possibility of infection (e.g., shave, scrub as ordered).
      7. Discuss postoperative expectations.
   B. Goal: *promote healing postoperatively.*
      1. Monitor respiratory status q1–4h and prn: rate, depth of respiration; auscultate for signs of congestion; question client about chest pain (*pulmonary emboli* common complication).

2. Monitor for hemorrhage; keep tourniquet at bedside; keep Ace wrap secure.

3. Medicate for pain as ordered—client may have phantom limb pain.

4. Support stump on pillow for first 24 h to reduce edema; **remove pillow** after 24 h to prevent contracture.

5. *Position: turn client onto stomach* to prevent hip contracture.

6. ROM exercises for joint above amputation to prevent joint immobilization; strengthening exercises for arms, unaffected limbs, abdominal muscles.

7. Stump care:
   a. Early postoperative dressings changed prn.
   b. As incision heals, bandage is applied in cone shape to prepare stump for prosthesis: prevent edema.
   c. Inspect for blisters, redness, abrasions.
   d. Remove stump sock daily and prn.

8. Assist in rehabilitation program.

C. Goal: **health teaching** *for prosthesis care*:

1. Clean socket with damp cloth to prevent infection

2. Instruct to wear prosthesis when out of bed to prevent swelling

3. Follow up appointment with prosthetist yearly.

V. **Evaluation/outcome criteria**

A. Begins rehabilitation program.

B. No hemorrhage, infection.

C. Adjusts to altered body image.

Gout

Disorder of purine metabolism; genetic disease believed to be transmitted by a dominant gene, characterized by recurrent attacks of acute pain and swelling of one joint (usually the great toe).

I. **Pathophysiology**: urate crystals and infiltrating leukocytes appear to damage the intracellular phagolysosomes → leakage of lysomal enzymes into the synovial fluid → tissue damage, joint inflammation.

II. **Risk factors/causes:**

A. Men.

B. Age (>50 yr).

C. Genetic/familial tendency.

D. Prolonged hyperuricemia (*elevated* serum uric acid level).

III. **Assessment**

A. *Subjective data*:

1. Pain: excruciating.

2. Fatigue.

3. Anorexia.

B. *Objective data*:

1. Joint: erythema (redness), hot, swollen, difficult to move; skin stretched and shiny over joint.

2. Subcutaneous nodules, trophi (deposits of urate) on hands and feet.

3. Weight loss.

4. Fever.

5. Sensory changes, with cold intolerance.

6. Lab data:
   a. Serum uric acid; *increased significantly* (6.5/dL in women, 7.5/dL in men) in *chronic* gout; only *slightly increased* in *acute* gout.
   b. WBC: 12,000–15,000/mm³.
   c. Erythrocyte sedimentation rate: >20 mm/h.
   d. 24-h urinary uric acid: *slightly elevated*.
   e. Proteinuria (*chronic* gout).
   f. Azotemia (presence of nitrogen-containing compounds in blood) in *chronic* gout.

IV. **Analysis/nursing diagnosis**

A. *Pain* related to inflammation and swelling of affected joint.

B. *Impaired physical mobility* related to pain.

C. *Knowledge deficit* related to diet restrictions and increased fluid needs.

D. *Altered urinary elimination* related to kidney damage.

V. **Nursing care plan/implementation**

A. Goal: *decrease discomfort*.

1. Administer antigout medications as ordered:
   a. Treatment of *acute attacks*: colchicine, phenylbutazone (*Butazolidin*), indomethacin (*Indocin*), allopurinol (*Zyloprim*).
   b. *Preventive* therapy: probenecid (*Benemid*), sulfinpyrazone (*Anturane*).

2. Absolute rest of affected joint, then gradual increase in activities, to prevent complications of immobilization; at the same time, rest for comfort.

B. Goal: *prevent kidney damage*.

1. *Increase fluid* intake to 2000–3000 mL/d.

2. Monitor urinary output.

C. Goal: **health teaching**.

1. Need for *low purine diet* during acute attack (see Purine-restricted diet in **Appendix B**.

2. Importance of *increased fluid in diet*.

3. Signs and symptoms of increased disease.

4. Dosage and side effects of prescribed medications.

VI. **Evaluation/outcome criteria**

A. Swelling decreased.

B. Discomfort alleviated.

C. Mobility returned to status before attack.

D. Lab values return to normal.

🦴 Summary of Key Points

1. Impaired musculoskeletal function affects a client's ability to perform basic activities of daily living.

2. A nursing priority in clients with many medical-surgical disorders includes maintaining the ROM of the affected joints.

3. The greatest risk associated with a fracture is not the break itself, but the potential for it to injure nerves, blood vessels, and muscles that surround it. *Bone infection* is another risk.

4. Traction is applied *continuously* unless the physician orders that it be intermittent. *Suspension traction* allows for more movement and activity than running (straight) traction.

5. Regardless of the type of traction, the nurse must regularly assess the *circulation* and *sensation* in and *motor* function of the limb (CSM).

6. The ability to bear weight after surgery for a hip fracture is determined by the fixation procedure used.

7. Dislocation is more common in clients with a prosthesis as compared to those with fixation using a pin, nail, or screw. Remember *abduction*, not adduction, should be employed because bringing the limb closer to the body or "adding" to the body causes dislocation.

8. There are *three types of arthritis*—rheumatoid, osteo, and gouty. The causes are all *different*. However, all *cause* pain and joint immobility, and all are improved with weight loss and treatment with anti-inflammatory agents.

9. Osteoarthritis does not entail the *systemic* involvement of rheumatoid arthritis.

10. The greatest concern after a total hip and knee replacement is *contractures*. Maintaining limb extension or continuous passive motion is done to prevent this.

11. The nursing priorities after an amputation are: preventing *edema*, observing for *bleeding*, and then preventing limb *contractures*.

⩗ Diagnostic Studies/Procedures

Arthroscopy—examination of a joint through a fiberoptic endoscope called an *arthroscope*. Usually done in the operating room (same-day surgery) under aseptic conditions using a local anesthetic, although a general anesthetic may be used. A tourniquet is applied to reduce blood flow to the area while the scope is introduced through a cannula. Saline is used as the viewing medium. Biopsy or removal of loose bodies from the joint may be done. A compression dressing (e.g., Ace bandage) is applied afterward. Restrictions vary according to surgeon preference and nature of procedure. Weight bearing may be immediate or restricted for 24 h. Teach client to observe for signs of infection.

Magnetic Resonance Imaging (MRI)—noninvasive, nonionic technique produces cross-sectional images by exposure to magnetic energy sources. Provides superior contrast of soft tissue, including healthy, benign, and malignant tissue, along with veins and arteries; utilizes no contrast medium; takes 30–90 min to complete; client must *stay still* for periods of 5–20 min at a time. *Client preparation*: client can take food and medications except when undergoing low abdominal and pelvic studies (food/ fluids withheld 4–6 h to decrease peristalsis). *Restrictions*: clients who have metal implants, permanent pacemakers, or implanted medication pumps such as insulin, or who are pregnant or on life support systems. Clients who are obese may not be able to undergo full-body MRI because they may not fit in the scanner tunnel.

💡 Study and Memory Aids

Compartment Syndrome—Characteristics: "Five P's"

Pain
Pale color
Pulselessness
Paralysis
Paresthesias

(Modified from Rogers P: *The Medical Students' Guide to Top Board Scores.* Boston: Little, Brown)

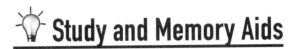 Traction—Nursing Care Plan: "TRACTION"

Trapeze bar overhead to raise and lower upper body
Requires free-hanging weights for body alignment
Analgesia for pain, prn
Circulation (check color and pulse)
Temperature (check extremity)
Infection prevention
Output (monitor)
Nutrition (alteration related to immobility)

Diet

Fractures: Diet to Promote Healing

↑ Bulk
Fluid
Fruits
Iron
Protein
Vitamins

Drug Review

Fractures

Analgesics
Acetaminophen/codeine (*Tylenol* #1, #2, #3): 1–2 tablets q3–4h, as needed
Meperidine HCl (*Demerol*): IM or SC, 50–150 mg
Morphine sulfate: IM or SC, 5–20 mg
Oxycodone/acetaminophen (*Tylox, Percocet*): 5 mg q3–6h, as needed

Anticoagulants
Aspirin: 1.3 g/daily in 2–4 divided doses
Enoxaparin (*Lovenox*): SC, 30-40 mg bid, for 7-10 days
Heparin sodium: IV, 1000 U/h; SC, 8000–10,000 U q8h, adjusted according to partial thromboplastin time (PTT)
Warfarin (*Coumadin*): 10–15 mg/d adjusted according to prothrombin time (PT)

Stool softener
Docusate (*Colace*): 50–500 mg/d

Osteoarthritis

Anti-inflammatories
Aspirin (*Ecotrin*): 2.6–6.2 g/d in divided doses
Ibuprofen (*Motrin*): 300–800 mg 3–4 times/d, *not to exceed* 3200 mg/d
Indomethacin (*Indocin*): 25–50 mg 2–4 times/d

Total Joint Replacement: Hip or Knee

Analgesics
Acetaminophen/codeine (*Tylenol* #1, #2, #3): 1–2 tablets q3–4h, as needed
Meperidine HCl (*Demerol*): IM or SC, 50–150 mg
Morphine sulfate: IM or SC, 5–20 mg
Oxycodone/acetaminophen (*Tylox, Percocet*): 5 mg q3–6h, as needed

Anticoagulants
Aspirin: 1.3 g/d in 2–4 divided doses
Enoxaparin (*Lovenox*): SC, 30-40 mg bid, for 7-10 days
Heparin sodium: IV, 1000 U/h; SC, 8000–10,000 U q8h, adjusted according to PTT
Warfarin (*Coumadin*): 10–15 mg/d, adjusted according to PT

Amputation

Analgesics
Acetaminophen/codeine (*Tylenol* #1, #2, #3): 1–2 tablets q3–q4h, as needed
Meperidine HCl (*Demerol*): IM or SC, 50–150 mg
Morphine sulfate: IM or SC, 5–20 mg
Oxycodone/acetaminophen (*Tylox, Percocet*): 5 mg q3–6h, as needed

Gout (some of the drugs used)

Allopurinol (*Zyloprim*): 200–800 mg/d
Colchicine: *acute*—0.5–2 mg injected IV over several minutes, then 0.5–10 mg q6h until relief obtained; total dose should *not exceed* 4 mg during any 24-h period; prophylaxis, up to 1–1.8 mg/d
Probenecid (*Benemid*): 250 mg bid for one wk; increase to 500 mg bid. Do *not* exceed 3 g/d.
Sulfinpyrazone (*Anturane*): 100–200 mg bid; increase to 800 mg/d in 2 divided doses

Questions

1. The nurse tells the client that to minimize claustrophobia in an MRI scanner, the technician will:
   1. Leave the client alone in the room.
   2. Keep the air flow in the scan room cool.
   3. Give the client a "Walk-man" to listen to music.
   4. Ask the client to keep the eyes open so that the client can see the room.

2. The most important exercise for rebuilding hip muscles to teach a client who has undergone total hip replacement is to:
   1. Press the knee firmly backward into the bed.
   2. Alternately adduct and abduct the hip.
   3. Ride a stationary bicycle 20 to 30 minutes a day.
   4. Do slow deep-knee bends while holding onto a rail.

3. In the immediate period after a total knee replacement, it would be a priority for the nurse to assess the client's:
   1. Bowel sounds.
   2. Pedal pulses.
   3. Urine output.
   4. Gag reflex.

4. Which nursing diagnosis would it be most important to identify when preparing to discharge a client who has undergone a total hip replacement?
   1. Risk for injury.
   2. Impaired adjustment.
   3. Sleep pattern disturbance.
   4. Impaired physical mobility.

5. A client who has fractured the left foot will be using crutches until a walking cast is applied. When teaching the client the correct technique for the three-point gait, the instructions would include:
   1. Advancing the left crutch, then the right foot, followed by the right crutch, then the left foot.
   2. Moving the left crutch and right foot forward together, then the right crutch and left foot.
   3. Advancing both crutches forward, then swinging both legs forward.
   4. Moving both crutches and the injured leg forward, then moving the other leg.

6. A client fractured the femur 3 days ago. The nurse would recognize the signs and symptoms of a fat embolism if the client experienced:
   1. Disorientation, dyspnea, and tachycardia.
   2. Petechiae over the chest and bradycardia. *↓ tachycardia*
   3. Pain, swelling, and redness in the extremity.
   4. Cyanosis and Cheyne-Stokes breathing.

7. A client is temporarily placed in Buck's extension traction while awaiting surgery for a fractured hip. The nurse would recognize a complication of the treatment if the following was noted:
   1. Redness and drainage at the pin site.
   2. Dusky color of the toes of the affected leg.
   3. Flushed skin over the fracture site.
   4. Dorsiflexion of the affected foot.

8. The nurse can tell a client with degenerative joint disease that the most frequent side effect of the ibuprofen often used in its treatment can be minimized by:
   1. Taking the drug with meals.
   2. Drinking cranberry juice.
   3. Taking the drug at regular intervals.
   4. Taking the drug before meals.

9. During an acute flare-up of osteoarthritis, the client should be advised to:
   1. Immobilize the affected joints.
   2. Continue passive range-of-motion exercises.
   3. Decrease the doses of prescribed medications.
   4. Stay out of the sun.

10. After removal of the dressing on a below-the-knee amputation, the nurse would wash the well-healed stump with:
    1. Soap and water.
    2. Lotion and water.
    3. Dilute hydrogen peroxide.
    4. Betadine solution.

11. Correct instructions on the use of a cane would include the importance of:
    1. Holding the cane on the same side as the affected leg.
    2. Moving the cane and the unaffected leg in unison.
    3. Using the cane on the side opposite the affected leg.
    4. Keeping the elbow flexed while bearing weight on the hand grip.

12. The nurse can explain to the client that the purpose of wrapping an above-the-knee amputation with an elastic bandage 10 days after surgery is to:
    1. Promote muscle relaxation and comfort.
    2. Shape the stump in preparation for the prosthesis.
    3. Reduce edema in the thigh.
    4. Prevent bleeding from the incision.

13. A client with osteoarthritis asks the nurse why she is not receiving prednisone as her friend with arthritis is. The best response for the nurse to make is that:
    1. Orally administered prednisone is not indicated for the treatment of osteoarthritis.
    2. Addiction to the drug is likely to occur.
    3. Weight gain is a side effect, and this may worsen her condition.
    4. Her friend's treatment is irrelevant.

14. Which crutch-walking gait should the nurse teach a client who cannot put any weight on the affected leg?
    1. Two-point.
    2. Three-point.
    3. Four-point.
    4. Swing-through.

Answers/Rationale

1. **(2)** A client undergoing MRI scanning must be able to tolerate very close surroundings. Keeping the room cool often helps reduce the closed-in feeling. Leaving the client alone (1) may increase the feeling of claustrophobia. Talking to the technologist may help distract the client from the claustrophobia during the procedure. *No metal*, such as that in a radio headset (3), can be in the area, or it may be pulled into the powerful magnet. Closing the eyes, *not* keeping them open (4), may help to decrease the client's sense of closeness. **IMP, APP, 3, SECE, Management of care**

2. **(1)** Pressing the knee firmly backward into the bed strengthens the quadriceps. Any exercise that involves adduction (2) or acute flexion of the hip (3 and 4) may cause the prosthesis to dislocate. **IMP, APP, 3, PhI, Reduction of risk potential**

3. **(2)** Pedal pulses, as well as skin color, capillary refill, warmth, movement, sensation, and ability to dorsiplantar flex the foot, are all assessment priorities, because the circulatory, sensory, and motor status of the operated limb is of the greatest importance to the success of the procedure. Bowel sounds (1), urine output (3), and the gag reflex (4) are all affected by general anesthesia and need to be assessed, but they are *not* as much of a *priority*. **AS, ANL, 6, PhI, Reduction of risk potential**

4. **(1)** The priority in such a client is to prevent injury. The ability to ambulate, get into and out of bed, and sit and stand without dislocating the prosthesis or falling must be determined before

discharge. Problems adjusting (2) or sleeping (3) are not expected problems in such a client. If they are present at discharge, they would probably only become a serious concern if they were prolonged. Immobility (4) would also be a concern at discharge, but the risk for injury as a result of the immobility would be a *more specific choice*. **AN, ANL, 3, SECE, Management of care**

5. (4) Moving both crutches is the first point; moving the injured leg is the second point; and moving the good leg is the third point. The other three options are the three other common types of crutch gaits: the four-point gait (1), the two-point gait (2), and the swing-through gait (3). **IMP, RE/KN, 3, HPM, Health promotion and maintenance**

6. (1) Fat emboli form when fat droplets are forced into the systemic circulation as pressure changes occur in the interior of the fracture; this causes pulmonary effusion and defective gas exchange, resulting in the signs and symptoms of hypoxia and tissue death. Petechiae (2) would be present, but *not* bradycardia. The fractured limb (3) would *not* be *directly* affected by the emboli. Cyanosis (4) would be present, but *not* Cheyne-Stokes breathing, which is an irregular breathing pattern often seen in elderly or clients who are head-injured. **AS, APP, 6, PhI, Physiological adaptation**

7. (2) Buck's traction involves skin traction, and if it is too tight, there would be indications of circulatory impairment. There are *no pins* (1) with skin traction. Skin traction is usually applied distal to the fracture site, so there would be *no visible changes* at the site (3). If there were a problem with the foot position, it might be plantar flexion (foot drop), but *not dorsiflexion* (4). **AN, COM, 3, PhI, Reduction of risk potential**

8. (1) Taking the drug with food will minimize the gastrointestinal (GI) tract irritation that is a side effect of ibuprofen because the food protects the GI mucosa. Another less common side effect is renal toxicity. Drinking cranberry juice (2) would be part of the treatment for *urinary* tract infection to make the urine more acidic. It is important to take most

medication at a regular interval (3), but this does *not prevent* side effects. Taking it before meals (4) would *not minimize* the GI distress. **IMP, COM, 1, PhI, Pharmacological and parenteral therapies**

9. (2) To preserve joint function even during a flare-up, the joint must be exercised. Pain medication should be taken before passive exercise, however. Osteoarthritis is the most common form of arthritis. Joint rest is important, but complete immobilization (1) would *contribute* to joint immobility. The doses of medications would more likely be *increased* than decreased (3). Avoiding sunlight (4) is called for in a client with *systemic lupus erythematosus* who has joint pain. **IMP, APP, 3, PhI, Reduction of risk potential**

10. (1) No special cleansing agents are used, just soap and water. Lotion and water (2) may be used if there is dry skin. Hydrogen peroxide (3) is *not* used as a wound cleansing agent. *Betadine* (4) is used to clean the skin before invasive procedures. **IMP, APP, 3, PhI, Reduction of risk potential**

11. (3) The cane is used on the side *opposite* the affected leg providing better balance and support. It should *not* be used on the *same* side as the affected leg (1). The affected leg, *not* the unaffected leg (2), moves with the cane, and the weight is placed on the unaffected leg. The cane needs to be long enough to allow for elbow extension, *not* flexion (4). **IMP, RE/KN, 3, SECE, Management of care**

12. (2) The purpose of wrapping the stump changes during the postoperative period. The shape of the stump is now important to ensure the proper fit of the prosthesis. A change in the client's position in bed and sitting in a chair would prevent contractures and increase comfort (1); a *bandage would not*. Elevation and wrapping would have been done to relieve edema (3) and minimize bleeding (4) in the *early* postoperative period. **PL, RE/KN, 3, PhI, Reduction of risk potential**

13. (1) Orally administered steroids are generally not indicated for the treatment of osteoarthritis, which is *not a systemic* condition, unless it is severe or life-threatening case. The drug of choice for the relief of arthralgia and joint inflammation is *aspirin* or NSAID, although a steroid may be injected locally. (The friend may have rheumatoid arthritis, which is a *systemic, autoimmune condition*.) Addiction (2) is *not* a concern with steroids. Weight gain (3) is a side effect of steroids and would aggravate the osteoarthritis, but that is *not* the *particular reason* it is not used. The response in option 4 does *not answer* the client's question of why the treatment is different. **IMP, RE/KN, 3, PhI, Pharmacological and parenteral therapies**

14. (4) In the swing-through crutch gait, the weight is either on the unaffected limb or on both crutches, never on the affected limb. In the two-point gait (1), there is some weight placed bilaterally as the client moves a crutch and the opposite limb together;

Key to Codes

Nursing process: **AS**, assessment; **AN**, analysis; **PL**, planning; **IMP**, implementation; **EV**, evaluation. (See **Appendix M** for explanation of nursing process steps.)

Cognitive level: **RE/KN**, recall/knowledge; **COM**, comprehension; **APP**, application; **ANL**, analysis; **EVL**, evaluation; **SYN**, synthesis. (See **Appendix M** for explanation.)

Category of human function: 1, protective; 2, sensory-perceptual; 3, comfort, rest, activity, and mobility; 4, nutrition; 5, growth and development; 6, fluid-gas transport; 7, psychosocial-cultural; 8, elimination. (See **Appendix O** for explanation.)

Client need: **SECE**, safe, effective care environment; **PhI**, physiological integrity; **PsI**, psychosocial integrity; **HPM**, health promotion and maintenance. (See **Appendix P** for explanation.)

Client subneed: (See **Appendix P** for explanation)

however, most of the weight is on the crutch. In the three-point gait (2) there is partial weight bearing on both legs, but if necessary, there could be no weight on the affected leg. The four-point gait (3) involves weight bearing on both limbs, because the crutches and the limbs move independently. **IMP, COM, 3, HPM, Health promotion and maintenance**

Neurologic Disorders

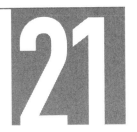

Chapter Outline

- Aphasia
- Traumatic Injuries to the Brain
  - Levels of consciousness
  - Glasgow coma scale
  - Positioning the client who is unconscious
- Increased Intracranial Pressure
- Craniotomy
- Epilepsy
  - Generalized seizures
    - Tonic-clonic (grand mal)
    - Absence (petit mal)
    - Minor motor seizures
  - Partial focal seizures
- Transient Ischemic Attacks
- Brain Attack (Stroke)
  - Bowel/bladder management

- Bacterial Meningitis
- Encephalitis
- Summary of Key Points
- Study and Memory Aids
  - Diagnostic Studies/Procedures
    - Cerebral Angiography
    - Brain Scan
    - EEG
    - Echoencephalography (EEG)
    - Skull X-ray
    - CAT (CT)
    - Lumbar Puncture
  - Drug review
- Questions
- Answers/Rationale

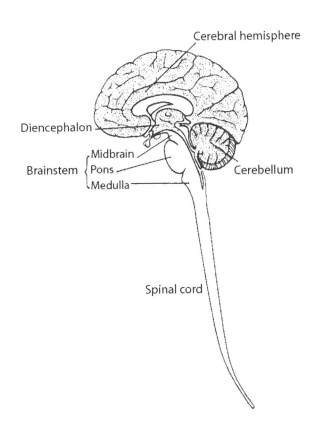

Major Divisions of the Central Nervous System (CNS)

Aphasia

Impaired ability to understand or use commonly accepted words or symbols; interferes with ability to speak, write, and/or read; usually occurs with right-sided hemiplegia in a stroke (brain attack).

I. **Types and pathophysiology:**
   A. *Receptive (sensory)*—lesion usually in Wernicke's area of temporal lobe; difficulty understanding spoken word (*auditory* aphasia) or written word (*visual* aphasia).
   B. *Expressive (motor)*—lesion usually in Broca's area of frontal lobe; difficulty expressing thoughts in speech or writing (*motor* aphasia).

II. **Risk factors/causes:**
   A. Vascular disease of the brain (stroke—also called *brain attack*).
   B. Alzheimer's disease.
   C. Sickle cell anemia.

III. **Analysis/nursing diagnosis**
   A. *Impaired verbal communication* related to cerebral cortex disorder.
   B. *Powerlessness* related to inability to express needs/ concerns.
   C. *Impaired social interaction* related to difficulty communicating.

IV. **Nursing care plan/implementation:** Goal: *assist with communication.*
   A. Assess comprehension: use simple requests, write questions or use picture cards.

B. Stand on client's unaffected side (stay within client's visual field).

C. Talk slowly, clearly; do *not* shout or "talk down" (there is *no* intellectual impairment).

D. Use short, simple phrases; repeat words; ask questions needing one-word answers.

E. Use alternative ways to communicate: hand gestures, picture cards.

F. *Avoid* frustration for client: do *not* force client to repeat words, allow ample time to respond; anticipate needs.

G. Respond to client's speech; if do not understand, tell client; encourage client to use other words.

H. Reinforce techniques taught by speech therapist.

I. Maintain one-way communication: receptive aphasia does *not* always accompany expressive aphasia.

V. **Evaluation/outcome criteria**

A. Communication reestablished.

B. Minimal frustration exhibited.

C. Participates in speech therapy.

Traumatic Injuries to the Brain

I. **Types:**

A. *Concussion*—transient disorder due to injury in which there is brief loss of consciousness due to paralysis of neuronal function; recovery is usually total.

B. *Contusion*—structural alteration of brain tissue characterized by extravasation of blood cells (bruising); injury may occur on side of impact or on opposite side (when cranial contents shift forcibly within the skull with impact).

C. *Laceration*—tearing of brain tissue or blood vessels caused by a sharp bone fragment or object or a tearing force.

D. *Hematomas*:
   1. *Subdural*—blood from ruptured or torn vein collects between arachnoid and dura mater; may be acute, subacute, or chronic.
   2. *Extradural* (epidural)—blood clot located between dura mater and inner surface of skull; most often results from tearing of middle meningeal artery; **emergency condition.**

II. **Pathophysiology** of impaired central nervous system (CNS) functioning:

A. Depressed neuronal activity in reticular activating system → depressed *consciousness* (**Table 21.1**).

B. Depressed neuronal functioning in lower brain stem and spinal cord → depression of reflex activity → decreased eye movements, unequal pupils → decreased response to light stimuli → widely dilated and fixed *pupils*.

C. Depression of respiratory center → altered respiratory pattern → decreased rate → *respiratory arrest.*

III. **Risk factors/causes**: accidents—automobile, industrial and home, motorcycle, military.

TABLE 21.1 LEVELS OF CONSCIOUSNESS

Stage	Characteristics
Alertness	Aware of time and place; responds to voice; appropriate spontaneous activity
Automation	Aware of time and place but demonstrates abnormal mood (euphoria to irritability)
Confusion	Inability to think and speak in coherent manner; responds to verbal requests but is unaware of time and place
Delirium	Restlessness and violent activity; may not comply with verbal instructions
Stupor	Quiet and uncommunicative; may appear unconscious—sits or lies with glazed look; unable to respond to verbal instructions; bladder and rectal incontinence may occur; responds to pain
Semicoma	Unresponsive to verbal instructions but responds to vigorous or painful stimuli; purposeful movement varies
Coma	Unresponsive to vigorous or painful stimuli; may be flaccid or may exhibit posturing

TABLE 21.2 GLASGOW COMA SCALE

Response	Description	Score
Best eye-opening response	Purposeful and spontaneous	4
	To voice	3
	To pain	2
	No response	1
	Untestable	U
Best verbal response	Oriented, alert	5
	Disoriented, confused	4
	Inappropriate words	3
	Incomprehensible sounds	2
	No response	1
	Untestable	U
Best motor response	Obeys commands	6
	Localizes pain	5
	Withdraws from pain	4
	Flexion to pain (decorticate posturing)	3
	Extension to pain (decerebrate posturing)	2
	No response	1
	Untestable	U

⋈ **IV. Assessment**

    A. *Subjective data*:

       1. Headache.

       2. Dizziness, loss of balance.

       3. Double vision.

       4. Nausea.

    B. *Objective data*:

       1. Laceration or abrasion around face or head; scalp vascular, *bloody* appearance with minor injuries.

       2. Drainage from ears or nose.

       3. Projectile vomiting, hematemesis.

       4. Vital signs indicating increased intracranial pressure (ICP) (see **Increased Intracranial Pressure, p. 283-284**).

       5. *Neurologic*:

          a. *Altered level of consciousness*; a numerical assessment, such as the *Glasgow Coma Scale* (**Table 21.2**), may be used. Generally, the lower the score, the poorer the prognosis.

          b. *Pupils*—equal, round, react to light, or unequal, dilated, unresponsive to light.

          c. *Extremities*—paresis or paralysis.

          d. *Reflexes*—hypo- or hypertonia; *Babinski* present (flaring of great toe when sole is stroked).

          e. See **Diagnostic Studies** box, **p. 290**.

⋈ **V. Analysis/nursing diagnosis**

    A. *Altered thought processes* related to brain trauma.

    B. *Sensory/perceptual alteration* related to depressed neuronal activity.

    C. *Risk for injury* related to impaired CNS functioning.

    D. *Risk for aspiration* related to respiratory depression.

    E. *Self-care deficit* related to altered level of consciousness.

    F. *Risk for disuse syndrome* related to paresis or paralysis.

⋈ **VI. Nursing care plan/implementation**

    A. Goal: *sustain vital functions and minimize or prevent complications*

       1. Patent airway: *endotracheal* tube or tracheostomy may be ordered.

       2. *Oxygen*: as ordered (because hypoxia increases cerebral edema).

       3. *Position*: semiprone or prone (*coma* position) with head level to prevent aspiration (*keep off back*); turn side to side to prevent stasis in lungs (see **Positioning** box below).

       4. Vital signs as ordered.

       5. *Neurologic check*: pupils, level of consciousness, muscle strength; report changes.

       6. *Seizure precautions*: padded siderails.

       7. Medications, as ordered:

          a. *Steroids* (dexamethasone [*Decadron*]).

          b. *Anticonvulsants* (phenytoin [*Dilantin*], phenobarbital).

          c. *Analgesics* (**morphine contraindicated**).

       8. Cooling measures or hypothermia to reduce elevated temperature.

       9. Assist with *diagnostic tests*:

          a. *Lumbar puncture* (**contraindicated** with increased ICP).

          b. *Electroencephalogram* (EEG).

      10. *Diet*: NPO for 24 h, progressing to clear liquids if awake.

      11. *Fluids*: IVs, *nasogastric tube* feedings, intake and output (I&O).

      12. Monitor blood chemistries: sodium imbalance common with head injuries.

    B. Goal: *provide emotional support and use comfort measures.*

       1. Comfort: skin care, oral hygiene; sheepskins; wrinkle-free linen.

       2. Eyes: lubricate q4h with artificial tears if periocular edema present.

       3. Range of motion (ROM) exercises—passive, active; physical therapy as tolerated.

       4. *Avoid* restraints.

       5. Encourage verbalization of concerns about changes in body image, limitations.

       6. Encourage family communication.

⋈ **VII. Evaluation/outcome criteria**

    A. Alert, oriented—no residual effects (e.g., cognitive processes intact).

    B. No signs of increased ICP (e.g., decreased respirations, increased systolic pressure with widening pulse pressure, bradycardia).

    C. No paralysis—regains motor/sensory function.

    D. Resumes self-care activities.

Increased Intracranial Pressure

Intracranial hypertension associated with altered states of consciousness.

I. **Pathophysiology**: increases in intracranial blood volume, cerebrospinal fluid (CSF), and/or brain

---

POSITIONING THE CLIENT WHO IS UNCONSCIOUS

Condition	Key Point	Rationale
Coma	Turn on side with head slightly *lowered*—"coma" position.	1. Important to let secretions drain out by gravity. 2. Must prevent aspiration.

Source: Jane Vincent Corbett, RN, MS, EdD, Professor Emerita, School of Nursing, University of San Francisco (reprinted with permission).

tissue mass → cerebral distortion → increased ICP → impaired neural impulse transmission → cellular anoxia, atrophy.

II. **Risk factors/causes:**
   A. Congenital anomalies (hydrocephalus).
   B. Space-occupying lesions (abscesses or tumors).
   C. Trauma (hematomas or skull fractures).
   D. Circulatory problems (aneurysms, emboli).
   E. Inflammation (meningitis, encephalitis).

⋈ III. **Assessment**
   A. *Subjective data*:
      1. Headache.
      2. Nausea.
   B. *Objective data*:
      1. Changes in level of consciousness.
      2. Pupillary changes—unequal, dilated (side opposite to injury), unresponsive to light (*late sign*).
      3. Vital signs—changes are variable (opposite of shock).
         a. *Blood pressure*—gradual or rapid elevation, widened pulse pressure.
         b. *Pulse*—bradycardia (*early*), tachycardia (*late*); significant sign is *slowing of pulse as blood pressure rises*.
         c. *Respiration*—pattern changes (*Cheyne-Stokes*, apneusis, *Biot's*), deep and sonorous.
         d. *Temperature*—moderate elevation.
      4. Projectile vomiting.
      5. See **Diagnostic Studies** section at the end of the chapter.

⋈ IV. **Analysis/nursing diagnosis**
   A. *Altered cerebral tissue perfusion* related to increased ICP.
   B. *Altered thought processes* related to cerebral anoxia.
   C. *Ineffective breathing pattern* related to compression of respiratory center.
   D. *Risk for aspiration* related to unconsciousness.
   E. *Self-care deficit* related to altered level of consciousness.
   F. *Impaired physical mobility* related to abnormal motor responses.

⋈ V. **Nursing care plan/implementation:** *promote adequate oxygenation and limit further impairment.*
   A. Vital signs: report changes **immediately**.
   ☞ B. Patent *airway*; keep alkalotic, to prevent increased ICP resulting from elevated CO_2; brief periods of hyperventilation may be useful to decrease $PaCO_2$, which causes vasoconstriction → ↓ in ICP; aggressive hyperventilation is *contraindicated*.
   ⊂▭ C. Give medications as ordered:
      1. *Hyperosmolar diuretics* (*mannitol*, urea) to reduce brain swelling.

   2. *Steroids* (dexamethasone [*Decadron*]) for anti-inflammatory action (may be of limited value).
   3. *Antacids* or H_2 antagonist or proton pump inhibitors to prevent stress ulcer.
   4. High-dose barbiturates (pentobarbital [*Nembutal*], thiopental [*Pentothal*]) may be used in clients with IICP refractory to other treatments.
   D. *Position*: elevate head of bed 30 degrees; *avoid* flexion/rotation of neck.
   E. Fluids: *maintain normovolemia;*, strict I&O; monitor fluid and electrolytes.
   ☞ F. Cooling measures to reduce temperature, as fever increases ICP.
   G. Prepare for surgical intervention (see **Craniotomy, below**).

⋈ VI. **Evaluation/outcome criteria**
   A. No irreversible brain damage—regains consciousness.
   B. Resumes self-care activities.

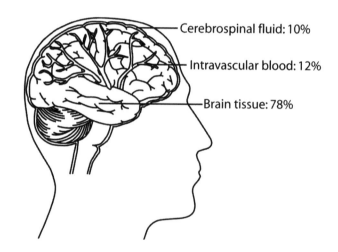

Cerebrospinal fluid: 10%
Intravascular blood: 12%
Brain tissue: 78%

Components of the Brain

Craniotomy

Excision of a part of the skull (burr hole to several centimeters) for exploratory purpose and biopsy; to remove neoplasms, evacuate hematomas or excess fluid, control hemorrhage, repair skull fractures, remove scar tissue, repair or excise aneurysms, drain abscesses; produces minimal neurologic deficit.

⋈ I. **Analysis/nursing diagnosis**
   A. *Altered cerebral tissue* perfusion related to edema.
   B. *Altered thought processes* related to disorientation.
   C. *Self-care deficit* related to continued neurologic impairment.
   D. Also see **analysis/nursing diagnosis** for Traumatic Injuries to the Brain (**p. 282**), Increased Intracranial Pressure (**p. 283**), and Perioperative Nursing, (**p. 127, 131**).

II. Nursing care plan/implementation

A. Preoperative care:

1. Goal: *obtain baseline measurements.*
   a. Vital signs.
   b. Level of consciousness.
   c. Mental, emotional status.
   d. Pupillary reactions.
   e. Motor strength, functioning.
2. Goal: *provide psychological support:* listen; give accurate, brief explanations.
3. Goal: *prepare for surgery.*
   a. Cut hair, shave scalp (may be done in operating room).
   b. Cover scalp with clean towel.
   c. Administer *enema* and/or cathartics, as ordered.
   d. Insert indwelling *Foley catheter,* as ordered.

B. Postoperative care:

1. Goal: *prevent complications and limit further impairment.*
   a. *Vital signs* (**indications of complications**):
      (1) Decreased blood pressure—*shock.*
      (2) Widened pulse pressure—*increased ICP.*
      (3) Respiratory failure—*compression* of medullary *respiratory* centers.
      (4) Hyperthermia—disturbance of heat-regulating mechanism, *infection.*
   b. *Neurologic:*
      (1) *Pupils*—ipsilateral dilatation (increased ICP), visual disturbances.
      (2) *Altered level of consciousness.*
      (3) *Altered cognitive or emotional status*—disorientation common.
      (4) *Motor function and strength*—hypertonia, hypotonia, seizures.
   c. Blood gases, to monitor adequacy of ventilation.
   d. Dressings: check frequently, aseptic technique, reinforce as necessary.
   e. Observe for:
      (1) CSF leakage (glucose-positive drainage from nose, mouth, ears)—**report immediately.**
      (2) Periorbital edema—apply light ice compresses as necessary—remove crusts from eyelids.
   f. Check integrity of seventh cranial nerve (facial)—incomplete closure of eyelids.
   g. *Position:*
      (1) *Supratentorial surgery* (cerebrum)—semi-Fowler's (*30-degree elevation*); may *not* lie on operative side.
      (2) *Infratentorial* (brain stem, cerebellum)—*flat* in bed (prone),

may turn to either side but *not* onto back.
   h. Fluids: NPO for 24–48 h.
   i. Medications as ordered:
      (1) *Osmotic diuretics* (mannitol).
      (2) *Corticosteroids* (dexamethasone [*Decadron*]).
      (3) *Mild analgesics* (do *not* mask neurologic or respiratory depression).
   j. Orient frequently to person, time, place—to reduce restlessness, confusion.
   k. Siderails up for safety.
   l. *Avoid* restraints (may increase agitation and ICP).
   m. Ice bags to head to reduce headache.
   n. Activity: assist with ambulation.
2. Goal: *provide optimal supportive care.*
   a. Cover scalp once dressings are removed (scarves, wigs).
   b. Deal realistically with neurologic deficits—facilitate acceptance, adjustment, independence.
3. Goal: **health teaching.**
   a. Prepare for physical, occupational, and/or speech therapy, as needed.
   b. Activities of daily living.

III. Evaluation/outcome criteria

A. Regains consciousness—is alert, oriented.

B. Resumes self-care activities within limits of neurologic deficits.

Epilepsy

Seizure disorder characterized by sudden, transient aberration of brain function; associated with motor, sensory, autonomic, or psychic disturbances.

I. Seizure: involuntary muscular contraction and disturbances of consciousness resulting from abnormal electrical activity.

II. Risk factors/causes:

A. Brain injury.

B. Infection (meningitis, encephalitis).

C. Water and electrolyte disturbances.

D. Hypoglycemia.

E. Tumors.

F. Vascular disorders (hypoxia or hypocapnia).

G. Congenital abnormalities.

H. Degenerative diseases.

III. Generalized seizures:

A. *Tonic-clonic (grand mal)* seizures:
   1. **Pathophysiology:** increased excitability of a neuron → possible activation of adjacent neurons → synchronous discharge of

impulses → vigorous involuntary sustained muscle spasms (*tonic* contractions). Onset of neuronal fatigue → intermittent muscle spasms (*clonic* contractions) → cessation of muscle spasms → fatigue.

2. **Assessment**

a. *Subjective data*—aura: flash of light; peculiar smell, sound; feelings of fear; euphoria.

b. *Objective data*:

(1) *Convulsive stage*—tonic and clonic muscle spasms, loss of consciousness, breathholding, frothing at mouth, biting of tongue, urinary or fecal incontinence; lasts 2–5 min.

(2) *Postconvulsion*—*subjective data*: headache, fatigue (postictal sleep); malaise, sore muscles, *objective data*: vomiting, choking on secretions, aspiration.

(3) See **Diagnostic Studies** box, **p. 290.**

B. *Absence* (petit mal) seizures:

1. **Pathophysiology**: unknown etiology, momentary loss of consciousness (10–20 sec); usually no recollection of seizure; resumes previously performed action.

2. **Assessment**–*objective data*:

a. Fixation of gaze, blank facial expression.

b. Flickering of eyelids.

c. Jerking of facial muscle or arm.

C. *Minor motor seizures*:

1. *Myoclonic*—involuntary jerking contraction of major muscles, may throw person to the floor.

2. *Akinetic*—momentary loss of muscle movement.

3. *Atonic*—total loss of muscle tone; person falls to the floor.

IV. **Partial (focal) seizures**:

A. *Partial motor*—arises from region in motor cortex (posterior frontal lobe); most commonly begins in upper extremities, spreading to face and lower extremities (*jacksonian march*); noting *progression* is important in identifying area of cortex involved.

B. *Partial sensory*—sensory symptoms occur with partial seizure activity; vary with region in brain—transient.

C. *Partial complex* (psychomotor)—arises out of anterior temporal lobe; frequently begins with an aura; characteristic feature is *automatism* (lip smacking, chewing, patting body, picking at clothes); lasts from 2–3 to 15 min; do *not* restrain.

V. **Analysis/nursing diagnosis**

A. *Risk for injury* related to convulsive disorder.

B. *Anxiety* related to sudden loss of consciousness.

C. *Self-esteem disturbance* related to chronic illness.

D. *Impaired social interaction* related to self-consciousness.

VI. **Nursing care plan/implementation** (*generalized* seizures)

A. Goal: *prevent injury during seizure.*

1. Do *not* force jaws open during convulsion.

2. Do *not* restrict limbs—protect from injury, place something soft under head (towel, jacket, hands).

3. Loosen constrictive clothing.

4. Note time, level of consciousness, type and duration of seizure.

B. Goal: *postseizure care*:

1. *Turn on side* to drain saliva and facilitate breathing.

2. *Suction* as necessary.

3. Orient to time and place.

4. Administer oral hygiene if tongue or cheek injured.

5. Check vital signs, pupils, level of consciousness.

C. Goal: *prevent or reduce recurrences of seizure activity.*

1. Encourage client to identify precipitating factors.

2. Moderation in diet and exercise.

3. Medications as ordered: phenytoin (*Dilantin*); phenobarbital; carbamazepine (*Tegretol*); primidone (*Mysoline*); trimethadione (*Tridione*)—*petit mal only.*

D. Goal: **health teaching.**

1. Medications:

a. Actions, side effects (apathy, ataxia, hyperplasia of gums).

b. Complications with sudden withdrawal (*status epilepticus*).

2. Attitude toward life and treatment, adhere to medication regimen.

3. Clarify misconceptions, fears—especially about insanity, bad genes.

4. Maintain activities, interests—*except* no driving until seizure-free for period of time specified by state Department of Motor Vehicles.

5. *Avoid*: stress, lack of sleep, emotional upset, alcohol.

6. Relaxation techniques, stress-management techniques.

7. Wear MedicAlert band or tag.

8. Appropriate community resources.

VII. **Evaluation/outcome criteria**

A. Avoids precipitating stimuli—achieves seizure control.

B. Complies with medication regimen.

C. Retains independence.

Transient Ischemic Attacks (TIAs)

Temporary, complete, or relatively complete cessation of cerebral blood flow to a localized area of brain, producing symptoms ranging from weakness and numbness to monocular blindness; an important *precursor* to a stroke (brain attack). Surgical intervention includes *carotid endarterectomy*; most common postoperative cranial nerve damage causes vocal cord paralysis or difficulty managing saliva and tongue deviation (cranial nerves VII, X, XI, XII); usually temporary; stroke may also occur.

Brain Attack (Stroke)

Brain lesions resulting from damage to blood vessels supplying brain.

I. **Pathophysiology**: reduced or interrupted blood flow → interruption of nerve impulses down corticospinal tract → decreased or absent voluntary movement on one side of the body (fine movements are more affected than coarse movements); later, autonomous reflex activity → spasticity and rigidity of muscles.

II. **Risk factors/causes**:
   A. Cerebral thrombosis (most common), embolism, hemorrhage.
   B. Prior ischemic episodes (transient ischemic attacks [TIAs]).
   C. Hypertension.
   D. Oral contraceptives.
   E. Emotional stress.
   F. Family history.
   G. Age.
   H. Diabetes mellitus.
   I. Smoking.
   J. Hyperlipidemia.
   K. Obesity.
   L. Heavy alcohol consumption.
   M. Atrial fibrillation.
   N. Sickle cell disease.

III. **Assessment**
   A. *Subjective data*:
      1. Weakness; sudden or gradual loss of movement of extremities on one side.
      2. Difficulty forming words.
      3. Difficulty swallowing (dysphagia).
      4. Nausea, vomiting.
      5. History of TIAs.
   B. *Objective data*:
      1. *Vital signs*:
         a. Blood pressure—*elevated*, widened pulse pressure.
         b. Temperature—*elevated*.
         c. Pulse—normal, slow.
         d. Respiration—tachypnea, altered pattern, deep, sonorous.
      2. *Neurologic*:
         a. *Altered level of consciousness*.
         b. *Pupils*—unequal; vision—*homonymous hemianopsia*.
         c. Ptosis of *eyelid*, drooping *mouth*.
         d. Paresis or paralysis (hemiplegia).
         e. Loss of *sensation* and *reflexes*.
         f. Incontinence of urine or feces.
         g. Aphasia (see **p. 281-282**).
      3. See **Diagnostic Studies** box, **p. 290**.

IV. **Analysis /nursing diagnosis**
   A. *Impaired physical mobility* related to hemiplegia.
   B. *Impaired swallowing* related to paralysis.
   C. *Impaired verbal communication* related to aphasia.
   D. *Risk for aspiration* related to unconsciousness, impaired gag reflex.
   E. *Sensory/perceptual alterations* related to altered cerebral blood flow, visual field blindness.
   F. *Altered thought processes* related to cerebral edema.
   G. *Self-care deficit* related to paresis or paralysis.
   H. *Body image disturbance* related to hemiplegia.
   I. *Total incontinence* related to interruption of normal nerve transmission.
   J. *Impaired social interaction* related to aphasia or neurologic deficit.
   K. *Risk for impaired skin integrity* related to immobility.
   L. *Unilateral neglect* related to cerebral damage.

V. **Nursing care plan/implementation**
   A. Goal: *reduce cerebral anoxia*.
      1. Patent **airway**.
         a. *Oxygen* therapy, as ordered; suctioning to prevent aspiration.
         b. Turn, cough, deep breathe q2h to prevent aspiration pneumonia (high incidence).
      2. Activity: bed rest, progressing to out of bed as tolerated.
      3. *Position*:
         a. Maximize ventilation.
         b. Support with pillows when on side, use hand rolls and arm slings as ordered.
   B. Goal: *prevent complications and maintain functioning*.
      1. Vital signs, neurologic checks.
      2. Medications, as ordered:
         a. *Antihypertensives* to prevent rupture.
         b. *Anticoagulants* to prevent thrombus.
      3. *Fluids*: IVs to prevent hemoconcentration, I&O, weigh daily.
      4. ROM exercises to prevent contractures, muscle atrophy, phlebitis.
      5. Skin care, position changes to prevent decubitus ulcers

TABLE 21.3 BOWEL AND BLADDER MANAGEMENT PROGRAM FOR CLIENTS RECOVERING FROM STROKE

🍎 **Diet**—unless contraindicated
- Fluid intake of 2500 to 3000 mL daily
- Prune juice
- Cooked fruit three times daily.
- Cooked vegetables three times daily. Whole-grain cereal or bread three to five times daily.

Bowel Management
- Place client on bedpan or bedside commode, or take to bathroom at regular time every day.
- Preferred time: approximately 30 minutes after breakfast.
- Stool softeners prn.
- Glycerin suppository may be inserted 15 to 30 minutes before sitting on commode.

Bladder Management
- Assess for bladder distention.
- Offer bedpan urinal, commode, or toilet every 2 hours while awake; every 3-4 hours during sleeping hours.
- Focus client on need to urinate.
- Assist with clothing and mobility.
- Schedule majority of fluid intake during the day, less in the evening and at night.
- Encourage sitting position for women and standing position for men

C. Goal: *provide for emotional relaxation*.
   1. Identify grief reaction to changes in body image.
   2. Encourage expression of feelings, concerns.
D. Goal: *client safety*.
   1. Identify existence of *homonymous hemianopsia* (visual field blindness) and *agnosia* (disturbance in sensory information).
   2. Use siderails and assist as needed.
   3. Remind to walk slowly, take adequate rest periods; ensure good lighting; look where client is going.
E. Goal: **health teaching**.
   1. Exercise routines.
   2. Diet: self-feeding, but assist as needed.
   3. Resumption of self-care activities.
   4. Use of supportive devices, transfer techniques.
   5. Bowel and bladder management (see **Table 21.3**)
VI. **Evaluation/outcome criteria**
   A. No complications (e.g., pneumonia).
   B. Regains functional independence—resumes self-care activities.
   C. Return of control over body functions (e.g., bowel, bladder, speech).

*Modified from Colombraro GC. Nursing Care of Children and Families. In *Little, Brown's NCLEX-RN® Examination Review*, SL Lagerquist (ed). Philadelphia, Lippincott Raven (out of print).

Bacterial Meningitis*

I. **Pathophysiology:**
   A. Bacterial organism, commonly *H. influenza*, *S. pneumoniae*, *Neisseria meningitis*, or *S. aureus*, crosses blood–brain barrier into CNS. Organism migrates via subarachnoid space, producing an inflammatory response to the foreign substance in the pia mater, the arachnoid, the CSF, and the cerebral ventricles.

II. **Risk factors/causes:**
   A. High population density (e.g., crowded living conditions).
   B. Basilar skull fracture.
   C. Brain or spinal surgery.
   D. Sinus or upper respiratory infection.
   E. Use of nasal sprays after sinus infection.
   F. Compromised immune system.

III. **Assessment**
   A. *Subjective data*:
      1. Headache.
      2. Neck pain.
      3. Photophobia.
   B. *Objective data*:
      1. Abrupt onset: initial sign may be a seizure following an episode of upper respiratory tract infection/acute otitis media.
      2. Chills and fever.
      3. Vomiting.
      4. Alterations in level of consciousness: delirium, stupor, increased ICP.
      5. Nuchal rigidity.
      6. Opisthotonos: head is drawn backward into overextension.
      7. Hyperactive reflexes related to CNS irritability.

IV. **Analysis/nursing diagnosis**
   A. *Risk for infection* related to communicability of meningitis.
   B. *Risk for injury* related to CNS irritability and seizures.
   C. *Pain* related to nuchal rigidity, opisthotonos, increased muscle tension.
   D. *Sensory/perceptual alterations* related to seizures and changes in level of consciousness.
   E. *Altered nutrition, less than body requirements*, related to fever and poor oral intake.
   F. *Knowledge deficit* regarding diagnostic procedures, condition, treatment, prognosis.

V. **Nursing care plan/implementation**
   A. Goal: *prevent spread of infection*.
      1. Institute transmission-based (droplet) precautions. (See **p. 153-155** for **CDC guidelines**).
      2. Enforce strict handwashing.

⚠ 3. Institute and maintain *respiratory isolation* (wear a mask when working within 3 feet of client) for minimum of 24 h after starting IV antibiotics, at which time client is no longer considered to be communicable and client can come off isolation.

4. Instruct family when using isolation techniques.

〰 5. Identify family members and others at high risk: do cultures (e.g., *Haemophilus influenzae, Escherichia coli*); possibly begin

⬭ prophylactic *antibiotics* (e.g., *rifampin*).

⬭ 6. Treat with IV *antiinfectives*, as ordered, as soon as possible after admission (after culture specimens are obtained); continue

〰 10–14 d (until CSF culture is negative and there is clinical improvement). (See **diagnostic studies** for lumbar punctures **p. 290.**)

7. Anticipate large IV doses of medications only—administer slowly in dilute form to prevent phlebitis.

☞ 8. Maintain IV.

B. Goal: *promote safety and prevent injury/seizures.*

☞ 1. Maintain seizure precautions.

2. Place client near nurses' station for maximum observation; provide private room for isolation.

3. Minimize stimuli: quiet, calm environment.

4. Restrict visitors to immediate family.

5. *Position*: head of bed *slightly elevated* to decrease ICP. (For opisthotonos: *side-lying*, for comfort and safety.)

🍎 C. Goal: *maintain adequate nutrition.*

1. NPO or clear liquids initially; supplement with IVs.

2. Diet as tolerated—client may experience anorexia (due to disease) or vomiting (due to increased ICP).

3. Monitor I&O, daily weights.

▶ VI. Evaluation/outcome criteria

A. No spread of infection noted.

B. Safety maintained.

C. Adequate nutrition and fluid intake maintained.

D. Client recovers without permanent neurologic damage (e.g., seizure disorders).

Encephalitis

Inflammation of the brain and its coverings, which usually results in prolonged coma.

I. **Pathophysiology**: brain tissue injury → release of enzymes that increase vascular dilatation, capillary permeability → edema → increased ICP → depression of CNS function.

II. **Risk factors/causes**:

A. Syphilis.

B. Lead or arsenic poisoning.

C. Carbon monoxide.

D. Typhoid fever.

E. Measles, chickenpox.

F. Viruses (most common cause).

▶ III. **Assessment**

A. *Subjective data*:

1. Headache—severe.

2. Nausea.

3. Photophobia

4. Difficulty concentrating.

B. *Objective data*:

1. Altered level of consciousness.

2. Nuchal rigidity.

3. Tremors, facial weakness.

4. Nystagmus.

5. Elevated temperature (sudden fever).

6. Vomiting.

〰 7. *Lumbar puncture*—fluid cloudy; *increased* neutrophils, protein. See **Diagnostic Studies** box at end of the chapter.

8. Lab data: blood—slight to moderate leukocytosis (about 14,000/mm^3).

▶ IV. **Analysis/nursing diagnosis**

A. *Self-care deficit* related to altered level of consciousness.

B. *Risk for injury* related to coma.

C. *Sensory/perceptual alteration* related to brain tissue injury.

D. *Altered thought processes* related to increased ICP.

▶ V. **Nursing care plan/implementation**

A. Goal: *support physical and emotional relaxation.*

☞ 1. Vital signs, neurologic signs, as ordered.

☞ 2. Seizure precautions.

☞ 3. *Position*: to maintain patent airway, prevent contractures; ROM exercises.

⬭ 4. Medications as ordered:

a. *Analgesics* for pain.

b. *Antipyretics* for fever.

c. *Sedatives* for agitation.

d. *Anticonvulsants* for seizures.

e. *Antiinfectives* for infection.

f. *Osmotic diuretics* (mannitol) to reduce cerebral edema.

5. *No* isolation.

🏠 B. Goal: **health teaching**: self-care activities with residual motor and speech deficits, physical therapy.

▶ VI. **Evaluation/outcome criteria**

A. Regains consciousness; is alert, oriented.

B. Performs self-care activities with minimal assistance.

✍ Summary of Key Points

1. Clients who are aphasic *can hear.* Speaking louder does not improve their comprehension.

2. With a client who is aphasic, use nonverbal techniques, face the client directly, speak slowly, repeat words, be patient and kind, and anticipate client's needs to reduce his or her frustration.

3. Learn a mnemonic to help remember the cranial nerves.

4. Scalp wounds are very bloody but may actually be minor injuries.

5. With suspected head trauma, assess for signs of *hypoxia* and increasing *ICP.* The vital sign changes in increased ICP are the *opposite* of those seen in hypovolemic shock.

6. Pupil dilatation is a *late sign* of increased ICP. *A change of level of consciousness is the first indication* of a worsening of the client's condition. Even a client who is comatose will show a change in responsiveness. Use the *Glasgow Coma scale* to assess objectively.

7. The greatest concern with increased ICP is the amount of distortion and *anoxia* caused by the pressure.

8. *Pupil dilation* occurs first in the pupil *opposite* the *side* of injury or hematoma.

9. Check any drainage from nose or ears for the presence of glucose, indicating a *CSF leak.*

10. Positioning and head elevation is determined by the type of surgery—*above or below the tentorium.*

11. The nursing priority *during* a seizure is to *protect the client* from *injury.* Maintaining a patent airway is usually not possible. *Clearing the airway after* the seizure ends is important.

12. *Aspiration pneumonia* is a concern during the period *immediately after* a brain attack (stroke). Positioning and careful observation of swallowing are important.

13. The amount of permanent disability is often not known for weeks after a brain attack (stroke). Nursing care focuses on prevention of complications and maintenance of optimal functioning.

14. *Homonymous hemianopsia* (visual field blindness) may be present, leading to accidents and behavior changes.

15. A *spinal headache* resulting from a lumbar puncture can be easily prevented by keeping the client *flat* and *well hydrated.*

⩗ Diagnostic Studies/Procedures

Cerebral Angiography—fluoroscopic visualization of the brain vasculature after injection of a contrast medium into the carotid or vertebral arteries; *used to:* localize lesions (tumors, abscesses, intracranial hemorrhages, occlusions) that are large enough to distort cerebrovascular blood flow.

Brain Scan—intravenous injection of a radioactive substance, followed by scanning that detects radioactivity.

1. *Increased* radioactivity at site of abnormality.

2. *Used to* detect: brain tumors, abscesses, hematomas, and arteriovenous malformation

Electroencephalography (EEG)—graphic record of the electrical potentials generated by the physiologic activity of the brain; *used to:* detect surface lesions or tumors of the brain and epilepsy.

Echoencephalography—beam of pulsed ultrasound is passed through the head, and returning echoes are recorded graphically; *used to:* detect shifts in cerebral midline structures caused by subdural hematomas, intracerebral hemorrhage, or tumors.

Skull X-ray Studies—outline configuration and density of brain tissues and vascular markings; *used to* determine the size and location of: skull fractures, intracranial calcifications, tumors, abscesses, or vascular lesions.

Computerized Axial Tomography (CAT or CT scan)—an x-ray beam sweeps around the body, allowing measurement of various tissue densities; provides clear radiographic definition of structures that are not visible by other techniques, permitting earlier diagnosis and treatment and more effective and efficient follow-up. Initial scan may be followed by "contrast enhancement," involving the IV injection of a contrast agent (iodine), followed by a repeat scan. *Client preparation:* instructions for eating before test vary. *Clear liquids* up to 2 h before are usually permitted.

Lumbar Puncture—puncture of the lumbar subarachnoid space of the spinal cord with a needle to withdraw samples of cerebral spinal fluid (CSF); *used to:* evaluate CSF for infections and determine presence of hemorrhage. *Not done if* ↑ *ICP suspected.*

💡 Study and Memory Aids

Transient Ischemic Attacks: Assessment—"3 T's"

T emporary unilateral visual loss
T ransient paralysis (one side)
T innitus → vertigo

Source: Modified from Zerwekh J D, et al. *Memory Notebook of Nursing*. Dallas: Nursing Education Consultants.

💊 Drug Review

Traumatic Brain (Head) Injury

Analgesics (NO MORPHINE)
Acetaminophen/codeine (*Tylenol* #1, #2, #3): 1–2 tablets q3–4h, as needed
Meperidine HCl (*Demerol*): IM or SC, 50–75 mg
Oxycodone/acetaminophen (*Tylox*, *Percocet*): 5 mg q3–6h, as needed

Anticonvulsants
Phenobarbital: 60–250 mg/d in single or divided doses
Phenytoin (*Dilantin*): loading dose, 1 g or 20 mg/ kg; maintenance dose, 300–400 mg

Steroids (should **never** be abruptly discontinued; gradually taper dose to prevent complications)
Dexamethasone (*Decadron*): 0.5–9 mg/d in single or divided doses
Methylprednisolone (*Medrol*): 4–48 mg/d
Prednisone (*Deltasone*): 5–60 mg/d

Increased Intracranial Pressure

Antiulceratives
Aluminum hydroxide gel (*Amphojel*): 5–10 mL q2–4h or 1h pc
Calcium carbonate (*Titralac*): 1–2 g with water pc and hs
Magnesium and aluminum hydroxides (*Maalox* suspension): 5–30 mL pc and hs
Sucralfate (*Carafate*): 1 g qid

Histamine antagonists
Cimetidine (*Tagamet*): 300–600 mg q6h
Ranitidine (*Zantac*): 150 mg bid

Osmotic diuretic
Mannitol (*Osmitrol*): IV, 0.25–2 g/kg as 15%–25% solution over 30–60 min

Proton pump inhibitors
Lansoprazole (*Prevacid*): 15 mg PO qd
Omeprazole (*Prilosec*): 20 mg PO qd

Steroids (should **never** be abruptly discontinued; gradually taper dosage to prevent complications)
Dexamethasone (*Decadron*): 0.5–9 mg/d in single or divided doses

Craniotomy

Analgesics (NO MORPHINE)
Acetaminophen/codeine (*Tylenol* #1, #2, #3): 1–2 tablets q3–4h, as needed
Meperidine HCl (*Demerol*): IM or SC, 50-75–mg
Oxycodone/acetaminophen (*Tylox*, *Percocet*): 5 mg q3–6h, as needed

Osmotic diuretic
Mannitol (*Osmitrol*): IV,0.25–2 g/kg as 15%–25% solution over 30–60 min

Steroids (should **never** be abruptly discontinued; gradually taper dose to prevent complications)
Dexamethasone (*Decadron*): 0.5–9 mg/d in single or divided doses

Epilepsy

Carbamazepine (*Tegretol*): 800–1200 mg/d in divided doses q6–8h
Phenobarbital: 60–250 mg/d in single or divided doses
Phenytoin (*Dilantin*): loading dose, 1 g or 20 mg/kg; maintenance dose, 30–400 mg
Primidone (*Mysoline*): 250 mg 3–4 times daily, *not to exceed* 2 g/d
Trimethadione (*Tridione*)—for *petit mal seizures only*: 900 mg in 3–4 divided doses with increases weekly of 300 mg to a total of 2400 mg per day.

Encephalitis

Analgesics
Acetaminophen/codeine (*Tylenol* #1, #2, #3): 1–2 tablets q3–4h, as needed
Meperidine HCl (*Demerol*): IM or SC, 50–75 mg
Oxycodone/acetaminophen (*Tylox*, *Percocet*): 5 mg q3–6h, as needed

Anticonvulsants
Phenobarbital: 60–250 mg/d in single or divided doses
Phenytoin (*Dilantin*, diphenylhydantoin): loading dose, 1 g or 20 mg/kg; maintenance dose, 300–400 mg

Antiinfectives
Cephalexin (*Keflex*): 250–500 mg q6h
Cephalothin (*Keflin*): IV, 0.5–2 g q4–6h
Erythromycin: 250–500 mg q6–12h
Gentamicin (*Garamycin*): 3–5 mg/kg/d in divided doses
Penicillin G: 1.2 million U in single IM dose

Antipyretic
Aspirin: 325–1000 mg q4–6h, *not* to exceed 4 g/d

Osmotic diuretic
Mannitol (*Osmitrol*): IV, 0.25–2 g/kg as 15%–25% solution over 30–60 min

Sedative
Phenobarbital: 30–120 mg/d in divided doses

Tranquilizers
Chlordiazepoxide HCl (*Librium*): 5–25 mg 3–4 times daily
Diazepam (*Valium*): 2–10 mg 2–4 times daily

Transient Ischemic Attacks

Anticoagulant
Warfarin (*coumadin*) 10 mg/d, adjusted according to INR.

Antiplatelets
Aggrenox: aspirin 25 mg/dipyridamole 200 mg
Aspirin: 1–3 g/d in 2–4 divided doses
Clopidogrel (*Plavix*): 75 mg qd
Dipyridamole (*Persantine*): 75-107 mg qid.
Ticlopidine (*Ticlid*): 250 mg bid with food.

Brain Attack (Stroke)

Anticoagulants
Heparin sodium: IV, 1000 U/h; SC, 8000–10,000 U q8h, adjusted according to partial thromboplastin time
Warfarin (*Coumadin*): 10 mg/d, adjusted according to INR.

Antihypertensive
Angiotensin-converting enzyme inhibitor (ACE)—
Captopril (*Capoten*): 12.5–25 mg tid

Antiplatelets
Aggrenox: aspirin 25 mg/dipyridamole 200 mg
Aspirin: 1–3 g/d in 2–4 divided doses
Clopidogrel (*Plavix*): 75 mg qd
Dipyridamole (*Persantine*): 75-107 mg qid.
Ticlopidine (*Ticlid*): 250 mg bid with food.

Questions

1. Which of the following respiratory changes would the nurse see in a client with increasing intracranial pressure (ICP)?
   1. Nasal flaring and sternal retractions.
   2. Slow, irregular respirations.
   3. Rapid, shallow respirations.
   4. Paradoxical chest movements.
2. Which nursing measure would prevent a further increase in ICP in a client with a head injury?
   1. Positioning the client flat in bed.
   2. Turning the client and having the client cough and deep breathe every 3 hours.
   3. Asking the client to exhale while turning in bed.
   4. Preventing the complications of immobility.
3. If a client who has suffered a brain attack is found to have homonymous hemianopsia, the nurse would know that the client has:
   1. Paralysis of limbs on one side of the body.
   2. Visual field blindness.
   3. Perceptual neglect of one side of body.
   4. Deafness in one ear.
4. The nurse tells the daughter of a client who has had a stroke that the most important aspect of rehabilitation after a stroke is:
   1. Return of bowel and bladder continence.

2. Family or support persons' involvement.
   3. Setting realistic goals for the client.
   4. Return of the long-term memory needed for learning.
5. The best way for the nurse to approach a client with left homonymous hemianopsia following a stroke would be to:
   1. Speak to the client while approaching from the left.
   2. Stand at the foot of the client's bed when talking.
   3. Speak to the client while approaching from the right.
   4. Stand directly in front of the client when talking.
6. A client who has suffered a stroke pays little attention to a roommate and seems withdrawn. When the nurse enters the room, the client is awake but does not respond until spoken to. The best explanation for this behavior is:
   1. The client does not remember the nurse's name.
   2. The client is angry because of having the stroke.
   3. Strokes frequently cause hearing impairment.
   4. The client may have visual field blindness.
7. While caring for a client in the postanesthesia recovery room after a craniotomy, the nurse observes signs of increasing ICP. The first nursing action would be to:
   1. Give the client dexamethasone (*Decadron*) IV, as ordered.
   2. Elevate the head of the client's bed 30 degrees.
   3. Contact the neurosurgeon for orders.
   4. Assess the client's bilateral pupillary reaction.
8. In providing health care teaching to a client who is being discharged on dexamethasone (*Decadron*) therapy, the nurse should inform the client that during long-term therapy the diet should be:
   1. High in carbohydrates, sodium, and protein.
   2. Low in carbohydrates and sodium and high in protein.
   3. High in protein, calcium, and carbohydrates.
   4. Low in potassium, protein, and carbohydrates.
9. The nurse knows that gentamycin, an aminoglycoside, may cause eighth cranial nerve damage. Which assessment finding would alert the nurse to this adverse effect?
   1. Drooping eyelid.
   2. Diplopia.
   3. Tinnitus.
   4. Dysphagia.

Answers/Rationale

1. (2) The respiratory change that occurs in the presence of increased ICP is often called ataxic or *Biot's breathing*, and it is a very irregular pattern that occurs with brainstem involvement. The

other respiratory changes are characteristic of *other* potentially life-threatening conditions. Left ventricular *failure* would likely produce nasal flaring and sternal retractions (1). Rapid, shallow breathing (3) would be seen with *acute respiratory distress*. Paradoxical movements (4) occur in *flail chest*. **AS, COM, 6, PhI, Physiological adaptation**

2. (3) When such clients turn, they instinctively hold their breath (Valsalva maneuver); this increases the intrathoracic pressure and the ICP. Exhaling or breathing through the mouth prevents the *maneuver*. The head of the bed should be elevated 30 degrees, *not flat* (1). Preventing respiratory complications is important, but *coughing* (2) would only *increase* the ICP. Preventing the complications of immobility (4) is *too vague*; many such complications would not have any bearing on ICP. **IMP, APP, 2, PhI, Reduction of risk potential**

3. (2) *Homonymous hemianopsia* means defective vision or visual loss in the same half of the visual field of both eyes. Frequently the optic nerve is affected in clients with a stroke, and this causes visual field blindness. The nasal field of one eye and the temporal field of the other eye would be blind, as if a curtain had been drawn across half of each eye. Paralysis on one side (1) is *hemiplegia*, not hemianopsia. Clients with a stroke may also fail to perceive one side of the body (3), and this is *unilateral neglect*. Deafness or loss of hearing in one ear (4) *is hemianacusia*, and this may occur with damage to the eighth cranial nerve (the auditory/acoustic nerve). **AN, COM, 2, PhI, Physiological adaptation**

4. (2) Rehabilitation requires the help of family or support persons, because they can help provide the encouragement and assistance the client needs during the process. The question does not provide any data about bowel and bladder control (1), so the rehabilitation needs in this regard are *not known*. However, the family would be critical to regaining control. Goals are set *with* the client, not for the client (3). There is also *no information* in the question about the client's memory (4), but if there were a problem, the family would be the key to successful rehabilitation. **IMP, APP, 2, HPM, Health promotion and maintenance**

5. (3) The client has left visual field blindness and can only see in the right visual fields of both eyes. Once the nurse is seen or heard approaching from the right, the client can more easily turn the head to the right to see than if approached from the left. The client would *not see* anyone approaching *from the left* (1) or any item placed to the left side of the bedside table or on the left side of the bed. Options 2 and 4 do not explain how to approach the client to avoid startling. **PL, APP, 2, SECE, Management of care**

6. (4) There is decreased sensory stimulation as a result of visual field blindness, and the client may appear withdrawn. Positioning the client's bed so that the door and/or roommate are visible will enable the client to be more responsive. The other explanations (1, 2, and 3) are possible, but visual field blindness should be ruled out before they are considered. **AN, ANL, 2, PhI, Physiological adaptation**

7. (2) Head elevation of 30 degrees is considered the optimal position after supratentorial surgery, such as a craniotomy. ICP is not affected by atmospheric pressure in this position. The other measures may be taken if the signs and symptoms of increased ICP continue. *Decadron* (1) would reduce the cerebral *edema*. Contacting the MD (3) turns the decision-making process over to the MD and is usually *not* the *first nursing action*. Changes in pupillary reaction (4) would be a *late* sign of increased ICP. **IMP, ANL, 2, PhI, Reduction of risk potential**

8. (2) The diet should be low in carbohydrates and sodium and high in protein, calcium, and potassium to counter the adverse effects of the drug. Option 1 is incorrect because CHO and sodium should be *low*. Option 3 is incorrect because CHO should be *low*. Option 4 is incorrect because potassium and protein should be *increased* in the diet. **IMP, COM, 4, PhI, Basic care and comfort**

9. (3) Tinnitus, or ringing in the ears, occurs if there is damage to the acoustic (auditory) nerve, or cranial nerve VIII. Drooping eyelid (1) is due to damage to cranial nerve III (the oculomotor nerve), which also affects the pupillary response. Diplopia (2), or double vision, occurs as a result of weakness of the eye muscles; extraocular movements are controlled by cranial nerves III (oculomotor), IV (trochlear), and VI (abducens). Dysphagia, or difficulty swallowing (4), occurs with damage to cranial nerve X (the vagus nerve). **AS, RE/KN, 2, PhI, Physiological adaptation**

Key to Codes

Nursing process: **AS,** assessment; **AN,** analysis; **PL,** planning; **IMP,** implementation; **EV,** evaluation. (See **Appendix M** for explanation of nursing process steps.)

Cognitive level: **RE/KN,** recall/knowledge; **COM,** comprehension; **APP,** application; **ANL,** analysis; **EVL,** evaluation; **SYN,** synthesis. (See **Appendix M** for explanation.)

Category of human function: 1, protective; 2, sensory-perceptual; 3, comfort, rest, activity, and mobility; 4, nutrition; 5, growth and development; 6, fluid-gas transport; 7, psychosocial-cultural; 8, elimination. (See **Appendix 0** for explanation.)

Client need: **SECE,** safe, effective care environment; **PhI,** physiological integrity; **PsI,** psychosocial integrity; **HPM,** health promotion and maintenance. (See **Appendix P** for explanation.)

Client subneed: (See **Appendix P** for explanation)

Disorders of the Spinal Cord

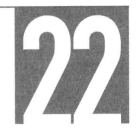

Chapter Outline

- Herniated/Ruptured Disk (Ruptured Nucleus Pulposus)
  - Lumbar injuries
  - Cervical injuries
- Laminectomy
- Spinal Cord Injuries
- Spinal Shock
- Autonomic Hyperreflexia (Autonomic Dysreflexia)
- Summary of Key Points
- Study and Memory Aids
  - Diagnostic Studies/Procedures

- Electromyography (EMG)
- Myelogram
  - Diet
  - Drug review
- Questions
- Answers/Rationale

Herniated/Ruptured Disk (Ruptured Nucleus Pulposus)

Strain or injury to a weakened cartilage between vertebrae can result in herniation of the nucleus, causing pressure on nerve roots in spinal canal, pain, and disability.

I. **Pathophysiology**: pulpy substance of disk interior (nucleus pulposus) bulges or ruptures through the outer annulus fibrosus → irritation and pressure on nerve endings in the spinal ligaments → muscle spasm and distortion of the joints of vertebral arches.

II. **Risk factors/causes**:
   A. Strain as result of poor body mechanics.
   B. Trauma.
   C. History of back injuries.
   D. Sneezing, sudden head or neck movement.

III. **Assessment**
   A. *Lumbar injuries* (90% of herniations):
      1. *Subjective data*:
         a. *Pain*: low back, radiating to buttocks, posterior thigh, calf; *relieved* by recumbency; *aggravated by* sneezing, coughing, flexion; sciatic pain continues even when back pain subsides.
         b. Numbness, tingling.
      2. *Objective data*:
         a. Muscle weakness: leg and foot.
         b. Inability to flex leg.
         c. Sensory loss: leg and foot.
         d. Alterations in posture: leans to side, unable to stand up straight.
         e. Edema: leg and foot.
         f. Positive *Lasègue's sign*: straight leg raising with hip flexed and knee extended produces sciatic pain.
      g. *Diagnostic tests* for cervical injuries (see **Diagnostic Studies** box).
         (1) Spinal x-rays.
         (2) Computerized axial tomographic (CAT) scan.
         (3) Magnetic resonance imaging (MRI)
         (4) Myelography (less preferred than CAT scan or MRI).
         (5) Electromyography.
         (6) *Neurologic exam*: special attention to *sensory* status, including pain, touch, and temperature identification; and to *motor* status, including strength, gait, and reflexes.
   B. *Cervical injuries* (10% of herniations):
      1. *Subjective data*:
         a. *Pain*: upper extremities, radiating to hands and fingers; aggravated by coughing, sneezing, straining; sharp pain between scapula and spine.
         b. Tingling, burning sensation in upper extremities and back of neck.
         c. History of sneezing followed by sharp pain.
      2. *Objective data*:
         a. Upper extremities: weakness, atrophy.
         b. Neck: restricted movement.
         c. Same *diagnostic tests* as for lumbar injury (see above).

IV. **Analysis/nursing diagnosis**
   A. *Pain* related to pressure on nerve roots.
   B. *Fear* related to disease progression and/or potential surgery.
   C. *Knowledge deficit* related to correct body mechanics.

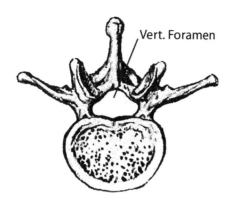

Vert. Foramen

Cross-section of Lumbar Vertebra from Above

D. *Impaired physical mobility* related to continued pain.

E. *Sleep pattern disturbance* related to difficulty finding comfortable position.

V. Nursing care plan/implementation

A. Goal: *relieve pain and promote comfort.*

1. *Bed rest* with bedboard.

2. *Position—avoid* twisting.

   a. *Lumbar disk: William's* (head elevated 30 degrees, knee gatch elevated to flatten the lumbosacral curve).

   b. *Cervical:* low-Fowler's.

3. Medications as ordered:

   a. *Analgesics.*

   b. *Muscle relaxants.*

   c. *Anti-inflammatories.*

   d. *Stool softeners.*

4. Moist heat.

5. Fracture bedpan.

6. Gradual increase in activity.

7. Apply brace for support.

8. Apply traction prn for comfort.

9. Prepare for surgery if medical regimen unsuccessful.

B. Goal: **health teaching.**

1. Correct body mechanics, keep back straight.

2. Exercise program as symptoms decrease.

VI. Evaluation/outcome criteria

A. Reports pain decreased.

B. Mobility increased, normal body posture attained.

Laminectomy

Excision of dorsal arch of vertebrae with or without spinal fusion of two or more vertebrae with a bone graft from iliac crest, to stabilize spine.

I. Analysis/nursing diagnosis

A. *Pain* related to edema resulting from surgery.

B. *Impaired physical mobility* related to pain and discomfort resulting from surgery.

II. Nursing care plan/implementation

A. Goal: *relieve anxiety.*

1. Answer questions, explain routines.

2. See **General Postoperative Nursing Care, Chap. 9.**

B. Goal: *prevent injury postoperatively.*

1. Monitor *vital signs:*

   a. *Neurologic signs* (e.g., check sensation, motor strength of limbs).

   b. Respiratory status (risk for *respiratory depression* with cervical laminectomy).

2. Monitor intake and output (1&O) (*urinary retention* common, especially with cervical laminectomy); may need catheterization.

   a. Encourage fluids.

3. Monitor bowel sounds (*paralytic ileus* common with lumbar laminectomy).

4. Monitor dressing for possible bleeding.

5. Bed *position* as ordered:

   a. *For lumbar laminectomy: head of bed flat*; supine with slight flexion of legs, with pillow between knees for turning and side-lying position.

   b. *For cervical laminectomy: head of bed elevated*, neck immobilized with collar or sand bags.

6. Encourage deep breathing to prevent respiratory complications.

7. Prevent strain or flexion at surgical site: log-rolling with spinal fusion.

C. Goal: *promote comfort:*

1. Administer *analgesics* because sciatic-type pain continues after lumbar surgery (arm pain after cervical surgery), due to edema resulting from trauma of surgery.

D. Goal: *prepare for early discharge:* Clients having microsurgery for repair of herniated disk are usually discharged from the hospital 1 d postoperative; teaching regarding allowed and restricted activities must be done early.

E. Goal: **health teaching.**

1. How to *turn and move* from side to side in one motion, *sit up*, and *get out of bed without twisting spine*; to get out of bed: raise head of bed while in side-lying position, then put feet over edge of bed, and stand.

2. Proper positioning and *ambulation* techniques.

3. Correct posture, *body mechanics*, activities to prevent further injury; increase activities according to tolerance.

4. Physiotherapy; encourage compliance for full rehabilitation.

III. Evaluation/outcome criteria

A. No respiratory, bowel, bladder complications noted.

1. Lung sounds clear.

2. Bowel sounds present; able to pass gas and feces.

3. Urinary output adequate.
B. Regains mobility.
C. Comfort level increases: reports leg and back pain decreased.
D. Demonstrates protective positioning and ambulation techniques.

Spinal Cord Injuries

Trauma from hyperextension, hyperflexion, axial compression, lateral flexion, or shearing of the spine.

I. **Types:**
   A. *C-1 and C-2 injury level*—resulting deficit:
      1. Phrenic nerve involvement.
      2. Diaphragmatic paralysis.
      3. Respiratory difficulties (require permanent ventilatory support).
      4. Possible quadriplegia.
      5. Possible death.
   B. *C-4 through T-1 injury level*—resulting deficit: possible quadriplegia.
   C. *Thoracic-lumbar injury level*—resulting deficit: possible paraplegia.

II. **Pathophysiology**: trauma → vertebral dislocation or fractures → cord trauma, compression or severance of the cord.

III. **Risk factors/causes:**
   A. Motor vehicle accidents.
   B. Athletic accidents (e.g., diving, surfing, contact sports).
   C. Falls.
   D. Gunshot wounds.

IV. **Assessment**
   A. *Subjective data*:
      1. Pain at the level of injury.
      2. Numbness/weakness, loss of sensation *below* level of injury.
      3. Psychological distress related to severity of injury and its effects.
   B. *Objective data*:
      1. Findings depend on extent of injury to spinal cord/spinal nerves.
      2. Paralysis: motor, sphincter.
         a. Initially a period of *flaccid paralysis* and loss of reflexes, called *spinal* or *neural shock*.
         b. *Incomplete injuries* may lead to loss of voluntary movement and sensory deficits below injury level (symptoms vary depending on injury).
         c. *Complete injury* leads to loss of function and all voluntary movement below level of injury.
      3. Respiratory distress.
      4. Alterations in temperature control.
      5. Alterations in bowel and bladder function.
      6. Involved muscles become spastic and hyperreflexic within days or weeks.
      7. Documentation via x-rays of the spine, CAT scan and neurological examination.

V. **Analysis/nursing diagnosis**
   A. *Ineffective breathing pattern* related to high-level injury.
   B. *Impaired physical mobility* related to injuries affecting lower limbs.
   C. *Fear* related to uncertain future health status.
   D. *Anxiety* related to loss of control over own activities of daily living.
   E. *Bathing/hygiene self-care deficit* related to injuries above T-1.
   F. *Impaired home maintenance management* related to quadriplegia or paraplegia.
   G. *Risk for altered body temperature* related to absence of sweating below level of injury.
   H. *Risk for injury* related to equipment necessary to accomplish daily activities.
   I. *Tactile sensory/perceptual alterations* related to injury level.
   J. *Body image disturbance* related to permanent change in physical status.

VI. **Nursing care plan/implementation**
   A. Goal: *maintain patent airway*.
      1. *Suction*, cough, *tracheostomy* care, prn.
      2. *Oxygen, ventilator care*.
      3. Monitor blood gas levels.
   B. Goal: *prevent further damage*.
      1. Immobilize spine.
      2. Firm mattress, *Stryker frame, Foster frame, CircO-electric bed*, traction, casts, braces.
      3. Skeletal traction via tongs: Crutchfield, Gardner-Wells (see Fractures, **p. 254, 255, 260**).
      4. Halo traction (see Fractures, **p. 254, 255, 260-261**).
   C. Goal: *relieve edema: anti-inflammatories, corticosteroids*.
   D. Goal: *relieve discomfort: analgesics, sedatives, muscle relaxants*.
   E. Goal: *promote comfort*:
      1. Maintain fluid intake: PO/IV, I&O.
      2. Increase nutritional intake.
      3. Prevent contractures and decubitus ulcers.
      4. Help client deal with psychosocial issues (e.g., role changes).
      5. Begin rehabilitation plan.
   F. Goal: *prevent complications*.
      1. Monitor for spinal shock during initial phase of injury (see Spinal Shock, **p. 298-299**).
      2. Monitor for hyperreflexia with severed spinal cord injuries (see Autonomic Hyperreflexia, **p. 299-300**).
   G. Goal: *Functional goals in rehabilitation*. (see **Table 22.1**)

TABLE 22.1 REHAB GOALS IN SPINAL CORD INJURY

Specific Level of Injury	Functional Goals
Cervical levels 1–2	1. *Limited* head and neck movement 2. Ventilator dependent 3. Wheelchair with breath, head and shoulder controls
Cervical levels 3-4	1. *Good* head and neck control 2. May need ventilator 3. Same as #3 above 4. Dependent in ADLs
Cervical level 5	1. *Full* head, neck, shoulder and diaphragm control 2. Some elbow flexion → feed self with adaptive devices 3. Major assistance with ADLs 4. Needs electric wheelchair with hand controls
Cervical level 6	1. Strong elbow flexion with some wrist extension 2. Independent in eating, grooming, bathing; bowel and bladder care with adaptive devices 3. Needs minor assistance with dressing and transfers 4. Able to drive manual wheelchair with hand controls, on level surfaces
Cervical level 7	1. Full elbow flexion with elbow extension, wrist flexion, and some finger control 2. Independent in ADLs with aids 3. Can use manual wheelchair on most surfaces
Cervical level 8 to thoracic level 1	1. Moderate to full arm, wrist and finger control 2. Independent in all ADLs; may need adaptive devices
Thoracic level 1 to lumbar level 2	1. Full use of arms; independent in ADLs 2. May have limited ability to walk short distances with crutches and orthoses; needs wheelchair
Lumbar level 2 and below	1. Full use of arms; independent in ADLs 2. Good candidate for walking with or without orthoses

H. Goal: **health teaching**.
1. Self-care techniques for highest level of independence; include significant others in teaching.
2. How to use ambulation-assistive devices (battery-operated wheelchair controlled by mouthpiece or hand controls, depending on level of paralysis).
3. Identify community resources for follow-up care and career counseling.
4. Signs and symptoms of autonomic hyperreflexia (see **p. 299**).
5. Methods to prevent skin breakdown, infections of respiratory, urinary tract.
6. Bowel, bladder program.

VII. **Evaluation/outcome criteria**
A. Complications avoided.
B. Accomplishes self-care to greatest ability for level of injury.
C. Participates in rehabilitation plan.
D. Grieves over loss and begins to integrate self into society.

Spinal Shock

Temporary flaccid paralysis and areflexia following a severe injury to the spinal cord.

I. **Pathophysiology**: squeezing or shearing of the spinal cord due to fractures or dislocation of vertebrae, interruption of sensory tracts, loss of conscious sensation, interruption of motor tracts, loss of voluntary movement, loss of facilitation, loss of reflex activity, loss of *muscle* tone, loss of stretch reflexes → bowel and bladder retention. Injury between T-1 and L-2, → loss of sympathetic tone and decrease in blood pressure. *Afferent* impulses are unable to *ascend* from below the injured site to the brain, and *efferent* impulses are unable to *descend* to points below the site.

II. **Risk factors/causes**:
A. Automobile/motorcycle accidents.
B. Athletic accidents (e.g., diving in shallow water).
C. Gunshot wounds.

III. **Assessment**
A. *Subjective data*:
1. Loss of sensation below level of injury.
2. Inability to move extremities.
3. Pain at level of injury.
B. *Objective data*:
1. *Neurologic*:
a. *Absent*: pinprick, pressure, vibratory sensations below level of injury; reflexes below level of injury.
b. Muscles: flaccid.

2. *Vital signs*:
   a. Blood pressure (BP) *decreased* (loss of vasomotor tone below level of injury).
   b. Bradycardia.
   c. *Elevated* temperature.
   d. Respirations: may be *depressed*; possible respiratory failure if diaphragm involved.
3. Absence of sweating below level of injury.
4. Urinary retention.
5. Abdominal distention: retention of feces, paralytic ileus.
6. *Skin*: cold, clammy.

IV. Analysis/nursing diagnosis
   A. *Decreased cardiac output* related to loss of vasomotor tone below level of injury.
   B. *Ineffective breathing pattern* related to injuries involving diaphragm.
   C. *Impaired physical mobility* related to loss of voluntary movement of limbs.
   D. *Urinary retention* related to loss of stretch reflexes.
   E. *Fear* related to serious physical condition.
   F. *Risk for injury* related to potential organ damage if shock continues.

V. Nursing care plan/implementation
   A. Goal: *prevent injury related to shock*.
      1. Maintain patent airway: *intubation* and *mechanical ventilation* may be necessary with cervical spinal injuries because of involvement of diaphragm.
      2. Monitor vital signs; **profound hypotension** and **bradycardia** are **most dangerous aspects of spinal shock.**
      3. Administer blood/IV fluids, as ordered.
      4. Nutrition and hydration:
         a. NPO in acute stage: maintain nutrition by IV infusions as ordered.
         b. When allowed to eat: *high* protein, *high* calorie, *high* vitamin diet.
      5. Maintain proper *position* to prevent further injury.
         a. Backboard is necessary to transport from place of injury.
         b. Support head in neutral alignment and prevent flexion.
         c. Skeletal traction is applied once diagnosis is made.
      6. Monitor urinary output q1h; may have Foley catheter while in shock; later, *intermittent* catheterization used as needed.
      7. Relieve bowel distention; use lubricant containing *anesthetic*, as necessary, when checking for or removing impaction.

VI. Evaluation/outcome criteria
   A. Complications are prevented.
   B. Body functions are maintained.

Autonomic Hyperreflexia (Autonomic Dysreflexia)

A group of spinal cord autonomic responses (symptoms) activated simultaneously; may occur when cord lesions are *above the sixth thoracic* vertebra; it is *most commonly* seen with cervical and high thoracic cord injuries; may occur up to 6 yr after injury. It is a pathologic reflex condition, which is an acute **medical emergency**, characterized by *extreme hypertension* and *exaggerated* autonomic responses to stimuli.

I. **Pathophysiology**: Stimulation of sensory receptors below the level of the cord lesion. The intact autonomic nervous system reflexively responds with an arteriolar spasm → increases blood pressure. When the hypertension is evident, the parasympathetic system is activated → heart rate decreases; but *visceral* and *peripheral* vessels do *not* dilate because efferent impulses cannot pass through the cord. The source of the stimulation, e.g., most commonly, distended bladder or rectum, must be corrected for autonomic hyperreflexia to be reversed.

II. **Risk factors/causes**:
   A. Distention of bladder or rectum.
   B. Stimulation of skin (e.g., decubitus ulcers, wrinkled clothing).
   C. Stimulation of pain receptors.

III. **Assessment**
   A. *Subjective data*:
      1. Severe headache.
      2. Blurred vision.
      3. Nausea.
      4. Restlessness.
      5. Flushed feeling.
   B. *Objective data*:
      1. *Severe hypertension* (systolic BP may reach 300 mm Hg).
      2. Bradycardia (30–40 beats/min).
      3. Profuse diaphoresis.
      4. *Flushing* of skin *above* level of injury.
      5. *Pale skin below* level of injury.
      6. Pilomotor spasm (goose flesh).
      7. Nasal congestion.
      8. Distended bladder, bowel.
      9. Skin breakdown.

IV. **Analysis/nursing diagnosis**
   A. *Hyperreflexia* related to high spinal cord injury.
   B. *Risk for injury* related to complications of hypertension, stroke (brain attack).
   C. *Visual sensory/perceptual alteration* related to blurred vision.
   D. *Urinary retention* related to inability to empty bladder due to spinal injury.
   E. *Constipation* related to inability to establish successful bowel-training program.
   F. *Impaired skin integrity* related to immobility.

V. Nursing plan/implementation

A. Goal: *decrease symptoms to prevent serious side effects.*

1. Identify and correct source of stimulation if possible; notify physician.
2. *Elevate head of bed*: lowers BP in persons with high spinal cord injuries.
3. Monitor BP q15min and prn; uncontrolled hypertension can lead to stroke, (brain attack), blindness, death.
4. Give medications as ordered: nitrates, nifedipine (*Procardia*), or hydralazine (*Apresoline*).

B. Goal: *maintain patency of catheter.*

1. Monitor output, palpate for distended bladder.
2. Check for tubing kinks, irrigate catheter prn.
3. Insert new catheter *immediately* if blocked.
4. Culture if infection suspected.

C. Goal: *promote regular bowel elimination.*

1. Bowel training program. (See box: **Bowel and Bladder Management for Clients with Spinal Cord Injury**)
   a. Establish a time schedule
   b. Increase *bulk* in diet
2. Administer suppository, enemas, *laxatives* as ordered and prn.
3. When checking for and/or *removing impaction*, first use *anesthetic* ointment (e.g., dibucaine [*Nupercainal*] ointment) to decrease irritation.

D. Goal: *prevent decubitus ulcers.*

1. Meticulous skin care.
2. *Position*: change q1-2h.
3. Flotation pads; alternating-pressure mattress on bed, wheelchair.

E. Goal: **health teaching**.

1. Risk factors that could trigger this condition.
2. Methods to prevent situations that increase risk (e.g., bowel program, bladder program, skin care, position change schedule).

VI. Evaluation/outcome criteria

A. BP remains within normal limits.
B. No complications occur.

☞ BOWEL AND BLADDER MANAGEMENT FOR CLIENTS WITH SPINAL CORD INJURY

Bowel Management

- Use rectal stimulant, e.g. suppository or mini-enema daily at same time.
- Follow with digital stimulation (gently!) and manual evacuation. Use topical *anesthetic* to prevent autonomic dysreflexia.
- Initially, procedure may be done in bed in *side-lying position*.
- When client is able to resume sitting position, procedure should be done on a commode or toilet in upright position.

Bladder Management

- Indwelling urinary catheter is usually preferred immediately after injury.
- When stable, client is usually started on intermittent catheterization program (ICP).
- Monitor output closely.
- Catheterize every 3-4 hours to prevent bacterial overgrowth and autonomic dysreflexia.
- Cranberry juice or cranberry extract tablets may be helpful to prevent UTI.
- Encourage *sitting* position for women and *standing* position for men, if able.

⩓ Diagnostic Studies/Procedures

Electromyography (EMG) provides information necessary in diagnosing neuromuscular diseases. It measures and documents electrical currents produced by skeletal muscles. Needle electrodes are inserted into muscles, which then document electrical potential of each muscle on a screen and paper. The client should *avoid* all stimulants for 24 h before the test. There may be some discomfort when the needles are inserted.

Myelogram—a contrast medium is injected through a lumbar-puncture needle into the subarachnoid space of the spinal column to visualize the spinal cord; *used to:* detect herniated or ruptured intervertebral disks, tumors, or cysts that compress or distort spinal cord.

☞ *Nursing responsibilities*: with *water-soluble* contrast, *elevate* head of bed; with *oil* contrast, head of bed should be *flat*; check for bladder distention with metrizamide (water-soluble contrast agent); check vital signs every 4 h for 24 h.

🔑 Summary of Key Points

1. Slight *back elevation* (10-30 degrees) and slight *knee flexion* are often most comfortable for a client with severe lumbar disk pain.

2. Surgery is done when the pain of a herniated disk is unrelieved and neurologic deficits increase. Microsurgery is now available, causing less trauma than the traditional laminectomy and spinal fusion.

3. *Log-rolling* is safest for turning the client who has undergone back surgery, unless otherwise advised by the surgeon. It prevents twisting of the spine and pulling on the incision.

4. Assessment of *breathing effectiveness* is the *first priority* with a suspected spinal cord injury.

5. The client must be observed initially for *spinal shock* after complete cord transection because *hypotension* can occur. Spinal shock may last days or months.

6. Autonomic hyperreflexia is a *life-threatening syndrome* for any client with cord injuries from T-7 up. Reportedly this exaggerated sympathetic response can arise during at least the first 5 years after injury.

7. Although bladder and bowel distention are the most common causes of autonomic hyperreflexia, any noxious stimuli can cause a response.

💡 Study and Memory Aids

🍎 Diet

Spinal Shock

NPO/IV → ↑ Calories
Protein
Vitamins

Drug Review

Herniated Intervertebral Disk

Analgesics
Acetaminophen/codeine (*Tylenol* #1, #2, #3): 1–2 tablets q3–4h, as needed
Meperidine HCl (*Demerol*): IM or SC, 50–75 mg
Oxycodone/acetaminophen (*Tylox, Percocet*): 5 mg q3–6h, as needed

Anti-inflammatories
Aspirin/ecotrin: 2.6–6.2 g/d in divided doses
Ibuprofen (*Motrin*): 300–800 mg 3–4 times daily (*not to exceed*) 3200 mg/d
Indomethacin (*Indocin*): 25–50 mg 2–4 times daily

Muscle relaxants
Baclofen (*Lioresal*): 5 mg 3 times daily, up to maximum of 80 mg/d
Carisoprodol (*Soma*): 350 mg 3–4 times daily
Cyclobenzaprine (*Flexeril*): 10 mg tid 20–40 mg/d, (*not to exceed*) 60 mg/d
Diazepam (*Valium*): 2–10 mg 2–4 times daily

Stool softener: Docusate (*Colace*): 50–500 mg/d

Laminectomy

Analgesics
Acetaminophen/codeine (*Tylenol* #1, #2, #3): 1–2 tablets q3–4h, as needed
Meperidine HCl (*Demerol*): IM or SC, 50–75 mg
Oxycodone/acetaminophen (*Tylox, Percocet*): 5 mg q3–6h, as needed

Spinal Cord Injury

Analgesics
Acetaminophen/codeine (*Tylenol* #1, #2, #3): 1–2 tablets q3–4h. as needed
Meperidine HCl (*Demerol*): IM or SC, 50–75 mg
Oxycodone/acetaminophen (*Tylox, Percocet*): 5 mg q3–6h. as needed

Anti-inflammatories
Aspirin/ecotrin: 2.6–6.2 g/d in divided doses
Ibuprofen (*Motrin*): 300–800 mg 3–4 times daily (*not to exceed* 3200 mg/d)
Indomethacin (*Indocin*):25–50 mg 2–4 times daily

Muscle relaxants
Baclofen (*Lioresal*): 5 mg 3 times daily, up to maximum of 80 mg/d
Carisoprodol (*Soma*): 350 mg 3–4 times daily
Cyclobenzaprine (*Flexeril*): 10 mg tid 20–40 mg/d, (*not to exceed 60 mg/d*)

Sedatives
Chlordiazepoxide HCl (*Librium*): 5–10 mg 3–4 times daily
Diazepam (*Valium*): 2–10 mg 2–4 times daily

Steroids (should **never** be abruptly discontinued; gradually taper dose to prevent complications):
Dexamethasone (*Decadron*): 0.5–9 mg/d in single or divided doses

Autonomic Hyperreflexia

Hydralazine HCl (*Apresoline*): 10–50 mg qid
Nifedipine (*Procardia*): 10–30 mg tid
Nitroglycerin: 0.25–0.6 mg repeated q5min for 15 min for severe hypertension

Questions

1. A 72-year-old woman has undergone a lumbar laminectomy with spinal fusion 3 days earlier. The nurse teaches her that the correct way to get onto the bedpan is to:
   1. Lift herself up with an overhead trapeze and swing onto the bedpan.
   2. Turn to her side, then log-roll onto the bedpan.
   3. Have two nurses lift her onto the bedpan.
   4. Push down on the bed to raise herself onto the bedpan.

2. During a lumbar puncture the nurse's role is to:
   1. Hold the client in the desired position.
   2. Check the client's vital signs every 15 minutes.
   3. Remind the client to breathe deeply to relax.
   4. Assess for indications of nerve damage.

3. Sciatic nerve involvement is suspected in a client with a herniated disc. Which test would confirm the nerve problem?
   1. Straight-leg raising.
   2. Gluteal contraction.
   3. Pinprick over the gluteal area.
   4. Plantar flexion of the foot.

4. Which observations made by a client preoperatively would provide the most useful information for the planning of care after a spinal fusion?
   1. Fears about surgery.
   2. Memories of previous hospitalizations.
   3. Preferred pain therapy.
   4. Currently experienced pain, muscle spasms, and numbness.

5. Which nursing action would be most helpful the first time a client sits in a chair after surgery for a herniated disc?
   1. Teaching the client relaxation techniques to use when getting out of bed.
   2. Using two people to transfer the client to the chair.
   3. Bracing the client's back with a rib support before the client gets out of bed.
   4. Giving the client the prescribed pain medication 30 minutes before getting out of bed.

6. An indication of adequate respiratory function in a client with a cervical spinal cord injury would be:
   1. Use of accessory muscles.
   2. Nasal flaring.
   3. Diaphragmatic breathing.
   4. Swallowing air.

Answers/Rationale

1. (2) Log-rolling would not be required for a lumbar laminectomy alone, but the spinal fusion would require that a shearing motion be avoided during turning. The client would therefore be taught to log-roll, and the nurse, or nurses, would assist her as needed. The key is having the client roll as a single unit, avoiding the placement of stress on any particular area of the body. An *older* woman may *not* have the *arm strength* to lift herself up (1) and may end up twisting. Lifting, even by the nurses (3), would *not* ensure proper body mechanics. Pushing down on the bed (4) would again rely on arm strength and *may not be possible* for an *older* client. **IMP, APP, 3, PhI, Basic care and comfort**

2. (1) The client is placed on the side with the back arched, neck flexed, and knees drawn up; holding the client still will ensure a safe procedure. Vital signs (2) would be assessed *before* and *after* the procedure, but it is not necessary to assess them every 15 minutes. Relaxation (3) would *not* reduce any discomfort, which is minimal, and deep breathing might cause too much movement. The site of a lumbar puncture is low enough that there is no danger of spinal cord injury, so assessment for nerve damage (4) is *unnecessary*. **IMP, COM, 3, SECE, Management of care**

3. (1) The sciatic nerve is the longest nerve in the body and is subjected to more trauma than any other nerve; any movement of the lower extremities stretches the nerve and would cause pain. Although the pain usually starts at the buttocks, contraction of the gluteal muscle (2) would *not* induce pain. Pinprick (3) is *too superficial* a stimulus. *Dorsiflexion*, rather than plantar flexion (4), might elicit pain. **AS, APP, 2, PhI, Reduction of risk potential**

4. (4) Postoperative care in this client would include assessing the effectiveness of the surgery by comparing the degree of any postoperative discomfort with the client's preoperative status. The observations in options 1 and 2 would be a source of increased preoperative anxiety, and this might influence the amount of anesthetic needed during surgery but would have less effect on the nature of postoperative care. If the surgery is successful, the degree of pain after surgery will be less, thus the client would require a different approach to pain management (3). **AN, ANL, 1, PsI, Psychosocial integrity**

5. (**4**) Once the anesthetic wears off, there will be pain resulting from swelling; administering pain medication before the client gets out of bed is recommended for any surgical client. Relaxation techniques (**1**) do reduce pain, but the client may be *too anxious* the *first time* out of bed to focus on such a technique. One nurse can assist the client in transferring to a chair (**2**) but should be careful that this not involve twisting. A metal brace, corset, or cast may be used temporarily to support the client's spine (**3**), but it would *not be used the first time* the client gets out of bed. **IMP, ANL, 3, PhI, Pharmacological and parenteral therapies**

6. (**3**) The diaphragm is a strong muscle and important to effective ventilation. The use of accessory muscles (**1**), nasal flaring (**2**), and swallowing air (**4**) would indicate *ineffective* breathing and respiratory difficulty. **EV, EVL, 6, PhI, Physiological adaptation**

Key to Codes

Nursing process: AS, assessment; AN, analysis; PL, planning; IMP, implementation; EV, evaluation. (See **Appendix M** for explanation of nursing process steps.)

Cognitive level: RE/KN, recall/knowledge; COM, comprehension; APP, application; ANL, analysis; EVL, evaluation; SYN, synthesis. (See **Appendix M** for explanation.)

Category of human function: 1, protective; 2, sensory-perceptual; 3, comfort, rest, activity, and mobility; 4, nutrition; 5, growth and development; 6, fluid-gas transport; 7, psychosocial-cultural; 8, elimination. (See **Appendix 0** for explanation.)

Client need: SECE, safe, effective care environment; **PhI**, physiological integrity; **PsI**, psychosocial integrity; **HPM**, health promotion and maintenance. (See **Appendix P** for explanation.)

Client subneed: (See **Appendix P** for explanation)

Degenerative Neurologic Disorders

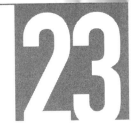

Chapter Outline

- Multiple Sclerosis
- Myasthenia Gravis
- Parkinson's Disease
- Amyotrophic Lateral Sclerosis
- Summary of Key Points

- Study and Memory Aids
  - Diets
  - Drug review
- Questions
- Answers/Rationale

Multiple Sclerosis

Progressive neurologic disease, common in temperate climates, such as northern United States, northern Europe, southern Canada and southern Australia; characterized by demyelination of brain and spinal cord, leading to degenerative neurologic function; chronic remitting and relapsing disease; cause unknown, but thought to be an autoimmune disease.

I. **Pathophysiology**: multiple foci (patches) of nerve degeneration throughout brain, spinal cord, optic nerve, and cerebrum → interruption (blockade) or distortion (slowing) of nerve impulses. Exacerbations aggravated by fatigue, chilling, and emotional distress.

II. **Risk factors/causes:**
   A. Northern climate.
   B. Onset age: 20–40 yr.
   C. Affects men and women equally.
   D. Heredity.

III. **Assessment**
   A. *Subjective data:*
      1. Extremities: numb, decreased sensation.
      2. Emotional: instability, apathy, irritability, mood swings, fatigue.
      3. Eyes: diplopia (double vision), spots before eyes (*scotomas*), potential blindness.
   B. *Objective data:*
      1. Nystagmus (involuntary rhythmic movements of eyeball), decreased visual acuity.
      2. Inappropriate outbursts of laughing or crying (sometimes related to ingestion of *hot food*).
      3. Disorders of speech.
      4. Susceptibility to infections.
      5. Tremors to severe muscle spasms and contractures.
      6. Dysphagia
      7. Changes in muscular coordination; *gait*: ataxic, spastic.
      8. Changes in bowel habits (e.g., constipation).
      9. Urinary frequency, urgency.
      10. Incontinence: urine and feces.
      11. Lab tests: cerebrospinal fluid contains gamma globulin, IgG.

IV. **Analysis/nursing diagnosis**
   A. *Impaired physical mobility* related to changes in muscular coordination.
   B. *Self-esteem disturbance* related to chronic, debilitating disease.
   C. *Altered health maintenance* related to spasms and contractures.
   D. *Risk for impaired skin integrity* related to contractures.
   E. *Constipation* related to immobility.
   F. *Impaired swallowing* related to tremors.
   G. *Visual-sensory/perceptual alteration* related to nystagmus and decreased visual acuity.

V. **Nursing care plan/implementation**
   A. Goal: *maintain normal routine as long as possible.*
      1. Maintain mobility—encourage walking as tolerated, active and passive range of motion (*ROM*); exercises, splints to decrease spasticity.
      2. *Avoid* fatigue, infections.
      3. Frequent position changes to prevent skin breakdown, contractures; *position at night*: prone to minimize flexor spasms of knees and hips.
      4. Bowel/bladder training program to minimize incontinence.
      5. *Avoid* stressful situations.
   B. Goal: *decrease symptoms*—medications as ordered:
      1. Baclofen (*Lioresal*) for alleviating spasticity; *avoid* sudden withdrawal (which may cause hallucinations, rebound spasticity).
      2. *Steroids* during exacerbations.
      3. *Skeletal muscle relaxants*: Diazepam (*Valium*), dantrolene (*Dantrium*) to relieve muscle spasm.

4. *Anticonvulsants* and *antidepressants* for dysesthesias or neuralgias: carbamazepine (*Tegretol*), phenytoin (*Dilantin*), amitriptyline HCl, (*Elavil*).

5. *Immunomodulators* for exacerbations: ß interferon (*Betaseron, Avonex*), glatiramer acetate (*Copaxone*).

6. *Cholinergics* for urinary retention due to flaccid bladder: bethanechol (*Urecholine*), neostigmine (*Prostigmin*).

7. *Anticholinergics* for urinary frequency and urgency (spastic bladder): probanthine (*Pro-Banthine*), oxybutynin (*Ditropan*).

C. Goal: **health teaching to** *prevent complications.*

1. Signs and symptoms of disease; measures to prevent exacerbations.

2. The way to monitor respiratory status to prevent infections.

3. Importance of physical therapy to prevent contractures.

4. Possible counseling or community support group for assistance in accepting longterm condition.

5. Teach special skin care to prevent decubitus ulcers.

6. Teach use of assistive devices to maintain independence.

VI. Evaluation/outcome criteria

A. Establishes daily routine; adjusts to altered lifestyle.

B. Injuries prevented; no falls.

C. Urinary and bowel routines established; incontinence decreased.

D. Infections prevented.

E. Symptoms minimized by medications.

Myasthenia Gravis

Neuromuscular disease characterized by weakness and easy fatigability of facial, oculomotor, pharyngeal, and respiratory muscles.

I. Pathophysiology: inadequate acetylcholine or excessive or altered cholinesterase → impaired transmission of nerve impulses to muscles at myoneural junction.

II. Risk factors/causes:

A. Possible autoimmune reaction.

B. Thymus tumor.

C. Thyrotoxicosis.

D. Lupus.

E. Rheumatoid arthritis.

F. Age: 20–40 yr; affects more women than men.

G. Older age groups: affects men and women equally.

III. Assessment

A. *Subjective data:*

1. Diplopia (double vision).

2. Severe generalized fatigue.

B. *Objective data*:

1. Muscle weakness: hands, arms affected first.

2. Ptosis (drooping of eyelids), expressionless facies.

3. Hypersensitivity to: narcotics, barbiturates, tranquilizers.

4. Abnormal speech pattern, with high-pitched nasal voice.

5. Difficulty chewing/swallowing food.

6. Decreased ability to cough and deep breathe, vital capacity.

7. Positive *Tensilon* test (administration of edrophonium chloride, 10 mg IV, produces relief of symptoms within 30 sec).

8. Positive *Prostigmin* test (neostigmine methylsulfate, 1.5 mg SC, produces relief of symptoms within 15 min, increased muscle strength within 30 min).

IV. Analysis/nursing diagnosis

A. *Ineffective breathing pattern* related to weakness.

B. *Risk for injury* related to muscle weakness.

C. *Activity intolerance* related to severe fatigue.

D. *Bathing/dressing self-care deficit* related to progressive disease.

E. *Impaired physical mobility* related to decrease in strength.

F. *Anxiety* related to physical symptoms and disease progression.

G. *Knowledge deficit* related to medication administration and expected effectiveness.

V. Nursing care plan/implementation

A. Goal: *promote comfort.*

1. Passive and active ROM exercises, as tolerated, to increase strength.

2. *Mouth care*: before and after meals.

3. *Diet*: as tolerated; soft, pureed, or tube feedings.

4. *Skin care* to prevent decubitus ulcers.

5. *Eye care*: remove crusts, patch on affected eye prn.

6. Monitor *respiratory* status: *suction* airway prn.

B. Goal: *decrease symptoms.*

1. Administer medications, as ordered:

a. *Anticholinesterase* (neostigmine [*Prostigmin*], pyridostigmine) to elevate concentration of acetylcholine at myoneural junction.

b. Give *before* meals to aid in chewing, *with* milk or food to decrease gastrointestinal (GI) symptoms; may be given parenterally.

C. Goal: *prevent complications.*

1. Respiratory assistance if breathing pattern not adequate.

2. Monitor for choking/increased oral secretion.

3. *Avoid: narcotics, barbiturates, tranquilizers.*

D. Goal: *promote increased self-concept.*
   1. Encourage independence when appropriate.
   2. Encourage communication; provide alternative methods when speech pattern impaired.

E. Goal: **health teaching.**
   1. Medication information:
      a. Adjust dosage to maintain muscle strength.
      b. Medication must be taken at prescribed time to *avoid:*
         (1) *Myasthenic crisis* (too little medication).
         (2) *Cholinergic crisis* (too much medication).
   2. Signs and symptoms of crisis: dyspnea, severe muscle weakness, respiratory distress, difficulty swallowing.
   3. Importance of preventing upper respiratory tract infections.
   4. Determine methods to conserve energy, maintain independence as long as possible, while *avoiding* overexertion.
   5. Refer to Myasthenia Gravis Foundation and other community agencies for assistance in reintegration into the community and plans for follow-up care.

VI. **Evaluation/outcome criteria**
   A. Independence maintained as long as possible.
   B. Respiratory arrest avoided.
   C. Infection avoided.
   D. Medication regimen followed and crisis avoided.

Parkinson's Disease

Progressive disease of the brain occurring in later life; characterized by stiffness of muscles, tremors, slowing of movement (bradykinesia).

I. **Pathophysiology**: degeneration of the substantia nigra of basal ganglia → decreased dopamine (neurotransmitter necessary for proper muscle movement) → decreased, slowed voluntary movement; wooden facies; difficulty initiating ambulation. Decreased inhibitions of alpha-motorneurons → increased muscle tone → rigidity of flexor and extensor muscles, tremors at rest.

II. **Risk factors:**
   A. Age of onset: 50–60 yr.
   B. Affects men and women equally.
   C. Cause unknown, possibly connected to arteriosclerosis or viral infection.
   D. Drug-induced parkinsonian syndromes have been linked to:

1. Phenothiazines.
2. Reserpine (*Serpasil*).
3. Butyrophenones (*Haloperidol*).
4. Methamphetamines.

III. **Assessment**
   A. *Subjective data*:
      1. Insomnia.
      2. Depression.
      3. Defects in judgment, emotional instability; intelligence *not* impaired.
   B. *Objective data*:
      1. Limbs, shoulders: stiff, resistant to passive ROM.
      2. Loss of coordination, muscular weakness with rigidity.
      3. Shuffling gait: difficulty initiating, then propulsive walking; trunk bent forward.
      4. Tremors: pillrolling of fingers, to-and-fro head movements.
      5. Loss of postural reflexes.
      6. Weight loss, constipation.
      7. Difficulty maintaining social interactions because of impaired speech, lack of facial affect, drooling.
      8. Facies: wide-eyed, eye blinking, decreased facial expression.
      9. Akinesia (abnormal absence of movement).
      10. Excessive salivation, drooling.
      11. Dysphagia.
      12. Speech: slowed, slurred.
      13. Heat intolerance.

IV. **Analysis/nursing diagnosis**
   A. *Impaired physical mobility* related to loss of coordination.
   B. *Altered health maintenance* related to defective judgment.
   C. *Risk for injury* related to altered gait.
   D. *Dressing/grooming self-care deficit* related to muscular rigidity.
   E. *Sleep pattern disturbance* related to insomnia.
   F. *Body image disturbance* related to tremors and drooling.
   G. *Social isolation* related to altered physical appearance.
   H. *Altered nutrition, less than body requirements,* related to lack of appetite, dysphagia.
   I. *Impaired swallowing* related to excessive drooling.
   J. *Constipation* related to dietary changes.

V. **Nursing care plan/implementation**
   A. Goal: *promote maintenance of daily activities.*
      1. ROM exercises, skin care, physical therapy.
      2. Encourage ambulation, discourage sitting for long periods.

3. Assist with meals—*high protein, high calorie; soft diet*; small, frequent feedings; encourage increased fluids. Provide thickened liquids, and soft solids.

4. Encourage compliance with medication regimen:

   a. *Dopamine agonists*:

      (1) Levodopa: given in increasing doses until symptoms are relieved; given *with food* to decrease GI symptoms. *Side effects*: nausea, vomiting, anorexia, postural hypotension, mental changes, cardiac arrhythmias. Levodopa helps restore dopamine in striated muscle.

      (2) *Sinemet* (carbidopa and levodopa): limits the metabolism of levodopa peripherally and provides more levodopa for the brain.

   b. *Anticholinergics*: effective in lessening muscle rigidity; trihexyphenidyl (*Artane*), benztropine (*Cogentin*), biperiden (*Akineton*).

   c. *Antihistamines*: have mild central anticholinergic properties; diphenhydramine (*Benadryl*), chlorphenoxamine (*Phenoxene*).

5. Prepare for possible surgical intervention; used in clients who are unresponsive to drug therapy or who have developed severe motor complications.

   a. *Deep brain stimulation* (DBS)—places an electrode in the thalamus, globus pallidus or subthalamic nucleus; attached to device that delivers specific current to a particular brain location.

   b. *Pallidotomy*—stereotactic ablation of globus pallidus.

   c. *Thalamotomy*—stereotactic ablation of areas in thalamus.

B. Goal: *protect from injury*.

   1. Monitor blood pressure, side effects of medications (e.g., orthostatic hypotension).

   2. Monitor for GI disturbances.

   3. *Avoid* pyridoxine (*vitamin B_6*): cancels effect of levodopa.

   4. Levodopa *contraindicated* with:

      a. Glaucoma (causes increased intraocular pressure).

      b. Monoamine oxidase inhibitors (causes possible hypertensive crisis).

C. Goal: **health teaching**.

   1. Teach client, family about medications: dosage range, side effects, not discontinuing medications abruptly.

   2. Exercise program to maintain ROM and normal body posture; also get adequate rest to prevent fatigue.

3. *Dietary adjustment and precautions* regarding cutting food in small pieces to prevent choking, taking fluid with food to facilitate swallowing.

4. Importance of adding *roughage* to diet to prevent constipation.

5. Help client, family adjust to this chronic debilitating illness.

VI. **Evaluation/outcome criteria**

A. Activity level maintained.

B. Symptoms relieved by medications, no drug interactions.

C. Complications prevented.

Amyotrophic Lateral Sclerosis (ALS; Lou Gehrig's Disease)

Progressive degeneration of motorneurons within the brain and/or spinal cord, leading to death within 2–5 yr, usually from pneumonia resulting from respiratory or bulbar paralysis.

I. **Pathophysiology**: myelin sheaths destroyed, replaced by scar tissue; involves lateral tracts of spinal cord, eventually medulla and ventral tracts.

II. **Risk factors/causes**:

A. Affects more men than women.

B. Onset usually in middle age.

C. Viral infection possible causal agent.

D. Possible familial or genetic component.

III. **Assessment**

A. *Subjective data*:

   1. Early symptoms: fatigue, awkwardness.

   2. Alert, no sensory loss.

B. *Objective data*:

   1. Symptoms depend on which motorneurons affected.

   2. Dysphagia, dysarthria.

   3. Decreased fine finger movement.

   4. Progressive muscular weakness, atrophy.

   5. Spasticity of flexor muscles; one side of body becomes more involved than other.

   6. Progressive respiratory difficulties → diaphragmatic paralysis.

   7. Progressive disability of upper and lower extremities.

   8. Tongue fasciculations.

IV. **Analysis/nursing diagnosis**

A. *Ineffective airway clearance* related to difficulty coughing.

B. *Ineffective breathing pattern* related to progressive respiratory difficulties and eventually respiratory paralysis.

C. *Impaired swallowing* related to disease progression.

D. *Impaired physical mobility* related to progressive muscular weakness.

E. *Bathing/hygiene and dressing/grooming self-care deficit* related to neuromuscular impairment.

F. *Powerlessness* related to progressive physical helplessness.

G. *Altered health maintenance* related to inability to perform self-care activities

V. Nursing care plan/implementation

A. Goal: *maintain independence as long as possible.*

1. Assistance with activities of daily living (ADL); *splints, prosthetic devices* to support weak limbs and maintain mobility.

2. Skin care to prevent decubitus.

3. *Soft/liquid diet* to aid in swallowing, prevent choking; *suction* prn; *head of bed elevated* when eating.

4. *Respiratory* assistance as needed, ventilators as disease progresses and diaphragm becomes involved.

5. Arrange long-term care if home maintenance no longer feasible.

6. Emotional support, when client is alert; continue involving client in decisions regarding care.

7. Drug therapy: Riluzole (*Rilutek*) slows progression of ALS and may delay need for tracheostomy and death for several months.

B. Goal: **health teaching.**

1. Skin care to prevent decubitus.

2. Ramifications of disease, so client and family can make decisions regarding future care, whether client will remain at home as disease progresses or enter a long-term care facility.

3. The way to use suction apparatus to clear airway.

4. Care of nasogastric or gastrostomy feeding tube.

VI. Evaluation/outcome criteria

A. Obtains physical and emotional support.

B. Complications prevented in early stage of disease.

C. Remains in control of ADL as long as possible.

D. Skin breakdown prevented.

E. Peaceful death.

💡 Study and Memory Aids

🍎 Diets

Myasthenia Gravis

Pureed
Soft
or
Tube feed

Parkinson's Disease

↑ Calories
Fluids
Frequent feeding   +   soft and bland
Protein
Roughage

↓ Size of feedings
Size of pieces of food

🔑 Summary of Key Points

1. Several degenerative disorders occur in young adults as early as 20-30 yr of age. Parkinson's disease is *more* common in adults over 60 yr.

2. *Visual* problems are often the *first indication* of multiple sclerosis.

3. Treatment for multiple sclerosis is *symptomatic* and designed to prevent complications, which may be fatal. Disease progression is *unpredictable.*

4. Muscle weakness resulting from myasthenia gravis increases with exercise and diminishes after rest.

5. Myasthenia gravis, like multiple sclerosis, often presents with *ocular* symptoms. The clinical course can vary greatly and may progress slowly or rapidly.

6. The nurse must be able to distinguish between a *myasthenic* and *cholinergic crisis.*

7. Parkinson's disease causes disability as a result of *tremors* and *rigidity.* Intellectual ability is usually *not* affected.

8. The *bowel* and *bladder-related side* effects of anticholinergic drugs used to treat Parkinson's disease may be distressing to older adults.

9. ALS ends in death 2–5 yr after diagnosis. The cause of death is usually *pneumonia* secondary to ineffective respiratory function.

10. Nursing actions for a client with ALS are *supportive.* Even after total debilitation the client's *mental status* is *intact.*

Drug Review

Multiple Sclerosis

Anticonvulsants
Carbamazepine (*Tegretol*): 200 mg bid; maintenance dose 800–1200 mg daily.
Phenytoin (*Dilantin*): 100 mg tid; maximum dose 600 mg daily.

Antidepressant
Amitriptyline HCl (*Elavil*): 75–100 mg in 1–4 divided doses; maintenance dose 40–100 mg daily.

Skeletal muscle relaxants
Baclofen (*Lioresal*): 5 mg 3 times daily, up to maximum of 80 mg/d (20 mg 4 times daily); optimal effect between 40–80 mg
Dantrolene (*Dantrium*): 25 mg/d; increase to 25 mg 2–4 times daily up to 100 mg 2–4 times daily (*not* to exceed 40 mg/d)
Diazepam (*Valium*): 2–10 mg 2–4 times daily

Steroids (should **never** be abruptly discontinued; gradually taper dose to prevent complications)
Dexamethasone (*Decadron*): 0.5–9 mg/d in single or divided doses
Methylprednisolone (*Medrol*): 4–48 mg/d
Prednisone: 5–60 mg/d.

Myasthenia Gravis

Anticholinesterase agents (Cholinergic)
Neostigmine (*Prostigmin*): 15 mg q3–4h; increase daily until optimal response achieved; usual maintenance dose, 150 mg/d (up to 375 mg may be needed)
Pyridostigmine (*Mestinon*): 60 mg 3 times/d; maintenance dose 60–1500 mg/d.

Parkinson's Disease

Anticholinergics
Benztropine (*Cogentin*): 0.5–6 mg/d in 1–2 divided doses
Biperiden (*Akineton*): 2 mg 3–4 times daily, *not* to exceed 16 mg/d
Trihexyphenidyl (*Artane*): 1–2 mg/d; increase by 2 mg q3–5 days; usual maintenance dose, 5–15 mg/d in 3–4 divided doses

Antihistamines
Chlorpheniramine maleate (*Chlor-Trimeton*): 2–4 mg tid
Diphenhydramine (*Benadryl*): 25–50 mg bid

Dopamine Agonists
Carbidopa/levodopa (*Sinemet*): 25–250 mg/d in 3–4 divided doses; can increase to 200/8000 mg/d
Levodopa (*L-dopa*): 500–1000 mg/d in divided doses q6–12h; increase by 100–750 mg/d q3–7 d until response reached; usual maintenance dose, should *not* exceed 8 g/d.

NO PYRIDOXINE (B₆)

Questions

1. A 30-year-old woman with suspected myasthenia gravis is admitted to undergo testing to confirm or rule out the diagnosis. Which physical change would the nurse likely observe in the woman?
   1. Intention tremor.
   2. Muscle rigidity.
   3. Drooping eyelids.
   4. Hemiplegia.

2. Although the *Tensilon* (edrophonium) test is frequently used to establish the diagnosis of myasthenia gravis, the nurse should know that a more conclusive diagnosis is possible using neostigmine (*Prostigmin*) because:
   1. The desired effect occurs more rapidly.
   2. The desired effect lasts hours rather than minutes.
   3. The improvement is generalized, not just localized.
   4. The improvement is permanent, not temporary.

3. Which nursing diagnosis would be the greatest concern during the hospitalization of a client with myasthenia gravis?
   1. Risk for activity intolerance.
   2. Pain.
   3. Impaired adjustment.
   4. Impaired memory.

4. Which drug would be contraindicated in a client with myasthenia gravis?
   1. Nifedipine (*Procardia*).
   2. Furosemide (*Lasix*).
   3. Atropine.
   4. Potassium penicillin.

Answers/Rationale

1. **(3)** Myasthenia gravis is an autoimmune disease that presents with muscular weakness and fatigue resulting from a loss of acetylcholine receptors in the postsynaptic neurons of the neuromuscular junction. As a result, affected clients are often unable to keep their eyes open, chew, or swallow. Intention tremor (**1**) and muscle rigidity (**2**) would be seen in a client with *Parkinson's* disease. Hemiplegia (**4**) would be seen in a client who has had a stroke. **AS, COM, 3, PhI, Physiological adaptation**

2. **(2)** Neostigmine's effects last 2 to 4 hours, and edrophonium's effects only last 30 minutes. Testing with neostigmine would therefore permit more time to observe for an alleviation or worsening of symptoms. The onset of neostigmine's effects is slower, *not* more rapid (**1**). *Both* drugs produce generalized effects (**3**), and improvement is *temporary*, *not* permanent (**4**). **AN, COM, 3, PhI, Reduction of risk potential**

3. **(1)** The muscle weakness and fatigue, if not controlled with drug therapy, will interfere with basic activities, such as eating. The condition is *painless* (2). There may be problems with adjustment (3) to the chronic illness, but the *priority* would be the activity intolerance. There is *no* memory impairment (4) in myasthenia. **AN, ANL, 3, SECE, Management of care**

4. **(2)** The loss of potassium ions resulting from diuretic therapy may cause the muscle weakness to worsen. Nifedipine (1) may cause muscle cramping, but *not* weakness. Atropine (3) affects cardiac function, *not* skeletal muscle strength. Potassium penicillin (4) does *not* affect the potassium ion concentration. **IMP, APP, 6, PhI, Pharmacological and parenteral therapies**

Key to Codes

Nursing process: **AS**, assessment; **AN**, analysis; **PL**, planning; **IMP**, implementation; **EV**, evaluation. (See **Appendix M** for explanation of nursing process steps.)

Cognitive level: **RE/KN**, recall/knowledge; **COM**, comprehension; **APP**, application; **ANL**, analysis; **EVL**, evaluation; **SYN**, synthesis. (See **Appendix M** for explanation.)

Category of human function: **1**, protective; **2**, sensory-perceptual; **3**, comfort, rest, activity, and mobility; **4**, nutrition; **5**, growth and development; **6**, fluid-gas transport; **7**, psychosocial-cultural; **8**, elimination. (See **Appendix 0** for explanation.)

Client need: SECE, safe, effective care environment; **PhI**, physiological integrity; **PsI**, psychosocial integrity; **HPM**, health promotion and maintenance. (See **Appendix P** for explanation.)

Client subneed: (See **Appendix P** for explanation)

Neoplastic Disorders

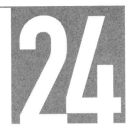

Chapter Outline

The Client with Cancer

Cancer is a multisystem stressor. Regardless of the specific type of cancer, certain aspects of the disease and of nursing care are the same. The following principles apply universally and should be referred to when studying individual kinds of cancer.

I. **Pathophysiology**: result of altered cellular mechanisms. Several theories about causation, but current thinking is multiple causation. Alterations result in a progressive, uncontrolled multiplication of cells, with selective ability to invade and metastasize. **(Figure 24.1)**

II. **Risk factors/causes:**
    A. Heredity (e.g., retinoblastoma).
    B. Familial susceptibility (e.g., breast cancer).
    C. Acquired diseases (e.g., ulcerative colitis).
    D. Virus (e.g., Burkitt's tumor).
    E. Environmental factors:
        1. Tobacco.
        2. Alcohol.
        3. Radiation.
        4. Occupational hazards.
        5. Drugs (e.g., *immunosuppressive*, *cytotoxic*).
    F. Age.
    G. Air pollution.
    H. Diet (e.g. high animal protein)
    I. Chronic irritation.
    J. Precancerous lesions (e.g. gastric ulcers).
    K. Stress.

III. **Assessment**
    A. Specific symptoms depend on the anatomic and functional characteristics of the organ or structure involved.

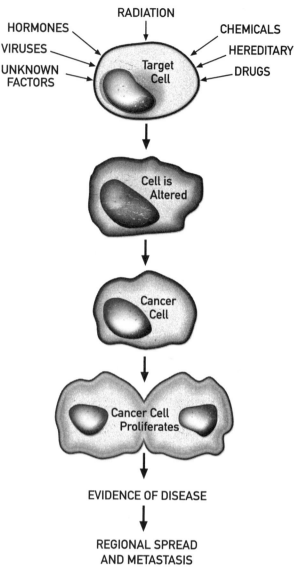

FIGURE 24.1 CANCER DEVELOPMENT

Diagram text: RADIATION, HORMONES, VIRUSES, UNKNOWN FACTORS, CHEMICALS, HEREDITARY, DRUGS → Target Cell → Cell is Altered → Cancer Cell → Cancer Cell Proliferates → EVIDENCE OF DISEASE → REGIONAL SPREAD AND METASTASIS

1. Warning signs—"CAUTION"
   a. **C**hange in bowel/bladder habits.
   b. **A** persistent sore throat.
   c. **U**nusual discharge/bleeding.
   d. **T**hickening or lump.
   e. **I**ndigestion, dysphagia.
   f. **O**bvious change in mole, work.
   g. **N**odes, with hoarse voice, cough.

B. Mechanical effects:
   1. *Pressure*—tumors growing in confined areas such as bone produce pain early, whereas tumors growing in expandable areas such as the abdomen may be undetected for some time.
   2. *Obstruction*—tumors that compress tubular structures such as the esophagus, bronchi, or lymph channels may cause symptoms such as swallowing difficulties, shortness of breath, edema. Symptoms depend on location of tumor and on the particular organ or structure being compressed.

3. *Interruptions of blood supply*—compression of blood vessels or diversion of blood supply may cause necrosis or ulceration or may precipitate hemorrhage.

C. Systemic effects:
   1. Anorexia, weakness, weight loss.
   2. *Metabolic* disturbances—malabsorption syndrome.
   3. *Fluid and electrolyte* imbalances.
   4. *Hormonal* imbalances—*increased* antidiuretic hormone (ADH), adrenocorticotropic hormone (ACTH), thyrotropin, or parathyroid hormone.
   5. *Diagnostic tests:*
      a. *Biopsy*—excision of part of tumor.
      b. *Needle biopsy*—aspiration of cells from subcutaneous masses or organs such as liver.
      c. *Exfoliative cytology*—scraping of any endothelium (cervix, mucous membranes) applied to slide.
      d. *X-rays*—detect tumor growth in gastrointestinal (GI), respiratory, renal systems.
      e. *Endoscopy*—visualization of body cavity through endoscope.
      f. *Computerized axial tomography* (CAT)—visualization of a body part whereby layers of tissue can be seen utilizing the very narrow beams of this type of x-ray equipment.
      g. *Magnetic resonance imaging* (MRI)—a scanning device using a magnetic field for visualization.
   6. Lab data:
      a. *Blood and urine tests*—refer to **Appendix G** for normal values.
      b. *Alkaline phosphates*—greatly *increased* in osteogenic carcinoma (>92 U/L).
      c. *Calcium*—*elevated* in multiple myeloma bone metastases (>10.5 mg/dL).
      d. *Sodium*—*decreased* in bronchogenic carcinoma (<135 mEq/L).
      e. *Potassium*—*decreased* in extensive liver carcinoma (<3.5 mEq/L).
      f. *Serum gastrin*—gauges gastric secretions. *Decreased* in gastric carcinoma. Normal value: 40–150 pg/mL.
      g. *Neutrophilic leukocytosis*—tumors.
      h. *Eosinophilic leukocytosis*—brain tumors, Hodgkin's disease.
      i. *Lymphocytosis*—chronic lymphocytic anemia.

IV. **Analysis/nursing diagnosis**
   A. *Pain* related to diagnostic procedures, pressure, obstruction, interruption of blood supply, or side effects of drugs.
   B. *Anxiety* related to fear regarding diagnosis or disease progression, treatment, and its known or expected side effects.

C. *Altered nutrition, less than body requirements,* related to anorexia.

D. *Risk for injury* related to radioactive contamination of excreta.

E. *Body image disturbance* related to loss of body parts, change in appearance as a result of therapy.

F. *Powerlessness* related to diagnosis and own perception of its meaning.

G. *Self-esteem disturbance* related to impact of cancer diagnosis.

H. *Risk for infection* related to immunosuppression resulting from radiation and chemotherapy.

I. *Altered urinary elimination* related to dehydration.

J. *Risk for injury* related to damage of normal tissue resulting from radiation source.

K. *Fluid volume deficit* related to nausea and vomiting.

L. *Diarrhea* related to irradiation of bowel.

M. *Constipation* related to dehydration.

N. *Anticipatory grief* related to poor prognosis.

V. **Nursing care plan/implementation—*general care*** of the client with cancer:

A. Goal: *promote psychosocial comfort.*

1. Assist with diagnostic workup by providing psychological support and information about diagnostic tests, diagnosis, treatment options.

2. Reduce anxiety by listening, making referrals for special problems (peer support groups, self-help groups such as Reach to Recovery), supplying information, or correcting misinformation, as appropriate.

3. Stress-management techniques.

4. Nursing management related to client who is depressed.

B. Goal: *minimize effects of complications.*

1. *Anorexia/anemia*:

a. *Decrease anemia* by:

(1) Providing well-balanced, *iron-rich*, small, frequent meals.

(2) Administering supplemental vitamins and iron, as ordered.

(3) Administering *packed red blood cells*, as ordered.

(4) Maintaining *hyperalimentation*, as ordered.

b. *Enhance nutrition* by providing nutritional supplements and a diet *high in protein*, necessary because of increased metabolism related to metastatic process. *Consult* with dietitian for suggestions about best food for individual client.

2. *Hemorrhage*: monitor *platelet* count and maintain platelet infusions, as ordered. Teach client to monitor for any signs of bleeding.

3. *Infection*: observe for signs of sepsis (changes in: vital signs, temperature of skin, mentation, urinary output, or pain), monitor laboratory values, administer *antiinfectives* as ordered.

4. *Pain and discomfort*: alleviate by frequent position changes, diversions, conversations guided imagery, relaxation, back rubs, *narcotics*, as ordered.

5. Assist in adjusting to altered body image by encouraging expression of fears and concerns. *Don't* ignore client's questions; give honest answers; be available.

C. Goal: **general health teaching.**

1. Self-care skills to maintain independence, e.g., client who has a colostomy should know how to manage the colostomy before going home.

2. Importance of follow-up care and routine physical examinations to monitor for general health and possible signs of further disease.

3. Dietary instructions, adjustments necessary to maintain nutrition during and after treatment.

4. Health maintenance programs: teach hazards of tobacco and alcohol use; *avoid: high* fat, *low* roughage diet.

5. Risk factors: family history, stress, age, diet, occupation, environment.

VI. **General surgical intervention**: surgery may be *curative* (when the lesion is localized or metastases to the lymph nodes are minimal) or *palliative* (to decrease symptomatology). (Also see **The Perioperative Experience**, **Chapter 9**, and specific types of cancer, following.)

A. **Nursing care plan/implementation**

1. **Preoperative care:**

a. Goal: *prevent respiratory complications.*

(1) Coughing and deep-breathing techniques.

(2) *No* smoking for 1 wk before surgery.

b. Goal: *counteract nutritional deficiencies.*

(1) *Diet*:

(a) High *protein*, high *carbohydrate* for tissue repair.

(b) *Vitamin* and *mineral* supplements.

(c) Hyperalimentation, as ordered.

(2) Blood transfusions may be needed if counts are low.

c. Goal: *reduce apprehension.*

(1) Clarify postoperative expectations.

(2) Explain care of ostomies or tubes.

(3) Answer client's questions honestly.

2. **Postoperative care:**

a. Goal: *prevent complications.*

(1) Monitor respiratory and hemodynamic status.

☞ (2) *Wound* care; active and passive *exercises* as allowed; *respiratory* hygiene; coughing, deep breathing, turning; fluids (see **Postoperative Experience, p. 131-141**).

b. Goal: *alleviate pain and discomfort*.
(1) Encourage early ambulation, depending on surgical procedure.
(2) Administer prescribed medications, as needed.
▭ (3) Administer *stool softeners* and *enemas*, as ordered.

c. Goal: **health teaching**.
(1) Involve client, significant others, family members in rehabilitation program.
(2) Prepare for further therapies, such as radiation or chemotherapy.
(3) Support groups, as appropriate: Reach to Recovery, Ostomy Associates, Laryngectomy Association.
(4) Develop skills to deal with disease progression if cure not realistic or metastasis evident (see **X. Palliative care, p. 320-321**).

▭ **VII. Chemotherapy:** used as single treatment or in combination with surgery and irradiation, for early or advanced diseases. Antineoplastic agents' primary mode of action involves interfering with the supply and utilization of building blocks of nucleic acids as well as interfering with intact molecules of DNA or RNA, which are needed for replication and growth. *Bone marrow, hair follicles*, and the *GI tract* are three areas of the body in which cells are actively dividing; this is why *most side effects* are related to these areas of the body.

A. *Types*: alkylating agents, antimetabolites, antitumor anti- infectives, plant-derived alkaloids, enzymes, hormones. See **Appendix D, Table D.6**.

B. *Major problem*: lacks specificity, thus affecting normal as well as malignant cells.

C. *Major side effects*: bone marrow depression, stomatitis, nausea and vomiting, GI ulcerations, diarrhea, alopecia (**Table 24.1**).

D. *Routes of administration*: oral, intramuscular, intravenous (*Hickman or Groshong catheter*), subclavian lines, porta caths, peripheral, intraarterial (may have infusion pump for continuous or intermittent flow rate), intracavity (e.g., bladder through cystoscopy, Omaya reservoir). (See **p. 111** for information about administration of *IV chemotherapeutic agents*.)

E. **Nursing care plan/implementation**
1. Goal: *assist with treatment of specific side effects*.
▭ **a.** *Nausea and vomiting*—*antiemetic* drugs (before treatment) and *antacid* therapy as ordered and scheduled; withhold food 4–6 h before chemotherapy; small, frequent, *high calorie, high potassium, high protein* meals; include milk and milk products when tolerated for *increased calcium*; carbonated drinks; frequent mouth care; rest after meals; *avoid* food odors during preparation of meals; pleasant environment during meals; appropriate distractions; IV therapy; *nasogastric* tube for control of severe nausea or as route for *tube feeding* if unable to take food by mouth; *hyperalimentation*.

b. *Diarrhea*—clear liquids → *low residue diet; increased potassium; increased fluids*; atropine sulfate-diphenoxylate HCl (*Lomotil*) or kaolin-pectin *Kaopectate*), as ordered; *avoid* hot or cold foods/liquids; monitor electrolytes.

c. *Stomatitis* (painful mouth)—soft toothbrushes or sponges (toothettes); *mouth care* q2–4h; *viscous lidocaine* HCl (*Xylocaine*), as ordered, before meals. Oral salt and soda mouth rinses; *avoid* commercial mouthwashes that contain high level of alcohol, which could be very irritating to mucous membranes. *Avoid* hot foods/liquids; include *bland* foods at cool temperatures; offer popsicles as a source of moisture for cracked lips; remove dentures if sores are under dentures; moisten lips with petroleum jelly (water-soluble lubricant).

d. *Skin care*—*avoid* soap, wash with plain water and pat dry; use cornstarch or olive oil; *avoid* talcum powder and powder with zinc oxide; monitor: wounds that do not heal, infections (client receives frequent sticks for blood tests and therapy); *avoid* sunlight; use sunblock, especially if receiving doxorubicin (*Adriamycin*).

☞ **e.** *Alopecia*—ice caps during therapy or tourniquet around forehead for 20 min before, during, and after infusion of a few drugs (as ordered by physician); be gentle when combing or lightly brushing hair; use wigs, night caps, scarves; provide frequent linen changes. Advise client to have hair cut short before treatment with drugs known to cause alopecia (bleomycin, cyclophosphamide, dactinomycin, daunorubicin HCl, doxorubicin HCl, 5-fluorouracil, ICRF-159, hydroxyurea, methotrexate, mitomycin, VP 16-213, vincristine).

TABLE 24.1 ⊂⊃ COMMON TOXICITIES OF ANTINEOPLASTIC AGENTS

	Nausea and Vomiting	Mucositis	Diarrhea	Skin Reactions	Lung	Neurologic
Antimetabolites						
Cytosine arabinoside (low dose)	+	+	0	Rash	0	0
(moderate dose)	++	++	+	Alopecia	0	0
(high dose)	+++	+++	+	Alopecia	0	Cerebellar
Fludarabine	+	+	+	0	+	0
5-Fluorouracil (low dose)	+	+	+	Phlebitis	0	Cerebellar
(moderate dose)	++	+++	+++	Phlebitis	0	Cerebellar
(high dose)	+++	++	+	Hand-foot syndrome	0	0
(with leucovorin)	+	++	+++	Hand-foot syndrome	0	0
Methotrexate	+++	+++	+++	Dermatitis	+	0
(with leucovorin)	+	+	+	Dermatitis	+	0
2-Deoxycoformycin	+	+	+	Erythema	0	Lethargy, coma
6-Mercaptopurine	+	+	+	Rash	0	0
Thioguanine	+	0	0	0	0	0
2-Chlorodeoxyadenosine	+	+	+	0	0	0
Alkylating agents						
Busulfan	+	+	+	Alopecia	0	0
Chlorambucil	0	0	0	0	+	0
Cyclophosphamide (low dose)	+	+	+	0	+	0
(moderate dose)	++	+	+	Alopecia	+	0
(high dose)	+++	+++	+++	Alopecia	+	0
DTIC	+++	0	0	0	0	0
Ifosfamide	+++	0	0	Alopecia	0	Encephalopathy
Mechlorethamine	+++	+	+	Alopecia, rash	0	0
Melphalan	+	0	0	0	0	0
Nitrosoureas						
Carmustine (BNCU)	+++	0	+	0	+	0
Lomustine (CCNU)	+	0	0	0	0	0
Streptozocin	+++	0	0	0	0	0
Thiotepa	++	+++	+++	Alopecia, rash	0	0
Plant alkaloids						
Etoposide	+	0	0	0	0	0
Vinblastine	+	+	0	Alopecia, vesicant	0	+ Numbness, tingling
Vincristine	0	0	0	Vesicant, alopecia	0	++ Neuropathy
Taxol	+	0	0	Alopecia	0	Neuropathy
Tumor antimicrobials						
Bleomycin	+	+	0	Erythema, alopecia	+	0
Dactinomycin	++	++	++	Alopecia, rash	0	0
Daunorubicin	++	+	+	Alopecia, vesicant	0	0
Doxorubicin	++	+	+	Alopecia, vesicant	0	0
Idarubicin	++	++	+	Alopecia, vesicant	0	0
Mitomycin C	++	+	0	Vesicant, alopecia	+	0
Mitoxantrone	+	+	+	Alopecia, vesicant	0	0
Other agents						
Carboplatin	++	0	+	0	0	0
Cisplatin	+++	0	+	0	0	+
Hydroxyurea	0	0	0	Skin atrophy	0	0
L-Asparaginase	+	0	0	0	0	Encephalopathy
Procarbazine	++	0	+	Rash, alopecia	0	Encephalopathy

0 = none; + = mild; ++ = moderate; +++ = severe.

Source: Adapted from Ewald G, McKenzie C (eds). *Manual of Medical Therapeutics*. Boston: Little, Brown. and: www.cancer.org (2006)

2. Goal: **health teaching**.
   a. Educate client and family to purpose of proposed drug regimen and anticipated side effects.
   b. Advise that frequent checks of hematologic status will be necessary (client will undergo frequent IV sticks, lab tests).
   c. Advise client and family of increased risk for infection (*avoid* uncontrolled crowds and individuals with upper respiratory tract infections or childhood diseases).
   d. Monitor injection site for signs of extravasation (infiltration) (site must be changed if leakage suspected, and guidelines to neutralize must be followed according to drug protocol).

F. **Nursing precautions with chemotherapy**:
   1. Nurse should wear *gloves* and *mask* when preparing chemotherapeutic agents for administration.
   2. Drugs are toxic substance; nurses must take every precaution to handle them with care.
   3. When expelling air bubbles from syringes, care must be taken that the drugs are *not* sprayed into the atmosphere.
   4. Contaminated needles and syringes should be disposed of intact (to prevent aerosol generation) in plastic-lined box and incinerated. Disposable equipment should be used whenever possible.
   5. If skin becomes contaminated with a drug, wash under running water.
   6. Nurses should know the half-life and excretion route of the drugs being administered and take the special precautions necessary. For example, while the drug is actively being excreted, use *gloves* when touching *client, stool, urine, dressings, vomitus*, etc.
   7. Nurses who are in the early phase of pregnancy should exercise caution when caring for clients receiving chemotherapeutic agents.

VIII. **Radiation therapy**: used in high doses to kill cancer cells or palliatively for pain relief. Side effects depend on site of therapy (vary in each person): nausea, vomiting, stomatitis, esophagitis, dry mouth, diarrhea, depression of bone marrow, suppression of immune response, decreased life span, sterility.
   A. **External radiation**: cobalt or linear accelerator machine.
      1. *Procedure*: daily treatments, Monday through Friday, for prescribed number of times according to size and location of tumor (duration of treatment is usually 4–6 wk). Client remains alone in room during treatment. (Nurse, therapist, family members cannot stay in room with client during treatment due to radiation exposure). Client instructed to lie still, so exactly same area irradiated each treatment. Marks (tattoos or permanent-ink marks) are made on skin to delineate area of treatment; marks must *not* be removed during entire treatment course.
      2. **Nursing care plan/implementation**
         a. Goal: *prevent tissue breakdown*.
            (1) Do *not* wash off site-identification marks (tattoos cannot be removed); dosage area is carefully calculated and must be exact for each treatment.
            (2) Assess skin daily and teach client to do same (most radiation therapy is done on outpatient basis, so client needs skills to manage independently).
            (3) Keep skin dry; cornstarch is usually the only topical application allowed.
            (4) *Contraindicated measures*:
               (a) Talcum powders, due to potential to alter radiation dose.
               (b) Lotions, due to increased moistening of skin.
               (c) Aloe preparations with alcohol, due to drying of skin. Check ingredients.
            (5) Reduce skin friction by *avoiding* constricting bedclothes or clothing, and by using electric shaver.
            (6) Dress areas of skin breakdown with nonadherent dressing and paper tape.
         b. Goal: *decrease side effects of therapy*.
            (1) Provide meticulous oral hygiene.
            (2) If diarrhea occurs, may need IV infusions, *antidiarrheal* medications; monitor bowel movements, possible adhesions resulting from surgery and radiation treatments.
            (3) Monitor vital signs, particularly respiratory function and blood pressure (sloughing of tissues puts client at *risk for hemorrhage*).
            (4) Monitor hematologic status—bone marrow depression can cause fatal toxicosis and sepsis.
            (5) Institute *protective isolation* as necessary to prevent infections (protective isolation usually instituted if <50% neutrophils).
         c. Goal: **health teaching**.
            (1) Instruct client to *avoid*:

(a) *Strong sunlight*; must wear sunblock lotion, protective clothing over radiation site.

(b) *Extremes in temperature* to the area (hot-water bottles, ice caps).

(c) Synthetic, *nonporous* clothes *or tight* constrictive clothing over area.

(d) Eating 2–3 h *before* treatment and 2 h *after*, to decrease nausea; *do* give small, frequent meals *high* in *protein* and *carbohydrates* and *low* in *residue*.

(e) Strong *alcohol-base mouthwash*; use daily salt and soda mouthwash.

(f) *Fatigue*, an overwhelming problem. Need to pace themselves, nap; may need someone to drive them to therapy; can continue with usual activities as tolerated.

(g) *Crowds* and persons with upper respiratory tract infections or any other infections.

(2) Provide appropriate birth control information for clients of childbearing age.

B. **Internal radiation: sealed** (radium, iridium, cesium).

1. Used for localized masses (e.g., mouth, cervix, breast, testes). Due to exposure from radiation source, precautions must be taken while it is in place. Health care personnel and family must adhere to *principles of time, distance, and shielding to decrease exposure* (*shortest* amount of time possible, stay as *far away* as possible from the source of radiation, and wear *protective* lead apron, gloves). If source of radiation accidentally falls out, it should be picked up only with *forceps*. Radiation officer should be notified **immediately**. Client should be in *private* room, and bed should be in the center of the room, if possible, to protect others. Unless the walls are lead lined, radiation will penetrate them; placing the bed in *center of room* will decrease exposure. Once the source of radiation has been removed, there is no radiation exposure from client, excretions, or linens.

2. **Nursing care plan/implementation**

a. Goal: *assist with cervical radium implantation* (cervical radium is used here as the most common example of an internal radiation source).

(1) *Prior to insertion*—give douche, enema; perform perineal preparation; insert Foley catheter, as ordered.

(2) *After implantation—check* position of applicator q24h.

(a) Keep client on bed rest in *flat position* to prevent displacing applicator (may turn to side for eating).

(b) Notify physician if temperature increases, nausea and/or vomiting occurs (indicate *radiation reaction* or *infection*).

(c) *After removal* of implant (48–144 h)—bathe and douche client; remove catheter as ordered.

b. Goal: **health teaching**.

(1) Explain that nursing care will be limited to essential activities during postinsertion period.

(2) Signs and symptoms of complications, so client can notify staff if something unusual happens (e.g., bleeding, radiation source falls out, fever).

3. **Nursing precautions for sealed internal radiation:**

a. **Never handle radium directly**—if applicators should accidentally be removed, pick up applicator by strings with long-handled forceps and **notify radiation officer**.

b. Linen must remain in client's room and *not* be sent to laundry until source of radiation has been accounted for and returned to its container.

c. **Time, distance, and shielding** are factors that increase or decrease potential effects on personnel. Need to minimize exposure of nursing staff, client's family, other health professionals. Nurses who may be *pregnant* should *not* care for clients with a radiation implant because of possible damage to the fetus from the radiation.

C. **Internal radiation: unsealed** (radioisotope/radionuclide).

1. Source of radiation is given orally or intravenously or instilled into a cavity as a liquid.

2. **Nursing care plan/implementation:** Goal: *reduce radiation exposure of others*.

a. *Isolate* client, tag room with radioactivity symbol.

b. *Rotate* personnel to *avoid* overexposure (principles of *time*, *distance*, and *shielding*). Staff should use good handwashing technique. Client should be in a room with running water. (Nurse who may be pregnant should *not* care for client while radiation source still active.)

c. Encourage family to maintain telephone contact or use intercom, to decrease exposure to others.

d. Plan independent diversional activities.

⚡ 3. **Specific nursing precautions** (post in chart, on client's door).

a. *Radioactive iodine* (^{131}I): half-life—8.1 d; excreted in urine, saliva, perspiration, vomitus, feces.

(1) Wear *gloves* and isolation *gowns* when handling client, excreta, or dressings directly.

(2) Collect *paper* plates, eating utensils, dressings, linen in impermeable bags; label and dispose of according to agency protocol.

(3) Collect excreta in *shielded* container and send to lab daily to monitor excretion rate and disposal.

b. *Radioactive phosphorus* (^{32}P): half-life—14 d; injected into cavity or given IV or orally.

☞ (1) If injected into cavity, turn client q10–15min for 2 h to ensure distribution.

(2) *No* radiation hazard unless leakage from instillation site or from client's excreta, which are collected in *lead-lined containers* and brought to the radioisotope laboratory for disposal. Linen is collected in container, marked *radioactive*, and brought to the radioisotope lab for special handling.

(3) Seepage will stain linens *blue*; wear *gloves* when handling contaminated linens, dressings. Excreta disposed of as in **3. a. (3)** above.

c. *Radioactive gold* (^{198}Au): half-life—2.7 d; usually injected into pleural or abdominal cavity.

(1) May seep from instillation site or drainage tubes in cavity; stains *purple*.

☞ (2) Turn client q15min for 2 h to ensure distribution.

(3) Same precautions regarding handling excreta as in **3. a. (1)** and **3. b. (2)**.

⚡ D. **Precautions for nurses:**

1. Use principles of *time*, *distance*, and *shielding* when caring for clients who are undergoing active radiation therapy.

2. Nurses who may be pregnant should *not accept* an assignment caring for clients who have an active radiation source in place.

3. Always use *gloves, gowns* to protect skin and clothing.

4. Wear detection *badge* to determine exposure to energy source.

IX. **Immunotherapy:** it has been hypothesized that clinical malignancy may occur as a result of failure of the immunologic surveillance system of the body to fight off cancer cells as they develop. The goal of immunotherapy is to immunize clients against their own tumors.

A. *Nonspecific* immunotherapy—encourages a host-immune response by use of an unrelated agent. *BCG* (bacillus Calmette-Guérin) vaccine and *Corynebacterium parvum* are the two agents used for this type of immunotherapy.

B. *Specific* immunotherapy—uses substances that are antigenically related to the tumor that stimulate a specific host-immune response.

C. *Side effects*—malaise, chills, nausea, vomiting, diarrhea; local reaction at site of injection, such as pruritus, scabbing.

D. **Nursing care plan/implementation**

1. Goal: *decrease discomfort associated with side effects of therapy.*

a. Identify measures to lessen side effects (see **V. Nursing care plan/implementation**—general care of the client with cancer, **p. 315**).

b. Know type of immunotherapy being used, adverse and desirable effects of therapy.

c. Administer fluids, encourage rest.

d. Administer acetaminophen, as ordered, to decrease flulike symptoms.

e. Administer *antiemetics*, as ordered, to control nausea.

f. Monitor for respiratory distress.

g. Administer *analgesics*, as ordered, to relieve pain.

2. Goal: **health teaching**.

a. Comfort measures to decrease side effects of therapy.

b. Expected and side effects of therapy.

c. Investigational nature of therapy.

d. Care of administration site.

e. Answer questions honestly.

X. **Palliative care:** When treatment has been ineffective in controlling the disease, the nurse must plan palliative, terminal care. Cure is not possible for such clients in an advanced phase of malignancy. Symptoms increase in severity; clients and family have many special problems.

A. **General problems of client with terminal cancer:**

1. *Cachexia*: progressive weakness, wasting, weight loss.

2. *Anemia*: leukopenia, thrombocytopenia, hemorrhage.

3. *GI tract disturbances*: anorexia, constipation.

4. *Tissue breakdown* leading to decubitus, seeping wounds.

5. *Urine*: retention, incontinence, renal calculi, tumor obstruction of ureters.

6. *Hypercalcemia* occurs in 10%–30% of clients.
7. *Pain* due to: tumor growth, obstruction, vertebral compression, or secondarily to complications (e.g., decubitus, stiffened joints, stomatitis). Also neuropathy due to prolonged use of neurotoxic chemotherapeutic agents such as vincristine.
8. *Fatigue*: major and debilitating problem.

B. **Nursing care plan/implementation**
1. Goal: *make client as comfortable as possible*; involve nursing staff, family, support personnel, clergy, volunteers, support groups, hospice, etc.
   a. *Nutrition*: obtain nutritional consultation; *high calorie, high protein diet*; small, frequent meals; blenderized or strained; commercial nutritional supplements (*Ensure, Vivonex, Sustacal*).
   b. Prevent tissue breakdown and vascular complications: frequent turning, massage, air mattress, active and passive range of motion (ROM) exercises.
   c. GI tract disturbances: observe for toxic reactions to therapy, particularly vomiting and diarrhea; administer medications: *antiemetics, antidiarrheal* agents, as ordered.
   d. Relieve pain.
      (1) Use supportive measures such as massage, relaxation techniques, guided imagery, drugs for *pain* relief: administer codeine, fentanyl, aspirin–oxycodone HCl (*Percodan*), pentazocine (*Talwin*), morphine, methadone, as ordered.
      (2) Monitor for side effects of narcotics: depressed respiratory status, constipation, anorexia.
2. Goal: *assist client to maintain self-esteem and identity*.
   a. Encourage self-care.
   b. Spend time with client; isolation is a great fear for the client who is dying.
3. Goal: *assist client with psychological adjustment*.

XI. **General evaluation/outcome criteria**
A. Tolerates treatment—complications of surgery are prevented, tolerates chemotherapy, completes radiation therapy.
B. Side effects of treatment are managed by effective nursing care and health teaching.
C. Maintains good nutritional status.
D. Uses effective coping mechanisms or seeks appropriate assistance to deal with psychosocial concerns.
E. Makes choices for follow-up care based on accurate information.
F. Finds methods to control pain and minimize discomfort.

G. Dignity maintained until death and/or during dying.

Lung Cancer

I. **Pathophysiology**: *squamous cell carcinoma*: undifferentiated, pleomorphic; accounts for 45%–60% of all cases of lung cancer; *small-cell (oat-cell) carcinoma*: small, dark cells located between cells of mucosal surfaces; characterized by early metastasis and poor prognosis; *large-cell (giant-cell) carcinoma*: located in the peripheral areas of the lung, has poor prognosis; *adenocarcinoma*: found in men and women; not necessarily related to smoking.

II. **Risk factors/causes**:
A. Heavy cigarette smoking, 20-yr smoking history.
B. Exposure to certain industrial substances, such as *asbestos*.
C. Increased incidence in women during the last decade of life.

III. **Assessment**
A. *Subjective data*:
1. Dyspnea.
2. Pain: on swallowing; dull and poorly localized chest pain, referred to shoulders.
3. Anorexia.
4. History of: cigarette smoking over a period of years; recurrent respiratory tract infections with chills and fever, especially pneumonia or bronchitis.
B. *Objective data*:
1. Wheezing, dry to productive persistent cough, hemoptysis.
2. Weight loss.
3. Positive diagnosis: cytology report of cells in tissue specimen obtained during bronchoscopy.
4. Signs of metastasis.

IV. Annual incidence: 178,100 new cases; 160,400 estimated deaths.

V. **Analysis/nursing diagnosis**
A. *Ineffective breathing pattern* related to pain.
B. *Impaired gas exchange* related to tumor growth.
C. *Pain* related to disease progression.
D. *Fear* related to uncertain future.
E. *Powerlessness* related to inability to control symptoms.
F. *Knowledge deficit* related to disease and treatment.

VI. **Nursing care plan/implementation**
A. Goal: *make client aware of diagnosis and treatment options*.
1. Allow time to talk and to discuss diagnosis.
2. Client makes informed decision regarding treatment.

B. Goal: *prevent complications related to surgery* for client whose cancer is diagnosed early and for whom surgery is an option: wedge or segmental resection, lobectomy, or pneumonectomy are usual procedures.
   1. See **Nursing care plan/implementation** for the client undergoing thoracic surgery, **p. 82.**
   2. Monitor vital signs, including accurate respiratory assessment for respiratory congestion, blood loss, infection.
   3. Assist client to deep breathe, cough, change position.
C. Goal: *assist client to cope with alternative therapies* when surgery is deemed not possible.
   1. *Radiation therapy*: megavoltage x-ray, cobalt—usual form of radiation. (See **Nursing care plan/implementation** for the client undergoing radiation therapy, **p. 318.**)
   2. *Chemotherapy*:
      a. Cyclophosphamide (*Cytoxan*), doxorubicin (*Adriamycin*), CCNU, methotrexate, vincristine sulfate (*Oncovin*) are the usual drugs given for lung cancer.
      b. See **Nursing care plan/implementation** for the client undergoing chemotherapy **p. 316.**
D. Goal: **health teaching**.
   1. Encourage client to stop smoking to ensure best possible air exchange.
   2. Encourage *high protein, high calorie diet* to counteract weight loss.
   3. *Force fluids* to liquefy secretions so they can be expectorated.
   4. Encourage adequate rest and activity to prevent problems of immobility.
   5. Desired effects and side effects of medications prescribed for therapy and pain relief.
   6. Coping mechanisms for maximal comfort and advanced disease (see X. **Palliative care**, p. 320-321).

VII. **Evaluation/outcome criteria**
   A. Copes with disease and treatment.
   B. Side effects of treatment are minimized by proper nursing management.
   C. Acid-base balance is maintained by careful management of respiratory problems.
   D. Client is aware of the seriousness of the disease.

Colon and Rectal Cancer

I. **Risk factors/causes:**
   A. Men.
   B. Middle age.
   C. Personal or family history of colon and rectal cancer.

D. Personal or family history of polyps in the rectum or colon.
E. Ulcerative colitis.
F. Diet *high in beef* and *low in fiber.*
G. *Gardner's syndrome* (multiple colonic adenomatous polyps, osteomas of the mandible or skull, multiple epidermoid cysts, or soft-tissue tumors of the skin).

II. Annual incidence: 131,200 new cases, 54,900 estimated deaths.

III. **Assessment**
   A. *Subjective data*:
      1. Change in bowel habits.
      2. Anorexia.
      3. Weakness.
      4. Abdominal cramping or vague discomfort with or without pain.
      5. Chills.
   B. *Objective data*:
      1. Diarrhea (pencil-like or ribbon-shaped feces) or constipation.
      2. Weight loss.
      3. Rectal bleeding, anemia.
      4. Fever.
      5. Signs of intestinal obstruction: obstipation, distention, pain, vomiting, fecal oozing.
      6. *Diagnostic tests*:
         a. Digital examination reveals palpable mass if lesion is in ascending or descending colon.
         b. Slides of stool specimen, for occult blood.
         c. Proctoscopy.
         d. Sigmoidoscopy.
         e. Barium enema.
      7. Lab data: occult blood, blood serotonin level *increased*, carcinoembryonic antigen; (CEA); *positive* radioimmunoassay of serum or plasma indicates presence of carcinoma or adenocarcinoma of colon; *positive* results after resection indicate return of tumor.

IV. **Analysis/nursing diagnosis**
   A. *Constipation or diarrhea* related to presence of mass.
   B. *Altered health maintenance* related to care of stoma.
   C. *Sexual dysfunction* related to possible nerve damage during radical surgery.
   D. *Body image disturbance* related to colostomy.

V. **Nursing care plan/implementation** (see **also V. Nursing care plan/implementation**—general care of the client with cancer, **p. 315-316**).
   A. *Radiation therapy*: to reduce tumor or for palliation.
   B. *Chemotherapy*: to reduce tumor mass and metastatic lesions.

1. *Antitumor anti-infectives*—mitomycin C, doxorubicin HCl (*Adriamycin*).
2. *Alkylating agents*—methyl-CCNU.
3. *Antimetabolites*—5-fluorouracil.
4. *Steroids and analgesics* for symptomatic relief.
C. Prepare client for surgery (colostomy), if necessary.

◄ VI. Evaluation/outcome criteria
A. Return of peristalsis and formed stool following resection and anastomosis.
B. Adjusts to alteration in bowel elimination route following abdominoperineal resection (e.g., no depression, resumes lifestyle).
C. Demonstrates self-care skills with colostomy.
D. Makes dietary adjustments that affect elimination, as indicated.
E. Identifies alternative methods of expressing sexuality, if needed.

Breast Cancer

I. Risk factors/causes:
A. Women >age 50 yr.
B. Family history of breast cancer.
C. Never bore children, or bore first child after age 30 yr.
D. Had breast cancer in other breast.
E. Menarche before age 11 yr.
F. Menopause after age 50 yr.
G. Excessive animal fat in diet.
H. Exposure to endogenous estrogens.

II. Annual incidence: 181,600 new cases, 44,190 estimated deaths.

◄ III. Assessment
A. *Subjective data*:
1. Burning, itching of nipple.
2. Reported usually painless lump.
B. *Objective data*:
1. Firm, nontender lump or mass.
2. Asymmetry of breast.
3. Nipple—retraction, discharge.
4. Alteration in breast skin—redness, dimpling, ulceration.
5. Palpation reveals lump.
6. *Diagnostic tests*: *mammography, needle biopsy, excisional biopsy*—level of estrogen-receptor protein predicts response to hormonal manipulation of metastatic disease and may represent a *prognostic* indicator for *primary* cancer; measurement of *carcinoembryonic antigen* useful for client with *metastatic* disease of the breast (see **Diagnostic Studies** box at end of chapter, **p. 338**).

◄ IV. Analysis/nursing diagnosis
A. *Risk for injury* related to surgical intervention.

B. *Body image disturbance* related to effects of surgery, radiation therapy, or chemotherapy.
C. *Altered sexuality patterns* related to loss of breast.
D. *Decisional conflict* related to treatment options.

◄ V. Nursing care plan/implementation (see also **V. Nursing care plan/implementation**—general care of the client with cancer, **p. 315**). Treatment depends on clinical and pathological staging.
A. Goal: *assist through treatment protocol*.
1. *Radiation therapy*—adjunctive, external, or implantation to primary lesion site or nodes.
2. *Chemotherapy*:
a. *Cytotoxic* agents to destroy tumor and control metastasis.
b. *Alkylating* agents: cyclophosphamide (*Cytoxan*); damages cell DNA by causing breaks in double strand helix.
c. *Antitumor anti-infectives*: doxorubicin (*Adriamycin*); modifies function of DNA and interferes with transcription of RNA.
d. *Antimetabolites*: fluorouracil, methotrexate (*Amethopterin*); mimics specific cellular metabolites and interferes with synthesis of DNA.
e. *Plant alkaloids*: vincristine sulfate (*Oncovin*); interrupts cellular replication.
f. *Hormones* to control metastasis, provide palliation: androgens, fluoxymesterone (*Halotestin*), testolactone (*Teslac*).
g. *Antiestrogens*: tamoxifen citrate (*Nolvadex*); suppresses cellular mitosis.
h. *Cortisols*: cortisone, prednisolone (*Delta-Cortef*), prednisolone acetate (*Meticortelone*), prednisone (*Deltasone, Deltra*); disrupts cell membrane, inhibit synthesis of protein, decrease circulating lymphocytes, inhibit mitosis, depress immune system.
i. *Estrogens*: diethylstilbestrol; stimulates cellular differentiation, decreases cellular proliferation.
3. *Surgery*—primary treatment.
a. **Preoperative care**:
(1) Goal: *prepare for surgery—types*:
(a) *Lumpectomy* (with or without radiation therapy)—used when lesion is small; section of breast is removed (often accompanied by radiation therapy and then radium interstitial implant).
(b) *Simple mastectomy*—breast removed, no alteration in nodes.
(c) *Modified radical mastectomy*—breast, some axillary nodes, subcutaneous tissue removed; pectoralis minor muscle removed.
(continued on p.325)

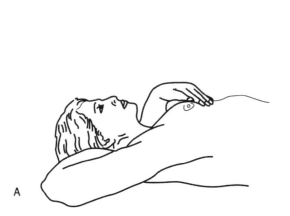
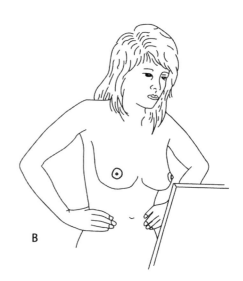

FIGURE 24.2 HOW TO EXAMINE THE BREASTS

Source: Adapted from © Lagerquist, SL: *Little, Brown's NCLEX-RN® Examination Review*. Boston: Little, Brown, (out of print)

Figure 24.2 A:

- *Lie down* and place right arm behind head; when lying down the breast tissue spreads evenly over the chest wall and is as thin as possible, making it much easier to feel all the breast tissue.

- Use the finger pads of the 3 middle fingers on left hand to feel for lumps in the right breast. Use *overlapping dime-sized circular* motions of the finger pads to feel the breast tissue.

- Use *3 different levels of pressure* to feel all the breast tissue: *light* pressure to feel the tissue closest to the skin; *medium* pressure to feel a little deeper; and *firm* pressure to feel the tissue closest to the chest and ribs. A firm ridge in the lower curve of each breast is normal. Use each pressure level to feel the breast tissue before moving on to the next spot.

- Move around the breast in an *up and down* pattern, starting at an imaginary line drawn straight down the side from the underarm and moving across the breast to the middle of the chest bone (sternum). (There is some evidence to suggest that the up and down pattern—sometimes called the *vertical pattern*—is the most effective pattern for covering the entire breast and not missing any breast tissue.) Check the entire breast area going down until only ribs are felt and up to the neck or collarbone (clavicle).

- Repeat the exam on the left breast, using the finger pads of the right hand.

Figure 24.2 B:

- While standing in front of a mirror with hands pressing firmly down on hips, look at the breasts for any changes of size, shape, contour, or dimpling. (The pressing down on the hips position contracts the chest wall muscles and enhances any breast changes.)

- Examine each underarm while sitting up or standing and with arm only slightly raised. (Raising the arm straight up tightens the tissue in this area and makes it difficult to examine.)

- If a change occurs, e.g. a lump or swelling, skin irritation or dimpling, nipple pain or retraction (turning inward), redness or scaliness of the nipple or breast skin, or a discharge other than breast milk, a health-care provider should be seen as soon as possible for evaluation.

This procedure for doing breast self-exam represents changes in previous procedure recommendations, based on an extensive review of the medical literature and input from an expert advisory group. There is evidence that the woman's *position* (lying down), *area felt, pattern of coverage* of the breast, and use of *different amounts of pressure* increase the sensitivity of BSE.

Adapted from American Cancer Society, 2004. Also see the American Cancer Society's Web site for more information: www.cancer.org.

(d) *Radical mastectomy*—breast, axillary nodes, and pectoralis major and minor muscles removed.

(e) *Reconstructive surgery*—done at time of initial mastectomy or (most often) later, when other adjuvant therapy has been completed.

(2) Goal: *promote comfort.*

   (a) Allow client and family to express fears, feelings.

   (b) Provide correct information about diagnostic tests, surgical procedure, postoperative expectations.

☞ b. **Postoperative care:**

(1) Goal: *facilitate healing.*

   (a) Observe pressure dressings for bleeding; will appear under axilla and toward the back.

   (b) Report if dressing becomes saturated; reinforce dressing as needed; monitor drainage from *Hemovac* or *suction pump.*

   (c) *Position*: semi-Fowler's to facilitate venous and lymphatic drainage; use pillows to *elevate affected arm* above right atrium, to prevent edema if nodes removed.

(2) Goal: *prevent complications.*

   (a) Monitor vital signs for shock.

   (b) Use gloves when emptying drainage.

   (c) Maintain joint mobility—flexion and extension of fingers, elbow, shoulder.

   (d) ROM exercises, as ordered, to prevent ankylosis.

   (e) If skin graft done, check donor site and limit exercises.

(3) Goal: *facilitate rehabilitation.*

   (a) Encourage client, significant others, family to look at incision.

   (b) Involve client in incisional care, as tolerated.

   (c) Refer to Reach to Recovery program of the American Cancer Society

   (d) Exercise program, hydrotherapy for clients who are postmastectomy, to reduce lymphedema.

(4) Goal: **health teaching.**

   (a) Ways to avoid injury to affected area; ways to prevent lymphedema.

(b) Exercises to gain full ROM.

(c) Availability of prosthesis, reconstructive surgery.

(d) Correct breast self-examination (BSE) technique (is at risk for breast cancer in remaining breast) (**Figure 24.2**). Best time for exam: women who are premenopausal, seventh day of cycle; women who are postmenopausal, same day each month.

◄ VI. **Evaluation/outcome criteria**

A. Identifies feelings regarding loss.

B. Demonstrates postmastectomy exercises.

C. Gives rationale for avoiding fatigue and avoiding constricting garments on affected arm; necessity for avoiding injury (cuts, bruises, burns) while carrying out activities of daily living.

D. Describes signs and symptoms of infection.

E. Demonstrates correct BSE technique.

Uterine (Endometrial) Cancer

Originates from epithelial tissues of the endometrium; second only to cervical cancer as cause of pelvic cancer. Slow growing, metastasizes late; responsive to therapy with early diagnosis, Pap test *not* as effective—more effective to have endometrial tissue sample (**Tables 24.2 and 24.3**). **Table 24.4** summarizes the staging and other aspects of cervical cancer.

I. **Risk factors/causes:**

A. History of infertility (nulliparity).

B. Failure of ovulation.

C. Prolonged estrogen therapy.

D. Obesity.

E. Menopause after age 52 yr.

F. Diabetes.

II. **Annual incidence:** 34,900 new cases; 6000 estimated deaths.

◄ III. **Assessment**

A. *Subjective data*:

   1. History of risk factor(s).

   2. Pain (late symptom).

B. *Objective data*:

   1. Obese.

   2. Abnormal cells obtained by aspiration of endocervix or endometrial washings.

   3. Postmenopausal uterine bleeding.

   4. Abnormal menses, intermenstrual or unusual discharge.

   5. See **Diagnostic Studies** box, **p. 338**.

◄ IV. **Analysis/nursing diagnosis**

A. *Pain* related to surgery.

B. *Risk for injury* related to surgery.

C. *Body image disturbance* related to loss of uterus.

D. *Risk for infection* related to immunosuppression caused by radiation treatment or chemotherapy.

◄ V. **Nursing care plan/implementation** (see also **nursing care plan/implementation**—general care of the client with cancer, **p. 315**):

A. Goal: *assist client through treatment protocol.*

1. *Radiation therapy*—external and/or internal with client who is a poor surgical risk.

⬬ 2. *Chemotherapy*—to reduce tumors and produce remission of metastasis. *Antineoplastic* drugs: dacarbazine (DTIC), doxorubicin (*Adriamycin*), medroxyprogesterone acetate (*Provera*), megestrol acetate (*Megace*).

B. Goal: *prepare client for surgery—types*:

1. *Subtotal hysterectomy*: removal of the uterus; cervical stump remains.

2. *Total hysterectomy*: removal of entire uterus, including cervix (abdominally—approximately 70% of clients—or vaginally).

3. *Total hysterectomy with bilateral salpingo-oophorectomy*: removal of entire uterus, fallopian tubes, ovaries.

C. Goal: *reduce anxiety and depression*: allow for expression of feelings, concerns about femininity, role, relationships.

D. Goal: *prevent postoperative complications.*

☞ 1. *Catheter* care—temporary bladder atony may be present as a result of edema or nerve trauma, especially when vaginal approach is used.

TABLE 24.2 PAPANICOLAOU SMEAR CLASSES

Class	Recommended Actions
I Normal	None
II Atypical cells, nonmalignant	Treat vaginal infections; repeat Pap smears
III Suspicious cells	Biopsy; dilatation & curettage
IV Abnormal cells; suspicious of malignancy	Biopsy; dilatation & curettage; conization
V Malignant cells present	See **Table 24.3** for recommended treatment according to stage of invasion.

Source: ©Lagerquist SL: *Little, Brown's NCLEX-RN® Examination Review.* Boston: Little, Brown (out of print).

TABLE 24.3 UTERINE CANCER: RECOMMENDED TREATMENT, BY STAGE OF INVASION

Stage of Invasion	Recommended Treatment
0 (In situ) Atypical hyperplasia	Cryosurgery, conization
I Uterus is of normal size	Hysterectomy
II Uterus slightly enlarged, but tumor is undifferentiated	Radiation implant, x-ray; hysterectomy 4–6 wk after radiation therapy
III Uterus enlarged, tumor extends outside uterus	Radiation implant, total hysterectomy 4–6 wk after radiation therapy
IV Advanced metastatic disease	Radiation therapy, chemotherapy; ⬬ progestin therapy to reduce pulmonary lesions

Source: ©Lagerquist SL: *Little, Brown's NCLEX-RN® Examination Review.* Boston: Little, Brown (out of print).

TABLE 24.4 INTERNATIONAL SYSTEM OF STAGING FOR CERVICAL CARCINOMA

Stage	Location	Prognosis	Treatment
0	*In situ*	Highly curable	Conization
1	Cervix	Cure rate decreases as stage progresses	Radiation therapy
II	Cervix to upper vagina		Radiation therapy
III	Cervix to pelvic wall or lower third of vagina		Surgical procedures: 1. Panhysterectomy, wide vaginal excision with removal of lymph nodes; ileal conduit.
IV	Cervix to true pelvis, bladder, or rectum		2. Pelvic exenteration: a. *Anterior*: removal of vagina and bladder; ileal conduit b. *Posterior*: removal of rectum and vagina; colostomy c. *Total*: both anterior and posterior ⬬ 3. Chemotherapy

Source: ©Lagerquist SL: *Little, Brown's NCLEX-RN Examination Review.* Boston: Little, Brown (out of print).

☞ 2. Observe for abdominal distention and hemorrhage:
   a. Auscultate for bowel sounds.
   b. Measure abdominal girth.
   c. Utilize *rectal tube* to decrease flatus.
3. *Decrease pelvic congestion and prevent venous stasis.*
   a. *Avoid* high Fowler's position.
   b. *Antiembolic* stockings, as ordered.
   c. Institute *passive leg* exercises.
   d. Apply *abdominal support*, as ordered.
   e. Encourage early ambulation.
E. Goal: *support coping mechanisms* to prevent psychosocial response of depression: allow for verbalization of feelings.
F. Goal: **health teaching** to prevent complication of hemorrhage, infection, thromboemboli.
   1. *Avoid*:
      a. Douching or coitus until advised by physician.
      b. Strenuous activity and work, for 2 mo.
      c. Sitting for long time and wearing constrictive clothing, which tend to increase pelvic congestion.
   2. Explain hormonal replacement therapy, if applicable; correct dosage, desired and side effects of prescribed medications.
   3. Explain:
      a. Menstruation will no longer occur.
      b. Importance of reporting symptoms (e.g., fever, increased or bloody vaginal discharge, hot flashes).

VI. Evaluation/outcome criteria
   A. Adjusts to altered body image.
   B. No complications—hemorrhage, shock, infection, thrombophlebitis.

Prostate Cancer

I. **Risk factors/causes**:
   A. African-American men.
   B. Age >50 yr.
   C. Familial history.
   D. Geographical distribution (northern areas), environmental (e.g., industrial exposure to cadmium).
   E. Diet high in *animal fat, dairy* products (e.g. butter, whole milk).
II. Annual incidence: 334,500 new cases; 44,800 estimated deaths; number two cause of death in men (number one is lung cancer)
III. **Assessment**
   A. *Subjective data*:
      1. Difficulty in starting urinary stream, frequency, urgency.

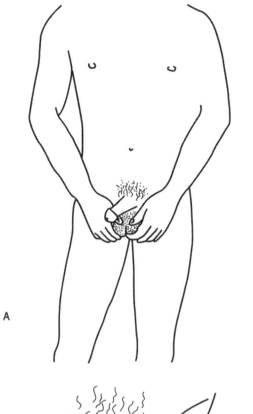

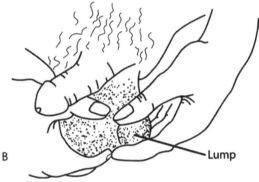

FIGURE 24.3 TESTICULAR SELF–EXAMINATION.
(A) Grasp testis with both hands; palpate gently between thumb and fingers. **(B)** Abnormal lumps or irregularities are reported to physician.

Source: ©Lagerquist SL: *Little, Brown's NCLEX-RN® Examination Review.* Boston: Little, Brown (out of print).

   2. Pain due to metastasis in lower back, hip (advanced cancer).
   3. Symptoms of cystitis.
B. *Objective data*:
   1. Urinary: smaller, less forceful stream; terminal dribbling; nocturia; *retention* (inability to void after ingestion of alcohol or exposure to cold).
   2. *Ultrasound*, needle biopsy: tissue specimen shows type of cancer cells (Gleason grade; stage).
   3. Lab data: *elevated*: prostate-specific antigen (PSA).

IV. **Analysis/nursing diagnosis**

A. *Altered urinary elimination* related to incontinence

B. *Altered sexuality pattern* related to surgery (nerve damage).

C. *Body image disturbance* related to erectile dysfunction (ED).

D. *Anxiety* related to fear about diagnosis.

E. *Pain* related to surgery

V. **Nursing care plan/implementation** (see also **nursing care plan/implementation**—general care of the client with cancer, **p. 315**).

A. Goal: *assist client in decision-making about choices of treatment.*

1. *Radiation therapy*—3D conformal or radiation seed implant (brachytherapy).

2. *Adrenocortical* hormones to limit production of androgens.

3. *Surgery*—see **Prostatectomy, p. 222.**

VI. **Evaluation/outcome criteria: see Prostatectomy, p. 222.**

Bladder Cancer

The bladder is most common site of urinary tract cancer.

I. **Risk factors/causes:**

A. Contact with certain dyes and solvents.

B. Cigarette smoking.

C. Excessive coffee intake.

D. Prolonged use of analgesics with *phenacetin*.

E. Three times more common in men.

II. Annual incidence: 54,500 new cases; 11,700 estimated deaths.

III. **Assessment**

A. *Subjective data*:

1. Frequency, urgency.

2. Pain: flank, pelvic; dysuria.

B. *Objective data*:

1. Painless hematuria (initially).

2. *Diagnostic tests*:

a. Cystoscopy, intravenous pyelography—mass or obstruction.

b. Bladder biopsy, urine cytology—malignant cells.

3. Lab data: urinalysis—*increased* red blood cells (men, >4.8 mm³; women, >4.3 mm³; erythrocytes (>30 mg/dL).

IV. **Analysis/nursing diagnosis**

A. *Risk for injury* related to surgical intervention.

B. *Altered urinary elimination* related to surgery.

V. **Nursing care plan/implementation** (see also **care of the client with cancer, p. 315**).

A. Goal: *assist client through treatment protocol.*

1. *Radiation therapy*—cobalt, radioisotopes, radon seeds; often before surgery to slow tumor growth.

2. *Chemotherapy*:

a. *Antitumor anti-infectives*: doxorubicin HCl (*Adriamycin*).

b. *Antimetabolites*: 5-fluorouracil.

c. *Alkylating* agents: thiotepa.

d. *Sedatives, antispasmodics.*

B. Goal: *prepare client for surgery—types*:

1. *Transurethral fulguration or excision*: used for small tumors with minimal tissue involvement.

2. *Segmental resection*: up to half the bladder may be resected.

3. *Cystectomy with urinary diversion*: complete removal of the bladder, performed when disease appears curable.

C. Goal: *assist with acceptance of diagnosis and treatment.*

D. Goal: *prevent complications during postoperative period.*

1. *Transurethral fulguration* or *excision*:

a. Monitor for clots, bleeding, spasms.

b. Maintain patency of *Foley catheter*.

2. *Urinary diversion with stoma*:

a. Protect skin, ensure proper fit of appliance—because constantly wet with urine (see also **Ileal conduit, p. 220-221**, and **ostomies** and **stoma care, p. 202-203**).

b. Prevent infection by *increasing acidity* of urine and *increasing fluid* intake.

E. Goal: **health teaching**.

1. Self-care of stoma and appliance.

2. Expected and side effects of medications.

3. Importance of follow-up visits for early detection of metastasis.

VI. **Evaluation/outcome criteria**

A. Accepts treatment.

B. Utilizes prescribed measures to decrease side effects of surgery, radiation therapy, chemotherapy.

C. Plans follow-up visits for further evaluation.

D. Maintains dignity.

Laryngeal Cancer

I. **Risk factors/causes:**

A. Eight times more common in men.

B. Occurs most often after age 60 yr.

C. Cigarette smoking.

D. Alcohol.

E. Chronic laryngitis, vocal abuse.

F. Family predisposition to cancer.

II. Annual incidence: 10,900 new cases; 4230 estimated deaths.

⋈ III. **Assessment**
   A. *Subjective data*:
      1. Dysphagia—pain in area of Adam's apple that radiates to ear.
      2. Dyspnea.
   B. *Objective data*:
      1. Persistent hoarseness.
      2. Cough and hemoptysis.
      3. Enlarged cervical nodes.
      4. General debility and weight loss.
      5. Foul breath.
      6. Diagnosis made by: history, laryngoscopy with biopsy and microscopic study of cells.

⋈ IV. **Analysis/nursing diagnosis**
   A. *Impaired verbal communication* related to removal of larynx.
   B. *Body image disturbance* related to radical surgery.
   C. *Ineffective airway clearance* related to increased secretions through tracheostomy.

⋈ V. **Nursing care plan/implementation** (see also **Nursing care plan/implementation**—general care of client with cancer, **p. 315**): treatment primarily surgical (see **Laryngectomy, p. 84, 86,**); radiation therapy may also be indicated.

⋈ VI. **Evaluation/outcome criteria**: see **Laryngectomy, p. 86**.

Additional Types of Cancer

See **Table 24.5**.

Table 24.5 Selected Cancer Problems

⧗ Assessment

	Subjective Data	Objective Data	Risk Factors	Annual Incidence	Specific Treatment
BLOOD AND LYMPH TISSUES					
Hodgkin's disease	Fatigue, generalized pruritus, anorexia. Night sweats	Painless enlargement of lymph nodes, especially in cervical area; fever; hepatosplenomegaly; anemia; peak age of incidence, ⟩⟩⟩ 15–35 yr; *diagnostic tests*—biopsy shows presence of *Reed-Sternberg cells; x-rays; scans, laparotomy.*	For young adults 15–35 yr old, not clearly defined, some relationship to socioeconomic status; male-female ratio is 1.5:1; increased frequency among whites.	7,500 new cases, 1,480 estimated deaths.	*Staging and treatment:* *Stage I*—involvement of a *single* node or a single node region; excision of lesion, and total nodal irradiation (see **nursing care plan/implementation** for client having radiation therapy, **p. 318-320).** *Stage II*—involvement of *two or more* lymph node regions on *same* side of diaphragm; excision of lesion and irradiation (see **nursing care plan/implementation** for client having radiation therapy, **p. 318-320).** *Stage III*—involvement of lymph node regions on *both* sides of the diaphragm, which may include the spleen; combination of radiation and chemotherapy. *Stage IV*—involvement of one or more *extralymphatic organs or tissues,* with or without lymphatic involvement; treated with chemotherapy alone, radiation therapy alone, or both. Presence or absence of symptoms of night sweats, significant fever, and weight loss; treated with *chemotherapy.* 💊 MOPP protocol—*Mustargen* (mechlorethamine HCl, alkylating agent), *Oncovin* (vincristine, plant alkaloid), *procarbazine* (antineoplastic), *prednisone* (corticosteroid) (see **nursing care plan/implementation** for client having chemotherapy, p. 316, 318).

(continued)

Table 24.5 Selected Cancer Problems

| | ⋈ Assessment | | | |
	Subjective Data	Objective Data	Risk Factors	Annual Incidence	Specific Treatment
BLOOD AND LYMPH TISSUES (continued)					
Non-Hodgkin's lymphoma	Night sweats.	Nontender lymphadenopathy, hepatomegaly, splenomegaly, fever of unknown origin, weight loss.	Age, 50–60 yr.	53,600 new cases; 23,800 estimated deaths.	*Stage I*—rarely observed, but remission possible with radiotherapy. *Stage II*—radiotherapy. *Stage III and IV*—combination chemotherapy with or without radiation therapy.
Multiple myeloma	Weakness; history of frequent infections, especially pneumonias; severe bone pain on motion; neurologic symptoms, paralysis.	Fractures of long bones; deformity of sternum, ribs, vertebrae, pelvis; hepatosplenomegaly; renal calculi, renal insufficiency; ⁓ anemia and bleeding tendencies; elevated uric acid.	Exposure to ionizing radiation; middle-aged or older women.	13,800 new cases; 10,900 estimated deaths.	*Surgery:* relieve spinal cord compression; orthopedic procedures to relieve or support bone problems (see **nursing care plan/ implementation** for clients with internal fixation for fractures, **Chap. 20 p. 261;** client with spinal cord injuries when paralysis occurs, **p. 297-298**). *Radiation:* for some lesions (see **nursing care plan/implementation** for the client having radiation therapy, **p. 318-320**). ⌾ *Chemotherapy: alkylating agents, antitumor anti-infectives, plant alkaloids, hormones*—melphalan and prednisone (see **nursing care plan/ implementation** for client having chemotherapy, **p. 316, 318**).
ENDOCRINE					
Thyroid cancer	Painless nodule, dysphagia, dyspnea.	Enlarged thyroid nodule; palpable thyroid, lymph nodes; hoarseness; hypofunctional nodule seen on ⁓ isotopic imaging; needle biopsy for cytology studies.	Radiation exposure in childhood.	16,100 new cases; 1,230 estimated deaths.	*Surgery:* total thyroidectomy, possible radical neck dissection (see **Thyroidectomy,** p. 232). *Radiation:* external or with radioactive iodine (^{131}I) (see **nursing care plan/ implementation** for client having radiation therapy, **p. 318-320**). ⌾ *Chemotherapy:* chlorambucil, doxorubicin, vincristine (*Leukeran, Adriamycin, Oncovin,* respectively) (see **nursing care plan/ implementation** for client having chemotherapy, **p. 316, 318**).

(continued)

Table 24.5 Selected Cancer Problems

| | ▶ Assessment | | | | |
	Subjective Data	Objective Data	Risk Factors	Annual Incidence	Specific Treatment
GASTROINTESTINAL TRACT					
Esophageal cancer	Dysphagia—difficulty swallowing, discomfort described as lump in throat, pressure in chest, pain; fatigue; lethargy, apathy, depression; anorexia.	Weight loss; regurgitation, vomiting; *diagnostic tests—barium swallow, esophagoscopy, biopsy.*	Age >50 yr, alcoholism, use of tobacco; increasing risk in nonwhite women, in people with achalasia (inability to relax lower esophagus with swallowing) or hiatal hernias.	12,500 new cases; 11,500 estimated deaths.	*Surgery:* resection with anastomosis or removal with gastrostomy. *Radiation:* best form of therapy. *Chemotherapy:* antineoplastic drugs *ineffective;* medications to reduce pain, discomfort, anxiety; **see nursing care plan/ implementation** for client for client with cancer (p. 315); having radiation therapy (p. 318-320); having chemotherapy (p. 316, 318); having surgery (p. 315-316).
Oral cancer	Difficulty chewing, swallowing, moving tongue or jaws; history of heavy smoking, drinking, or chewing tobacco.	Sore that bleeds and does not heal, persistent red or white patch; *diagnosis by biopsy;* early detection: dental checks.	Heavy smoking and drinking, user of chewing tobacco, men age >40 yr (affects twice as many men as women).	30,750 new cases; 8,440 estimated deaths.	*Surgery,* with reconstructive surgery, useful for cure and palliatively (see **nursing care plan/ implementation** for client with cancer, p. 315). *Radiation* using simulated computer localization to avoid destruction of normal tissue (see **nursing care plan/implementation** for client having radiation therapy, **p. 318-320**).

(continued)

Table 24.5 Selected Cancer Problems

▶ *Assessment*

	Subjective Data	Objective Data	Risk Factors	Annual Incidence	Specific Treatment
GASTROINTESTINAL TRACT *(continued)*					
Pancreatic cancer	Anorexia, nausea; pain in upper abdomen, radiating to back; dyspnea.	Jaundice, vomiting, weight loss; determination of solid mass in area of pancreas by *computed tomographic scanning and ultrasound;* tissue identification by thin-needle percutaneous *biopsy.*	Excessive intake of alcohol; exposure to dry cleaning chemicals, gasoline, coffee and decaffeinated coffee; possibly diabetes and chronic pancreatitis.	27,600 new cases; 28,100 estimated deaths.	*Surgery:* removal (must then have supplemental *pancreatic enzymes;* some clients become diabetics who are insulin-dependent) or bypass to relieve obstruction (see nursing **care plan/implementation for client with diabetes, pp. 168.**) *Radiation:* intraoperative high dose to pancreatic tumors with external high beam; palliative radiation therapy for pain (see **nursing care plan/implementation for client** having radiation therapy, **p. 318-320**; see **nursing care plan/ implementation for client with cancer, p. 315).** *Chemotherapy: pain relief, antiemetics, insulin, pancrelipase, 5-fluorouracil, cyclophosphamide, methotrexate, vincristine, mitomycin C* (see **nursing care plan/implementation for client** having chemotherapy, **p. 316, 318).**
Stomach cancer	Vague feeling of fullness, pressure, or epigastric pain following ingestion of food; anorexia, nausea, intolerance of meat; malaise.	Eructation, regurgitation, vomiting; melena, hematemesis, anemia; jaundice, diarrhea, ascites; big belly, upper gastric area; often palpable mass.	Men, lower socioeconomic classes, colder climates, early exposure to dietary carcinogens; *blood group A,* pernicious anemia, atrophic achlorhydric gastritis.	22,400 new cases; 14,000 estimated deaths.	*Surgery:* gastrectomy (see **Gastric surgery, p. 192,** for nursing care) *Radiation: not* as useful because dosage needed would cause side effects unlikely to be tolerated by client. *Chemotherapy* alone or in conjunction with surgery; *antitumor anti-infectives, antimetabolites, nitrosoureas, hematinics* (see **nursing care plan/implementation for client** having chemotherapy, **p. 316, 318).**

(continued)

Table 24.5 Selected Cancer Problems

	⧗ Assessment			
	Subjective Data	Objective Data	Risk Factors	Annual Incidence	Specific Treatment

GENITAL ORGANS

	Subjective Data	Objective Data	Risk Factors	Annual Incidence	Specific Treatment
Cervical cancer	Vague pelvic or low back discomfort, pressure, pain.	Intermenstrual postcoital, or postmenopausal bleeding; vaginal discharge— serosanguineous and malodorous hypermenorrhea; abdominal distention with urinary frequency; abnormal *Pap smear* (see **Table 24.2**); *Note:* recommended guidelines by American Cancer Society: Pap test annually; after 3 consecutive normal tests, MD may recommend less frequent testing; pelvic/uterine exam every 3 yr.	Early age at first intercourse; multiple sex partners; low socioeconomic status; exposure to herpes virus 2.	14,500 new cases; 4,800 estimated deaths.	*Staging* (see **Table 24.4**): *Stage 0*—carcinoma *in situ*; no distinct tumor observable; stage may last 8–10 yr; cure rate 100% following wedge or cone resection of cervix during childbearing years, or simple hysterectomy. *Stage I*—malignant cells infiltrate cervical mucosa; lesion bleeds easily; cure rate 80% with hysterectomy. *Stage II*—neoplasm spreads through cervical muscular layers, involves upper third of vaginal mucosa; cure rate 50% with radical hysterectomy. *Stage III*—neoplasm involves lower third of vagina; cure rate 25% with pelvic exenteration. *Stage IV*—involves metastasis to bladder, rectum and surrounding tissues; considered incurable. *Radiation:* external and/or internal, in conjunction with surgery or alone, depending on stage of disease or condition of client (see **nursing care plan/implementation** for client having radiation therapy, **p. 318-320**). ⊂ *Chemotherapy:* progestin, antineoplastics, megestrol (*Megace*), medroxyprogesterone (*Curretab, Provera*); alkylating agents— dacarbazine (DTIC).

(continued)

Table 24.5 Selected Cancer Problems

	⧗ Assessment				
	Subjective Data	Objective Data	Risk Factors	Annual Incidence	Specific Treatment
GENITAL ORGANS (*continued*)					
Testicular cancer	Aching or dragging sensation in groin, usually painless.	Gynecomastia; enlargement, swelling, lump, hardening of testes; young adult men; early diagnosis—monthly testicular self-exam; see **Figure 24.3.**	Second most common malignancy among men between 25 and 40 yr; possibly exposure to chemical carcinogens; trauma, orchitis; gonadal dysgenesis; cryptorchidism (undescended testicles).	7,200 new cases; 350 estimated deaths; 95%–100% 5-yr survival rate for early detected non-metastatic lesions.	*Surgery:* orchiectomy (see **nursing care plan/implementation for the pre- and postop client, p. 127-129 & 132-141**). *Radiation:* see **nursing care plan/ implementation for client having radiation therapy, p. 318-320.** ⊟ *Chemotherapy:* chlorambucil (*Leukeran*), methotrexate, *steroids* (see **nursing care plan/ implementation for client having chemotherapy, p. 316, 318**).
NERVOUS SYSTEM					
Brain	*Headache:* steady, intermittent, severe (may be intensified by physical activity); nausea; lethargy; easy fatigability; forgetfulness; disorientation; impaired judgment; visual disturbances; blackouts.	Vomiting, may be projectile; sight loss, auditory changes; signs of increased intracranial pressure; seizures; paresthesia; behavior changes; *diagnostic studies*—computed tomography scan, arteriography, cytology of cerebrospinal fluid.	None known for primary tumors; brain is common site for metastasis.	17,600 new cases (brain and spinal cord); 13,200 estimated deaths.	*Surgery:* craniotomy with excision of lesion; ventricular shunt to allow for drainage of fluid (see **nursing care plan/implementation—general care of the client with cancer, p. 315.**) *Radiation:* cobalt (local or entire central nervous system); total brain irradiation causes alopecia, which may be permanent (see **nursing care plan/implementation for client having radiation therapy, p. 318-320**); could be used alone, with surgery, or with chemotherapy. ⊟ *Chemotherapy: antineoplastic alkylating agents; nitrosoureas* (cross blood-brain barrier to reduce tumor)—carmustine (BCNU), lomustine (CCNU), semustine (methyl-CCNU); *cerebral diuretics* to reduce edema; *anticoagulants; analgesics; sedatives* (see **nursing care plan/ implementation for client having chemotherapy, p. 316, 318**).

(continued)

Table 24.5 Selected Cancer Problems

	⧗ Assessment				
	Subjective Data	*Objective Data*	*Risk Factors*	*Annual Incidence*	*Specific Treatment*
SKIN					
Skin cancer: *basal cell*	Reported painless lesion.	Scaly plaques, papules that ulcerate; pale, waxy, pearly nodule or red, sharply outlined patch; unusual skin condition, change in size or color, or other darkly pigmented growth or mole.	Exposure to: sun, coal tar, pitch, arsenic compounds, creosote, radium; fair complexion.	900,000 new cases (40,300 of these are malignant melanoma; 7,300 estimated deaths).	*Surgery:* electrodesiccation (dehydration of tissue by use of needle electrode) cryosurgery (destruction of tissue by application of extreme cold) (see **nursing care plan/implementation**—general care of the client with cancer, **p. 315**). *Radiation therapy* (see **nursing care plan/implementation** of client having radiation therapy, **p. 318-320**). *Prevention: avoid* sun from 10 am to 3 pm; use protective clothing, sunblock lotion.
Melanoma	Reported increase in size or color of an existing mole or nevus.	Irregular color, surface, and border; sometimes as small as 1 cm. Varied colors: red, white, black, blue, gray, brown. May be flat or elevated. Occurs most frequently on the back and in women on the chest and lower legs.	Sun exposure via occupation or recreational activities; UV radiation; skin sensitivity; genetic, hormonal, and immunologic factors; spontaneous mutation in gene (B-RAF).	Constitutes 11% of all skin cancers and causes 40,000 deaths per year. Can metastasize to any organ, including heart and brain; if detected early, before it has penetrated beyond epidermis, it is almost 100% curable.	Surgery is first choice: full thickness removal with wide excision. If lesion has spread to lymph nodes or other sites: will most likely require *chemotherapy, biological therapy, and/or radiation therapy.*

(continued)

Table 24.5 Selected Cancer Problems

	▼ Assessment			
	Subjective Data	Objective Data	Risk Factors	Annual Incidence	Specific Treatment
URINARY ORGANS				
Kidney cancer	Anorexia, nausea, fatigue, abdominal or flank pain.	Painless, gross hematuria; firm nontender, palpable kidney; vomiting and weight loss; *complications*— hypertension, nephrotic syndrome, lung metastasis; *lab and diagnostic tests*: intravenous pyelography; *urinalysis*—presence of red blood cells and albumin; *complete blood count—decrease in red blood cells and leukocytes, reduction in serum albumin, elevation in alpha-globulin.*	More common among men than women, whites than blacks; radiation exposure; possible familial influence; common site of metastasis from lung, breast.	28,800 new cases; 11,300 estimated deaths.	*Surgery:* nephrectomy (see pre/ **postoperative nursing care, p. 219**). *Radiation:* local as well as irradiation of metastatic sites when tumor is radiosensitive (see **nursing care plan/implementation** for client having radiation therapy, **p. 318-320**). *Chemotherapy: plant alkaloids—* vincristine (*Oncovin*); *antitumor anti-infectives*—dactinomycin (*Actinomycin D*), doxorubicin (*Adriamycin*); *alkylating agents*— cyclophosphamide (*Cytoxan*) (see **nursing care plan/ implementation** for client having chemotherapy, **p. 316, 318**).

🔑 Summary of Key Points

1. The most important nursing function for a client with cancer is teaching regarding prevention and detection, and, if treatment is necessary, symptom management.

2. Symptoms of cancer often do not appear until there is sufficient disease to produce *pressure, distortion, obstruction*, or *metabolic alterations*.

3. Side effects from radiation therapy are related to the size of the area being treated, the actual *part* of the body being irradiated, and the *total dose* of radiation.

4. Body excretions are *not radioactive* in clients undergoing treatment with a *sealed* source of radiation.

5. Skin redness is common with radiation therapy. Teach the client how to care for the skin. *Avoid* products containing alcohol, even some aloe products.

6. Assure the client fatigue is common during radiation and chemotherapy.

7. The carcinogenic risk to the nurse giving chemotherapy has not been proved conclusively, and suggested handling is controversial. However, antineoplastic agents are excreted in the client's body fluids and feces, so *gloves* should definitely be worn.

8. Side effects from chemotherapy are numerous and vary depending on the antineoplastic agent. The most common is *decreased white blood cell* and *platelet count*, leading to *infection* and *bleeding*.

9. Nausea and vomiting are thought to be the side effects most dreaded by clients.

10. The negative impact cancer has on *body image* and *self-concept* is an area where the nurse can have a positive effect.

〰️ Diagnostic Studies/Procedures

Breast Biopsy—needle aspiration or incisional removal of breast tissue for microscopic examination; *used to* differentiate among: benign tumors, cysts, and malignant tumors in the breast.

Cervical Biopsy and Cauterization—removal of cervical tissue for microscopic examination and cautery; *used to*: control bleeding or obtain additional tissue samples.

Culdoscopy—surgical procedure in which a culdoscope is inserted into the posterior vaginal cul-de-sac; *used to* visualize: uterus, fallopian tubes, broad ligaments, and peritoneal contents.

Hysterosalpingography—x-ray examination of uterus and fallopian tubes after insertion of a radio paque substance into the uterine cavity; *used to*: determine patency of fallopian tubes and detect abnormality in uterine cavity.

Mammography—examination of the breast with or without the injection of radiopaque substance into the ducts of the mammary gland; *used to* determine the presence of tumors or cysts. *Client preparation: no* deodorant, perfume, powders, or ointment in underarm area on day of x-ray. May be uncomfortable.

Thermography—a picture of the surface temperature of the skin using infrared photography (not ionizing radiation) detects the circulation pattern of areas in the breasts. Tumors produce more heat than normal breast tissue. Useful in clients with large tumors but may not detect small or deep lesions. Requires expensive equipment, and picture is difficult to interpret accurately.

Uterotubal insufflation (Rubin's test)—injection of carbon dioxide into the cervical canal; *used to* determine fallopian tube patency.

💡 Study and Memory Aids

Cancer: Focus of Client Care—"CANCER"

Chemotherapy
Assess body image disturbance (related to alopecia, ostomy, or mastectomy)
Nutritional needs when nausea and vomiting are present
Comfort from pain
Effective response to treatment (Evaluate)
Rest (for client and family)

Source: Modified from Zerweth, et al. *Memory Notebook of Nursing.* Dallas: Nursing Education Consultants.

🍎 Diets

Cancer—Prior to Surgery

↓ Fat	↑ Carbohydrates
	Iron
	Protein
	Roughage

After Chemotherapy—To Combat Nausea

| ↑ Calcium |
| Calories |
| Potassium |
| Protein |

After Chemotherapy—To Combat Diarrhea

↑ Fluids	Foods with odors
Potassium	Hot foods
	↓ Residue

Cancer—Palliative Care

↑ Blenderized foods
Calories
Protein
Supplements

Radiation Therapy—To Decrease Nausea

Do **not** eat 2–3 hours *before* and 2 hours *after* treatment; then

↑ Carbohydrates
Frequency
Protein

↑ Residue
↓ Size of feedings (small)

Drug Review

Cancer

Antineoplastic medications listed in **Appendix D.6.**

Questions

1. In which position should the nurse place the arm of a client after a radical mastectomy of the right breast?
   1. Any position of comfort.
   2. Close to the chest.
   3. Elevated above the heart.
   4. Hyperextended to the side.

2. Postoperative exercises performed by the client during the first 24 hours after a radical mastectomy of the left breast would include:
   1. Brushing her own hair with her left arm.
   2. Squeezing a rubber ball in her left hand.
   3. Pulling herself up in bed with a trapeze.
   4. Using her left hand to blow her nose.

3. The client asks if she will be able to have visitors while receiving internal radiation therapy for cervical cancer. The best response is that:
   1. The threat to others is too great to allow visiting.
   2. Visiting is permitted on a limited basis, usually 30 minutes per day.
   3. There is no threat to the visitors, and therefore no restrictions.
   4. Only her husband may visit briefly every 24 hours.

4. What common systemic side effect of chemotherapy will the nurse observe in a client receiving it?
   1. Ascites.
   2. Dysphagia.
   3. Polycythemia.
   4. Leukopenia.

5. A desired long-term goal of arm exercises after a mastectomy would include being able to:
   1. Squeeze a tennis ball with the affected hand.
   2. Brush the hair with the nonaffected arm.
   3. Cut meat on plate at meals.
   4. Raise both arms above head.

6. After a mastectomy the client verbalizes concern about being unattractive to her husband. The best response to her concern would be:
   1. "Don't worry. After reconstruction you'll look like new."
   2. "Your feeling is normal after this kind of surgery."
   3. "I know he'll love you just the same as he did before the surgery."
   4. "Why do you feel so unattractive?"

7. The best nursing intervention for a client who is having trouble accepting a mastectomy for removal of a malignant mass would be to:
   1. Ask the MD to talk to her about all the benefits of surgery.
   2. Tell her husband to tell her he still loves her as much as he did before the surgery.
   3. Have a member from a mastectomy support group visit her.
   4. Suggest that a psychiatric consultation be scheduled.

8. A client receiving radiation therapy shows that he understands the nurse's teaching when he states:
   1. "I'll wash the area with soap and water."
   2. "I'll apply lotion to the affected area."
   3. "I'll massage the area vigorously."
   4. "I'll wear loose clothing over the area."

9. After chemotherapy, the client's hematocrit is 25%, the hemoglobin level is 8.6 g/dL, the WBC is 600/mm^3 and the platelet count is 10,000/mm^3. The nurse would be alert to which manifestations of these laboratory findings?
   1. Mental confusion, headache, and blurred vision.
   2. Fatigue, alopecia, and stomatitis.
   3. Convulsions, tremors, and chills.
   4. Infection, respiratory arrest, and anorexia.

10. The client returns from the post anesthesia recovery room (PAR) after a radical mastectomy of the right breast. An IV is running into the antecubital space of the left arm. Which technique is appropriate for drawing a blood sample needed for hemoglobin and hematocrit testing?
    1. Apply a tourniquet to the right arm and draw the sample.
    2. Do a fingerstick on the client's left hand.
    3. Do a fingerstick on the client's right hand.
    4. Call the MD to do an arterial stick.

Answers/Rationale

1. **(3)** To prevent lymphedema after a mastectomy and removal of the lymph nodes, the arm should be elevated to facilitate lymph drainage. In *none* of the other positions (**1, 2,** and **4**) would the affected arm be placed *above the level of the heart.* **IMP, APP, 3, PhI, Basic care and comfort**

2. **(2)** During the early postoperative period, squeezing a ball in the hand of the affected arm would be done to begin strengthening the limb. Other exercises would be done *progressively,* from blowing her nose (**4**) to brushing her hair (**1**). The arm should *not* be raised *above* the shoulder until the drains are removed. Pulling herself up with a trapeze (**3**) would *not* be done during hospitalization because sufficient healing would not have occurred yet. *Mobility, not straining,* is the focus of exercises at this time. **IMP, COM, 1, PhI, Basic care and comfort**

3. **(2)** Radiation precautions include time, distance, and shielding; visitors to clients undergoing radiation therapy are protected in terms of the duration of exposure as well as distance from the client, so limited visitation *is* permitted. Shielding is not routinely provided. No visitation (**1**) is an *extreme* restriction; no restrictions (**3**) is *unsafe;* and permitting only the husband to visit (**4**) is *too restrictive.* **IMP, COM, 1, SECE, Management of care**

4. **(4)** Chemotherapeutic agents suppress the body's normal immune response, resulting in a depressed white blood cell count (WBC), or leukopenia. This leaves the client vulnerable to infection. Ascites (**1**) is associated with *liver* failure. Dysphagia (**2**), or difficulty swallowing, may occur in association with a *stroke* or *tumor.* Polycythemia (**3**), or an excessive number of immature *red* blood cells (RBCs), may be due to a primary problem in the *spleen* or a secondary problem stemming from *hypoxia.* **AS, APP, 1, PhI, Pharmacological and parenteral therapies**

5. **(4)** Exercises done after a mastectomy *progress* from squeezing a tennis ball, to brushing the hair, to being able to raise the arm, or arms, above the head, the latter signifying *maximum* mobility. Squeezing a tennis ball (**1**) is the *first* step, not the desired outcome. A *secondary* step would be brushing the hair with the *affected* arm, *not* the unaffected arm (**2**). Cutting meat (**3**) would *not* demonstrate the desired use of the affected arm. **EV, EVL, 3, PhI, Reduction of risk potential**

6. **(2)** The best response is to let the client know that such feelings are normal and she may even feel depressed or angry. Allow clients time to verbalize their fears and anxieties; do not rush them if they show a desire to talk about their feelings regarding their surgery. Encourage them to ask questions. The nurse should *not* offer *uncertain* assurances (**1** and **3**). Even the most secure woman will experience a sense of loss and altered body image, so asking her why she feels this way (**4**) is *not therapeutic.* **IMP, APP, 7, PsI, Psychosocial integrity**

7. **(3)** A group such as Reach for Recovery is designed to help women who have undergone a mastectomy meet common psychosocial, physical, and cosmetic needs. A hospital visit from the member of such a group may need to be authorized by the client's physician, however. The difficulty accepting the mastectomy is normal. Knowing the benefits (**1**) does *not* compensate for the loss. Even with a supportive spouse (**2**), the woman must grieve the loss over time. Because the grief is normal in the immediate postoperative period, a psychiatric consultation period (**4**) would be *unnecessary* at *this* time. **IMP, APP, 7, SECE, Management of care**

8. **(4)** The client should avoid wearing any clothing that will rub on the skin and cause it to break down. If washing of the skin is needed (**1**), lukewarm water is used, as well as a hypoallergenic soap that is free of alcohol or perfume, to avoid possible irritation of reddened skin. Many lotions (**2**), including some aloe products, contain alcohol, which is drying. Massaging or rubbing the radiated skin (**3**) may contribute to skin breakdown. **EV, EVL, 1, PhI, Basic care and comfort**

9. **(1)** The client has anemia (low RBC count), thrombocytopenia (low platelet count), and leukopenia (low WBC). The severe anemia and thrombocytopenia are the cause of the symptoms. Fatigue (**2**) would also be explained by the laboratory findings, *but* alopecia and stomatitis would be related to *drug toxicity.* Convulsions, tremors, and chills (**3**) would be seen if the client had a fever resulting from a *severe infection.* Although the client has an extremely low WBC and the risk of infection is great, the *low WBC alone would not* cause the symptoms. Anorexia (**4**) occurs as a result of chemotherapy, but *respiratory arrest* and, as already noted, *infection* are *not* related to the laboratory findings alone. **AS, ANL, 6, PhI, Reduction of risk potential**

10. **(2)** Capillary tubes of blood can be drawn from a fingerstick for these tests; in this case, the fingerstick should be done on the left hand. *No* blood pressure measurements, injections, IVs, or blood draws should be done or placed on the *right* arm (**1** and **3**), because these can cause circulatory impairment or infection in the limb. An arterial stick (**4**) is painful and *not* done for routine laboratory tests such as hemoglobin measurements and hematocrit determinations. **IMP, RE/KN, 1, PhI, Reduction of risk potential**

Key to Codes

Nursing process: **AS**, assessment; **AN**, analysis; **PL**, planning; **IMP**, implementation; **EV**, evaluation. (See **Appendix M** for explanation of nursing process steps.)

Cognitive level: **RE/KN**, recall/knowledge; **COM**, comprehension; **APP**, application; **ANL**, analysis; **EVL**, evaluation; **SYN**, synthesis. (See **Appendix M** for explanation.)

Category of human function: **1**, protective; **2**, sensory-perceptual; **3**, comfort, rest, activity, and mobility; **4**, nutrition; **5**, growth and development; **6**, fluid-gas transport; **7**, psychosocial-cultural; **8**, elimination. (See **Appendix 0** for explanation.)

Client need: **SECE**, safe, effective care environment; **PhI**, physiological integrity; **PsI**, psychosocial integrity; **HPM**, health promotion and maintenance. (See **Appendix P** for explanation.)

Client subneed: (See **Appendix P** for explanation)

Emergency Nursing

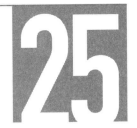

Chapter Outline

- Burns
- Primary Survey of Trauma Client: A, B, C, D, E, F, G
- Principles of Triage
- Emergency Nursing Procedures
  - *Abdominal emergencies*
    - Aortic aneurysm
    - Blunt injuries—spleen
  - *Cardiovascular emergencies*
    - Myocardial infarction
    - Cardiac arrest (CPR)
    - Shock
  - *Eye and ear emergencies*
    - Blunt injuries secondary to flying missiles
    - Sharp ocular trauma
    - Foreign bodies in ears
  - *Respiratory emergencies*
    - Choking
    - Acute respiratory failure
    - Near-drowning
  - *Systemic injuries*
    - Multiple traumas
    - Maxillofacial injuries
    - Spinal injuries
    - Chest injuries
    - Abdominal injuries
    - Fractures
    - Burns (care by degree of burn)
    - Chemical burns
    - Burns of eye-acid
    - Burns of eye-alkali
- Selected Geriatric Emergencies
- Selected Infectious Diseases and Agents of Bioterrorism
- Summary of Key Points
- Study and Memory Aid
  - Trauma care–complications
- Questions
- Answers/Rationale

Burns

Wounds caused by exposure to: excessive heat, chemicals, fire, steam, radiation, or electricity; most often related to carelessness or ignorance; 10,000–12,000 deaths annually; survival best at ages 15–45 yr and for burns covering less than 20% of total body surface.

I. **Pathophysiology**:
   A. *Emergent phase* (injury to 72 h): shock due to pain, fright, or terror → fatigue, failure of vasoconstrictor mechanisms → hypotension. Capillary dilatation, increased permeability → plasma loss to blisters, edema → hemoconcentration → hypovolemia → hypotension → decreased renal perfusion → renal shutdown.
   B. *Acute phase* (3–5 days): interstitial-to-plasma-fluid shift → hemodilution → hypervolemia → heart failure → pulmonary edema.

▶◀ II. **Assessment**
   A. *Subjective data*: how the burn occurred.
   B. *Objective data*:
      1. Extent of body surface involved: *"rule of nines"*—head and both upper extremities, 9% each; front and back of trunk, 18% each; lower extremities, 18% each; perineum, 1%. Requires adjustment for variation in size of head and lower extremities according to age. See **Figure 25.1**.
      2. *Location*—facial, perineal, hand and foot burns associated with potentially more scomplications and fatalities because of poor vascularization.
      3. *Depth* of burn (**Table 25.1**).
         a. *First degree (superficial)*—epidermal tissue only; not serious unless large areas involved.
         b. *Second degree (shallow or deep partial thickness)*—epidermal and dermal tissue; hospitalization required if over 25% of body surface involved (major burn).
         c. *Third degree (full thickness)*—destruction of all skin layers; requires immediate hospitalization; involvement of 10% of body surface considered major burn.
         d. *Fourth degree (deep penetrating)*—skin and structures underneath.
      4. Indications of *airway burns* (e.g., singed nasal hair, brassy cough, sooty expectoration → increased mortality), edema may occur in 1 h.
      5. Poorer prognosis—*infants*, due to immature immune system and effects of fluid loss; *elderly* due to degenerative diseases and poor healing.
      6. Medical history—presence of hypertension, diabetes, alcohol abuse, or chronic obstructive pulmonary disease increases complication rate.

TABLE 25.1 BURN CHARACTERISTICS ACCORDING TO DEPTH OF INJURY

Classification	Tissue Damage	Appearance	Pain	Clinical Course
Superficial (*first* degree)	Epidermis	Mild to fiery red erythema; no blisters	Very painful	Ordinarily heals in 3–7 d
Partial thickness: superficial or deep (*second* degree)	Epidermis and dermis	*Superficial*: mottled moist, pink or red; may or may not blanch with pressure; usually blisters *Deep*: dry	*Superficial*: extreme pain and hypersensitivity to touch *Deep*: may or may not be painful	Healing takes 10–18d; if infection develops in deep burn, it converts to full-thickness burn
Full thickness (*third* degree)	All layers of skin and subcutaneous tissue	Charred and leathery or pale and dry	Usually absent	Heals only with grafting or scarring
Fourth degree	All layers of skin and subcutaneous tissue, muscle, and bone	Black	Usually absent	Heals only with grafting or scarring

*Used in some classification systems. May require several days after a severe burn to determine fourth degree.

Source: ©Lagerquist SL: *Little, Brown's NCLEX-RN® Examination Review*. Boston: Little, Brown (out of print).

III. Analysis/nursing diagnosis

A. *Impaired skin integrity* related to thermal injury.

B. *Pain* (depending on type of burn) related to exposure of sensory receptors.

C. *Fluid volume excess or deficit* related to hemodynamic changes.

D. *Risk for infection* related to destruction of protective skin.

E. *Impaired gas exchange* related to airway injury.

F. *Body image disturbance* related to scarring, disfigurement.

G. *Ineffective individual or family coping* related to traumatic experience.

IV. Nursing care plan/implementation

A. Goal: *alleviate pain, relieve shock, and maintain fluid and electrolyte balance.*

1. Medications: give *narcotic* while physical exam is being completed and removing burned clothing.

2. Fluids: *IV* therapy (see **Chap. 7, p. 109, 110-111**), colloids, crystalloids, or 5% dextrose according to burn formula.

3. Monitor hydration status:
   a. Insert indwelling *catheter*.
   b. Note color, odor, amount of urine; report fixed specific gravity—may indicate kidney problems.
   c. *Strict* intake and output (I&O).
   d. Check hematocrit (normal: men >40%; women >37%).
   e. Weigh daily.

4. Soak: small burns may be soaked in cool saline.

B. Goal: *prevent physical complications.*

1. Vital signs: hourly; central venous pressure (CVP) for signs of shock or fluid overload.

2. Assess respiratory function (particularly with head, neck burns), patent airway, breath sounds.

3. Give medications, as ordered—*tetanus booster; antiinfectives* to prevent infection; *sedatives* and *analgesics; steroids; antipyretics—avoid* aspirin.

4. Isolation: *protective; strict* surgical asepsis (handwashing, protective clothing).

5. *Positioning*: turn q2h; prevent contractures—*Stryker frame* or circle bed if circumferential trunk burns present.
   a. Head and neck burns—use pillows under shoulders only for *hyperextension* of neck.
   b. Hand burns—use towel rolls or sandbags to align hands.
   c. Upper-body burns—keep arms at 90-degree angle from body and slightly above shoulders.
   d. Ankle and foot burns—allow feet to hang at 90-degree angle from ankles in *prone* position; use footboards to maintain angle in *supine* position, *elevate* to prevent edema.
   e. *Traction and splints* to maintain positions.
   f. Range of motion exercises according to therapy guidelines, usually several times per day; active exercises most beneficial.

6. *Diet*: initially NPO; begin oral fluids after bowel sounds return; do *not* give ice chips or free water, as these may contribute to electrolyte imbalance; food as tolerated—high *protein*, high *calorie* for energy and tissue repair (promote positive nitrogen balance).

6. Point out signs of progress (e.g., decreased edema, healing), as client and family tend to become discouraged and cannot see progress.
7. Encourage self-care to highest level tolerated.
8. Anticipate psychological changes:
   a. *Acute period*—severe anxiety, mental confusion: orient to person, place, time; maintain eye contact; explain procedures.
   b. *Intermediate period*—reactions associated with pain, dependency, depression, anger: give medications to decrease *pain*; explain procedures; use other clients as models; have open, nonjudgmental attitude; use consistent approaches to care; contract with client regarding division of responsibilities; encourage self-care.
   c. *Recuperative period*—grief process reactivated: anxiety, depression, anger, bargaining, as client tries to cope with altered body image, leaving security of hospital, finances. Encourage verbalization; refer to self-help group to assist with adaptation.
D. Goal: *promote wound healing*—wound care:
   1. *Open method*—exposure of burns to drying effect of air; useful for burns of neck, face, trunk, perineum; eliminates painful dressing changes; *protective isolation* may be required.
   2. *Closed method*—pressure dressings applied to burned areas, particularly extremities; changed 1–3 times/d; if ordered, give *pain* medication 30 min before change; tubbing facilitates removal.
   3. *Topical antimicrobial therapies* (**Table 25.2**).
   4. *Tubbing and debridement*:
      a. Hydrotherapy—body temperature bath water; loosens dressings so they float off; soak 20–30 min; encourage limb exercises; do *not* leave unattended; loss of body heat may occur, with chilling and poor perfusion resulting.
      b. Removal of eschar (*debridement*)—done with forceps and curved scissors; medicate for pain before; use *sterile* technique; only loose eschar removed, to prevent bleeding; examine wound for infection, color change, decreased granulation—report changes **immediately.**
   5. Wound coverage, to decrease chances of infection:
      a. Temporary wound dressings (**Table 25.3**).
      b. *Autograft*—client donates skin for wound coverage.

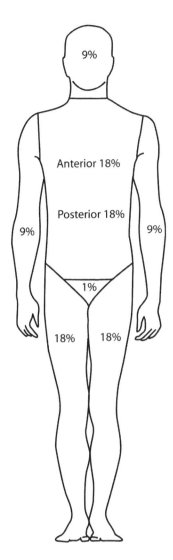

FIGURE 25.1 THE RULE OF NINES USED FOR ESTIMATING THE PERCENTAGE OF BODY BURNS IN THE ADULT.

7. Observe for:
   a. *Curling's (stress) ulcer*— sudden drop in hemoglobin, melena (give *antacids*, cimetidine, as ordered).
   b. Constriction due to *eschar* (circumferential or chest wall): prepare for *escharotomy* (lengthwise incisions)—painless procedure.
C. Goal: *promote emotional adjustment and provide supportive therapy.*
   1. Care by same personnel as much as possible, to develop rapport and trust.
   2. Involve client in care plans.
   3. Answer questions clearly, accurately.
   4. Encourage family involvement and participation.
   5. Provide diversional activities and change furnishings or room adornments when possible, to prevent perceptual deprivation related to immobility.

TABLE 25.2 ⬤ TOPICAL ANTIMICROBIALS USED IN BURN CARE

Agent	Advantages	Disadvantages	◄ Nursing Implications
Mafenide acetate (*Sulfamylon*) cream or solution	Eschar penetration Effective with *Pseudomonas* Topical agent of choice for electrical burns Suitable for open method of treatment (cream) Used for gram-negative organisms	Severe pain and burning (lasts 30 min) Metabolic acidosis Carbonic anhydrase inhibitor Ineffective against fungi May cause hypersensitivity rash	Administer pretreatment *analgesic* Monitor for metabolic acidosis and hyperventilation Check for allergy to sulfa, observe for rash
Silver nitrate	Low cost Broad spectrum Effective with *Candida*	Continuous wet soaks Superficial penetration Black staining Stinging Electrolyte imbalances (*low* sodium, *low* chloride, *low* calcium, *low* potassium); alkalosis	Check serum electrolytes daily Rewet dressing q2h
Silver sulfadiazine 1% (*Silvadene*)	Broad spectrum Antifungal Nonstaining Relatively painless Usable without dressings No systemic metabolic abnormalities	Less eschar penetration than mafenide acetate *Decreased* granulocyte formation; transient leucopenia Macular rash	Check for allergy to sulfa

Source: ©Lagerquist SL: *Little, Brown's NCLEX-RN® Examination Review*. Boston: Little, Brown (out of print).

(1) Types—free grafts (unattached to donor site), pedicle grafts (attached to donor site).

(2) Procedure—general anesthesia; donor sites shaved and prepared; graft applied to granulation bed; face, hands, and arms grafted first.

☞ (3) *Post–skin graft care*:

  (a) Roll cotton-tipped applicator over graft to remove excess exudates; maintain dressings; ⚠ use *aseptic* technique; apply heat lamps to dry donor sites.

  (b) Third to fifth day—graft looks pink if it has taken.

  (c) *Skeletal traction* may be applied, to prevent contractures.

  (d) Elastic bandages may be applied for 6 mo to 1 yr, to prevent hypertrophic scarring.

🏠 E. Goal: **health teaching**.

  1. Mobility needs: exercise, physical therapy, splints, braces

  2. Community resources: mental health practitioner or psychotherapist if needed for problems with self-image or sexual role, referrals as needed.

  3. Techniques to camouflage appearance: slacks, turtlenecks, long sleeves, wigs, makeup.

◄ V. Evaluation/outcome criteria

  A. Return of vital signs to preburn levels

  B. Minimal to no hypertrophic scarring

  C. Free of infection; demonstrates wound care.

  D. Maintains functional mobility of limbs; no contractures.

  E. Adjusts to changes in body image; no depression.

  F. Regains independence; returns to work, social activities.

Emergency Nursing Procedures

I. **Purpose**—to initiate assessment and intervention procedures that will speed total care of the client toward a successful outcome.

☼ II. **Primary survey of the trauma client**: A B C D E F G

  A. *Airway*

    1. Use jaw-thrust method, immobilize cervical spine.

    2. Clear blood and secretions.

    3. Insert airway, prn; **never** use nasal airway in facial trauma.

  B. *Breathing*

    1. Intubate (if *Glasgow coma scale* is <8).

    2. Give high flow oxygen (hyperventilate if have ↑ ICP).

TABLE 25.3 TEMPORARY BURN DRESSINGS

Example	Advantage	Disadvantage	⋈ Nursing Implications
Biologic			
Xenograft—pigskin	Promotes healing of clean wound; relieves pain; readily available; reduces water and heat loss	Easily digested by wound collagenase	Change q2–5d if over granulation tissue; overlap edges slightly, trim away when skin underneath has healed
Homograft—cadaver skin	Reduces water and heat loss; relieves pain; used with antimicrobial mesh, may be left in place for up to 8 d; debrides exudative wounds	May harbor disease	Observe for signs of infection
Amnion	Relieves pain; reduces water and heat loss; has bacteriostatic properties	Limited shelf life, requires special preparation for use	Change cover dressing q48h; leave on wound until it sloughs
Biosynthetic			
Biobrane	Protects from microbial penetration; decreases pain; promotes healing in partial-thickness burn	Not effective for preparing a granulation bed	☞ Must be secured to skin with sutures, closure straps, tape, or staples; wrap with gauze; after 48 h, check for adherence; once adherence has occurred, may be left open to air; check for signs of infection.
Artificial			
Integra	Useful when conventional autograft is not available or advisable	Temporary	Relatively new treatment

Source: ©Lagerquist SL: *Little, Brown's NCLEX-RN® Examination Review.* Boston: Little, Brown (out of print).

C. *Circulation*
1. Control hemorrhage.
2. Start chest compression, if indicated.
3. Place bilateral large-bore IVs.
4. Draw blood for type and cross-match.

D. *Disability*
1. Assess: neurological status, LOC, pupils.
2. For cervical spine injury: immobilize with cervical collar, backboard.

E. *Entire* body, head-to-toe assessment.

F. *Findings*
1. Document.
2. Order x-rays, labs.

G. *Glasgow coma scale*—assign and monitor score (see **p. 282**).

III. **Principles of Triage**—sort and categorize clients so that the most critical client is treated *first*. Levels of urgency:

A. *Emergent*
1. Needs *immediate* attention: life, limb or eye threatened.
2. Needs continuous re-evaluation.
3. Examples: trauma, chest pain, cardiac arrest, respiratory arrest, severe respiratory distress, chemicals in eyes, limb amputation.

B. *Urgent*
1. Needs treatment within *2 h.*
2. Re-evaluate every 30–60 min.
3. Examples: simple fracture, asthma with *no* respiratory distress; diastolic BP >130 mmHg; fever >104° F.

C. *Non-urgent*
1. Can wait *hours or days* for treatment.
2. Re-evaluate every 1–2 hours.
3. Examples: sprains, minor lacerations, simple headache, rash.

IV. **Emergency nursing procedures** for adults are detailed in **Table 25.4.**

TABLE 25.4 NURSING CARE OF THE ADULT IN MEDICAL AND SURGICAL EMERGENCIES

Condition	◄ Assessment: Signs and Symptoms	◄ Prehospitalization Nursing Care	◄ In-Hospital Nursing Care
Abdominal Emergencies			
Aortic aneurysm— rupture or dissection	Primarily men > age 60 yr. Sudden onset of excruciating pain: abdominal, lumbosacral, groin, or rectal. Orthopnea, dyspnea. Fainting, hypotension; if dissecting, marked hypertension may be present. Palpable, tender, pulsating mass in umbilical area. Femoral pulse present; dorsalis pedis—weak or absent.	1. Notify physician. 2. Lay client *flat* or *raise head* if in respiratory distress. 3. Cover—keep warm but *not* hot. ☞ 4. **Institute shock measures (see p. 122, 350-351).** 5. Calm client; reassure that help is on the way.	1. Assess respiratory and hemodynamic status. ☞ 2. Institute shock measures if indicated. 3. Evaluate and compare peripheral pulses. ⌇⌇ 4. Assist with x-rays. 5. Assist with emergency preoperative treatment.
Blunt injuries— spleen	Left upper quadrant pain, tenderness and moderate rigidity; left shoulder pain (*Kehr's sign*). Hypotension; weak, thready pulse; increased respirations (shock).	☞ 1. Lay client *flat.* ☞ 2. Institute shock measures.	1. Assess respiratory and hemodynamic status: ☞ a. Maintain airway and ventilation as indicated. ⌷ b. Institute infusions of colloids and/or crystalloids, as ordered. ☞ c. Insert both CVP and arterial monitoring lines. ☞ d. Insert Foley catheter. 2. Prepare for splenectomy.
Cardiovascular Emergencies			
Myocardial infarction— ischemia and necrosis of cardiac muscle *secondary* to: • insufficient • obstructed coronary blood flow	**Prehospital:** *Chest pain*: viselike choking, unrelieved by rest or nitroglycerin. *Skin*: ashen, cold, clammy. *Vital signs*: pulse—rapid, weak, thready; increased rate and depth of respirations; dyspnea. *Behavior*: restless, anxious. **In hospital:** *C/V*: blood pressure and pulse pressure *decreased*. *Heart sounds*: soft; S$_3$ may be present. *Respirations*: fine basilar crackles. ⌇⌇ *Lab*: ECG consistent with tissue necrosis (Q waves) and injury (ST segment elevation); serum enzymes *elevated*.	1. If coronary suspected, call physician, paramedic service, or emergency ambulance. 2. Calm and reassure client that help is coming. 3. Place in *semi-Fowler's position*. 4. Keep client warm but not hot. ⌷ 5. Administer aspirin 325 mg if available.	1. Rapidly assess hemodynamic and respiratory status. ⌷ 2. Start IV as ordered— usually 5% D/W per microdrip to establish lifeline for emergency drug treatment. 3. Draw blood for electrolytes, enzymes, as ordered. ☞ 4. Place on cardiac monitor. ⌷ 5. Relieve *pain*—morphine sulfate IV, as needed. ⌇⌇ 6. Take 12-lead *ECG*. 7. Once client is stable, transfer to CCU.

(continued)

TABLE 25.4 NURSING CARE OF THE ADULT IN MEDICAL AND SURGICAL EMERGENCIES (continued)

Condition	◄ *Assessment: Signs and Symptoms*	◄ *Prehospitalization Nursing Care*	◄ *In-Hospital Nursing Care*
Cardiac arrest— cardiac standstill or ventricular fibrillation *secondary to*: • rapid administration • overdose of anesthetics or narcotic drugs • obstruction of the respiratory tract (mucus, vomitus, foreign body) • acute anxiety • cardiac disease • dehydration • shock, electrical shock • emboli	*Respirations*: gasping, rapid, shallow, absent. *Pulse*: weak, thready, >120 beats/min, absent. *Muscle*: twitching. *Pupils*: dilated. *Skin*: cold, clammy, cyanotic Loss of consciousness.	☞ **CPR for Healthcare Providers** *Single rescuer:* 1. *In a witnessed sudden collapse* the rescuer should phone emergency medical services, obtain an Automatic External Defibrillator (AED) if available, then return to the victim to begin CPR. 2. *In a hypoxic cardiac arrest* (e.g. drowning, drug overdose), the rescuer should begin CPR first 3. *Position*: flat on back. 4. Shake vigorously— establish unresponsiveness. 5. Use head tilt-chin lift maneuver to open airway. 6. *If a trauma victim*, use jaw thrust maneuver *first*, *then* use head tilt-chin lift maneuver if jaw thrust fails to open airway. 7. Check for *adequate* breathing for 5-10 seconds. **Victim not breathing:** 1. Use head tilt-jaw thrust maneuver to open airway. 2. Pinch nostrils shut. Rescuer forms a complete seal with lips over victim's lips. 3. Taking a normal breath, rescuer breaths into victim's mouth, each breath over 1 second. 4. Rescuer should see victim's chest rise with each breath. 5. Check pulse. If victim has a pulse but no respirations, continue rescue breathing at rate of 1 breath every 5 seconds.	1. If monitored, note rhythm; call for help and note time. ☞ 2. Countershock if rhythm is ventricular fibrillation or ventricular tachycardia. ☞ 3. Begin CPR **immediately** after each shock. 4. Limit interuptions of chest compressions.

(continued)

TABLE 25.4 NURSING CARE OF THE ADULT IN MEDICAL AND SURGICAL EMERGENCIES (continued)

Condition	◄ *Assessment: Signs and Symptoms*	◄ *Prehospitalization Nursing Care*	◄ *In-Hospital Nursing Care*
		Victim has no pulse: 1. Use AED as soon as available, if rhythm indicates. 2. Begin chest compressions **immediately** after each shock. **One person and two-person rescue:** 1. Provide chest compressions at a rate of 100 compressions per minute. 2. Provide 2 breaths after every 30 compressions. *Note:* for *two-person CPR on infants and children only,* use a 15:2 chest compression-to-ventilation ratio.	**Two-person rescue:** *First person* on scene: begins CPR as described. *Second person:* 1. Page code (cardiac arrest) team. ☞ 2. Bring defibrillator to bedside. Deliver shock if indicated. 3. Bring emergency cart to bedside. ☞ 4. *Suction* airway, if obstructed with secretions or vomitus. ☞ 5. Bag client with *100% O_2*. ☞ 6. Assist with *intubation* when arrest team arrives. ☞ 7. Establish *IV* line if one is not available.
Shock—cellular hypoxia and impairment of cellular function *secondary to:* • trauma • hemorrhage • fright • dehydration • cardiac insufficiency • allergic reactions • septicemia • impairment of nervous system • poisons	**Early shock:** *Sensorium:* conscious, apprehensive, restless; some slurring of speech. *Pupils:* dull but reactive to light. *Pulse:* <140 beats/min; amplitude full to mildly decreased. *Blood pressure:* normal to slightly decreased. *Neck veins:* normal to slightly flat in supine position; may be full in septic shock or grossly distended in cardiogenic shock. *Skin:* cool, clammy, pale. *Respirations:* rapid, shallow. *GI:* nausea, vomiting, thirst. *Renal:* urine output 20–40 mL/h.	☞ 1. Check breathing—clear airway if necessary; if not breathing, give *artificial respirations*; if breathing is irregular or labored, *raise* head and shoulders. ☞ 2. *Control bleeding* by placing pressure on the wound or at pressure points (proximal artery). 3. Make comfortable and reassure. 4. Cover lightly to prevent heat loss, but don't bundle up. 5. If neck or spine injury is suspected—do *not* move, unless victim in danger of more injury. If *client unconscious or has wounds of the lower face and jaw*—place on *side* to promote drainage of fluids; position client on *back* unless otherwise indicated.	1. Check vital signs rapidly—pulse, pupils respirations. 2. Check airway; clear if necessary; PO_2 should be maintained above 60 mm Hg; *elevated* PCO_2 indicates need for intubation and ventilatory assistance. ☞ 3. Control gross bleeding. ☞ 4. Prepare for insertion of *intravenous line* and *central lines*—if abdominal injuries present ☞ 5. *Peripheral line* should be placed in upper extremity if fluids being lost in abdomen. ☞ 1. Draw blood for specimens: Hgb, Hct, CBC, glucose, CO_2, sodium amylase, BUN, K^+; type and cross-match, blood gases, enzymes, prothrombin times. ⬭ 2. Prepare infusion of 5% D/NS *unless* hypernatremia suspected; ⬭ dextran if *blood loss*.

(continued)

TABLE 25.4 NURSING CARE OF THE ADULT IN MEDICAL AND SURGICAL EMERGENCIES (continued)

Condition	► Assessment: Signs and Symptoms	► Prehospitalization Nursing Care	► In-Hospital Nursing Care
Shock (continued)	**Severe or late shock:** *Sensorium*: confused, disoriented, apathetic, unresponsive; slow, slurred speech, often incoherent. *Pupils*: dilating, dilated, slow or nonreactive to light. *Pulse*: >150 beats/min, thready, weak. *Blood pressure*: 80 mm Hg or unobtainable. *Neck veins*: flat in a supine position—no filling; full to distended in septic or cardiogenic shock. *Skin*: cold, clammy, mottled; circumoral cyanosis, dusky, cyanotic. *Eyes*: sunken—vacant expression. *Renal*: urine output <20 mL/h	1. *Raise* feet 6–8 in. unless client has head or chest injuries; if victim becomes less comfortable, lower feet. 2. If client complains of thirst, do **not** give fluids unless you are more than 6 h away from professional medical help; under **no** conditions give water to clients who are: unconscious, convulsing, or vomiting; appearing to need general anesthetic; or with a stomach, chest, or skull injury. 3. Be calm and confident; reassure client help is on the way.	1. Assess and intervene as in early shock; then obtain information as to onset and past history. ☞ 2. *Catheterize* and monitor client urine output, as ordered. ⌇ 3. Take 12-lead ECG. ☞ 4. Insert *nasogastric tube* and assess aspirate for volume, color, and blood; save specimen if poison or drug overdose suspected. 5. *If CVP low*—infuse 200–300 mL over 5–10 min. *If CVP rises* sharply—fluid restriction necessary; if remains low, hypovolemia present. ⌇ 6. If client febrile—*blood cultures* and *wound cultures* will be ordered. 7. If urine output scanty or ⌐ absent—give mannitol as ordered.
Eye and Ear Emergencies			
Chemical burns	*See Burns*	*See Burns*	*See Burns*
Blunt injuries secondary to: • flying missiles (e.g. balls, striking face against car dashboard)	Decreased visual acuity, diplopia, blood in anterior chamber. Pain, conjunctiva reddened, edema of eyelids.	1. Prevent victim from rubbing eye. ☞ 2. Cover with patch to protect eye. 3. Seek medical help **immediately**.	⌇ 1. Test visual acuity of each eye using *Snellen* or *Jaeger* chart. ⌇ 2. Assist with *fluorescein* administration—to facilitate identifying breaks in cornea.
Sharp ocular trauma— secondary to: • small or larger foreign bodies	Reports of feeling something hit eye. Pain, tearing, reddened conjunctiva. Blurring of vision. Foreign object may be visible.	1. Keep victim from rubbing eye. ☞ 2. Cover very lightly—do **not** apply pressure.	⌇ 1. Check visual acuity in both eyes. 2. Check pupils. ⌐ 3. Instill 1% tetracaine HCl, as ordered, to relieve *pain*. ⌐ 4. Administer *antiinfective* drops or ointment, as ordered. ☞ 5. Apply eye patch. 6. Provide instructions for subsequent care and follow-up.

(continued)

TABLE 25.4 NURSING CARE OF THE ADULT IN MEDICAL AND SURGICAL EMERGENCIES (continued)

Condition	◄ Assessment: Signs and Symptoms	◄ Prehospitalization Nursing Care	◄ In-Hospital Nursing Care
Eye and Ear Emergencies (continued)			

Foreign bodies in ears—beans, peas, candy, foxtails, insects	Decreased hearing; pulling, poking at ear and ear canal; buzzing, discomfort.	1. Do *not* attempt to remove object.
		2. Seek medical assistance.
			1. Inspect ear canal.
			2. Assist with sedating client—*restraint* may be necessary.
			3. Assist with procedures to remove object.
			  a. Forceps or curved probe for *foxtails, irregularly shaped* objects
			  b. 10F or 12F catheter with tip cut squarely off and attached to suction to remove *round* object.
			4. Irrigate external auditory canal to flush out *insects*, materials that do not absorb water; do *not* irrigate if danger of perforation.

Respiratory Emergencies			
Choking— obstruction of airway *secondary to*: aspiration of a foreign object	Gasping, wheezing; looks panicky, but can still breathe, talk, cough. *Cough*: weak, ineffective; breathing sounds like high-pitched crowing. *Color*: white, gray, blue. Difficulty speaking; clutches throat.	Do not interfere if coughing; do *not* slap on back; watch closely; call for assistance. **Victim standing, sitting, and conscious:** Perform *obstructed airway maneuver* (formerly, *Heimlich*): stand behind victim, wrap arms around waist, place fist against abdomen, and with your other hand, press fist into the victim's abdomen with a quick upward thrust until the obstruction is relieved or the victim becomes unconscious. **Victim lying down:** Roll the victim onto his or her back; straddle the victim's thighs; place heel of hand in the middle of abdomen; place other hand on top of the first; stiffen arms and deliver 6–10 abdominal thrusts.	(As in **prehospital** care). (As in **prehospital** care).

(continued)

TABLE 25.4 NURSING CARE OF THE ADULT IN MEDICAL AND SURGICAL EMERGENCIES (*continued*)

Condition	◄ Assessment: Signs and Symptoms	◄ Prehospitalization Nursing Care	◄ In-Hospital Nursing Care
Choking (continued)		**Unconscious victim:** ☞ Try to ventilate; if unsuccessful, deliver abdominal thrusts using technique described for **conscious victim**; probe mouth for foreign objects; keep repeating above procedure until ventilation occurs; as victim becomes more deprived of air, muscles will relax and maneuvers that were previously unsuccessful will begin to work; when successful in removing obstruction, give two breaths; check pulse; start CPR if indicated. ☞ **Obese or pregnant victims:** Use *chest* thrusts instead of abdominal thrusts. **You are victim and alone:** ☞ Place your two fists for abdominal thrusts; bend over back of chair, sink, etc., and exert hard, repeated pressure on abdomen to force object up.	☞ As in *prehospital care*; when probing mouth for foreign object, *turn* head to side, unless client has neck injury; in event of neck injury, *raise* the arm opposite you and *roll* the head and shoulders as a unit, so that head ends up supported on the arm.
Acute respiratory failure—sudden onset of an abnormally low PO_2 (<60 mm Hg) and/or high PCO_2 (>60 mm Hg) *secondary to*: • lung disease • trauma • peripheral or central nervous system depression • cardiac failure • severe obesity • airway obstruction • environmental abnormality	*Hypoxia:* *Sensorium*: acute apprehension. *Respiration*: dyspnea; shallow, rapid respirations. *Skin*: circumoral cyanosis; pale, dusky skin and nailbeds. *C/V*: slight hypertension and tachycardia, or hypotension and bradycardia. *Hypercapnia:* *Sensorium*: decreasing mentation, headache. *Skin*: flushed, warm, moist. *C/V*: hypertension; tachycardia.	☞ If you suspect respiratory distress, call physician; calm and reassure client; place in a chair or *semisitting position*; keep warm but *not* hot; phone for ambulance; if respirations cease or client becomes unconscious, clear airway and commence *respiratory resuscitation*; check pulse; initiate *CPR* if necessary; continue resuscitation until help arrives.	Check client's ability to speak; maintain airway by placing in *high-Fowler's position*; check vital signs: BP, pulse rate and rhythm, temperature, skin color, rate and depth of respirations. *Prepare for intubation if*: 1. Client has flail chest. 2. Client is comatose without gag reflex. 3. Has respiratory arrest; maintain mouth to mouth until intubation. 4. PCO_2 >55 mm Hg. 5. PO_2 <60 mm Hg. 6. F_1O_2 >50% using nasal cannula, catheter, or mask. 7. Respiratory rate >36 breaths/min.

(*continued*)

TABLE 25.4 NURSING CARE OF THE ADULT IN MEDICAL AND SURGICAL EMERGENCIES (continued)

Condition	◄ Assessment: Signs and Symptoms	◄ Prehospitalization Nursing Care	◄ In-Hospital Nursing Care
Acute respiratory failure (continued)			☞ *After intubation*: 1. Check bilateral lung sounds. 2. Observe for symmetric lung expansion. ☞ 〰 3. Maintain humidified oxygen at lowest F_1O_2 possible to achieve PO_2 of 60 mm Hg. ☞ *Improve ventilation (decrease PCO_2) by*: 1. Liquefying *secretions*—oral and parenteral fluids; if intubated, frequent instillations of normal saline or sodium bicarbonate. 2. Frequent *suctioning*. 3. *IPPB* indicated if tidal volume ↓. 4. Chest *physiotherapy*. ▭ Administer drugs, as ordered: *sympathomimetics, xanthines, anti-infectives,* and *steroids.* 〰 Monitor: arterial blood gases, electrolytes, Hct, Hgb, and WBC. **Do not:** 1. Administer sedatives. 2. Correct acid-base problems without monitoring electrolytes. 3. Overcorrect PCO_2. 4. Leave client alone while oxygen therapy is initiated. Once client is stable, transfer to ICU.
Near-drowning—asphyxiation or partial asphyxiation *due to*: • immersion or • submersion in a fluid or liquid medium	**Conscious victim:** Acute anxiety, panic; Increased rate of respirations. Pale, dusky skin. **Unconscious victim:** Shallow or no respirations. Weak or no pulse.	**Conscious victim:** 1. Try to talk victim out of panic so can find footing and way to shore. 2. Utilize devices such as poles, rings, clothing to extend to victim; do *not* let panicked victim grab you; do *not* attempt swimming rescue unless specially trained.	**Nonsymptomatic near-drowning victim:** 〰 1. Draw blood for arterial blood gases with client breathing room air. 〰 2. PA and lateral chest *x-ray*. ☞ 3. Auscultate lungs. 4. Admit to hospital for further evaluation if: 〰 a. PO_2 <80 mm Hg. b. pH <7.35. c. Pulmonary infiltrates present, or auscultation reveals crackles.

(continued)

TABLE 25.4 NURSING CARE OF THE ADULT IN MEDICAL AND SURGICAL EMERGENCIES (*continued*)

Condition	▶◀ *Assessment: Signs and Symptoms*	▶◀ *Prehospitalization Nursing Care*	▶◀ *In-Hospital Nursing Care*

Near-drowning (*continued*)		3. If you suspect head or neck injury—handle carefully, floating victim back to shore with body and head as straight as possible; do **not** turn head or bend back.
		
		On shore:
		1. Check breathing.
		2. Lay victim *flat* on back; cover and keep warm.
		3. Calm and reassure victim.
		4. Do *not* give food or water.
		5. Get to medical assistance as soon as possible.
		☞ 6. *If unconscious and not breathing*: begin sequence for CPR; compress water from abdomen *only* if interfering with ventilation attempts.
		☞ 7. *If airway obstructed*: reposition head; attempt to ventilate; perform 6–10 abdominal thrusts; sweep mouth deeply; attempt to ventilate; repeat until successful.
		☞ 8. *Once ventilation established*: check pulse; if absent, begin chest compressions as in CPR, one-person or two-person rescue.
		9. Continue CPR until victim revives or help arrives.
		10. *If victim revives*: cover and keep warm; reassure victim help is on the way.
		11. Rescue personnel can further assist emergency room personnel by:
		  a. Documenting prehospital resuscitation methods used.
		☞ b. Immobilizing victims suspected of cervical spine injuries.
			d. Victim inhaled fluids containing: chlorine, hydrocarbons, sewage, or hypotonic or fresh water.
			Symptomatic near-drowning victim:
			☞ 1. Provide basic or advanced cardiac life support.
			☞ 2. Provide clear airway and adequate ventilation by:
			  a. *Suctioning* airway.
			  b. Inserting artificial *airway* and attaching it to *ventilator*, as indicated.
			  c. Inserting *nasogastric tube* to suction to minimize aspiration of vomitus.
			3. Monitor ECG continuously.
			▭ 4. Start IV infusion of 5% D/W at keep-open rate for *fresh water near-drowning*; 5% D/NS in *salt water near-drowning*.
			☞ 5. Assist with insertion of *CVP* and *pulmonary artery catheter* to guide subsequent infusion rates.
			▭ 6. Administer drugs, as ordered; *anticonvulsants, steroids, anti-infectives, stimulants, antiarrhythmics*.
			7. Provide rewarming if hypothermia present.
			☞ 8. Insert *Foley* to assess kidney output, as fresh water near-drowning causes renal tubular necrosis due to RBC hemolysis.
			Transfer to ICU when stabilized.

(*continued*)

TABLE 25.4 NURSING CARE OF THE ADULT IN MEDICAL AND SURGICAL EMERGENCIES *(continued)*

Condition	⋈ Assessment: Signs and Symptoms	⋈ Prehospitalization Nursing Care	⋈ In-Hospital Nursing Care
Near-drowning *(continued)*		c. Utilizing a sterile container to take a sample of immersion fluid. ☞ d. Taking on-scene arterial blood gas sample for later analysis.	
Systemic Injuries			
Multiple traumas	*Sensorium*: alert; disoriented, stuporous, comatose. *Respirations*: increased rate, depth; shallow; asymmetric; paradoxical breathing; mediastinal shift; gasping, blowing. *C/V*: signs of shock (see **p. 121-122**). *Abdomen*: contusions; pain; abrasions; open wounds; rigidity; increasing distention. *Skeletal system*: pain; swelling; deformity; inappropriate or no movement. *Neurologic*: pupils round, equal, reactive to light; ipsilateral dilatation and unresponsive; fixed and dilated bilaterally. Bilateral movement and sensation in all extremities. Progressive contralateral weakness. Loss of voluntary motor function. See *Sensorium* for level of consciousness.	1. *Don't* move client unless you must, to prevent further injury; send for help. ☞ 2. Check breathing—give *mouth-to-mouth* resuscitation if indicated. 3. Check for bleeding. ☞ 4. *Control bleeding* by applying pressure on wound or on pressure points (artery proximal to wound). ☞ 5. Use tourniquet *only* if above pressure techniques fail to stop severe bleeding. 6. Check for shock (pulse, pupils, skin color) and other injuries. 7. Fractures: keep open-fracture area clean. 8. Do *not* try to set bone. ☞ 9. If client must be moved—*splint* broken bones with splints that extend past the limb joints; tie splints on snugly but not so tight as to cut off circulation. ☞ 10. Check peripheral pulses. ☞ 11. If head or back injury suspected—keep body straight; move only with help. 12. Reassure client that help is on the way.	1. Assess vital functions. ☞ 2. Establish airway; *ventilate* with *Ambu-bag*, volume-cycled ventilator. 3. Draw arterial blood gases. ☞ 4. Control bleeding. ☞ 5. Support circulation by *closed-chest massage*. ⊂⊃ 6. Prepare *infusions* of dextran, blood, crystalloids. 7. Assess for other injuries: head injuries—suspect cervical neck injury with all head injuries. ☞ 8. Place sandbags to immobilize head and neck. ☞ 9. Do *mini-neurologic* exam: level of consciousness, pupils, bilateral movement, and sensation. 10. Get history—time of injury, any loss of consciousness, any drug ingestion. ☞ 11. Stop bleeding on or about head. ☞ 12. Apply ice to contusions and hematomas. 13. Check for bleeding from nose, pharynx, ears. 14. Check for cerebrospinal fluid from ears or nose. ☞ 15. Assist with spinal tap if ordered 16. Keep accurate I&O. 17. Protect from injury if restless; seizures: orient to time, place, person. ⊂⊃ 18. Administer *steroids, diuretics*, as ordered.

(continued)

TABLE 25.4 NURSING CARE OF THE ADULT IN MEDICAL AND SURGICAL EMERGENCIES (continued)

Condition	◄ Assessment: Signs and Symptoms	◄ Prehospitalization Nursing Care	◄ In-Hospital Nursing Care
Multiple traumas (continued)			☞ 19. *Check for signs of increasing intracranial pressure*: slowing pulse and respiration, widened pulse pressure, decreasing mentation.
Maxillofacial injuries		1. Clear and *open airway.* Remove obstructions (loose teeth, foreign objects) if possible. ☞ 2. Immobilize head and neck: *always* suspect head and cervical spine injury when trauma to the head or face. 3. Control bleeding if able.	1. Establish airway— ☞ *ventilate* with Ambu-bag. Intubate. (*Tracheotomy* or *cricothyroidotomy* may be performed if upper airway too obstructed.) ☞ 2. Suction if necessary. 3. If suspect cervical neck ☞ injury—*immobilize* head, neck and spine.

Spinal injuries			1. Assess and support vital functions as above.
			☞ 2. *Immobilize*—no flexion or extension allowed.
			☞ 3. **If in respiratory distress**—*nasotracheal intubation* or *tracheostomy* to *avoid* hyperextending neck.
			☞ 4. **Check for level of injury and function**, asking client to:
			   a. Lift elbow to shoulder height (C-5).
			   b. Bend elbow (C-6).
			   c. Straighten elbow (C-7).
			   d. Grip your hand (C8-T1).
			   e. Lift leg (L-3).
			   f. Straighten knee (L-4, L-5).
			   g. Wiggle toes (L-5).
			   h. Push toes down (S-1).
			5. If client **comatose**—rub sternum with knuckles:
			   a. If all extremities move, severe injury unlikely.
			   b. If one side moves and other does not, potential *hemiplegia.*
			   c. If arms move and legs don't, *lower spinal cord* injury.
			6. Administer *steroids,* as ordered.
			7. Assist with application of skull tongs—*Vinke* or *Crutchfield.*
			8. Maintain *IV* infusions.

(continued)

TABLE 25.4 NURSING CARE OF THE ADULT IN MEDICAL AND SURGICAL EMERGENCIES (continued)

Condition	⋈ Assessment: Signs and Symptoms	⋈ Prehospitalization Nursing Care	⋈ In-Hospital Nursing Care
Spinal injuries (continued)			☞ 9. Insert *Foley* as indicated. 10. Assist with *dressing* of open wounds.
Chest injuries			1. Note color and pattern of respirations, position of trachea. ☞ 2. Auscultate lungs and palpate chest for: crepitus, pain, tenderness, position of trachea. ☞ 3. Place gauze soaked in petroleum jelly over open pneumothorax (sucking chest wound) to seal hole and decrease respiratory distress. ☞ 4. Assist with tracheostomy if indicated. 5. Prepare for insertion of chest tubes if pneumothorax or hemothorax present.
Abdominal injuries			1. Observe for rigidity. 2. Check for hematuria. ☞ 3. Auscultate for bowel sounds. 4. Assist with *paracentesis* to confirm bleeding in abdominal cavity. 5. Prepare for exploratory laparotomy. ☞ 6. Insert *nasogastric tube*—to detect presence of UGI bleeding. 7. Monitor vital signs. ***If organs protruding:*** 1. *Flex* client's *knees*. ☞ 2. Cover intestines with sterile towel soaked in saline. 3. Do *not* attempt to replace organs.
Fractures			⊂⊃ 1. Administer *tetanus toxoid*, as ordered. 2. Observe for: pain, peripheral pulses, pallor, loss of sensation and/or movement. ☞ 3. Assist with: wound cleansing, casting, x-rays, reduction. 4. Prepare for surgery if indicated. 5. Monitor vital signs.

(continued)

TABLE 25.4 NURSING CARE OF THE ADULT IN MEDICAL AND SURGICAL EMERGENCIES (*continued*)

Condition	⋈ *Assessment: Signs and Symptoms*	⋈ *Prehospitalization Nursing Care*	⋈ *In-Hospital Nursing Care*
Burns—tissue trauma *secondary to*: • scalding fluid • flame, • electricity	**Superficial (first degree)** Erythema and tenderness. Usually sunburn.	☞ Relieve pain by applying cold wet towel or cold water (not iced).	☞ 1. Cleanse thoroughly with mild detergent and water. ☞ 2. Apply gauze or sterile towel. ⊂⊃ 3. Administer *sedatives, narcotics,* as ordered. 4. Arrange for follow-up care, or prepare for admission if burn ambulatory care impractical.

	Partial thickness (second degree)
	Swelling, blisters; moisture due to escaping plasma.
		1. Douse with cold water until pain relieved.
		2. Blot skin dry and cover with clean towel.
		3. Do **not** break blisters, remove pieces of skin, or apply antiseptic ointments.
		4. If arm or leg burned, keep *elevated.*
		5. Seek medical attention if *second-degree* burns:
		  a. Cover 15% of body surface in adult.
		  b. Cover 10% of body surface in children.
		  c. Involve hands, feet, or face.
			⊂⊃ 1. Check tetanus immunization status.
			⊂⊃ 2. Administer *sedatives* or *narcotics,* as ordered.
			☞ 3. Assess respiratory and hemodynamic status; *oxygen* or ventilatory assist as indicated; *IV* infusions as ordered to combat shock.
			4. Remove all clothing from burn area.
			⚠ 5. Using *aseptic technique,* cleanse burns with antiseptic followed by soap and water, and ☞ irrigate with normal saline.

	Full thickness (third degree)
	White, charred areas.
		1. *Don't* remove charred clothing.
		2. Cover burned area with clean towel, sheet.
		3. *Elevate* burned extremities.
		☞ 4. Apply cold pack to hand, face or feet.
		5. *Sit* up client with face or chest wound to assist respirations.
		☞ 6. Maintain *airway.*
		7. Observe for shock.
		8. **Do not:**
		  a. Put ice water on burns or immerse wounds in ice water—may increase shock.
		  b. Apply ointments.
		9. Calm and reassure victim.
			1. Do *not* break blebs or attempt debridement.
			☞ 2. Assist with application of *dressings,* as ordered.
			3. Maintain frequent checks of vital signs, urine output.
			4. Provide psychological support—explain procedures, orient, etc.
			☞ 5. Assist with application of *splints* as ordered.
			⊂⊃ 6. Administer *tetanus,* immune globulin or toxoid as ordered.
			7. Assist with transfer to hospital unit.

(continued)

TABLE 25.4 NURSING CARE OF THE ADULT IN MEDICAL AND SURGICAL EMERGENCIES (continued)

Condition	◄ Assessment: Signs and Symptoms	◄ Prehospitalization Nursing Care	◄ In-Hospital Nursing Care
Burns (continued)		10. Get medical help promptly. 11. *If client conscious*, not *vomiting, and medical assistance is more than 6 h away*: may give sips of weak solution of *salt, soda,* and *water.*	
	Fourth degree Black.	Same as *full thickness*.	
Chemical burns		☞ 1. Flush with copious amounts of water. 2. Get rid of clothing over burned area.	☞ 1. Flush with copious amounts of water. ⊂⊃ 2. Administer *sedatives* or *narcotics*, as ordered.
Burns of the eye—acid		☞ 1. Flush eye with water for at least 15 min. ☞ 2. Pour water from inside to outside of eye to *avoid* contaminating unaffected eye. 3. Cover—seek medical attention **at once**.	☞ 1. Irrigate with water; *never* use neutralizing solution. ⊂⊃ 2. Instill 0.5% tetracaine, as ordered. ☞ 3. Apply patch.
Burns of the eye— alkali (laundry detergent or cleaning solvent)		1. *Don't* allow client to rub eye. ☞ 2. Flush eye with water for at least 30 min. 3. Cover—seek medical attention **at once**.	As above for **acid**.

C/V cardiovascular; CPR = cardiopulmonary resuscitation; D/W = dextrose in water; ECG = electrocardiogram; CCU = cardiac care unit; Hgb = hemoglobin; Hct = hematocrit; CBC = complete blood count; BUN = blood urea nitrogen; D/NS = dextrose in normal saline; GI = gastrointestinal; CVP = central venous pressure; IPPB = intermittent positive-pressure breathing; WBC = white blood cell count; ICU = intensive care unit; PA = posteroanterior; RBC = red blood cell; I&O = intake and output; UGI = upper GI tract.

Source: ©Lagerquist SL: *Little, Brown's NCLEX-RN® Examination Review.* Boston: Little, Brown (out of print).

TABLE 25.5 SELECTED GERIATRIC EMERGENCIES

Condition	◄ Assessment	◄ Prehospital Care	◄ In-Hospital Care
Chest pain	*Typical s/sx:* Pressure or squeezing sensation in sternal area; may radiate to neck or jaw. *S/sx in the elderly:* • Restlessness. • Confusion. • Syncope. • GI upset, e.g. heartburn (especially in women); nausea. • Diaphoresis. • Dyspnea may also occur, but is more common in younger adults.	• *Obtain history:* – Location of discomfort, duration; what makes symptoms worse or better; shortness of breath; weakness, feeling faint; medications client is taking and when last taken. • If client has nitroglycerin, give 1 tablet sublingually every 5 min. for 3 doses. • If myocardial infarction is suspected, call 911. • In the meantime, make client comfortable; loosen restrictive clothing; prepare for going outdoors (e.g. warm clothing if weather is cold); collect all client's medications to take to hospital.	• Continuous cardiac monitoring. • IV fluids. • Supplemental oxygen. • Medications: *antianginal, antithrombotics, thrombolytic agents* (tissue plasminogen activator, streptokinase). *Lab and diagnostic tests:* cardiac enzymes, troponin, APTT, 12-lead EKG, chest x-ray, pulse oximetry.
Abdomen	*Typical s/sx:* Abdominal pain and rigidity; fever. *S/sx in the elderly:* • Changes in mental status. • Tachypnea. • Urinary urgency and frequency. • Abdomen tender, rigid.	• *Obtain history:* – Pain: location, onset, severity, duration, quality. – Pain radiating to *back:* may indicate cholecystitis. – Pain radiating to *shoulder:* may indicate irritated peritoneum or ruptured spleen (especially important if client was in motor vehicle accident). – Constipation, diarrhea, nausea or vomiting. • Assess abdomen for: distension, discolorations, surgical scars. • Auscultate abdomen for bowel sounds in 4 quadrants: rapid, high-pitched sounds may indicate early bowel obstruction. • Light palpation to assess for tenderness and rigidity.	• *No* medications until diagnosis is made, then pain medications. • IV fluids to replace volume and electrolytes. • Nasogastric tube. • Indwelling urinary catheter. *Lab and diagnostic tests:* abdominal ultrasound, x-rays, barium enema, CT scan, I&O, urine culture and sensitivity.

(continued)

TABLE 25.5 SELECTED GERIATRIC EMERGENCIES (*continued*)

Condition	◄ Assessment	◄ Prehospital Care	◄ In-Hospital Care
Musculoskeletal injuries	*Typical s/sx:* • History of fall (most common cause of m/s injury). • Bruising, and edema over site. • Deformity or shortening of limb. *S/sx in the elderly:* • Assess for signs of possible *internal injury*: increasing abdominal girth, abdominal pain and rigidity; labored breathing may be consistent with rib fractures. • Assess for s/sx of *abuse*: multiple bruises in various stages of healing, soft-tissue injury on wrists, poor hygiene, malnutrition.	• *Obtain history:* – Falls can be precipitated by: diminished vision and coordination, orthostatic hypotension or transient syncope from medications or vascular disease, osteoporosis. – Increased risk of tears and bruising due to: decreased skin elasticity and subcutaneous tissue. Do **not** move client; make client as comfortable as possible; keep client warm; stay with client until EMS arrives.	☞ • Immobilization of injured area. • NPO. ⊂⊃ • IV fluids. • Pain management. • Contact social services if abuse is suspected. 〰 *Lab and diagnostics tests:* x-rays, EKG, CT scan, baseline blood studies, e.g. CBC and electrolytes.
Delirium	*Typical s/sx—sudden onset of:* • Disorientation. • Decreased attention span. • Decreased recent memory. • Poor judgment. • Restlessness. • Altered LOC. • Altered perception. • Usually precipitated by an underlying condition (such as hypoglycemia, infection, pneumonia, trauma, dehydration, stroke, cerebral tumor).	• *Obtain history:* – Determine: onset and duration of symptoms, underlying conditions, and medications client takes. • Keep environment calm and quiet. *Avoid:* bright lights, sudden movement, extremes of temperature. • Remove any hazards from the area, (e.g. knives, scissors, decorative artificial fruit.) • Supervise carefully.	• Monitor VS. ☞ • Check for pulse deficit. ☞ • Cardiac monitoring. ☞ • Neuro assessment. ☞ • Check for carotid bruits. • Keep siderails up and bed in lowest position. • Calm reassurance. • Restraints as a last resort if client is in danger of harming self or others. 〰 *Lab and diagnostics tests:* CBC, ESR, electrolytes, glucose, BUN, creatinine, drug screen, arterial blood gas; urinalysis; chest x-ray, CT scan , EKG; mental status evaluation.

(*continued*)

TABLE 25.5 SELECTED GERIATRIC EMERGENCIES (*continued*)

Condition	◄ Assessment	◄ Prehospital Care	◄ In-Hospital Care

Thermal regulation	**Hyperthermia**—*typical s/sx:*
	• Altered level of consciousness.
	• Tachycardia.
	• Warm and dry skin.
	• Thirst.
	• Faintness.
	• Muscle cramps.
		• *Obtain history:*
		  – **Risk factors include:** decreased subcutaneous fat, decreased vascularity, fewer sweat glands, diminished reflexes, less total body water, and diminished thirst reflex.
		  – Anticholinergic or sedative medications may alter thermoregulation.
		  – Chronic diseases such as diabetes or stroke may alter intrinsic temperature regulation.
		Hyperthermia:
		• Open clothing.
		• Use fan to cool client.
		• Moist compresses to forehead, groin, neck, or axilla.
		• Do **not** give fluids if client is extremely lethargic or confused.
			Hyperthermia:
			• Isotonic IV fluids, e.g. Lactated Ringer's solution.
			• Supplemental oxygen.
			• Pulse oximetry.
			• Continuous cardiac monitoring.
			Lab and diagnostic tests: rectal temperatures, CBC, electrolytes, BUN, creatinine.

	Hypothermia—*typical s/sx:* • S/sx can mimic other conditions: dilated pupils, bradycardia, amnesia, slurred speech, muscle rigidity, cold skin.	**Hypothermia:** • If skin feels cold, institute warming measures (blanket; remove wet clothing).	**Hypothermia:** • 90–94°: start passive rewarming—blankets, stockinette cap for head, socks, heat lamps, warmed IV fluids. • <90°: peritoneal lavage with warmed isotonic fluids, intubation. *Lab and diagnostic tests:* rectal temperatures, pulse oximetry, continuous cardiac monitoring.

VI. **High protein, high carbohydrate diet:**

A. *Purpose*: corrects large protein losses and raises the blood albumin level. May be modified to include *low* fat, *low* sodium, *low* cholesterol diets.

B. *Use*: burns, hepatitis, cirrhosis, pregnancy, hyperthyroidism, mononucleosis, protein deficiency due to poor eating habits, geriatric clients with poor food intake, nephritis, nephrosis, liver and gall-bladder disorders.

C. *Foods allowed*: general diet with added protein. In adults, high-protein diets usually contain 135–150 g of protein.

D. *Foods avoided*: restrictions depend on modifications added to the diet. These modifications are determined by the client's condition.

VII. **Purine-restricted diet:**

A. *Purpose*: designed to reduce the amount of consumed uric acid–producing foods.

B. *Use*: high uric acid retention, uric acid renal stones, gout.

C. *Foods allowed*: general diet plus 2–3 quarts of liquid daily.

D. *Foods avoided*: cheese containing spices or nuts, fried eggs, meat, liver, seafood, lentils, dried peas and beans, broth, bouillon, gravies, oatmeal and whole wheats, pasta, noodles, alcoholic beverages. *Limited* quantities of meat, fish, seafood allowed.

VIII. **Bland diet:**

A. *Purpose*: provision of a diet low in fiber, roughage, mechanical irritants, chemical stimulants.

B. *Use*: ulcers (gastric and duodenal), gastritis, hyperchlorhydria, functional GI disorders, gastric atony, diarrhea, spastic constipation, biliary indigestion, hiatal hernia.

C. *Foods allowed*: varied to meet individual needs and food tolerances.

D. *Foods avoided*: fried foods, including eggs, meat, fish, seafood; cheese with added nuts or spices; commercially prepared luncheon meats; cured meats such as ham; gravies and sauces; raw vegetables; potato skins; fruit juices with pulp; figs; raisins; fresh fruits; whole wheats; rye bread; bran cereals; rich pastries; pies; chocolate; jams with seeds; nuts; seasoned dressings; caffeinated coffee; strong tea; cocoa; alcoholic and carbonated beverages; pepper.

IX. **Low fat, cholesterol-restricted diet:**

A. *Purpose*: reduce hyperlipidemia, provide dietary treatment for malabsorption syndromes and clients having acute intolerance to fats.

B. *Use*: hyperlipidemia, atherosclerosis, pancreatitis, cystic fibrosis, sprue, gastrectomy, massive resection of the small intestine, cholecystitis.

C. *Foods allowed*: nonfat milk; *low* carbohydrate, low-fat vegetables; most fruits; breads; pastas; cornmeal; lean meats; unsaturated fats such as corn oil; desserts made without whole milk; unsweetened carbonated beverages.

D. *Foods avoided*: whole milk and whole milk or cream products, avocados, olives, commercially prepared baked goods such as donuts and muffins, poultry skin, highly marbled meats, shellfish, fish canned in oil, nuts, coconut, commercially prepared meats, butter, ordinary margarines, olive oil, lard, pudding made with whole milk, ice cream, candies with chocolate, cream, sauces, gravies, commercially fried foods.

X. **Diabetic diet:**

A. *Purpose*: maintain blood glucose as near normal as possible, prevent or delay onset of diabetic complications.

B. *Use*: diabetes mellitus.

C. *Foods allowed*: composed of 15%–20% carbohydrates, less than 10% fats, 60%–75% protein. The American Diabetic Association no longer recommends a specific "ADA diet". Nutritional management of diabetes is based on a meal plan that is healthy for most people, such as the Food Guide Pyramid: 6–11 servings of bread, pasta, rice, cereal; 3–5 servings of vegetables; 2–4 servings of fruit; 2–3 servings of milk, yogurt, cheese; 2–3 servings of meat, poultry, fish, dry beans, eggs; minimal fats, oils, sweets..

D. *Foods avoided*: concentrated sweets or regular soft drinks.

XI. **Diet for preventing renal calculi:**

A. *Purpose*: provide a well-balanced diet that limits intake of foods high in purine, calcium, and/or oxalate.

B. *Use*: retard the formation of renal calculi. The type of diet chosen depends on laboratory analysis of the stones.

C. *Avoid* the following food groups:

1. Foods containing *purines*:
High: sardines, herring, mussels, liver, kidney, goose, venison, meat soups, sweetbreads.
Medium: chicken, salmon, crab, veal, mutton, bacon, pork, beef, ham.

2. Foods containing *calcium*: milk, cheese, ice cream, yogurt, sauces containing milk, all beans (except green beans), lentils, fish with fine bones, dried fruits, nuts, chocolate, cocoa, Ovaltine.

3. Foods containing *oxalate*: spinach, rhubarb, asparagus, cabbage, tomatoes, beets, nuts, celery, parsley, runner beans, chocolate, cocoa, instant coffee, Ovaltine, tea, Worcestershire sauce.

D. *Foods allowed*: all the client wants of the following.

1. Breads: any, preferably whole grain; crackers; rolls.

TABLE B.4 HOT–COLD THEORY OF DISEASE TREATMENT *

Hot Diseases or Conditions	Cold Foods	Cold Medicines and Herbs	Cold Diseases or Conditions	Hot Foods	Hot Medicines and Herbs
Infections	Fresh vegetables	Bicarbonate of soda	Cancer	Chocolate	Penicillin
Kidney diseases	Tropical fruits	Milk of magnesia	Earache	Cheese	Aspirin
Diarrhea	Dairy products	Sage	Rheumatism	Temperate-zone fruits	Castor oil
Rashes and other skin eruptions	Low-prestige meats (goat, fish, chicken)	Linden	Tuberculosis	Chili peppers	Cod liver oil
Sore throat	Honey	Orange flower water	Common cold	Cereal grains	Iron preparations
Warts	Raisins		Headache	Goat milk	Vitamins
Constipation	Bottled milk		Paralysis	High-prestige meats (beef, water-fowl, mutton)	Anise
Ulcer	Barley water		Stomach cramps		Cinnamon
Liver complaints	Cod		Teething		Garlic
			Menstrual period		Mint
			Joint pain	Oils	Ginger root
			Malaria	Hard liquor	Tobacco
			Pneumonia	Aromatic beverages	
				Coffee	
				Onions	
				Peas	
				Eggs	

*A Latin American, particularly Puerto Rican, approach to treating diseases. A "hot" disease is treated with "cold" treatments (foods, medicines) and vice versa.

Source: Reprinted with permission from Wilson HS, Kneisl CR. Psychiatric Nursing (2nd ed). Menlo Park, CA: Addison-Wesley. (out of print).

2. Cereals: any, preferably whole grain.
3. Desserts: angel food or sunshine cake; cookies made without baking powder or soda; cornstarch pudding; cranberry desserts; custards; gelatin desserts; ice cream; sherbet
4. Fats: any, such as butter, margarine, salad dressings, Crisco, Spry, lard, salad oils, olive oil.
5. Fluids: increase to 3 L/day.
6. Fruits: cranberries, plums, prunes.
7. Meat, eggs, cheese: any meat, fish, or fowl, two servings daily; at least one egg daily.
8. Potato substitutes: corn, hominy, lentils, macaroni, noodles, rice, spaghetti, vermicelli.
9. Soup: broth as desired; other soups from foods allowed.
10. Sweets: cranberry or plum jelly; sugar, plain sugar candy.
11. Miscellaneous: cream sauce, gravy, peanut butter, peanuts, popcorn, salt, spices, vinegar, walnuts.

E. *Restricted foods*: no more than the amount allowed each day.
  1. Milk: 1 pint daily (may be used in other ways than as beverage).
  2. Cream: 1/3 cup or less daily.
  3. Fruits: one serving of fruit daily (in addition to the prunes, plums, cranberries); certain fruits listed under Foods *avoided are not allowed at any time.*

4. Vegetables, including potatoes: two servings daily; certain vegetables listed under *Foods avoided are not allowed at any time.*

XII. **High fiber diet:**
A. *Purpose*: soften stool, exercise digestive tract muscles; speed passage of food through digestive tract to prevent exposure to cancer-causing agents in food; lower blood lipid levels; prevent sharp rise in blood glucose level after eating.
B. *Use*: diabetes, hyperlipidemia, constipation, diverticulosis, anticarcinogenic (colon).
C. *Foods allowed*: recommended intake about 6 g of crude fiber daily: all bran cereals; watermelon, prunes, dried peaches, apple with skin; parsnips, peas, brussels sprouts; sunflower seeds.

XIII. **Low residue (low fiber) diet:**
A. *Purpose*: reduce stool bulk and slow transit time.
B. *Use*: bowel inflammation during acute diverticulitis or ulcerative colitis, preparation for bowel surgery, esophageal and intestinal stenosis.
C. *Foods allowed*: eggs; ground or well-cooked tender meat, fish, poultry; milk; mild cheeses; strained fruit juice (except prune); cooked or canned apples, apricots, peaches, pears; ripe bananas; strained vegetable juice; canned, cooked, or strained asparagus, beets, green beans, pumpkin, acorn squash, spinach; white bread; refined cereals (Cream of Wheat).

XIV. **Low phosphate diet:**
A. *Purpose*: to reduce the amount of phosphate.
B. *Use*: chronic renal failure.
C. *Foods avoided*: dairy products (milk, cheese, ice cream, yogurt) and foods that contain dairy products (e.g., pudding).

TABLE B.5 PHYSIOLOGIC FUNCTIONS AND DEFICIENCY SYNDROMES OF COMMON VITAMINS

Nutrient	Functions	Signs of Deficiency
Fat-Soluble Vitamins		
Vitamin A	Essential for formation and maintenance of epithelial cells; essential for normal function of the *retina* and the synthesis of rhodopsin (visual purple)	Night blindness; xerosis and softening of the cornea; dry, bumpy skin
Vitamin D	Necessary for absorption and metabolism of calcium and phosphorus; important for the formation of normal *teeth* and *bones*	Rickets in children; osteomalacia in adults
Vitamin E	Antioxidant that protects red blood cells from hemolysis; utilized in epithelial tissue maintenance and prostaglandin synthesis	*Increased* hemolysis of red blood cells, macrocytic anemia, *increased* capillary fragility
Vitamin K	Essential for the formation of prothrombin and other clotting factors by the *liver*	Hypoprothrombinemia; hemorrhagic disease in newborns
Water-Soluble Vitamins		
Vitamin C	Essential for the formation of collagen; promotes healing of *wounds and fractures*; reduces susceptibility to infections; promotes the absorption of *iron*; necessary for the conversion of folic acid and folinic acid, tryptophan to serotonin, and cholesterol to bile salts; may play a role in resistance to certain types of cancer	Scurvy—petechiae and ecchymoses, joint pain, delayed wound healing, gingivitis, bleeding gums, loss of teeth
Vitamin B_1 (thiamine)	Coenzyme in carbohydrate metabolism; essential for normal *nerve* function	Beriberi—peripheral neuropathy, muscle cramping, paresthesia, muscle degeneration, and heart failure
Vitamin B_2 (riboflavin)	Coenzyme in cellular metabolism and respiration; essential for healthy *eyes*	Red conjunctivae; fissures at corners of mouth, around nose and ears, on tongue; magenta tongue
Vitamin B_3 (niacin)	Coenzyme in the metabolism of carbohydrates and amino acids; essential for the synthesis of fatty acids and cholesterol and the conversion of phenylalanine to tyrosine	Pellagra—cracks in skin and lips; red lesions of hands, feet, face, and neck; dementia
Vitamin B_6 (pyridoxine)	Coenzyme in protein metabolism and several other enzymatic reactions; necessary for the formation of: norepinephrine, epinephrine, tyramine, dopamine, serotonin	Seborrheic dermatitis, cheilosis, peripheral neuritis, convulsions
Vitamin B_9 (folic acid)	Essential for DNA synthesis and normal maturation of *red blood cells*	Megaloblastic and macrocytic anemia; reduced platelet levels
Vitamin B_{12} (cyanoco-balamin)	Coenzyme in protein metabolism; essential for *red blood cell* formation and maintenance of *myelin sheaths of nerves*	Pernicious anemia, progressive neuropathy owing to demyelination

Source: Adapted from: Shlafer M, Marieb E. *The Nurse, Pharmacology and Drug Therapy*. Menlo Park, CA: Addison-Wesley. (out of print) (reprinted with permission)

Food List for Ready Reference in Menu Planning

I. **High cholesterol foods**—over 50 mg/100 g portion: beef, butter, cheese, egg yolks, shellfish, kidney, liver, pork, veal.

II. **High sodium foods**—over 500 mg/100 g portion: *bacon*—cured, Canadian; *beef*—corned, cooked, canned, dried, creamed; biscuits, baking powder; bouillon cubes; bran with added sugar and malt; bran flakes with thiamine; raisins; *breads*—wheat, French, rye, white, whole wheat; butter; *cheese*—cheddar, Parmesan, Swiss, pasteurized American; cocoa; cookies—gingersnaps; corn flakes; cornbread; *crackers*—graham, saltines; margarine; *milk*—dry, skim; mustard; oat products; olives—green, ripe; peanut butter; pickles—dill; popcorn with oil and salt; *salad dressing*—blue cheese, Roquefort, French, Thousand Island; *sausages*—bologna, frankfurters; soy sauce; catsup; tuna in oil.

III. **High potassium foods**—more than 400 mg/100 g portion: almonds; bacon, Canadian; baking powder, low sodium; *beans*—white, lima; beef—hamburger; fruits, fruit juices; bran with sugar and malt; cake—fruitcake, gingerbread; cashew; chicken, white meat; cocoa; coffee, instant; cookies—gingersnaps; dates; garlic; *milk*—skim, powdered; peanuts, roasted; peanut butter; peas; pecans; potatoes, boiled in skin; scallops; tea, instant; tomato puree; turkey, white meat; veal; walnuts, black; yeast, brewers.

IV. **Foods high in B vitamins (see Table B.5):**
   A. *Thiamine*: pork, dried beans, dried peas, liver, lamb, veal, nuts, peas.
   B. *Riboflavin*: liver, poultry, milk, yogurt, whole-grain cereals, beef, oysters, tongue, fish, cottage cheese, veal.
   C. *Niacin*: liver, fish, poultry, peanut butter, whole grains and enriched breads, lamb, veal, beef, pork.

V. **Foods high in vitamin C (see Table B.5):** oranges, strawberries, dark-green leafy vegetables, potatoes, grapefruit, tomato, cabbage, broccoli, melons, liver.

VI. **Foods high in iron, calcium, and residue:**
   A. *Iron: breads*—brown, corn, ginger; fish, tuna; poultry; organ meats; whole-grain cereals; shellfish; egg yolk; *fruits*—apples, berries; *dried fruits*—dates, prunes, apricots, peaches, raisins; *vegetables*—dark-green leafy, potatoes, tomatoes, rhubarb, squash; molasses; dried beans and peas; peanut butter; brown sugar; noodles; rice.
   B. *Calcium: milk*—dry, skim, whole, evaporated, buttermilk; *cheese*—American, Swiss, hard; *vegetables*—kale; turnip greens; mustard greens; collards; tofu.
   C. *Residue*: whole-grain *cereals*—oatmeal, bran, shredded wheat; *breads*—whole wheat, cracked wheat, rye, bran muffins; *vegetables*—lettuce, spinach, Swiss chard, raw carrots, raw celery, corn, cauliflower, eggplant, sauerkraut, cabbage; *fruits*—bananas, figs, apricots, oranges.

VII. **Foods to be used in low protein and low carbohydrate diets**
   A. *Low protein**: milk—buttermilk, reconstituted evaporated, low sodium, skim, dry; *meat*—chicken, lamb, turkey, beef (lean), veal; *fish*—sole, flounder, haddock, perch; *cheese*—cheddar, American, Swiss, cottage; eggs; *fruits*—apples, grapes, pears, pineapple; *vegetables*—cabbage, cucumbers, lettuce, tomatoes; *cereals*—cornflakes, puffed rice, puffed wheat, farina, rolled oats.
   B. *Low carbohydrate: all meats; cheese*—hard, soft, cottage; eggs; *shellfish*—oysters, shrimp; *fats*—bacon, butter, French dressing, salad oil, mayonnaise, margarine; *vegetables*—asparagus, green beans, beet greens, broccoli, brussels sprouts, cabbage, celery, cauliflower, cucumber, lettuce, green pepper, spinach, squash, tomatoes; *fruits*—avocados, strawberries, cantaloupe, lemons, rhubarb.

VIII. **Food guide pyramid**—guide to daily food selection (**Figure B-1**).
   A. *Fats, oils*: use sparingly.
   B. *Milk group*: two to three servings.
   C. *Meat group*: two to three servings.
   D. *Fruit group*: two to four servings.
   E. *Vegetable group*: three to five servings.
   F. *Bread/cereal group*: six to 11 servings.

*These proteins are allowed in various amounts in controlled-protein diets for renal decompensation.

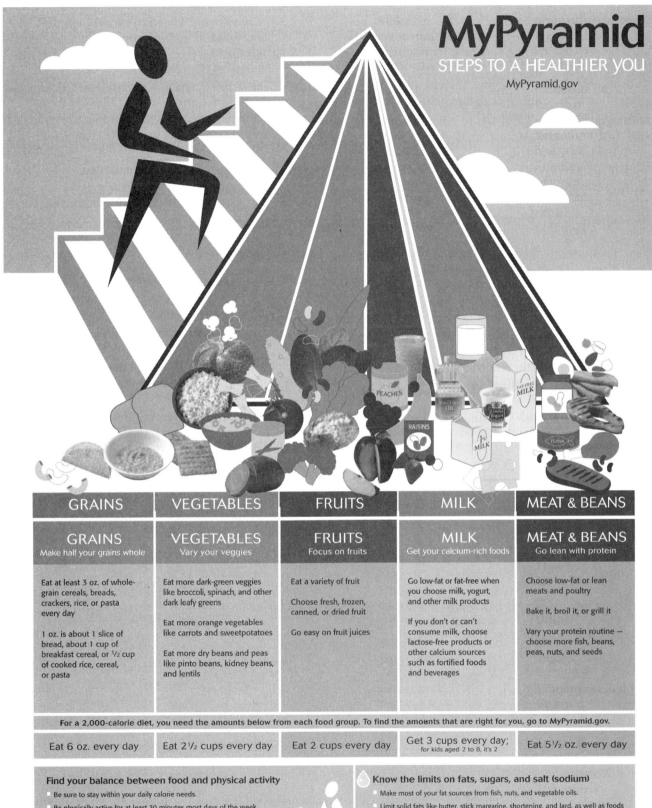

FIGURE B-1. FOOD GUIDE PYRAMID—GUIDE TO DAILY FOOD CHOICES. (From U.S. Department of Agriculture.)

Obesity

In the United States approximately 50% of adults are overweight, 15% are obese, 5% are seriously obese, and 3% are morbidly obese (see **Chapter 1, page 4** for calculation of body mass index [BMI]).

I. **Pathophysiology**: an abnormal increase in the proportion of fat cells. Speculation exists about the processes leading to obesity.

II. **Risk factors/causes:**
   A. Sedentary lifestyle.
   B. Unbalanced nutrition.
   C. Consuming more calories than what is expended.

III. **Assessment**
   A. *Subjective data*:
      1. Onset of obesity; family history of obesity.
      2. Presence of diseases related to obesity (e.g., hypertension, cardiovascular disease, diabetes type 2, chronic joint pain, gout, cholelithiasis.)
      3. Medications the client takes, (e.g., thyroid medications or diet pills.)
      4. Previous weight reduction programs, surgeries, or treatments.
   B. *Objective data*:
      1. Body mass index (BMI). (see **Chapter 1, page 4** for BMI parameters.)
      2. Hypertension.
      3. Hypoventilation.
      4. Joint pain and decreased mobility.
      5. Laboratory tests: *elevated* serum glucose; *elevated* cholesterol and triglycerides; polycythemia.

IV. **Analysis/nursing diagnosis**
   A. *Nutrition imbalance*: more than body requirements related to excessive intake compared to metabolic needs.
   B. *Impaired physical mobility* related to excessive body weight.
   C. *Ineffective breathing pattern* related to decreased lung expansion.
   D. *Disturbed body image* related to alterations in physical appearance and perceived unattractiveness.

V. **Nursing care plan/implementation**
   A. Goal: *develop plan to promote weight loss*.
      1. Meal plan should be well balanced, and restricted in calories.
      2. Identify exercise program appropriate for client.
      3. Develop strategies to maintain motivation for weight loss, such as, a system of rewards or attendance at a support group.
   B. Goal: **health teaching:**
      1. *Avoid* "fad" diets which produce loss of body water, rather than loss of fat.
      2. Refer to nutritionist for individualized plan.

VI. **Evaluation/outcome criteria**
   A. Long-term weight loss.
   B. Improvement in conditions related to obesity, (e.g., hypertension.)
   C. Adopt healthy lifestyle choices.
   D. Improved self-image.

Index to 🍎 Diets

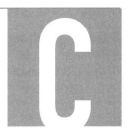

For a quick review, use this appendix to locate pages where **60+ special dietary** considerations are covered in this text as they pertain to specific medical conditions.

Review of Pharmacology

 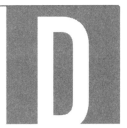

Administering Medication:

Common Injection Sites

Absorption Rates

Common Drugs

Adrenergics
Adrenocortical steroids
Analgesics
Antianemic
Antianginals
Antiarrhythmics
Antiasthmatic
Anticholinergics
Anticoagulants
Anticoagulant antidotes
Anticonvulsants
Antidiarrheals
Antiemetics
Antifungals
Antigouts
Antihistamines
Antihyperglycemics
    Insulins
Antihypertensives
Anti-infectives
Antilipemics
Antiplatelet
Antituberculosis
Antiulceratives
Antivirals
Bronchodilators
Calcium channel blockers
Cardiac glycosides
Cholinergic drugs
Cholinergic miotics
CNS stimulants
Decongestant
Diuretics
Emetic

Enzymes
Expectorants
Fibrinolytic agents
Fibrinolytic antidote
Mucolytic agent
Muscle relaxants
Narcotic antagonist
Sedatives and hypnotics
Thyroid hormone inhibitors
Thyroid hormone replacements

Guide to Important Food and Drugs Considerations

Common Herb/Drug Interactions

Classification of Anticancer Drugs

Properties of Selected Anti-inflammatory Agents

Classification of Drugs by Drug Name Endings

Common Drug Calculations

Onset, Peak, and Duration of Different Types of Insulin; Tips for Drawing Up and Giving Insulin

Common Patterns of Medication Use Among Elderly Clients

TABLE D. 1 COMMON INJECTION SITES

Injection Site	Major Nerves in Area	Major Blood Vessels in Area	Bone Landmarks	Anatomical Area	Client Position
Intramuscular injections					
Deltoid	Radial and ulnar nerves	Brachial artery	Find the lower edge of the acromion process. The injection site is three finger widths below the acromion process.	Upper arm	Sitting or Standing
Ventrogluteal Note: this site is preferred, and is especially useful for clients who are thin.	Free of major nerves	Free of major blood vessels	Use the hand opposite of the side on which the injection is to be given. Place the palm of the hand over the trochanter and the index finger on the anterior-superior iliac spine. The thumb should be pointing toward the groin and the rest of the fingers toward the client's head. Spread the middle finger away from the index finger along the client's iliac crest to make a 'V'. The injection site is in the middle of the 'V' [triangle].	Above the hip	Side-lying with knees bent Supine
Dorsal gluteal Note: this site is not a preferred site for IM injections because of the proximity of major nerve and blood vessel, and the inconsistency of the subcutaneous layer over the site.	Sciatic nerve	Gluteal artery	Imagine a diagonal line running from the posterior-superior iliac spine and the trochanter. The injection site is above and lateral to the diagonal line.	Upper outer aspect of the upper outer quadrant of the buttock	Prone or Side-lying
Vastus lateralis	Free of major nerves	Free of major blood vessels	1 handbreadth below the groin, 1 handbreadth above the knee, between the midline of anterior thigh and midline of the lateral thigh	Midline of anterior thigh	Supine with knee slightly flexed or sitting

TABLE D. 1 COMMON INJECTION SITES (*continued*)

Injection Site	Major Nerves in Area	Major Blood Vessels in Area	Bone Landmarks	Anatomical Area	Client Position
Subcutaneous Injections					
Arm	N/A	N/A	N/A	Outer aspects of upper arms, one handbreadth below shoulder and above elbow	Sitting Standing Supine
Thigh	N/A	N/A	N/A	Anterior surface of thighs, one handbreadth below groin and above knee	Sitting or Supine
Abdomen	N/A	N/A	N/A	Below the umbilicus, between the iliac crests, *avoiding* a 2-inch area around the umbilicus.	Semi-Fowler's or Supine
The scapular and upper ventral and dorsal gluteal areas can also be used.					
Intradermal injections					
Forearm	N/A	N/A	N/A	3-4 fingerwidths below antecubital space and one hand above wrist.	Sitting or Standing
The scapulae and upper ventral and dorsal gluteal areas can also be used if the forearm is not available.					

☞ **Steps for administering a medication using Z-track technique.**

1. After drawing up the medication, change the needle on the syringe.
2. Draw up 0.2 mL of air into the syringe to create an air lock.
3. Prep the site, then pull the overlying skin and subcutaneous tissue 2.5 to 3.5 cm (1-1 ½ inches) laterally.
4. While holding the skin taut, insert the needle deep into the muscle using a 90° angle; aspirate for at least 5 seconds, and inject the medication and air.
5. Wait 10 seconds for the medication to disperse before withdrawing the needle.

TABLE D.2 RATES OF ABSORPTION BY DIFFERENT ROUTES

Route of Administration	Time Until Drug Takes Effect *
Topical	Hours to days
Oral	30-90 min
Rectal	5-30 min (unpredictable)
Subcutaneous injection	15-30 min
Intramuscular injection	10-20 min
Sublingual tablet	3-5 min
Inhalation	3 min
Endotracheal	3 min
Intravenous	30-60 sec
Intracardiac	15 sec

*In a healthy person with normal perfusion.

Source: Adapted from: Caroline NL. *Emergency Care in the Streets* (5th ed). Boston: Little, Brown (out of print).

TABLE D.3 COMMON DRUGS

Drug and Dosage	Use	Action	▶◀ Assessment: Side Effects
ADRENERGICS			
Alpha and beta agonists Epinephrine (*Adrenalin*)—SC or IM 0.1-0.5 mg ; IV 0.1-0.5 mg, may be followed by 1-4 mcg/min infusion; intracardiac 0.3-0.5 mg; inhalation MDI 1 inhalatiion	Asystole, bronchospasm, anaphylaxis, glaucoma	Stimulates pacemaker cells; inhibits histamine and mediates bronchial relaxation	Ventricular arrhythmias, fear, anxiety, anginal pain, decreased renal blood flow, headache

NURSING IMPLICATIONS: Use *TB syringe* for greater accuracy; *massaging* injection site hastens action; repeated injections may cause tissue necrosis; *avoid* injection in buttocks because bacteria in area may lead to gas gangrene; may make mucous plugs in lungs more difficult to dislodge.

Norepinephrine (*Levophed*)—IV 0.5-1 mcg/min	*Acute* hypotension, cardiogenic shock	Increases rate and strength of heart beat; increases vasoconstriction	Palpitations, pallor, headache, hypertension, anxiety, insomnia, dilated pupils, nausea, vomiting, glycosuria, tissue sloughing

NURSING IMPLICATIONS: Observe vital signs, mentation, skin temperature, and color (earlobes, lips, nailbeds); tissue necrosis occurs with infiltration; *antidote is phentolamine* 5–10 mg in 10–15 mL normal saline.

Beta agonists			
Dobutamine (*Dobutrex*) —IV 2.5–15 mg /kg/min	Acute heart failure	Stimulates cardiac contractile force (positive inotropy); fewer changes in heart rate than dopamine or isoproterenol	Tachycardia, arrhythmias

NURSING IMPLICATIONS: Mix with 5% dextrose; do *not* dilute until ready to use; *protect from light*; administer with *infusion pump*; check vital signs *constantly; extravasation* can produce tissue necrosis, see Norepinephrine.

Dopamine (*Intropin*)—IV 0.5–5 mcg/kg/min titrated to desired response (10–30 min. intervals); maintenance at 10 mcg/kg/min or less	Acute heart failure	↑ Cardiac contractility; ↑ Renal blood flow	Ectopic beats, nausea, vomiting, tachycardia, anginal pain, dyspnea, hypotension

NURSING IMPLICATIONS: Monitor vital signs, urine output, and signs of peripheral ischemia; will cause *tissue sloughing* if infiltration occurs.

Isoproterenol (*Isuprel*)— Inhalation 1-2 inhalations x 4-6 daily; IV 0.5–5.0 mcg/min in solution	Cardiogenic shock, heart block, bronchospasm–asthma, emphysema	↑ Cardiac contractility; facilitates AV conduction and pacemaker automaticity; bronchodilation	Tachyarrhythmias, hypotension, headache, flushing of skin, nausea, tremor, dizziness

NURSING IMPLICATIONS: Monitor vital signs, ECG: oral inhalation solutions must *not* be injected.

ADRENOCORTICAL STEROIDS			
Cortisone acetate—PO or IM 20–100 mg qd in single or divided doses	ACTH insuffiency, rheumatoid arthritis, allergies, ulcerative colitis, nephrosis	Anti-inflammatory effect of unknown action	Moon facies, hirsutism, thinning of skin, striae, hypertension, menstrual irregularities, delayed healing, psychoses

NURSING IMPLICATIONS: Give oral form *pc*, with snack at bedtime; give deep IM (*never* deltoid); monitor vital signs; observe for behavior changes; skin care and activity to tolerance; 🍎 *diet*–salt restricted, high protein, KCl supplement; protect from injury.

(continued)

TABLE D.3 COMMON DRUGS

Drug and Dosage	Use	Action	⋈ Assessment: Side Effects
ADRENOCORTICAL STEROIDS (*continued*)			
Hydrocortisone—IM 100–500 mg q 2-6 hr; PO 20-240 mg/day in divided doses	Addison's disease, burns, surgical shock, adrenal surgery	Anti-inflammatory	Edema, hypertension, pulmonary congestion, hypokalemia
NURSING IMPLICATIONS: *Salt restriction* according to BP readings; monitor vital signs; *weigh* daily			
Dexamethasone (*Decadron*)—PO 0.75–9.0 mg qd; IM or IV 4–20 mg qd	Addison's disease, allergic reactions, leukemia, Hodgkin's disease, iritis, dermatitis, rheumatoid arthritis, cerebral edema	Anti-inflammatory effect	See Cortisone acetate
NURSING IMPLICATIONS: Contraindicated in tuberculosis; see Cortisone acetate for nursing implications.			
Methylprednisolone sodium (*Solu-Medrol*)—IV, IM 10–40 mg, slowly; PO 160 mg/d x 7 days, then taper	Same as Dexamethosone	See Dexamethasone	See Dexamethasone
NURSING IMPLICATIONS: See Dexamethasone.			
Prednisone—PO 5-60 mg qd	Rheumatoid arthritis, cancer therapy	Anti-inflammatory effect of unknown action	Insomnia, gastric distress
NURSING IMPLICATIONS: See Cortisone acetate.			
ANALGESICS			
Acetaminophen (*Tylenol, Datril, Panadol*)—PO 325–650 mg q4h	Simple fever or pain	Analgesic and antipyretic actions; *no* anti-inflammatory or anticoagulant effects	No remarkable side effects when taken for a short period
NURSING IMPLICATIONS: Consult with physician if no relief after 4 d of therapy.			
Aspirin (acetylsalicylic acid)—PO or rectal 325-500 mg q 3h for pain/fever; up to 5.4 g/day for inflammation; 1-1.3 g/daily to prevent TIA	Minor aches and pains, fever of colds and influenza, rheumatoid arthritis, anticoagulant therapy	Inhibits prostaglandin production; decreases platelet aggregation	Erosive gastritis with bleeding, coryza, urticaria, nausea, vomiting, tinnitus, impaired hearing, respiratory alkalosis
NURSING IMPLICATIONS: Administer *with food or after meals*; observe for nasal, oral or subcutaneous *bleeding*; push *fluids*; ⋙ check: *Hct, Hgb, prothrombin times* frequently; *avoid* use in children with flu.			
Codeine—PO, IM or SC 15–60 mg (gr ¼ to 1)	Control pain; may be used during the puerperium	Nonsynthetic narcotic analgesic	Of little use during labor; allergic response, constipation, GI upset
NURSING IMPLICATIONS: Note response to the medication; less respiratory depression; preferred for a client with head injury.			
Ecotrin (enteric-coated aspirin)	See Aspirin	See Aspirin	See Aspirin
NURSING IMPLICATIONS: See Aspirin.			
Etodolac (*Lodine*)—PO 400–1200 mg/d, 300–400 mg q6–8h	Management of osteoarthritis, mild to moderate pain	Inhibits prostaglandin synthesis, suppression of inflammation and pain (NSAID)	Dyspepsia, asthma, drowsiness, dizziness, rash, tinnitus, anaphylaxis
NURSING IMPLICATIONS: Give 30 min *before or 2 h after* meals for rapid effect; may be taken *with* food to decrease GI irritation			

(continued)

TABLE D.3 COMMON DRUGS

Drug and Dosage	Use	Action	▶◀ Assessment: Side Effects
ANALGESICS (continued)			
Fentanyl transdermal (*Duragesic*)—25–100 mcg /h	Chronic pain; *not* recommended for postoperative pain	Binds to opiate receptors in the CNS to alter response and perception of pain	Drowsiness, confusion, weakness, constipation, dry mouth, nausea, vomiting, anorexia, sweating

NURSING IMPLICATIONS: Apply to *upper* torso, flat, nonirritated surface; when applying, hold firmly with palm of hand 10–20 sec.

Hydromorphone (*Dilaudid*)— PO 2–4 mg q3–6h; IM 1–2 mg q3–6h up to 2–4 mg q4 mg q4–6h; IV 0.5–1.0 mg q3h	Moderate to severe pain; antitussive	Binds to opiate receptors in the CNS; alters perception and response to pain.	Sedation, confusion, hypotension, constipation

NURSING IMPLICATIONS: Give PO with *food or milk*; give 2 mg IV over 3–5 min; *fluids,* 🍎 *bulk*, and laxatives to minimize constipation.

Ibuprofen (*Motrin*—300–800 mg oral 3–4/d, *not to exceed* 3200 mg/d	Nonsteroidal anti-inflammatory, *antirheumatic* used for chronic arthritis pain	Inhibition of prostaglandin *synthesis or release*	GI upset, leukopenia, sodium/*water retention*

NURSING IMPLICATIONS: Give on *empty stomach* for best result; may mix with food if GI upset severe; teach caution when using other medications.

Indomethacin (*Indocin*)—PO 25 mg 3–4/d; increase to max 200 mg daily in divided doses	Rheumatoid arthritis, bursitis, gouty arthritis	Antipyretic/anti-inflammatory action, inhibits prostaglandin biosynthesis	GI distress, GI bleeding, rash, headache, blood dyscrasias, corneal changes

NURSING IMPLICATIONS: Monitor GI side effects; administer *after* meals for best effect or *with* food, milk, or antacids if GI symptoms severe.

Ketorolac (*Toradol*)—PO 10 mg q4–6h; IM 30–60 mg initially; then 15–30 mg q6h	Short-term management of pain	Inhibits prostaglandin synthesis producing peripherally mediated analgesia, antipyretic/anti-inflammatory	Drowsiness, dizziness, dyspnea, prolonged bleeding time, dyspepsia

NURSING IMPLICATIONS: May be given routinely or prn; *advise* dentist or MD before any procedure.

Meperidine HCl (*Demerol*)— PO or IM 50–100 mg q3–4h	Pain due to trauma or surgery; allays apprehension prior to surgery	Acts on CNS to produce analgesia, sedation, euphoria, respiratory depression	Palpitations, bradycardia, hypotension, nausea, vomiting, syncope, sweating, tremors, convulsions

NURSING IMPLICATIONS: Check *respiratory rate* and depth before giving drug; give IM, as *subcutaneous* administration is *painful* and can cause local irritation.

Morphine SO_4—PO 10–30 mg (*Roxanol, MS Contin*); SC 8–15 mg; IV 4–10 mg; rectal 10–20 mg	Control pain and relieve fear, apprehension, restlessness, as in pulmonary edema	Depresses CNS reception of pain and ability to interpret stimuli; depresses respiratory center in medulla	Nausea, vomiting, flushing, confusion, urticaria, depressed rate and depth of respirations, decreased blood pressure

NURSING IMPLICATIONS: Check rate and depth of *respirations* before administering drug; observe for gas pains and *abdominal distention*; smaller doses for aged; monitor vital signs; observe for *postural hypotension*.

(*continued*)

TABLE D.3 COMMON DRUGS

Drug and Dosage	Use	Action	◄◄ Assessment: Side Effects
ANALGESICS (*continued*)			
Naproxen (*Naprosyn*)—PO 250–500 mg bid	Mild to moderate pain, dysmenorrhea, rheumatoid arthritis, osteoarthritis (NSAID)	Inhibits prostaglandin synthesis; suppresses inflammation	Headache, drowsiness, dizziness, nausea, dyspepsia, constipation, bleeding
NURSING IMPLICATIONS: Take with a full glass of *water; avoid* exposure to sun.			
Oxycodone HC1 (*Percodan, Tylox*)—PO 3–20 mg; SC 5 mg	Controls pain; 5–6 times more potent than codeine	Less potent and addicting than morphine; for moderate pain—peak action 1h	See Morphine SO$_4$
NURSING IMPLICATIONS: Administer per order and observe for effect.			
Pentazocine (*Talwin*)—PO 50–100 mg; IM 30–60 mg q3–4h	Relief of moderate to severe pain	Narcotic antagonist, opioid antagonist properties, equivalent to codeine	Respiratory depression, nausea, vomiting, dizziness, light-headedness, seizures
NURSING IMPLICATIONS: Monitor *respirations*, BP; *caution* with clients: with MI, head injuries, COPD.			
ANTACIDS (see **Antiulceratives**)			
ANTIANEMIC			
Ferrous SO$_4$ (*Feosol, Fer-in-Sol*)—adults, PO 300 mg –1.2 g qd	Iron deficiency anemia; prophylactically during infancy, childhood, pregnancy	Corrects nutritional iron deficiency anemia	Nausea, vomiting, anorexia, constipation, diarrhea, yellow-brown discoloration of eyes, teeth
NURSING IMPLICATIONS: To minimize GI distress, give *with* meals; do *not* give with antacids or tea; liquid form should be taken through straw to prevent *staining* of teeth; *causes dark-green/black stool.*			
ANTIANGINALS			
Atenolol (*Tenormin*)—PO 50–150 mg daily; IV 5 mg initially; wait 10 min, then another 5 mg	Hypertension, angina, arrhythmias	Blocks beta$_1$, (cardiac) adrenergic receptors	Fatigue, weakness, bradycardia, heart failure, pulmonary edema
NURSING IMPLICATIONS: Give 1 mg/min IV; check vital signs; assess for signs of fluid *overload*.			
Isosorbide dinitrate (*Isordil, Isorbid*)—sublingual 2.5–10.0 mg q5–10min for 3 doses; PO 5–20 mg initially, 10–40 mg q6h	Acute angina, *long-term* prophylaxis for angina, heart failure	Produces vasodilation, decreases preload	Headache, dizziness, hypotension, tachycardia
NURSING IMPLICATIONS: *Avoid* eating, drinking, or smoking until sublingual tablets are dissolved; change positions *slowly*; aspirin or acetaminophen for headache.			
Nitroglycerin—sublingual 0.25–0.6 prn; transdermal (patch) 2.5–15.0 mg/d; topical 1-2 in. q8h; IV 10–20 mcg/min	Angina pectoris; adjunctive treatment in MI, heart failure, hypertension (IV form)	Directly relaxes smooth muscle, dilating blood vessels; lowers peripheral vascular resistance; increases blood flow	Faintness, throbbing headache, vomiting, flushing, hypotension, visual disturbances
NURSING IMPLICATIONS: Instruct client to *sit* or *lie* down when taking drug, to reduce *hypotensive* effect; onset 1–3 min; may take 1–3 doses at 5–min intervals to relieve pain; up to *10/d* may be allowed; if headache occurs, tell client to expel tab as soon as pain relief occurs; keep drug at bedside or on person; watch *expiration* dates—tabs lose potency with exposure to air and humidity; *alcohol* ingestion soon after taking may produce *shocklike syndrome* from drop in BP; *smoking* causes vasoconstricting effect; causes burning under tongue; may crush between teeth to ↑ absorption.			

(continued)

TABLE D.3 COMMON DRUGS

Drug and Dosage	Use	Action	⏴ Assessment: Side Effects
ANTIARRHYTHMICS			
Bretylium (*Bretylol*)—IV 0.5–10 mg/kg q6h; continuous IV infusion at 1-2 mg/min	Ventricular fibrillation, ventricular tachycardia	Inhibits norepinephrine release from sympathetic nerve endings; increased fibrillation threshold	Worsening of arrhythmia; tachycardia and increased BP *initially*; nausea, vomiting, hypotension *later*
NURSING IMPLICATIONS: Monitor BP and cardiac status closely; *rotate* IM injection sites; no more than 5 mL/site.			
Lidocaine HC1—IV 50–100 mg. bolus; 1–4 mg/kg/ min, IV drip	Ventricular tachycardia; PVCs	Depresses myocardial response to abnormally generated impulses	Drowsiness, dizziness, nervousness, confusion, paresthesias
NURSING IMPLICATIONS: *Check apical and radial pulses* for deficits; observe for signs of *CNS* toxicity; monitor ECG for *prolonged* PR interval.			
Procainamide HC1 (*Pronestyl*)—PO, IM 500– 1000 mg 4–6 times qd; IV 100 mg q 5 min until arrhythmia is suppressed or 100 mg have been given	Atrial and ventricular arrhythmias; PVCs, *overdose* of digitalis; general anesthesia	Depresses myocardium, lengthens conduction time between atria and ventricles	Polyarthralgia, fever, chills, urticaria, nausea, vomiting, psychoses, rapid decrease in BP
NURSING IMPLICATIONS: Check pulse rate *before* giving; monitor heart action during IV administration.			
Propranolol HC1 (*Inderal*)— 0.5–3.0 mg, IV push (up to 3 mg); 20–60 mg orally 3–4 times daily	Ventricular ectopy, angina *unresponsive* to nitrites, paroxysmal atrial tachycardia, hypertension	Beta-adrenergic blocker, ↓ cardiac contractility, ↓ heart rate, ↓ myocardial oxygen requirements	Bradycardia, hypotension, vertigo, paresthesia of hands
NURSING IMPLICATIONS: Instruct client to take pulse *before* each dose; do **not** give to clients with history of asthma or chronic obstructive pulmonary disease (COPD); *no* smoking, as hypertension may occur.			
ANTIASTHMATIC			
Cromolyn sodium—inhale, 1 cap 4 times qd, or 2 sprays qid	Perennial bronchial asthma (*not* acute asthma or status asthmaticus)	Inhibits release of bronchonconstrictors— histamine and SRS-A; suppresses allergic response	Cough, hoarseness, wheezing, dry mouth, bitter aftertaste, urticaria, urinary frequency
NURSING IMPLICATIONS: Instruct on *use of inhaler*—exhale; tilt head back; inhale rapidly, deeply, steadily; remove inhaler; exhale—repeat until dose is taken; gargle or drink water after treatment.			
ANTICHOLINERGICS			
Atropine SO_4—0.3–1.2 mg PO, SC, IM, or IV; ophthalmic 0.5%–1.0% up to 6 times qd	Peptic ulcer, spasms of GI tract, Stokes-Adams syndrome; control excessive secretions during surgery, bradyarrhythmias	Blocks parasympathomimetic effects of acetylcholine on effector organs	Dry mouth; tachycardia, blurred vision, drowsiness; skin flushing; urinary retention; *contraindications*: glaucoma, paralytic ileus
NURSING IMPLICATIONS: Observe for postural *hypotension* when ambulating clients; administer cautiously in elderly; monitor vital signs for *pulse* and *respiratory* rate changes.			
Propantheline bromide (*Pro-Banthine*)—PO 15 mg qid; IM or IV 30 mg	Decreases hypertonicity and hypersecretion of GI tract, ulcerative colitis, peptic ulcer	Blocks neural transmission at ganglia of autonomic nervous system and at parasympathetic effector organs	Nausea, gastric fullness, constipation, mydriasis
NURSING IMPLICATIONS: Give *before* meals; observe urinary output to *avoid retention*, particularly in elderly; mouth care pc will relieve dryness; **contraindicated** with glaucoma.			

(*continued*)

TABLE D.3 COMMON DRUGS

Drug and Dosage	Use	Action	⋈ Assessment: Side Effects
ANTICHOLINERGICS (*continued*)			
Tincture of belladonna—0.3–0.6 mL tid	Hypermotility of stomach; bowel, biliary, and renal colic; prostatitis	Blocks parasympathomimetic effects of acetylcholine	Dry mouth, thirst, dilated pupils, skin flushing, elevated temperature, delirium

NURSING IMPLICATIONS: Administer 30–60 min *before* meals; observe for side effects; *physostigmine salicylate* is antidote.

ANTICOAGULANTS			
Enoxaparin (*Lovenox*)—SC 30 mg qd-bid for 7-10 d	Prevents deep vein thrombosis and pulmonary embolus in clients with hip or knee replacements, or abdominal surgery	Prevents conversion of fibrinogen to fibrin and prothrombin to thrombin	Hypochromic anemia, thrombocytopenia, cardiac toxicity, hematuria, bleeding gums, black tarry stools

NURSING IMPLICATIONS: Use electric razor; pressure on injections and venipuncture sites, monitor ⋙ CBC and clotting times; antagonist is *protamine sulfure*.

Heparin—initial dose: IV 5,000 U followed by 20,000–40,000 U infusion over 24h	Acute thromboembolic *emergencies*	Prevents thrombin formation	Hematuria, bleeding gums, ecchymosis

NURSING IMPLICATIONS: Observe clotting times—should be 20–30 min; antagonist is *protamine sulfate*.

Warfarin sodium (*Coumadin*)—initial dose, PO 10–15 mg; maintenance dose, PO 2–10 mg qd	Venous thrombosis, atrial fibrillation with embolization, pulmonary emboli, myocardial infarction	Depresses liver synthesis of prothrombin and factors VII, IX, X	Minor or major hemorrhage, alopecia, fever, nausea, diarrhea, dermatitis

NURSING IMPLICATIONS: Drug effects last 3–4 d; antagonist is *vitamin K;* 🍎 *avoid* foods high in vitamin K; *no* aspirin.

ANTICOAGULANT ANTIDOTES			
Protamine SO₄ 1%—IV 10 mg/mL *slowly*; 1 mg/100 U heparin	*Overdose* of heparin	Positive electrostatic charge inactivates negatively charged heparin molecules	Excessive coagulation, hypotension, bradycardia, dyspnea

NURSING IMPLICATIONS: *Slow* IV; no more than 50 mg in 10–min period; monitor vital signs continuously; Check ⋙ activated partial thromboplastin time for effectiveness.

Vitamin K₁ (*AquaMEPHYTON, Konakion*)—PO, IM, SC 2.5–25.0 mg; 0.5–1.0 mg in newborns	Warfarin hypoprothrombinemia, hemorrhagic disease in newborns	Counteracts the inhibitory effects of oral anticoagulants on hepatic synthesis of vitamin K–dependent clotting factors	Flushing, hypotension, allergic reactions, reappearance of clotting problems (high doses)

NURSING IMPLICATIONS: Give IV only *if absolutely necessary* at a rate *not* to sxceed 1 mg/min; *dilute* with preservative-free 0.9% NaCl, D₅W, or D₅NaC1; protect solution *from ligh*t; repeated injection may cause redness and pain; check ⋙ PT for drug effect

ANTICONVULSANTS			
Clonazepam (*Klonopin*)—PO 1.5 mg in 3 doses initially, increase by 0.5–1.0 mg q third day	Absence (petit mal) seizures, myoclonic seizures	Produces anticonvulsant and sedative effects in the CNS; mechanism unknown	Drowsiness, ataxia, behavioral changes

NURSING IMPLICATIONS: Give *with* food; evaluate ⋙ liver, CBC, and *platelets; Avoid* abrupt withdrawal–may cause *status epilepticus*

(continued)

TABLE D.3   COMMON DRUGS

Drug and Dosage	Use	Action	►◄ Assessment: Side Effects
ANTICONVULSANTS *(continued)*			
Diazepam (*Valium*)—PO 2–10 mg bid–qid; IM or IV 5–10 mg	All types of seizures	Induces calming effect on limbic system, thalamus, hypothalamus	Drowsiness, ataxia, and paradoxical increase in excitability of CNS
NURSING IMPLICATIONS: IV may cause *phlebitis*; give IV injection *slowly*, as respiratory arrest can occur; inject IM *deeply* into tissue			
Ethosuximide (*Zarontin*)—PO 500 mg/d, increase by 250 mg/d until effective	Absence seizures	Depresses motor cortex and reduces CNS sensitivity to convulsive nerve stimuli	GI distress: nausea, vomiting, cramps, diarrhea, anorexia; blood dyscrasias
NURSING IMPLICATIONS: Administer *with* meals; ⌇⌇⌇ regular *CBC*; precautions to prevent injury from drowsiness.			
Magnesium SO_4—PO 1–5 g; IM or IV 4-5 g followed by 1-2 g/hr continuous infusioin	Control seizures in pregnancy, epilepsy; relief of acute constipation; reduces edema, inflammation, and itching of skin; may inhibit preterm contractions	Depresses CNS as well as smooth, cardiac, and skeletal muscle; promotes osmotic retention of fluid	Flushing, sweating, extreme thirst, complete heart block, dehydration, depressed or absent reflexes, ↓ respirations
NURSING IMPLICATIONS: If given IV, monitor vital signs *continuously*; I&O; do *not* give during the 2 h preceding delivery; observe mother and newborn for signs of toxicity if given near delivery.			
Phenytoin (*Dilantin*)—PO loading dose 1g or 20 mg/kg in 3-4 divided doses, the 300-400 mg qd; IV 15-20 mg/kg, *rate not to exceed 50 mg/min*, followed by 100 mg q 6h	Treatment and prevention of tonic-clonic (grand mal) seizures and complex partial seizures; ventricular arrhythmia (old use)	Depresses motor cortex by prventing spread of abnormal electrical impulses	Nervousness, ataxia, hypotension, gastric distress, nystagmus, slurred speech, hallucinations, gingival hyperplasia, agranulocytosis, aplastic anemia, Stevens-Johnson Syndrome
NURSING IMPLICATIONS: Gice *with* meals *or* pc; frequent and diligent mouth care; advise client that urine may turn *pink to red-brown*; teach client signs of adverse reactions; mix IV with normal saline (precipitaties with 5% D/W). IM route should be used as a *last resort*.			
Primidone (*Mysoline*)—PO 100–375 mg, increase over 10 d	Tonic-clonic, focal, or local seizures	Inhibits abnormal brain electrical activity, dose-dependent CNS depression	Excessive sedation or ataxia, vertigo
NURSING IMPLICATIONS: Careful neurologic, cardiovascular, and respiratory assessment; have resuscitation equipment available.			
Valproic acid (*Depakene*)—PO 15 mg/kg/d, increase up to 60 mg/kg/d	Absence, tonic-clonic, myoclonic, focal, or local seizures	Inhibits spread of abnormal charges through brain	Nausea, vomiting, diarrhea (disappear over time); drowsiness or sedation if taken with other anticonvulsants
NURSING IMPLICATIONS: Assess responses; monitor ⌇⌇⌇ *blood levels*; precautions against excessive sedation; *discourage* alcohol use.			

(continued)

TABLE D.3 COMMON DRUGS

Drug and Dosage	Use	Action	▶◀ Assessment: Side Effects
ANTIDIARRHEALS			
Diphenoxylate HC1 with atropine sulfate (*Lomotil*)—PO 50–10 mg tid–qid	Diarrhea	Increases intestinal tone and decreases propulsive peristalsis	Rash, drowsiness dizziness, depression, abdominal distention, headache, blurred vision, nausea

NURSING IMPLICATIONS: May *potentiate* action of barbiturates, opiates, and other depressants; closely observe clients receiving these drugs, and administer *narcotic antagonists* such as levallorphan (*Lorfan*) tartrate, naloxone HC1 (*Narcan*) and nalorphine HC1 (*Nalline*) as ordered; administer cautiously to clients with hepatic dysfunction—may precipitate *hepatic coma.*

Kaolin with pectin, (*Kaopectate*)—adults, PO 60–120 mL after each bowel movement	Diarrhea	Reported to absorb irritants and soothe	Granuloma of the stomach

NURSING IMPLICATIONS: Do *not* administer: for more than *2 d*; in presence of *fever*; or to children *younger than 3 yr.*

Paregoric or camphorated opium tincture–5–10 mL q2h, *not* more than qid	Diarrhea	Acts directly on intestinal smooth muscle to increase tone and decrease propulsive peristalsis	Occasional nausea; prolonged use may produce dependence

NURSING IMPLICATIONS: Contains approximately 1.6 mg morphine or 16 mg opium and is subject to federal narcotic regulations; administer with partial glass of *water* to facilitate passage into stomach; observe number and consistency of stools—discontinue drug as soon as diarrhea is controlled; keep in tight *light-resistant* bottles.

Drug and Dosage	Use	Action	Assessment: Side Effects
ANTIEMETICS			
Chlorpromazine (*Thorazine*)—preop IM 12.5–25.0 g 1–2 h before; IV 25–50 mg; PO 10–25 mg q4–6h; IM 25–50 mg q3–4h; suppository 50–100 mg q6–8h	Nausea, vomiting, hiccups, preoperative sedation, psychoses	Alters the effects of dopamine in the CNS; anticholinergic; alpha-adrenergic blocker	Sedation, extrapyramidal reactions, dry eyes, blurred vision, hypotension, constipation, dry mouth, photosensitivity

NURSING IMPLICATIONS: Keep *flat* 30 min after IM injection; change positions slowly; frequent mouth care; may turn urine *pink* to *red-brown.*

Prochlorperazine dimaleate (*Compazine*)—5–30 mg qid PO, IM, rectal	Nausea, vomiting, retching	See Trimethobenzamide HC1	Drowsiness, orthostatic hypotension, palpitations, blurred vision, diplopia, headache

NURSING IMPLICATIONS: Use *cautiously* in: children, women who are pregnant, and clients with liver disease.

Trimethobenzamide HC1 (*Tigan*)—250 mg qid, PO, IM rectal	Nausea, vomiting	Suppresses chemoreceptors in the trigger zone located in the medulla oblongata	Drowsiness, vertigo, diarrhea, headache, hypotension, jaundice, blurred vision, rigid muscles

NURSING IMPLICATIONS: Give *deep IM* to prevent escape of solution; can cause edema, pain, and burning.

ANTIFUNGALS			
Amphotericin B (*Fungizone*)—IV 5 mg/250 mL dextrose over 4–6h (to 1 mg/kg body weight)	*Severe* fungal infections, histoplasmosis	Fungistatic or fungicidal; binds to sterols in cell membrane, altering cell permeability	Febrile reactions: chills, nausea and vomiting, muscle/joint pain, renal damage; hypotension; tachycardia; arrhythmias, hypokalemia

NURSING IMPLICATIONS: Monitor for side effects; *thrombophlebitis* at IV site; ▟▙▙ BUN > 40 mg/dL; creatinine 3 mg/dL or >; stop drug because of *nephrotoxicity*

(continued)

TABLE D.3 COMMON DRUGS

Drug and Dosage	Use	Action	▶◀ Assessment: Side Effects
ANTIFUNGALS *(continued)*			
Ketoconazole (*Nizoral*)—oral 200–400 mg daily	Histoplasmosis, *systemic* fungal infections	Antifungal	Headache, fatigue, dizziness; nausea and vomiting; decreased libido, impotence; gynecomastia, esp. in men

NURSING IMPLICATIONS: Administer *with* food; *avoid* concomitant use of antacids, H_2 blockers; advise to report side effects.

Drug and Dosage	Use	Action	Assessment: Side Effects
Nystatin (*Nilstat, Mycostatin*)—PO, rectal, vaginal 100,000–1,000,000 U 3–4 times qd	Skin, mucous membrane infections (*Candida albicans*); oral thrush; vaginitis, intestinal candidiasis	Fungistatic and fungicidal; binds to sterols in fungal cell membrane	Nausea, vomiting, GI distress, diarrhea

NURSING IMPLICATIONS: *Oral* use—clear mouth of food; keep medication in mouth several minutes before swallowing; *vaginal*—usually requires 2-wk therapy; continue use during menses; consult physician before using anti-infective douches; determine predisposing factors to infection (diabetes, pregnancy, anti-infectives, tight-fitting nylon pantyhose).

Drug and Dosage	Use	Action	Assessment: Side Effects
ANTIGOUTS			
Allopurinol (*Lopurin, Zyloprim*)—PO 100 mg initially; 300 mg daily with meals or pc	Primary hyperuricemia, secondary hyperuricemia with cancer therapy	Lowers plasma and urinary uric acid levels; *no* analgesic, anti-inflammatory, or uricosuric actions	Rash, itching, nausea, vomiting, anemia, drowsiness

NURSING IMPLICATIONS: Report side effects, particularly *rash*, as drug must be stopped; *avoid* driving or other complex tasks until drug effects known; give at least *3000 mL* fluid daily; minimum urine output of *2000 mL/d*; keep urine neutral or *alkaline* with sodium bicarbonate or potassium citrate; use *cautiously* with: liver disease, impaired renal function, history of peptic ulcers, lower GI disease, or bone marrow depression.

Drug and Dosage	Use	Action	Assessment: Side Effects
Colchicine—PO 1.0–1.2 mg acute phase; 0.5–2.0 mg nightly with milk or food; IV 1–2 mg initially	Gouty arthritis, acute gout	Inhibits leukocyte migration and phagocytosis in gouty joints; nonanalgesic, nonuricosuric	Nausea, vomiting, diarrhea, abdominal pain, peripheral neuritis, bone marrow depression (sore throat, bleeding gums, sore mouth), tissue and nerve necrosis with IV use

NURSING IMPLICATIONS: Do *not* dilute IV form with normal saline or 5% dextrose—use *sterile water* to prevent precipitation; infuse over *3–5 min* IV; potentiate drug action with 🍎 *alkaline ash foods* (milk, most fruits and vegetables).

Drug and Dosage	Use	Action	Assessment: Side Effects
Probenecid (*Benemid*)—PO 0.25–0.50 g twice daily pc	*Chronic* gouty arthritis; *no* value in acute; adjuvant therapy with penicillin to increase plasma levels	Inhibits renal tubular resorption of uric acid; *no* analgesic or anti-inflammatory activity; competitively inhibits renal tubular secretion of penicillin and many weak organic acids	Headache, nausea, vomiting, anorexia, sore gums, urinary frequency, flushing

NURSING IMPLICATIONS: Give *with* food, milk, or prescribed antacid; *3000 mL/d* fluids; *avoid* alcohol, which increases serum urates; do *not* take with aspirin—inhibits action of drug; 〰 renal function and *hematology* should be evaluated frequently; during acute gout, give with colchicine.

(continued)

TABLE D.3 COMMON DRUGS

Drug and Dosage	Use	Action	▶◀ Assessment: Side Effects
ANTIHISTAMINES			
Chlorpheniramine maleate (*Chlor-Trimeton*)—PO 2–4 mg tid–qid; SC, IM, or IV 5-40 mg	Asthma, hay fever, serum reactions, anaphylaxis	Inhibits action of histamine	Nausea, gastritis, diarrhea, headache, dryness of mouth and nose, nervousness, irritability
NURSING IMPLICATIONS: IV may *drop BP*; give *slowly*; *caution* client about drowsiness.			
Diphenhydramine HC1 (*Benadryl*)—PO 25–50 mg tid–qid; IM or IV 10–20 mg	Allergic and pyrogenic reactions, motion sickness, radiation sickness, hay fever, Parkinson's disease	Inhibits the action of histamine on receptor cells; decreases action of acetylcholine	Sedation: dizziness, inability to concentrate, headache, anorexia, dermatitis, nausea, diplopia, insomnia
NURSING IMPLICATIONS: *Avoid* use in newborn or premature infants and clients with glaucoma; supervise ambulation; *caution* against driving or operating mechanical devices; excitation or hallucinations may occur in children.			
Fexofenadine (*Allegra*)—PO 60 mg bid	Rhinitis, allergy symptoms, chronic idiopathic urticaria	Competes with H_1-receptor site; blocks effects of histamine	Hemolytic anemia, thrombocytopenia, leukopenia, agranulocytosis, pancytopenia, dysrhythmias
NURSING IMPLICATIONS: Assess for urinary retention; provide hard candy, gum, frequent mouth rinses for dry mouth. ⩗ Monitor cell blood count			
ANTIHYPERGLYCEMICS			
Sulfonylureas			
Acetohexamide (*Dymelor*)— PO 200–1500 mg qd; 1–2/d; duration 12–24 h	*Oral* hypoglycemic, anti-diabetic	Lowers blood glucose by stimulating insulin release from beta cells; effective only if pancreas has ability to produce insulin	Hypoglycemia (profuse sweating, hunger, headache, nausea, confusion, ataxia, coma), skin rashes, bone marrow depression, liver toxicity
NURSING IMPLICATIONS: Drug therapy *must* be combined with *diet* therapy, *weight* control, and planned, graded *exercise*; *alcohol intolerance* may occur (*disulfiram reaction*—flushing, pounding headache, sweating, nausea, vomiting); should *not* be taken at bedtime unless specifically ordered (nocturnal hypoglycemia more likely); take at *same time* each day; **contraindicated** in: liver disease, renal disease, pregnancy.			
Chlorpropamide (*Diabinese*)—PO 100–1,000 mg; 1/d; duration 30–60 h	See Acetohexamide	See Acetohexamide	See Acetohexamide
NURSING IMPLICATIONS: See Acetohexamide.			
Tolazamide (*Tolinase*)—PO 100–500 mg; 1/d; duration 10-14 h	See Acetohexamide	See Acetohexamide	See Acetohexamide
NURSING IMPLICATIONS: See Acetohexamide.			
Tolbutamide (*Orinase*)—PO 500-3000 mg; 2-3 d; duration 6-12 h	See Acetohexamide	See Acetohexamide	See Acetohexamide
NURSING IMPLICATIONS: See Acetohexamide.			

(continued)

TABLE D.3 COMMON DRUGS

Drug and Dosage	Use	Action	▶ Assessment: Side Effects
ANTIHYPERGLYCEMICS (*continued*)			
Acarbose (*Precose*)—PO 25 mg tid initially, increasing to a max of 100mg tid	Control blood sugar in non-insulin-dependent diabetes mellitus (NIDDM)	Delays absorption of glucose form GI tract	Gas, abdominal pain, diarrhea

NURSING IMPLICATIONS: Most effective when taken with the *first bite* of the main meal. Tends not to cause hypoglycemia when used alone. When used in combination with other oral antihyperglycemices, hypoglycemia may occur.

Glipizide (*Glucotrol*)—PO 5 mg/day, increase as needed up to 40 mg/day	Control blood sugar in non-insulin-dependent diabetes mellitus (NIDDM)	Stimulates release of insulin from pancreatic islets; decreases glycogenolysis and gluconeogenesis; enhances cellular sensitivity to insulin	Weight gain, hypoglycemia

NURSING IMPLICATIONS: Administer 30 minutes *before* a meal. Observe for/teach client signs and symptoms of hypoglycemia, monitor ⌇⌇⌇ blood glucose.

Glyburide (*Micronase, DiaBeta*)—PO 2.5-5 mg daily, increase up to 20 mg/day	Control blood sugar in non-insulin-dependent diabetes mellitus (NIDDM)	See Glipizide	Weight gain, hypoglycemia

NURSING IMPLICATIONS: Administer 30 minutes *before* a meal. Observe for/teach client signs and symptoms of hypoglycemia, monitor ⌇⌇⌇ blood glucose.

Metformin (*Glucophage*)—PO 500 mg bid, increase by 500 mg weekly up to 2000 mg/day	Control blood sugar in non-insulin-dependent diabetes mellitus (NIDDM)	Decreases hepatic glucose production; increases sensitivity to insulin; decreases intestinal absorption of glucose	Diarrhea, lactic acidosis

NURSING IMPLICATIONS: Clients who develop illness or laboratory abnormalities should be assessed for *ketoacidosis* or *lactic acidosis.* Assess ⌇⌇⌇ *renal* function before starting therapy. May be used in combination with sulfonylureas.

Rosiglitazone (*Avandia*)—PO 4 mg daily, may increase to 8 mg daily	Control blood sugar in non-insulin-dependent diabetes mellitus (NIDDM)	Increased glucose uptake in muscle; decreases endogenous glucose production	Weight gain, edema

NURSING IMPLICATIONS: Monitor ⌇⌇⌇ *liver* function before initiating therapy and periodically throughout. May be used together with other oral antihyperglycemics. Because *Avandia* may cause edema, it should *not* be given to clients with *heart failure*.

INSULINS			
Insulin—rapid acting			
Regular (*Humulin R*) (clear)– onset 0.5–1.0 h; peak 2–4 h; duration 6–8 h	*Poorly controlled* diabetes, trauma, surgery, coma	Enhances transmembrane passage of glucose into cells; promotes carbohydrates, fat and protein metabolism	Hypoglycemia (profuse sweating, nausea, hunger, headache, confusion, ataxia, coma), allergic reaction at injection site

NURSING IMPLICATIONS: ⌇⌇⌇ Monitor blood and urine for *glucose* and *acetone* levels; insulin currently being used can be kept at *room temperature for 1 mo*;refrigerate stock insulin only; *rotate* injection sites; cold insulin leads to: *lipodystrophy*, reduced absorption, and local reaction; *only* form of insulin that is given IV.

Prompt insulin zinc suspension (Semilente) purified pork (cloudy)— onset 1–2 h; peak 4–10 h; duration 12–16 h	Clients *allergic* to Regular; used in combination with longer-lasting insulin	Regular Insulin	Regular Insulin

NURSING IMPLICATIONS: See Regular Insulin; compatible with all Lente preparations

(*continued*)

TABLE D.3 COMMON DRUGS

Drug and Dosage	Use	Action	◄ Assessment: Side Effects
INSULINS (*continued*)			
Insulin—intermediate acting NPH insulin (isophane insulin suspension) purified pork (*Humulin* N⁺) (cloudy)— onset 1–2 h; peak 5–12 h; duration 18–24 h	Clients who can be controlled by *one dose* per day	See Regular Insulin	See Regular Insulin
NURSING IMPLICATIONS: Gently rotate vial between palms, invert several times to mix; do *not* shake; see Regular Insulin.			
Insulin zinc suspension (**Lente** insulin) (cloudy)— onset 1–3 h; peak 6–12 h; duration 18–24 h	Clients *allergic* to NPH	See Regular Insulin	See Regular Insulin
NURSING IMPLICATIONS: See Regular Insulin.			
Insulin—slow acting PZI (*Protamine zinc* insulin suspension) (cloudy)— onset 4–8 h; peak 14–24 h; duration 24–36 h	*Rarely* used, only if uncontrolled by other types	See Regular Insulin	See Regular Insulin
NURSING IMPLICATIONS: Between-meal snacks may be necessary; *bedtime snacks* are essential; see Regular Insulin.			
Extended insulin zinc suspension (Ultralente) purified beef (cloudy)— onset 4–8 h; peak 12–24 h; duration 36 h	Often *mixed* with **Semilente** for 24–h curve	See Regular Insulin	See Regular Insulin
NURSING IMPLICATIONS: See Regular Insulin			
ANTIHYPERTENSIVES			
Captopril (*Capoten*)—PO 50 mg tid	Hypertension, heart failure	Prevents production of angiotensin II, vasodilation	Hypotension, loss of taste perception, proteinuria, rashes
NURSING IMPLICATIONS: Monitor vital signs and weight; take 1 h *before* and 2 h *after* meals; change positions slowly; *avoid* salt and salt substitutes.			
Guanfacine HC1 (*Tenex*)—PO 1 mg daily to maximum dose of 3 mg/d	Hypertension, in combination with thiazidelike diuretics	Centrally acting alpha₂— adrenergic receptor agonist	Drowsiness, weakness, dizziness, dry mouth, constipation, impotence
NURSING IMPLICATIONS: Warn client *not* to drive or perform activities requiring alertness; take at *bedtime* to minimize sedation; monitor BP and pulse.			
Guanethidine SO₄ (*Ismelin*)—PO 10–50 mg qd in divided doses	Severe to moderately severe hypertension	Blocks norepinephrine at postganglionic synapses	Orthostatic hypotension, diarrhea, inhibition of ejaculation
NURSING IMPLICATIONS: *Postural hypotension* is marked in the morning and *accentuated* by hot weather, alcohol, and exercise; teach to rise slowly, with assistance.			
Hydralazine HC1 (*Apresoline*)—PO 10–50 mg qid	Moderate hypertension	Dilates peripheral blood vessels, increases renal blood flow	Palpitations, tachycardia, angina pectoris, tremors, depression
NURSING IMPLICATIONS: Encourage moderation in exercise and identification of stressful stimuli.			

(continued)

TABLE D.3 COMMON DRUGS

Drug and Dosage	Use	Action	▶️ Assessment: Side Effects
ANTIHYPERTENSIVES (*continued*)			
Methyldopa (*Aldomet*)—PO 500 mg–2 g in divided doses	Severe to moderately severe hypertension	Inhibits formation of dopamine, a precursor of norepinephrine	Initial drowsiness, depression with feelings of unreality; edema, jaundice, dry mouth

NURSING IMPLICATIONS: Contraindicated in acute and chronic liver disease; encourage not to drive car if drowsy.

Phentolamine HC1 (*Regitine*)—IV, IM, or local 5–10 mg; diluted in minimum 10 mL normal saline	Prevents dermal necrosis; hypertensive crisis; diagnosis of pheochromocytoma	Blocks alpha-adrenergic receptors	Weakness, dizziness, orthostatic hypotension, nausea, vomiting, abdominal pain

NURSING IMPLICATIONS: When giving parenterally, client should be *supine*; monitor for overdose (precipitous *drop* in BP); do *not* give with epinephrine.

Timolol (*Timoptic*)—PO 20–40 mg/d; ophthalmic 1 gtt 1–2 times/d	Hypertension, migraine, glaucoma	Blocks stimulation of myocardial (beta$_1$), and pulmonary/vascular (beta$_2$) receptors	Fatigue, weakness, depression, insomnia, peripheral vasoconstriction, diarrhea, nausea, vomiting

NURSING IMPLICATIONS: Check vital signs and for evidence of heart failure; do *not* take if pulse <50 beats/min; *avoid*: over-the-counter cold remedies, coffee, tea, and cola.

ANTI-INFECTIVES			
Cefazolin (*Ancef, Kefzol*)—IM or IV 250 mg–1.5 g q6–12h	*Staphylococcus aureus, Escherichia coli, Klebsiella*, group A and B *Streptococcus; Pneumococcus*	Bactericidal	Allergic reaction, urticaria, rash, abnormal bleeding

NURSING IMPLICATIONS: See Penicillin; may cause, *false-positive* lab tests (Coombs', urine glucose); oral probenecid may be taken *concurrently* to prolong effects of drug.

Cephalexin (*Keflex*)—PO 1–4 g/d in 2–4 equally divided doses	Infections caused by gram-positive cocci; infections: respiratory, biliary, urinary, bone, septicemia, abdominal, surgical prophylaxis	Bactericidal effects on susceptible organisms; inhibition of bacterial cell wall synthesis	Nausea, vomiting, urticaria, toxic paranoid reactions, dizziness, increased alkaline phosphatase, nephrotoxicity, bone marrow suppression

NURSING IMPLICATIONS: Peak blood levels delayed when given with food; *report*: nausea, flushing, tachycardia, headache; monitor for 〰️ *nephrotoxicity* and for bleeding.

Cephalothin (*Keflin, Seffin*)—IM, IV 2–12 g/d in 4–6 equally divided doses	Same as Cephalexin except *not* recommended for biliary tract infections	Same as Cephalexin	Same as Cephalexin

NURSING IMPLICATIONS: Same as Cephalexin; *pain* at site of IM; given in *large* muscle; *rotate* sites.

Ciprofloxacin (*Cipro*)—PO 250–750 mg q12h; IV 200–400 mg q12h; ophthalmic 1–2 gtt q 15–30 min, then 4–6 times daily	Lower respiratory tract infections; skin, bone, joint infections; UTI	Inhibits bacterial DNA synthesis	Restlessness, nausea, diarrhea, vomiting, abdominal pain

NURSING IMPLICATIONS: Give PO on an *empty* stomach unless GI irritation occurs, then take with food; *do not* take with milk or yogurt; IV over 60 min.

(*continued*)

TABLE D.3 COMMON DRUGS

Drug and Dosage	Use	Action	▶◀ Assessment: Side Effects
ANTI-INFECTIVES (continued)			
Clarithromycin (*Biaxin*)—PO 250–500 mg q12h	Upper respiratory including streptococcal pharyngitis and sinusitis; lower respiratory tract bronchitis, pneumonia	Bacteriostatic; gram-positive and gram-negative bacteria. *Not* effective against MRSA.	Headache, diarrhea, nausea, abnormal taste, abdominal pain.
NURSING IMPLICATIONS: Give around the clock without regard for meals. Food slows but does *not* decrease absorption.			
Cloxacillin (*Tegopen*)—PO 250–500 mg q6h	Penicillinase-producing staphylococci infections: respiratory, sinus, skin	Binds to bacteria cell wall, leading to cell death	Nausea, vomiting, diarrhea, rashes, allergic reactions, seizures (high doses)
NURSING IMPLICATIONS: *Give around the clock* on an *empty* stomach; observe for signs of *superinfection* (black, furry tongue, vaginal itching, loose stools).			
Co-trimoxazole (*Bactrim, Septra*)—PO 160 mg twice daily or 20 mg/kg/d for *Pneumocystis carinii* pneumonia	Acute otitis media, urinary tract infection, shigellosis, *P. carinii* pneumonia, prostatitis	Bacteriostatic, anti-infective; antagonizes folic acid production; combination of sulfamethoxazole and trimethoprim	Hypersensitivity; see Sulfisoxazole
NURSING IMPLICATIONS: IV administration can cause phlebitis and *tissue damage* with extravasation			
Erythromycin—adults, PO 250 mg q6h; children, PO 30–50 mg/kg qd	Pneumonia; pelvic inflammatory disease, intestinal amebiasis; ocular infections; used *if allergic* to penicillin	Inhibits protein synthesis of microorganism; more effective against gram-positive organisms	Abdominal cramping, distention, diarrhea
NURSING IMPLICATIONS: Be sure culture and sensitivity done *before* treatment; give on *empty* stomach 1 h before or 3 h after meals; do *not* crush or chew tabs; do *not* give with fruit juice			
Gentamicin (*Garamycin*)—IM, IV 3–5 mg/kg/d in 3–4 divided doses; topical: skin, eye	Serious gram-negative bacillary infections; possible S. *aureus*, uncomplicated urinary tract infections	Bactericidal effects on susceptible gram-positive and gram-negative organisms and mycobacteria	Serious toxic effects; kidneys, ear; causes muscle weakness/paralysis
NURSING IMPLICATIONS: Monitor ⋙ *plasma* levels (peak is 4–10 mg/mL); clients with burns, cystic fibrosis may need higher doses.			
Penicillin–penicillin G, PO 125-500 mg q 6-8 hr; IM, IV 1-5 million units q 4-6 h	*Streptococcus; Staphylococcus; Neisseria gonorrhoeae, Treponema pallidum*	Primarily bactericidal	Dermatitis, delayed or immediate anaphylaxis
NURSING IMPLICATIONS: Clients in ambulatory care should be observed for *20 min after injection*; clients who are hospitalized should be observed at frequent intervals for 20 min after injection.			
Pentamidine (*Pentam*)—IV 4 mg/kg once daily; inhale 300 mg via nebulizer	Prevention or treatment of *P. carinii* pneumonia	Appears to disrupt DNA or RNA synthesis to protozoa	Anxiety, headache, bronchospasm, cough, hypotension, arrhythmias, nephrotoxicity, hypoglycemia, leukopenia, thrombocytopenia, anemia, chills
NURSING IMPLICATIONS: Assess ⋙ CBC for infection and respiratory status; unpleasant metallic taste may occur (not significant).			

(continued)

TABLE D.3 COMMON DRUGS

Drug and Dosage	Use	Action	▶◀ Assessment: Side Effects
ANTI-INFECTIVES (continued)			
Sulfisoxazole (*Gantrisin*), sulfamethizole (*Thiosulfil*), sulfisomidine (*Elkosin*)	Acute, chronic, and recurrent urinary tract infections	Bacteriostatic, bactericidal	Nausea, vomiting, oliguria, anuria, anemia, leukopenia, dizziness, jaundice, skin rashes, photosensitivity

NURSING IMPLICATIONS: ⌇⌇⌇ Maintenance of *blood levels* very important; encourage *fluids* to prevent crystal formation in kidney tubules–push up to *3000 mL/d.*

Tetracyclines— chlortetracycline (*Aureomycin*), doxycycline, (*Vibramycin* hyclate), oxytetracycline (*Terramycin*), and tetracycline HC1 (*Sumycin*)	Broad-spectrum antibiotic	Primarily bacteriostatic	GI upsets such as diarrhea, nausea, vomiting, sore throat; black, hairy tongue; glossitis; inflammatory lesions in anogenital region

NURSING IMPLICATIONS: *Phototoxic* reactions have been reported; clients should be advised to stay out of direct sunlight, and medication should *not* be given with milk or snacks, as food interferes with absorption of tetracyclines; do **not** give to women who are pregnant and children under 8 yr.

Trimethoprim (TMP)/ sulfamethoxazole (SMZ) (*Bactrim*)—PO 15–20 mg/ kg/d in 3–4 divided doses; IV 8–10 mg/kg TMP/40–50 mg/kg SMZ q6–12h	Bronchitis, *Shigella* enteritis, otitis media, *P. carinii* pneumonia, urinary tract infection, traveler's diarrhea	Combination inhibits the metabolism of folic acid in bacteria; bactericidal	Nausea, vomiting, rashes, phlebitis at IV site, aplastic anemia, hepatic necrosis

NURSING IMPLICATIONS: Check IV site frequently; do *not* give IM; give PO on *empty* stomach; take *around the clock*; *avoid* exposure to sun.

ANTILIPEMICS			
Cholestyramine (*Questran*)— PO 4 g 1–2 times/d	Hypercholesterolemia, pruritus from increased bile	Binds bile acids in GI tract; increased clearance of cholesterol	Nausea, constipation, abdominal discomfort

NURSING IMPLICATIONS: Take *before* meals; *do not* take with other medications; give others 1 h before or 4–6 h after.

Gemfibrozil (*Lopid*)—PO 1200 mg/d	Hypercholesterolemia	May inhibit peripheral lipolysis and reduce triglyceride synthesis in liver	GI upset: abdominal pain, epigastric pain, diarrhea, nausea, vomiting; rash; headache; dizziness; blurred vision

NURSING IMPLICATIONS: Use *caution* when driving or doing tasks requiring alertness; take *before* meals.

Lovastatin (*Mevacor*)—PO 20–80 mg/d with evening meal	Primary hypercholesterolemia	Inhibits enzyme that catalyzes synthesis of cholesterol; decreases synthesis of low-density lipoproteins (LDLs)	Headache, constipation, diarrhea, altered taste, blurred vision, muscle cramps

NURSING IMPLICATIONS: Give *with* food; *restrict* fat, cholesterol, carbohydrate, and alcohol in diet.

Niacin (vitamin B_3, nicotinic acid)—PO 1.5–6.0 g	Hypercholesterolemia	Decreases liver's production of LDLs and synthesis of triglycerides	GI upset, flushing, pruritus, hyperuricemia, hyperglycemia

NURSING IMPLICATIONS: Take the drug *with* meals; prevent flushing by taking an *aspirin 30 min* before; monitor closely during *first year* of therapy.

(continued)

TABLE D.3 COMMON DRUGS

Drug and Dosage	Use	Action	▶ Assessment: Side Effects
ANTIPLATELET			
Dipyridamole (*Persantine*)— PO 70–100 mg 4 times/d; IV 570 mg/kg	Prevent thromboembolism; surgical graft patency; *diagnostic* agent in myocardial perfusion studies	Decrease platelet aggregation; coronary vasodilator	Headache, dizziness, hypotension, nausea; MI, arrhythmias with IV

NURSING IMPLICATIONS: Take at *evenly* spaced intervals; *avoid* use of alcohol; if no GI irritation, take 1 h *before* or 2 h *after* meals

ANTITUBERCULOSIS			
First-line drugs			
Isoniazid—5–10 mg/kg up to 900 mg PO or IM 2-3 times weekly; or 300 mg/day	Tuberculosis	Suppresses or interferes with biosynthesis; bacteriostatic	Peripheral neuritis, hepatitis, hypersensitivity

NURSING IMPLICATIONS: Give pyridoxine (vitamin B_6) 10 mg as *prophylaxis* for neuritis; 50–100 mg as treatment.

Ethambutol—15–25 mg/kg PO			Optic neuritis (*reversible* with discontinuation of drug; very rare at 15 mg/kg); skin rash

NURSING IMPLICATIONS: Use with caution with *renal* disease or when *eye testing* is not feasible; used in combination *with* other drug.

Rifampin—10–20 mg/kg up to 600 mg PO			Hepatitis, febrile reaction, purpura (rare)

NURSING IMPLICATIONS: *Orange* urine color; *negates* effect of birth control pills.

Streptomycin—15–20 mg/kg up to 1 g IM			*Eighth cranial* nerve damage, *nephrotoxicity*

NURSING IMPLICATIONS: Use with caution in *older* clients or those with **renal** disease.

Pyrazinamide—15–30 mg/kg up to 3 g PO			Hyperuricemia, hepatotoxicity

NURSING IMPLICATIONS: Combination with an aminoglycoside is bactericidal.

ANTIULCERATIVES			
Aluminum hydroxide gel (*Amphojel*)—PO 5–10 mL of concentrated suspension q 2–4h or 1 h pc	Gastric acidity, peptic ulcer; phosphatic urinary calculi; ↓ phosphorus level in chronic renal failure	Buffers HC1 in gastric juices without interfering with electrolyte balance	Constipation and fecal impaction

NURSING IMPLICATIONS: *Shake well* before administering; encourage *fluids* to prevent impaction and milk-alkali syndrome.

Calcium carbonate (*Titralac*)—PO 1–2 g taken with H_2O after meals and at bedtime	Peptic ulcer and chronic gastritis	Reduces hyperacidity	Constipation or laxative effect

NURSING IMPLICATIONS: See Aluminum hydroxide gel.

Cimetidine (*Tagamet*)—PO 300–600 mg q6h qid; IM, IV 300 mg q6h	Duodenal ulcers, gastroesophageal reflux disease (GERD), gastric hypersecretion, esophagitis	Inhibits action of histamine at H_2 receptor site, inhibits gastric secretion; neutralizes and absorbs excess acid	Confusion, dizziness; nausea, rash, diarrhea, constipation; hypermagnesemia

NURSING IMPLICATIONS: Give *with* meals or immediately *after*; *avoid* smoking. *Avoid* prolonged administration in clients with renal insufficiency.

(continued)

TABLE D.3 COMMON DRUGS

Drug and Dosage	Use	Action	⬤ Assessment: Side Effects
ANTIULCERATIVES (continued)			
Magnesium and aluminum hydroxide (*Maalox* suspension)—PO 5–30 mL pc and hs	Gastric hyperacidity, peptic ulcer, heartburn	Neutralizes and binds acids	Constipation, fecal impaction
NURSING IMPLICATIONS: Encourage fluid intake; **contraindicated** for clients who are debilitated or those with renal insufficiency.			
Omeprazole (*Prilosec*)—PO 20 mg qd for 4–8 wk (maximum 40 mg /d)	Gastroesophageal reflux (GERD), duodenal ulcers, gastric hyperacidity	Prevents transport of hydrogen ions into gastric lumen.	Abdominal pain, acid regurgitation; headache; dizziness, drowsiness
NURSING IMPLICATIONS: Give *before* meals, preferably in morning. Do *not*: crush, open, or chew capsules. May give with antacids.			
Ranitidine (*Zantac*)—PO 150 mg bid; IM 50 mg q6–8h; IV 50 mg q6–8h	Duodenal ulcer, gastric ulcer, GERD, gastric hypersecretion	Inhibits action of histamine at H_2 receptor site, inhibits gastric acid secretion	Headache, malaise, nausea, constipation, diarrhea
NURSING IMPLICATIONS: Food does *not* affect absorption; give 1 h *apart* from antacids; *smoking* interferes with action			
Sucralfate (*Carafate*)—PO 1 g qid	Prevention and treatment of duodenal cancer	Reacts with gastric acid to form a thick paste that adheres to the ulcer surface	Constipation
NURSING IMPLICATIONS: Give 1 h *before* meals and at *bedtime*; *do not* crush or chew tablets; take *antacids* 30 min before or 1 h after sucralfate; increase *fluids and* 🍎 *dietary* bulk.			
ANTIVIRALS			
Acyclovir (*Zovirax*)—PO 200 mg, 3–5 times/d; IV 5 mg/ kg q8h over 1 h; topical 6 times daily for 1 wk	Herpes simplex (1) (2)	Converts to an active cytotoxic metabolite that inhibits viral DNA replication	Headache, nausea and vomiting, diarrhea; increased serum BUN and creatinine
NURSING IMPLICATIONS: Measure I&O q8h; ensure adequate *hydration*; ⬤ monitor BUN and creatinine levels; assess for common side effects; apply topical with *finger cot* or rubber glove; refer for counseling.			
Zidovudine (*AZT, Retrovir*)— PO 200 mg tid	AIDS and related disorders	Inhibits replication of HIV	Blood disorders, especially anemia and granulocytopenia; headache; nausea; insomnia; myalgia
NURSING IMPLICATIONS: Monitor for signs of *opportunistic infection* and ⬤ blood disorders and other adverse drug effects; drug must be taken *around* the clock; regular *blood tests* (q2wk).			
BRONCHODILATORS			
Albuterol (*Ventolin*)—PO 2–6 mg 3–4 times/d; inhale q4–6h or 2 puffs 15 min before exercise	Bronchodilator	Results in accumulation of cyclic adenosine monophosphate at beta-adrenergic receptors	Nervousness, restlessness, tremor, hypertension, nausea
NURSING IMPLICATIONS: Give *with* meals; allow 1 min *between* inhalations; rinse mouth with water *after* inhalation.			
Aminophylline—PO 250 mg bid–qid; rectal 250–500 mg; IV 250–500 mg over 10–20 min	*Rapid* relief of bronchospasm; asthma; pulmonary edema	Relaxes smooth muscles and increases cardiac contractility; interferes with resorption of Na^+ and Cl^- in proximal tubules	Nausea, vomiting, cardiac arrhythmias, intestinal bleeding, insomnia, restlessness, rectal irritation from suppository
NURSING IMPLICATIONS: Give orally *with or after meals*; monitor *vital signs* for changes in BP and pulse; *weigh* daily; IM injections are painful.			

(continued)

TABLE D.3 COMMON DRUGS

Drug and Dosage	Use	Action	► Assessment: Side Effects
BRONCHODILATORS (*continued*)			
Ephedrine SO$_4$—PO, SC, or IM 25 mg tid–qid	Asthma; allergies; bradycardia, nasal decongestant	Relaxes hypertonic muscles in bronchioles and GI tract	Wakefulness, nervousness, dizziness, palpitations, hypertension
NURSING IMPLICATIONS: Monitor vital signs; *avoid* giving dose near bedtime; *check urine* output in older adults.			
Isoproterenol HC1 (*Isuprel*)—inhalation 1-2 puffs x 4-6 daily	Mild to moderately severe asthma attack, bronchitis, pulmonary emphysema	Relaxes hypertonic bronchioles	Nervousness, tachycardia, hypertension, insomnia
NURSING IMPLICATIONS: Monitor vital signs *before and after* treatment; teach client how to use nebulizer.			
Theophylline—PO 400 mg/d in divided doses; max. adult dose: 900 mg divided dose	Treatment/prevention of emphysema, asthma (broncho-constriction); chronic bronchitis	Bronchodilation	Restlessness, increased respiration/heart rate, palpitations, arrhythmias, nausea and vomiting, increased urine output → dehydration
NURSING IMPLICATIONS: Monitor theophylline levels: *10–20 mg/mL*; monitor signs of toxicity; take with 8 oz water or *with* meals to decrease GI symptoms.			
Terbutaline (*Brethine*)—PO 2.5–5.0 mg q6h (*not to* exceed 20 mg/24 h); SC 0.25 mg, repeat 15–30 min (*not to exceed 0.5 mg/h*); inhalation—2 puffs (0.2 mg each) q4–6h	Bronchospasm	See Isoproterenol HC1	See Isoproterenol HC1
NURSING IMPLICATIONS: See Isoproterenol HC1.			
CALCIUM CHANNEL BLOCKERS			
Diltiazem (*Cardizem*)–PO 30–120 mg 3–4 times/d; 5–15 mg/h	Angina, hypertension, atrial arrhythmias	Inhibits excitation-contraction; decreased SA, AV node conduction	Headache, fatigue, arrhythmias, edema, hypotension, constipation, rash
NURSING IMPLICATIONS: May take *with* meals; take pulse; do *not* give drug if pulse <50 beats/min; change positions *slowly*; may take nitroglycerin sublingually concurrently.			
Nicardipine (*Cardene*)—PO 20–40 mg tid; IV 0.5-2.2 mg/hr continuous infusion	Angina, hypertension	Inhibits excitation-contraction	Dizziness, light-headedness, headache, peripheral edema, flushing
NURSING IMPLICATIONS: Give on an *empty* stomach; chest pain may occur 30 min after dose (temporary, from *reflex tachycardia*).			
Nifedipine (*Procardia*)—PO 10–30 mg tid (*not to* exceed 180 mg/d); sublingual 10 mg repeated in 15 min	Angina, hypertension	Vasodilation	Dizziness, light-headedness, giddiness, headache, nervousness, nasal congestion, sore throat, dyspnea, cough, wheezing, nausea, flushing, warmth
NURSING IMPLICATIONS: May take *with* meals; make position changes *slowly*; angina may occur 30 min after dose (temporary).			

(continued)

TABLE D.3 COMMON DRUGS

Drug and Dosage	Use	Action	►◄ Assessment: Side Effects
CALCIUM CHANNEL BLOCKERS (*continued*)			
Verapamil HC1 (*Calan, Isoptin*)—PO 240–480 mg, 3–4 times/d; IV 75–150 mcg/kg over 2 min	Angina, supraventricular arrhythmias, essential hypertension	Inhibits calcium movement into smooth-muscle cells; lowers pressure by reducing cardiac contractility	Constipation; AV block; hepatotoxicity
NURSING IMPLICATIONS: Monitor vital signs and ECG for *bradycardia* and *arrhythmias*; observe for *jaundice, abdominal pain*; encourage *fluids* and 🍎 *bulk-forming* foods.			
CARDIAC GLYCOSIDES			
Digitoxin—digitalizing dose; PO 200 mcg twice/d; IM or IV 200–400 mg; maintenance dose: PO 50–300 mcg qd	Heart failure, atrial fibrillation and flutter, supraventricular tachycardia	Increases force of cardiac contractility, slows heart rate, decreases right atrial pressures, promotes diuresis	Arrhythmias; nausea, vomiting, anorexia, malaise, color vision (yellow or blue)
NURSING IMPLICATIONS: Hold medication if pulse rate less than *60* or over *120* beats/min; encourage 🍎 foods high in *potassium* (e.g., bananas, orange juice); observe for signs of electrolyte depletion, apathy, disorientation, and anorexia. Teach client to monitor own pulse.			
Digoxin (*Lanoxin*)— digitalizing dose: PO 10–15 mcg/kg; IM or IV 0.6–1 mg/kg; maintenance dose: PO 0.125-0.5 mg/day	See Digitoxin	See Digitoxin	See Digitoxin
NURSING IMPLICATIONS: See Digitoxin.			
CHEMOTHERAPY (see **Tables 24.1, p. 317; D.6, p. 417**)			
CHOLINERGIC DRUGS			
Bethanechol CI (*Urecholine*)— PO, 25-50 mg tid; SC 5 mg x 3-4 daily	Postoperative abdominal atony and distension; bladder atony with retention; postsurgical or postpartum urinary retention; myasthenia gravis	Increases GI and bladder tone; decreases sphincter tone	Belching, abdominal cramps, diarrhea, nausea, vomiting, incontinence, profuse sweating, salivation, and respiratory depression
NURSING IMPLICATIONS: Check *respirations*; have urinal or bedpan close at hand and answer calls quickly; atropine SO_4 is the *antidote* for cholinergic drugs.			
Edrophonium (*Tensilon*)—IV 2mg; IM 10 mg	*Diagnosis* of myasthenia gravis; reversal of neuromuscular blockers	Inhibits breakdown of acetylcholine; anticholinesterase, cholinergic	Excess secretions, bronchospasm, bradycardia, abdominal cramps, nausea, vomiting, diarrhea, excess salivation, sweating
NURSING IMPLICATIONS: Effects last up to 30 min; give IV *undiluted* with *TB* syringe.			
Neostigmine (*Prostigmin*)— PO 15 mg q3–4h up to 375 mg/day; SC, IM 0.5 mg	Myasthenia gravis, postoperative bladder distention, urinary retention, reversal of neuromuscular blockers	Inhibits breakdown of acetylcholine; cholinergic	Excess secretions, bronchospasm, bradycardia, abdominal cramps, vomiting, diarrhea, excess salivation, sweating
NURSING IMPLICATIONS: Take oral form *with* food or milk; with chewing difficulty, take 30 min before eating.			

(*continued*)

TABLE D.3 COMMON DRUGS

Drug and Dosage	Use	Action	►◄ Assessment: Side Effects
CHOLINERGIC MIOTICS			
Pilocarpine HCl—1–2 gtts 1–2% solution up to 6 times/d. Physostigmine salicylate (*Eserine*)—0.1 mL of 0.25–10.00% solution; *not* more than qid	Chronic open-angle and acute angle-closure glaucoma	Contraction of the sphincter muscle of iris, resulting in miosis	Brow ache, headache, ocular pain, blurring and dimness of vision, allergic conjunctivitis, nausea, vomiting and profuse sweating; bronchoconstriction in clients with bronchial asthma

NURSING IMPLICATIONS: Initially the medication may be irritating; teach proper *sterile* technique for instilling drops— *wipe excess* solution to prevent systemic symptoms; *discard cloudy* solutions.

Pyridostigmine (*Mestinon*)— PO 60-1500 mg/d; IM, IV 2 mg q2–3h; maintenance: 60–150 mg/d	Myasthenia gravis, reversal of neuromuscular blockers	Inhibits breakdown of acetyl-choline and prolongs its effects	See Neostigmine

NURSING IMPLICATIONS: See Neostigmine.

CNS STIMULANTS			
Amphetamine SO$_4$–PO 5–60 mg qd in divided doses	Mild depressive states; narcolepsy; postencephalitic parkinsonism; obesity control; minimal brain dysfunction in children (attention deficit disorder)	Raises BP, decreases sense of fatigue, elevates mood	Restlessness, dizziness, tremors, insomnia; increases libido; suicidal and homicidal tendencies; palpitations; angina pain

NURSING IMPLICATIONS: Give *before* 4 P.M. to avoid sleep disturbance; *dependence* on drug may develop; **contraindicated** with: MAO inhibitors, hyperthyroidism, and psychotic states.

Methylphenidate hydrochloride (*Ritalin*)— PO 0.3 mg/kg/d or adults 20–60 mg in divided doses	Childhood hyperactivity; narcolepsy; ADD (Attention Deficit Disorder) in children	Mild CNS and respiratory stimulation	Anorexia, dizziness, drowsiness, insomnia, nervousness, BP and pulse changes

NURSING IMPLICATIONS: To avoid insomnia take last dose *4–5 h before* bedtime; monitor vital signs; check *weight* 2–3 times weekly and report losses.

DECONGESTANT			
Phenylephrine (*Neo-Synephrine, Sinex*)—SC, IM 2–5 mg q10–15 min (*not* to exceed 5 mg); IV 40–60 mcg/min; nasal 2–3 gtts or 1–2 sprays q3–4h; ophthalmic 3 gtt/d	Shock, hypotension, decongestant, adjunct to spinal anesthesia, mydriatic	Constricts blood vessels by stimulating alpha adrenergic receptors	Dizziness, restlessness, dyspnea, tachycardia, arrhythmias; ophthalmologic–burning photophobia, tearing

NURSING IMPLICATIONS: Check for correct concentration; protect eyes from *light sensitivity*: blow nose *before* using; *rebound congestion* will occur with prolonged use.

DIURETICS			
Acetazolamide (*Diamox*)—PO 250–1000 mg/d; IV 250-500 mg	Glaucoma; heart failure; convulsive disorders	Weak diuretic; produces acidosis; self-limiting effect; increases bicarbonate excretion	Electrolyte depletion symptomatology—lassitude, apathy, decreased urinary output, and mental confusion

NURSING IMPLICATIONS: Weigh *daily*; I&O; assess edema; give *early* in day to allow sleep at night; observe for side effects; replace electrolytes as ordered.

(continued)

TABLE D.3 COMMON DRUGS

Drug and Dosage	Use	Action	◄ Assessment: Side Effects
DIURETICS (continued)			
Furosemide (*Lasix*)—PO IV, IM 40–80 mg qd in divided doses	Edema and associated heart failure; cirrhosis; renal disease; nephrotic syndrome; hypertension	Inhibits Na^+ and Cl^- reabsorption in the loop of Henle	Dermatitis, pruritus, paresthesia, blurring of vision, postural hypotension, nausea, vomiting, diarrhea, dehydration, electrolyte depletion, and hearing loss (usually reversible)

NURSING IMPLICATIONS: ⌇⌇⌇ Monitor electrolytes and assess for: weakness, lethargy, leg cramps, anorexia; *peak* action in 1–2 h; duration 6–8 h; do *not* give at bedtime; supplementary KCl indicated; may induce *digitalis toxicity*.

Hydrochlorothiazide (*Hydro-DIURIL* and *Esidrix* 25–100 mg tid)—PO Diuril 0.5–1.0 g qd	Edema; heart failure; Na^+ retention in steroid therapy; hypertension	Inhibits sodium chloride and water reabsorption in the distal ascending loop and the distal convoluted tubule of the kidneys	Hypokalemia, nausea, vomiting, diarrhea, dizziness, and paresthesias; may accentuate diabetes

NURSING IMPLICATIONS: Watch for *muscle weakness*; give well-diluted *potassium chloride* supplement; ⌇⌇⌇ *monitor* urine for changes in sugar and acetone.

Mannitol (*Osmitrol*)—IV 0.25-2 g/kg over 30-60 min	Cerebral edema	Hypertonic solution that kidney tubules cannot reabsorb, thereby causing obligatory water loss	↑ Extracellular fluid volume

NURSING IMPLICATIONS: Usually *Foley* catheter required; monitor *cardiac and respiratory* status

Spironolactone (*Aldactone*)—PO 25 mg bid–qid	Cirrhosis of liver; when other diuretics are ineffective	Inhibits effects of aldosterone in distal tubules of kidney	Headache, lethargy, diarrhea, ataxia, skin rash, gynecomastia

NURSING IMPLICATIONS: Potassium-sparing drug; do *not* give supplemental KC1; monitor for signs of electrolyte imbalance.

EMETIC			
Ipecac syrup—PO 15–30 mL for emesis, followed by 1–2 glasses H_2O (adults)	Emergency emetic for poison ingestion	NH_4 ions cause gastric irritation	Violent emesis, tachycardia, decreased BP, and dyspnea

NURSING IMPLICATIONS: Contraindicated in liver and renal disease; if given for emesis, follow dose with as much *water* as client will drink

ENZYMES			
Pancrelipase (*Viokase*)—adults, PO 325 mg–1 g qd, during meals; children, PO 300–600 mg tid	Chronic pancreatitis; cystic fibrosis; gastrectomy; pancreatectomy; sprue	Assists in digestion of starch, protein, and fats; decreases nitrogen and fat content in stool	Anorexia, nausea, vomiting, diarrhea, buccal/anal soreness (infants), sneezing, skin rashes, diabetes

NURSING IMPLICATIONS: May be taken *with* antacid or cimetidine; do *not* crush or chew tabs; *monitor* I&O, weight; be alert for signs of diabetes; children may use sprinkle.

EXPECTORANTS			
Guaifenesin (*Robitussin*)—PO 100–400 mg q4h	Respiratory congestion	Increases expectoration by causing irritation of gastric mucosa; reduces adhesiveness/surface tension of respiratory tract fluid	Low incidence of GI upset; drowsiness

NURSING IMPLICATIONS: Encourage to stop smoking; increase *fluid* intake; respiratory hygiene.

(continued)

TABLE D.3 COMMON DRUGS

Drug and Dosage	Use	Action	▶ Assessment: Side Effects
EXPECTORANTS (*continued*)			
Terpin hydrate—PO 5–10 mL q3–4h	Bronchitis; emphysema	Liquefies bronchial secretions	Nausea, vomiting, and gastric irritation
NURSING IMPLICATIONS: Give undiluted; *push* fluids.			
FIBRINOLYTIC AGENTS			
Alteplase, recombinant (*Activase, tPA*)—IV bolus 15 mg over 1–2 min; then 50 mg over 30 min; then 35 mg over 60 min; 100 mg over 90 min	Acute MI; under investigation for pulmonary emboli, deep vein thrombosis, and peripheral artery thrombosis	Promotes conversion of plasminogen to plasmin, which is fibrinolytic	Internal or local bleeding; urticaria; dysrhythmias related to reperfusion; hypotension, nausea, and vomiting
NURSING IMPLICATIONS: Assess for signs of *reperfusion* (relief of chest pain, no ST segment elevation); observe for *bleeding; avoid* IM injection; *do not* mix other meds in line.			
Streptokinase IV—1.5 million IU diluted to 45 mL infused over 60 min	Lysis of pulmonary or systemic emboli or thrombi; acute MI	Reacts with plasminogen, dissolves fibrin clots	Prolonged coagulation; allergic reactions; mild fever
NURSING IMPLICATIONS: Monitor for signs of excessive *bleeding*, particularly at injection sites; *avoid* nonessential handling of client.			
Urokinase—IV 4400 IU/kg over 10 min; 1.0–1.8 mL of 5000 IU/mL into catheter	Massive pulmonary emboli, coronary artery thrombi, occluded IV catheter	Directly activates plasminogen	Bleeding, anaphylaxis, rash
NURSING IMPLICATIONS: Vital signs; check *q 15 min* for bleeding during first h; *q 15–30 min for 8 h*; have *epinephrine* ready.			
FIBRINOLYTIC ANTIDOTE			
Aminocaproic acid (*Amicar*)—PO, IV 5 g loading dose; 1 g/h to 30 g in 24 h	Management of streptokinase or urokinase overdose	Inhibits plasminogen activator and antagonizes plasmin	Hypotension, bradycardia; cardiac arrhythmias
NURSING IMPLICATIONS: Give *slowly* IV to prevent side effects; *not* recommended for DIC.			
MUCOLYTIC AGENT			
Acetylcysteine (*Mucomyst*)—1–10 mL of 20% solution per nebulizer tid	Emphysema; pneumonia; tracheostomy care; atelectasis; cystic fibrosis	Lowers viscosity of respiratory secretions by opening disulfide linkages in mucus	Stomatitis, nausea, rhinorrhea, bronchospasm
NURSING IMPLICATIONS: Observe *respiratory rate*; maintain open airway with suctioning as necessary; observe clients with asthma carefully for *increased bronchospasm*; discontinue treatment **immediately** if this occurs; odor disagreeable initially.			
MUSCLE RELAXANTS			
Baclofen (*Lioresal*)—5 mg tid up to 10–20 mg 4/d maintenance dose	Relief of spasticity of multiple sclerosis, spinal cord injury	Centrally acting skeletal-muscle relaxant; depresses polysynaptic afferent reflex activity at spinal cord level	Pruritus, tinnitus; N/V, diarrhea or constipation; drowsiness
NURSING IMPLICATIONS: Administer *with* food if GI symptoms; monitor for safety when ambulating; do *not* discontinue abruptly.			
Dantrolene sodium (*Dantrium*)—25 mg/day to 25 mg bid–qid to 100 mg qid max	See Baclofen	See Baclofen	See Baclofen
NURSING IMPLICATIONS: See Baclofen.			

(*continued*)

TABLE D.3 COMMON DRUGS

Drug and Dosage	Use	Action	◄ Assessment: Side Effects
NARCOTIC ANTAGONIST			
Naloxone (*Narcan*) HC1—IV 0.1–0.2 mg repeated	Reverses respiratory depression due to narcotics	Reverses respiratory depression of morphine SO$_4$, meperidine HC1, and methadone HC1; does not itself cause respiratory depression, sedation, or analgesia	No known side effects

NURSING IMPLICATIONS: Note time, type of narcotic, dosage received; *not* useful with *CNS depression from other* drugs; respiratory depression *may return*; monitor closely.

SEDATIVES AND HYPNOTICS			
Chlordiazepoxide (*Librium*) HC1—PO 50–100 mg; IM or IV 50–100 mg	Psychoneuroses; preoperative apprehension; chronic alcoholism; anxiety	CNS depressant resulting in mild sedation; appetite stimulant; and anticonvulsant	Ataxia, fatigue, blurred vision, diplopia, lethargy, nightmares, and confusion

NURSING IMPLICATIONS: Ensure anxiety relief by allowing client to verbalize feelings; advise client to *avoid* driving and alcoholic beverages.

Chloral hydrate—PO 250 mg tid; hypnotic: PO 0.5–1.0 g; rectal supplement 0.3–0.9 g	Sedation for elderly; delirium tremens; pruritus; mania, barbiturate and alcohol withdrawal	Depresses sensorimotor areas of cerebral cortex	Nausea, vomiting, gastritis; pinpoint pupils; delirium; rash; decreased BP, pulse, respirations, and temperature; hepatic damage

NURSING IMPLICATIONS: *Caution*—should *not* be taken in combination with *alcohol*; dependency is possible.

Diazepam (*Valium*)—PO 2–10 mg tid–qid; IM or IV 2–10 mg q3–4h	Anxiety disorders; alcohol withdrawal; adjunctive therapy in seizure disorders; status epilepticus; tetanus; preoperative or preprocedural sedation (also see Midazolam)	Induces calming effect on limbic system, thalamus, and hypothalamus	CNS depression—sedation or ataxia (dose related); dry mouth; blurred vision; mydriasis; constipation; urinary retention

NURSING IMPLICATIONS: Do *not* mix with other drugs; IM injection painful; observe for *phlebitis*; monitor response; measures to ensure client safety (e.g., falls); high potential for *abuse*; **contraindicated** in acute angle-closure glaucoma and porphyria.

Flurazepam (*Dalmane*)—PO >15 yr, 30 mg hs; elderly or debilitated, 15 mg hs	Hypnotic, short-term management of insomnia	Fastest acting; see Diazepam	See Diazepam

NURSING IMPLICATIONS: See Diazepam.

Hydroxyzine pamoate (*Vistaril*)—PO 25–100 mg qid	See Chlordiazepoxide (*Librium*); antiemetic in postoperative conditions; adjunctive therapy	CNS relaxant with sedative effect on limbic system and thalamus	Drowsiness, headache, itching, dry mouth, and tremor

NURSING IMPLICATIONS: Give *deep IM only; potentiates* action of warfarin (*Coumadin*), narcotics, and barbiturate.

Lorazepam (*Ativan*)—PO 1–2 mg bid–tid (up to 10 mg); 2–4 mg hs; IM 4 mg *max*; IV 2 mg *max*	Anxiety disorders; insomnia; alternative to diazepam for status epilepticus; preanesthesia	See Diazepam	See Diazepam

NURSING IMPLICATIONS: See Diazepam.

(continued)

TABLE D.3 COMMON DRUGS

Drug and Dosage	Use	Action	▶◀ Assessment: Side Effects
SEDATIVES AND HYPNOTICS (*continued*)			
Meprobamate (*Equanil, Miltown*)—PO 400 mg tid–qid	Anxiety; stress, absence seizures	See Hydroxyzine pamoate (*Vistaril*)	Voracious appetite, dryness of mouth, and ataxia

NURSING IMPLICATIONS: Older clients prone to drowsiness and hypotension; observe for *jaundice*.

Midazolam (*Versed*)—IM 0.05–0.08 mg/kg; IV 1–1.5 mg/kg	Preanesthesia; prediagnostic procedures; induction of general anesthesia	Penetrates blood-brain barrier to produce sedation and amnesia	Respiratory depression; apnea; disorientation and behavioral excitement

NURSING IMPLICATIONS: Monitor ventilatory status and oxygenation; prevent injuries from CNS depression; nonirritating to vein.

Phenobarbital Na—sedative, PO 20–30 mg tid; hypnotic, PO 50–100 mg hs; IV or IM 100–300 mg. Butabarbital Na (*Butisol*), pentobarbital Na (*Nembutal*), secobarbital Na (*Seconal*)	Preoperative sedation; emergency control of convulsions; absence seizures	Depresses CNS, promoting drowsiness	Cough, hiccups, restlessness, pain, hangover, and CNS and circulatory depression

NURSING IMPLICATIONS: Observe for *hypotension* during IV administration; put up siderails on bed of older clients; observe for increased *tolerance*.

Promethazine (*Phenergan*)— 10-25 mg IV, IM, PO q 4 h	Preoperative sedation; postoperative sedation, treat and prevent nausea and vomiting	Antihistaminic; sedative, antiemetic, antimotion sickness	Drowsiness, coma, hypo/hypertension; leukopenia; photosensitivity; irregular respirations; blurred vision; urinary retention; dry

NURSING IMPLICATIONS: Administer oral med *with* food, milk; IM *deep* into large muscles, rotate sites; verify compatibility with other drugs; *safety* concerns due to sedative effect.

THYROID HORMONE INHIBITORS			
Lugol's solution—PO 2–6 drops tid 10 d prior to thyroidectomy	To reduce size, vascularity of thyroid before thyroid surgery; emergency treatment of thyroid storm; or control of hyperthyroid symptoms after radioiodine (^{131}I) therapy	Inhibits thyroid hormone secretion, synthesis	GI distress, stains teeth; increased respiratory secretions; rashes, acne

NURSING IMPLICATIONS: *Dilute in juice*, give through *straw*; bloody diarrhea/vomiting indicates acute poisoning.

Propylthiouracil—PO 300–900 mg/d, divided initial dose; 100–600 mg/d maintenance dose; methimazole (*Tapazole*) 15–60 mg/d initial dose; 5–15 mg/d maintenance dose	Hyperthyroidism; return client to euthyroid state; also used preoperatively	Inhibits functional thyroid hormone synthesis by blocking reactions; responsible for iodide conversion to iodine; inhibition of T_4 conversion to T_3	Blood dyscrasias; hepatotoxicity; hypothyroidism

NURSING IMPLICATIONS: Teach importance of compliance with med protocol; 🍎 *avoid* iodine-rich foods (seafood, iodized salt); caution when using other drugs.

Saturated potassium iodide (*SSKI*)—50-250 mg tid–qid	Same as Lugol's solution	Same as Lugol's solution	Same as Lugol's solution

NURSING IMPLICATIONS: Same as Lugol's solution.

(*continued*)

TABLE D.3 COMMON DRUGS

Drug and Dosage	Use	Action	✕ Assessment: Side Effects
THYROID HORMONE REPLACEMENTS			
Levothyroxine (*Levothroid, Synthroid*)—PO 0.05–0.10 mg/d oral; 200–500 mcg IV	Hypothyroidism	Replacement therapy to alleviate symptoms	Symptoms of hyperthyroidism
	Myxedema coma	Emergency replacement therapy	

NURSING IMPLICATIONS: Teach signs and symptoms of hyper/hypothyroidism; monitor bowel activity; teach diet to combat constipation; keep meds in tight *light-proof* containers; 🍎 *avoid foods* that inhibit thyroid secretion (turnips, cabbage, carrots, peaches, peas, strawberries, spinach, radishes).

Liothyronine (*Cytomel*)—PO 25 mcg/d to maintenance dose 27–75 mcg	Mild hypothyroidism in adults	Replacement therapy	See Levothyroxine

NURSING IMPLICATIONS: See Levothyroxine.

TABLE D.4 GUIDE TO IMPORTANT FOOD AND DRUG CONSIDERATIONS

Key to Nursing Implications
(with codes for medication administration records):
1. Take with **food** or milk (F-M).
2. Take on **empty** stomach (1 hour ac or 2 to 3 hours pc).
3. **Don't drink** milk or eat other dairy products (M-D).
4. Take with full glass of **water** (+ H$_2$O).
5. Take **before** meals (1/2 hour ac).
6. May take **without** regard to meals (OK with meals).

A
acebutolol 6
Achromycin V   2, 3
allopurinol 1
Amcill 2
aminophylline 1
amiodarone 1
amoxicillin 6
amoxicillin/clavulanate 6
Amoxil 6
ampicillin 2
aspirin 1
Augmentin 6
Azo Gantrisin 4, 6
Azolid 1

B
Bactrim 4, 6
Benemid 4
bisacodyl 3
Butazolidin 1

C
Capoten 2
captopril 2
Carafate 2
Carprofen 1
Ceclor 6
cefaclor 6
Ceftin 6
cefuroxime axetil 6
cephalexin 6
chlorothiazide 1
cimetidine 1
Cipro 6
ciprofloxacin 6
Cleocin 4, 6
clindamycin 4, 6
cloxacillin sodium 2
Cloxapen 2
CoIBENEMID 1, 4
Cordarone 1
co-trimoxazole 4,6
Cuprimine 2

D
Declomycin 2, 3
Deltasone 1
demeclocycline 2, 3
Depen 2
Desyrel 1
dicloxacillin sodium 2
diflunisal 1
Diuril 1
Dolobid 1
Donnatal 5
Dopar 1
doxycycline hyclate 3, 6
Dulcolax 3
Dynapen 2

E
Ecotrin 3
E.E.S. 2
E-Mycin 6
enalapril 6
ERYC 2
Ery-Tab 6
Erythrocin 2
erythromycin estolate 6
erythromycin
    ethylsuccinate 6
erythromycin stearate 2
etretinate 1

F
famotidine 6
Feldene 1
ferrous sulfate 3
Flagyl 1
flecainide 6
fluoxetine 6
Fulvicin 1
Furadantin 1

G
Gantrisin 4, 6
glycopyrrolate 5
Grifulvin V 1
Grisactin 1
griseofulvin 1

H
Hydropres 1
Hytrin 6

I
Ilosone 6
Indocin/indomethacin 1
INH 2
isoniazid 2

K
Kaon 1
Kay Ciel 1

Keflex 6
ketoconazole 1
 ketoprofen 1
K-Lor 1
K-Lyte 1

L
Larodopa 1
Larotid 6
levodopa 1
Lincocin 2
lincomycin 2
lisinopril 6
Lorelco 1
lovastatin 1

M
Macrodantin 1
Marax 1
methysergide maleate 1
metronidazole 1
Mevacor 1
mexiletine 1
Mexitil 1
Minocin 3, 6
Minocycline 3, 6

N
nafcillin 2
nitrofurantoin 1
nitrofurantoin
    macrocrystals 1
Nizoral 1
norfloxacin 2, 4
Noroxin 2, 4

O
Omnipen 2
Orazinc 3
Orudis 1
oxacillin sodium 2
oxytetracycline 2, 3

P
penicillamine 2
penicillin G (oral) 2
penicillin V 6
Pen-Vee K 6
Pepcid 6
phenylbutazone 1
pindolol 6
piroxicam 1
Polycillin 2
potassium chloride 1
prednisone 1
Prinivil 6
Pro-Banthine 5
probenecid 4
probucol 1
procainamide 6
Pronestyl 6

propantheline bromide 5
Prostaphlin 2
Prozac 6

R
ranitidine 6
Raudixin 1
rauwolfia serpentina 1
Regroton 1
reserpine 1
Rifadin 2
rifampin 2
Rimactane 2
rimadyl 1
Robinul 5

S
Sansert 1
Sectral 6
Septra 4, 6
Ser-Ap-Es 1
Serpasil 1
Sinemet 1
Slow-K 1
Somophyllin 1
sucralfate 2
sulfisoxazole 4, 6
Sumycin 2, 3

T
Tagamet 1
Tambocor 6
Tedral 1
Tegison 1
terazosin 6
Terramycin 2, 3
tetracycline HC1 2, 3
Theobid 6
Theo-Dur 6

U
Unipen 2

V
Vasotec 6
V-Cillin K 6
Vibramycin 3, 6
Visken 6

Z
Zantac 6
Zestril 6
zinc sulfate 3
Zyloprim 1

Source: Adapted from: McGavin K. 10 Golden rules for administering drugs safely. *Nursing 88*, 18(8):40

TABLE D.5 COMMON HERB/DRUG INTERACTIONS: Caution

Herb	Interaction with:
Aloe	Cardiac glycosides: may *increase* risk of toxicity. Potassium–wasting drugs: may *increase* hypokalemic effect.
Anise	Anticoagulants, MAO inhibitors, hormone therapy
Arnica	None known
Brewer's yeast	MAO inhibitors: *increased* BP
Camphor tree	None known
Chamomile	None known
Comfrey	Coumadin (warfarin)
Dill	None known
Echinacea	Immunosuppressants, anabolic steroids, methotrexate, ketoconazole
Eucalyptus	Induces liver enzymes, which may increase metabolism of other drugs
Fennel	None known
Garlic	Anticoagulants, antiplatelet drugs, thrombolytics, anti-inflammatory drugs: *decreases platelet* aggregation
Ginger	Anticoagulants, antiplatelets
Ginkgo biloba	Anticoagulants, thrombolytics, antiplatelet agents, MAO inhibitors: may *potentiate* effects of these drugs Cephalosporins, valproic acid, NSAIDs: may increase risk of *bleeding*
Ginseng	Warfarin, heparin, aspirin, NSAIDs: may *decrease* anticoagulant activity Phenelzine: may cause *headache, tremulousness, manic* episodes Corticosteroids: may *potentiate* toxic effects Estrogens Other herbs with anticoagulant properties: *increased* risk of bleeding Coffee, tea, soft drinks: may *potentiate* effects of caffeine
Kava-kava	Alprazolam: *added* effect CNS depressants: *potentiates* effect Levodopa: *decreased* effectiveness Antiplatelet agents, MAO inhibitors: *additive* effects Herbs with sedative properties: *added* effect
Lemon verbena	None known
Ma-Huang (ephedra)	Antihypertensives, antidepressants, MAO inhibitors, caffeine: *potentiates sympathomimetic* effects Theophylline, cardiac glycosides: *increased* risk for toxicity from these drugs
Peppermint	Gastric acid-blocking drugs
Saw palmetto	Oral contraceptives, hormone therapy
St. John's Wort	Alcohol, antidepressants: increased risk of *adverse CNS reactions* Indinavir: *decreased* levels and effectiveness
Valerian	Alcohol, CNS depressants: *potentiates* effects

TABLE D.6 CLASSIFICATION OF THE ANTICANCER DRUGS

I. **Alkylating agents**
   A. *Alkyl sulfonate*
      1. Busulfan (*Myleran*)
   B. *Ethylenimine*
      1. Thiotepa
   C. *Nitrogen mustards*
      1. Chlorambucil (*Leukeran*)
      2. Cyclophosphamide (*Cytoxan*)
      3. Ifosfamide (*Ifex*)
      4. Mechlorethamine hydrochloride (*Mustargen*, HN_2, nitrogen mustard)
      5. Melphalan (*Alkeran, L-PAM,* L-phenylalanine mustard)
   D. *Nitrosoureas*
      1. Carmustine (BCNU, BiCNU)
      2. Lomustine (CCNU, CeeNU)
      3. Semustine (methyl-CCNU)
      4. Streptozocin (*Zanosar,* streptozotocin)
   E. *Triazene*
      1. Dacarbazine (*DTIC-Dome*)

II. **Antimetabolites**
   A. *Folate antagonist*
      1. Methotrexate (*Folex, Mexate*)
   B. *Purine analogues*
      1. Cladribine (2-chloro-deoxyadenosine, *Leustatin*)
      2. Fludarabine (*Fludara*)
      3. Mercaptopurine (6-MP, *Purinethol*)
      4. Pentostatin (deoxycoformycin, *Nipent*)
      5. Thioguanine (6-TG, 6-thioguanine)
   C. *Pyrimidine analogues*
      1. Cytarabine (cytosine arabinoside, *Cytosar-U,* ara-C)
      2. Fluorouracil (5-FU, 5-fluorouracil)

III. **Anti–infectives**
   A. *Anthracyclines*
      1. Daunorubicin (daunomycin, *Cerubidine*)
      2. Doxorubicin hydrochloride (*Adriamycin*)
      3. Idarubicin (*Idamycin*)
   B. *Bleomycin*
      1. Bleomycin sulfate (*Blenoxane*)
   C. Dactinomycin (actinomycin D, *Cosmegen*)
   D. Mitomycin (mitomycin C, *Mutamycin*)
   E. Plicamycin (*Mithracin*)

IV. **Plant-derived products**
   A. *Epipodophyllotoxins*
      1. Etoposide (VP-16, *VePesid*)
      2. Teniposide (VM-26, *Vumon*)
   B. *Taxane*: paclitaxel (*Taxol*)
   C. *Vinca alkaloids*
      1. Vinblastine (*Velban*)
      2. Vincristine (*Oncovin*)

V. **Enzyme**
   A. L-Asparaginase (*Elspar*)

VI. **Hormonal agents**
   A. *Androgen/antiandrogen*
      1. Flutamide (*Eulexin*)
   B. *Estrogens/antiestrogens*
      1. Estramustine phosphate sodium (*Emcyt*)
      2. Tamoxifen citrate (*Nolvadex*)
   C. *Glucocorticoid*
   D. *Luteinizing hormone-releasing hormone* (LH-RH) *antagonists*
      1. Buserelin (*Suprefact*)
      2. Leuprolide (*Lupron*)
   E. Octreotide acetate (*Sandostatin*)
   F. Progestins

VII. **Miscellaneous agents**
   A. Carboplatin (*Paraplatin*)
   B. Cisplatin (*cis*-platinum II, *Platinol*)
   C. Hexamethylmelamine (HMM)
   D. Hydroxyurea (*Hydrea*)
   E. Mitotane (o,p'-DDD, *Lysodren*)
   F. Mitoxantrone (*Novantrone*)
   G. Procarbazine (N-methylhydrazine, *Matulane, Natulan*)

VIII. **Monoclonal antibodies**

IX. **Immunomodulating agents**
   A. Interferons
      1. Interferon alfa-2a (*Roferon-A*)
      2. Interferon alfa-2b (*Intron A*)
   B. Interleukins: aldesleukin (interleukin-2, IL-2, *Proleukin*)
   C. Levamisole (*Ergamisol*)

X. **Cellular growth factors**
   A. Erythropoietin (*Epogen, Aranesp*)
   B. Filgrastim (G-CSF, *Neupogen*)
   C. Oprelvekin (*Neumega*)
   D. Sargramostim (GM-CSF, *Leukine, Prokine*)

Source: Adapted from: Craig C, Stitzel R. *Modern Pharmacology.* Boston: Little, Brown

TABLE D.7 PROPERTIES OF SELECTED ANTI–INFLAMMATORY AGENTS

Specific Group	Analgesic	Antipyretic	Anti-inflammatory	Uricosuric
Salicylate derivatives				
Acetylsalicylic acid (aspirin)	✳	✳	✳	✳
Pyrazolone derivatives				
Phenylbutazone	✳	✳	✳	✳
Oxyphenbutazone	✳	✳	✳	✳
Sulfinpyrazone	0	0	0	✳
Paraaminophenl derivatives				
Acetaminophen	✳	✳	0	0
Phenacetin	✳	✳	0	0
Propionic acid derivatives				
Ibuprofen	✳	✳	✳	0
Naproxen	✳	✳	✳	0
Fenoprofen	✳	✳	✳	0
Flurbiprofen	✳	✳	✳	0
Ketoprofen	✳	✳	✳	0
Newer drugs				
Indomethacin	✳	✳	✳	0
Sulindac	✳	0	✳	0
Mefenamic acid	✳	0	✳	0
Tolmetin	✳	✳	✳	0
Diflunisal	✳	0	✳	0
Piroxicam	✳	✳	✳	0
Diclofenac	✳	✳	✳	0
Etodolac	✳	0	✳	✳
Nabumetone	✳	✳	✳	0

✳ = possesses the property assigned; 0 = lacks the property assigned.

Source: Adapted from: Ebadi M. *Pharmacology* (2nd ed). Boston: Little, Brown,

Table D.8 CLASSIFICATION OF DRUGS BY DRUG NAME ENDINGS

Drug Classification	Drug with ending of:
Ace inhibitors	–pril
Anesthetics (local)	–caine
Antianxiety agents	–lam –pam
Antibiotics/anti-infectives	–cillin –micin –mycin –oxacin
Antihyperlipidemics	–statin
Antiulcer agents (histamine H2 blockers)	–dine
Antiviral agents	–vir
Beta blockers	–olol
Diuretics	–mide –zide
Neuromuscular blocking agents	–nium
Opioid analgesics	–done
Oral hypoglycemics	–ide
Steroids	–sone

TABLE D.9 COMMON DRUG CALCULATIONS

I. Ratio And Proportion

A. Use to calculate partial doses.

$$\frac{\text{Known dose}}{\text{Known volume}} = \frac{\text{Desired dose}}{\text{Unknown volume}}$$

B. Example:
The nurse needs to give Demerol 35mg intravenously. Demerol 50mg/mL is available. How many mL should the nurse draw up?

$$\frac{50\text{mg}}{1\text{mL}} = \frac{35\text{mg}}{X\text{mL}}$$

To solve this problem:
Cross-multiply the opposite sides of the equation

$$\frac{50\text{mg}}{1\text{mL}} \times \frac{35\text{mg}}{X\text{mL}}$$

50mg(XmL) = 35mg(1mL)

Divide each side of the equation by the number with the X

$$\frac{50\text{mg}(X\text{mL})}{50\text{mg}} = \frac{35\text{mg}(1\text{mL})}{50\text{mg}}$$

XmL = 35/50
      X = 0.7mL

II. IV Drip Rate Calculations

A. Need to know:
   (1) <u>Volume</u> of solution to be infused.
   (2) <u>Time</u> over which the quantity of solution is to be infused.
   (3) <u>Calibration factor</u> (drop factor) of the tubing, which can be found on the box of IV tubing

$$\frac{\text{volume} \quad \text{x} \quad \text{calibration factor}}{\text{time of infusion}}$$

B. Example:
The nurse needs to infuse an antibiotic via piggyback. The piggyback bag contains 50mL of solution; it needs to run over <u>30min</u>, and the calibration factor of the tubing is <u>15gtt/mL</u>.

$$\frac{50\text{mL} \quad \text{x} \quad 15\text{gtt/mL}}{30\text{min}} = \frac{750\text{gtt}}{30\text{min}}$$

Answer: 25gtt/min

TABLE D.10 ONSET, PEAK, AND DURATION OF DIFFERENT TYPES OF INSULIN

Type of Insulin	Onset	Peak	Duration
Lispro: rapid acting	15 minutes	60-90 minutes	3-4 hours
Regular: short acting	30-60 minutes	2-3 hours	4-6 hours
NPH or *lente*: intermediate acting	2 hours	6-8 hours	12-16 hours
Ultralente: long acting	2 hours	16-20 hours	24 + hours
Insulin glargine (Lantus): long acting	1-2 hours	No peak	24 + hours

Tips for Drawing Up and Giving Insulin

- The *lente* insulins (Semilente, Lente, Ultralente) may be mixed with each other.
- Mixing *regular* insulin with lente insulin is not recommended , unless the client is well-controlled on this mixture.
- *Insulin glargine* cannot be mixed with other insulins.
- No other medications should be mixed with any insulin.
- Mixing two kinds of insulin in the same syringe:
    - Inject appropriate amount of air into the intermediate-acting insulin (cloudy insulin) without touching the tip of the needle to the insulin. Remove the syringe from the vial.
    - Using the same syringe, inject appropriate amount of air into the rapid- or short-acting insulin (clear insulin). Without removing the syringe from the vial, withdraw the correct amount of insulin from the vial. Remove the syringe from the vial and eject any air bubbles in the syringe.
    - Still using the same syringe, withdraw the correct amount of insulin from the intermediate-acting vial (clear to cloudy). Do **not** draw up more, or less than is correct.
    - Remember: "clear to cloudy" when mixing 2 different kinds of insulin.

TABLE D.11 COMMON PATTERNS OF MEDICATION USE AMONG ELDERLY CLIENTS

Polypharmacy
The client takes many medications concurrently, prescribed or not, in an effort to treat multiple problems. Typical prescribed meds include: analgesics, antihypertensives, antacids, antiarthritics, cardiovascular agents, laxatives, sedatives, and tranquilizers.

Over-the-counter medications
Approximately 75% of older adults use over-the-counter meds, including analgesics, laxatives, sleeping medications, and antacids.

Self-prescribing of medications
Older adults experience a variety of symptoms (e.g., pain, indigestion, constipation) for which they self-prescribe over-the-counter medications, folk medicines, and herbs.

Misuse of medications
Typical misuse of medications by older adults includes *over-use, under-use, inconsistent use*, or use of *contraindicated* drugs.

Non-compliance
About 75% of older adults do not follow their medication regimen, either by not taking the medication or by altering the dose. Reasons for non-compliance include: (a) the drug is perceived as ineffective, (b) the drug has undesirable side effects, or (c) the cost of the drug is too high.

Quick Guide to Common Clinical Signs

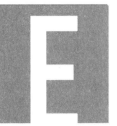

Many clinical signs have been named for the physicians who first described them or the phenomena they resemble. Following is a list of **25 of the most common clinical signs** for use as a quick reference as you review.

Babinski reflex dorsiflexion of the big toe after stimulation of the lateral sole; associated with *corticospinal* tract lesions.

Blumberg's sign transient pain in the abdomen after approximated fingers pressed gently into abdominal wall are suddenly withdrawn—rebound tenderness; associated with *peritoneal inflammation.*

Brudzinski's sign flexion of the hip and knee induced by flexion of the neck; associated with *meningeal* irritation.

Chvostek's sign facial muscle spasm induced by tapping on the facial nerve branches; associated with *hypocalcemia.*

Cheyne-Stokes respiration rhythmic cycles of deep and shallow respiration, often with apneic periods; associated with *central nervous system respiratory center dysfunction.*

Coppernail's sign ecchymoses on the perineum, scrotum, or labia; associated with *fracture* of the *pelvis.*

Cullen's sign bluish discoloration of the umbilicus; associated with acute *pancreatitis* or *hemoperitoneum*, especially *rupture of fallopian tube* in ectopic pregnancy.

Doll's eye sign dissociation between the movements of the head and eyes: as the head is raised, the eyes are lowered, and as the head is lowered, the eyes are raised; associated with global-diffuse disorders of the *cerebrum.*

Fluid wave sign transmission across the abdomen of a wave induced by snapping the abdomen; associated with *ascites.*

Goldstein's sign wide distance between the great toe and the adjoining toe; associated with *cretinism* and *trisomy* 21.

Homans' sign pain behind the knee, induced by dorsiflexion of the foot; associated with peripheral vascular disease, especially *venous thrombosis* in the calf.

Kehr's sign severe pain in the left upper quadrant, radiating to the top of the shoulder; associated with *splenic rupture.*

Kernig's sign inability to extend leg when sitting or lying with the thigh flexed on the abdomen; associated with *meningeal* irritation.

Knie's sign unequal dilatation of the pupils; associated with *Graves' disease.*

Kussmaul's respiration paroxysmal air hunger; associated with acidosis, especially *diabetic ketoacidosis.*

Lasègue's sign straight leg raising with hip flexed and knee extended will elicit sciatic pain; associated with *herniated lumbar disc.*

McBurney's sign tenderness at McBurney's point (located two-thirds of the distance from the umbilicus to the anterior-superior iliac spine); associated with *appendicitis.*

Murphy's sign pain on taking a deep breath when pressure is applied over the gallbladder; associated with *gallbladder disease.*

Osler's sign small painful erythematous swellings in the skin of the hands and feet; associated with *bacterial endocarditis.*

Psoas sign pain induced by hyperextension of the right thigh while lying on the left side; associated with *appendicitis.*

Setting-sun sign downward deviation of the eyes so that each iris appears to "set" beneath the lower lid, with white sclera exposed between it and the upper lid; associated with *increased intracranial pressure* or irritation of the brain stem.

Simian crease transverse palmar crease; associated with *Down syndrome*

Tinel's sign tingling sensation felt from light percussion on the radial side of the palmaris longus tendon; associated with *carpal tunnel syndrome.*

Trousseau's sign carpopedal spasm develops when BP cuff is inflated above systolic pressure for 3 minutes; associated with *hypocalcemia.*

Williamson's sign markedly diminished blood pressure in the leg as compared with that in the arm on the same side; associated with *pneumothorax* and *pleural effusions.*

Source: Adapted from Macklis RM, at al. *Introduction to Clinical Medicine*, Boston: Little, Brown.

Index to 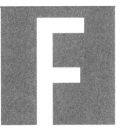 Common Diagnostic Tests and Procedures

APPENDIX F

For a quick review, use this index to locate **105 selected diagnostic tests and procedures** covered in this book as they relate to specific conditions

Test/Procedure	Condition	Page
Angiocardiography	Cardiovascular system (evaluation)	16, 51
Angiography	Arteriosclerosis obliterans	16
	CV system (evaluation)	28, 51
Ankle-arm pressure index (API)	Compartment syndrome	262, 263
Arthroscopy	Osteoarthritis	264, 275
Audiography/audiogram	Deafness	244
Audiometry	Otosclerosis	243
Babinski's sign	Brain injury (trauma)	283
	Pernicious anemia	61
Barium swallow	Esophageal cancer	332
	Hiatal hernia	191
Basal metabolic rate (BMR)	Immobility; adult and older adult	6, 263
	Myxedema	233
Bladder biopsy	Bladder cancer	328
Body mass index	Obesity	4
Bone marrow (iron)	Polycythemia vera	62
Bone marrow (aspiration)	Leukemia	62
Brain scan	AVM; brain abscesses and tumors	290
Breast biopsy	Breast cysts and tumors	323, 338
Bronchoscopy	Respiratory system evaluation; lung cancer	91, 321
Caloric stimulation test	Meniere's disease	248
Cardiac catherization	Angina pectoris	46
	Cardiac status evaluation	28, 33
Celiac angiography	Liver disease	182
Cerebral angiography	IICP	290
Cervical biopsy and cauterization	Cervical cancer, bleeding	326, 338
	Air embolus	115
Chest x-ray	ARDS	78
	Anthrax	366
	Atelectasis	71
	Delirium	362
	Emphysema	75
	Heart failure, chest pain	48, 361
	Hemothorax	80
	Hiatal hernia	191
	Histoplasmosis	72
	N-G tube placement	138
	Near drowning	354
	Pericarditis	32
	Pneumonia	70
	Pneumothorax	80, 81
	Pulmonary embolism	72
	Renal calculi	220
	Respiratory system assessment	5, 91

Laboratory Values

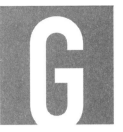
Use this chart as a quick overview of lab values: both normal and conditions that result in **high** or **low** values.

Test	Normal Values	Possible Significance	
		Increases	**Decreases**
HEMATOLOGY			
Aspartate amino-transferase (AST)—*formerly* called serum glutamic oxaloacetic transaminase (SGOT)	*Men*: 10–40 U/L *Women*: 9–25 U/L	Myocardial infarction, cardiac surgery, hepatitis, cirrhosis, trauma, severe burns, progressive muscular dystrophy, infectious mononucleosis, acute renal failure	Chronic dialysis Ketoacidosis Uremia
Bleeding time—indicator of hemostatic efficiency	1–9 min	Hemorrhagic purpura, acute leukemia, aplastic anemia, disseminated intravascular coagulation Anticoagulant therapy (oral)	
Hematocrit—volume of packed red blood cells per dL of blood	*Men*: 45% (38%–54%) *Women*: 40% (36%—47%)	Dehydration Polycythemia Congenital heart disease	Anemia, Leukemia, hemorrhage Dietary deficiencies
Hemoglobin—oxygen-combining protein	*Men*: 14–18 g/dL *Women*: 12–16 g/dL	Same as for **Hematocrit**	Same as for **Hematocrit**
International Normalized Ratio (INR)—test of coagulation	2.5—3.5	Anticoagulation therapy with warfarin (*Coumadin*)	
Partial thromboplastin time (PTT)—tests coagulation mechanism; stage I deficiencies	*APTT*: 30–40 sec *PTT*: 60–70 sec	Deficiency of Factors VIII, IX, X, XI, XII Anticoagulant therapy	Extensive cancer Disseminated intravascular coagulation
Platelets—thrombocytes	150,000–400,000/mm³	Polycythemia Postsplenectomy Anemia	Leukemia Aplastic anemia Cirrhosis, multiple myeloma Chemotherapy
Prothrombin time–tests extrinsic clotting; stages II and III	11–15 sec	Anticoagulant therapy Disseminated intravascular coagulation Hepatic disease Malabsorption	Digitalis therapy Diuretic reaction Vitamin K therapy
Red blood cell count—number of circulating erythrocytes in 1 mm³ of whole blood	*Men*: 4.5–6.2 million/mm³ *Women*: 4.0–5.5 million/mm³	Polycythemia vera Anoxia Dehydration	Leukemia Hemorrhage Anemias Hodgkin's disease
Sedimentation rate— speed at which red blood cells settle in uncoagulated blood	*Men*: 0–15 mm/h *Women*: 0–20 mm/h	Acute bacterial infection Cancer Infectious disease, numerous inflammatory states	Polycythemia vera Sickle cell anemia

Test	Normal Values	Possible Significance Increases	Possible Significance Decreases
White blood cell count—number of leukocytes in 1 mm³	5000–10,000/mm³	Leukemia Bacterial infection Severe sepsis	Viral infection, overwhelming bacterial infection, lupus erythematosus, Antineoplastic chemotherapy
White blood cell differential—enumeration of individual leukocyte distribution			
Basophils	25–100mL, or 0–1%	Myeloproliferative disease Leukemia	Anaphylactic reaction Hyperthyroidism Radiation therapy Infections Pregnancy Aging
Eosinophils	1%–4%	Allergic disorder Parasitic infestation Eosinophilic leukemia	Acute or chronic stress; Excess ACTH, cortisone or epinephrine Endocrine disorder
Lymphocytes	20–40%	Chronic and acute lymphocytic leukemia Infectious mononucleosis Chronic bacterial infection Viral infection	Systemic lupus erythematosus Immune deficiency disorders
Neutrophils	55%–70%	Bacterial infection, tumor, inflammation, stress, drug reaction, trauma, metabolic disorders	Acute viral infection, anorexia nervosa, radiation therapy, drug-induced, alcohol ingestion
BLOOD CHEMISTRY			
Alkaline phosphatase (ALP)	*men*: 45-115U/L *women*: 30-100U/L	Hyperparathyroidism, Paget's disease, cancer with bone metastasis, obstructive jaundice, cirrhosis, infectious hepatitis, rickets	Malnutrition, scurvy Celiac disease Chronic nephritis Hypothyroidism
Amylase	53–123U/L	Acute pancreatitis, mumps, duodenal ulcer, pancreatic cancer, perforated bowel, renal failure	Advanced chronic pancreatitis Chronic alcoholism
Bilirubin, serum	*Direct*: 0.1–0.3 mg/dL *Indirect*: 0.2–0.8 mg/dL *Total*: 0.1–1.0 mg/dL	Massive hemolysis, low-grade Hemolytic disease, cirrhosis, Obstructive liver disease, Hepatitis, biliary obstruction Erythroblastosis fetalis	
Calcium, serum	9–10.5 mg/dL, 4.5–5.6 mg/dL, ionized	Hyperparathyroidism, multiple myeloma, bone metastasis, bone fracture, thiazide diuretic reaction, milk-alkali syndrome	Hypoparathyroidism, renal failure, pregnancy, massive transfusion
Carbon dioxide	24–30 mEq/L	Emphysema Salicylate toxicity Vomiting	Starvation Diarrhea

Test	Normal Values	Possible Significance	
		Increases	Decreases
Chloride, serum	90–110 mEq/L	Hyperventilation Diabetes	Heart failure Pyloric obstruction, vomiting Hypoventilation, Chronic respiratory acidosis
Cholesterol (total serum)	<200 mg/dL	Hypercholesterolemia, hyperlipidemia, myocardial infarction, uncontrolled diabetes mellitus, high cholesterol diet, atherosclerosis, stress, glomerulonephritis (nephrotic stage), familial	Malnutrition Cholesterol-lowering medication Anemia Liver disease Hyperthyroidism
Creatinine, serum	*Men*: 0.6–1.2 mg/dL *Women*: 0.5–1.1 mg/dL	Chronic glomerulonephritis Nephritis Heart failure Muscle disease	Debilitation
Creatine kinase (CK) **(creatine phosphokinase** **[CPK])**	*Men*: 12–70 U/mL (55–170 U/L) *Women*: 10–55 U/mL (30–135 U/L)	Acute myocardial infarction Acute brain attack Convulsions Surgery Muscular dystrophy Hypokalemia	
Isoenzymes: CPK-MM/CK-MM/CKIII	95-100%	Muscular dystrophy, delirium tremens, surgery, hypokalemia, crush injuries, hypothyroidism	
CPK-MB/CK-MB/CKII	<3%	Acute myocardial infarction Cardiac defibrillation Myocarditis Cardiac ischemia	
CPK-BB/CK-BB	0%	Pulmonary infarction, brain surgery, brain attack, pulmonary embolism, seizures, intestinal ischemia	
Fibrinogen, serum	0.2–0.4 g/dL or 200–400 mg/dL	Pneumonia Acute infection Nephrosis Rheumatoid arthritis	Cirrhosis, toxic liver necrosis, anemia, disseminated intravascular coagulation, advanced carcinoma
Glucose (fasting) 12	80–120 mg/dL	Acute stress, Cushing's syndrome, hyperthyroidism, acute or chronic pancreatitis, diabetes mellitus, hyperglycemia	Addison's disease Liver disease Reactive hypoglycemia Pituitary hypofunction
Glycosylated hemoglobin **(HbA1$_c$)**	4.0%–7.0%	Newly diagnosed or poorly controlled diabetes mellitus	
Iron-binding capacity **(total)**	25–420 mg/L	Lead poisoning Hepatic necrosis	Iron deficiency anemia Chronic blood loss

Test	Normal Values	Possible Significance	
		Increases	Decreases
Lactate dehydrogenase (LDH)	40–90 U/L, 115–225 IU/L LDH-1: 17%–27% LDH-2: 27%–38% LDH-3: 18%–25% LDH-4: 3%–8% LDH-5: 0–5%	Myocardial infarction, pernicious anemia, chronic viral hepatitis, pneumonia, pulmonary emboli, brain attack, renal tissue destruction, leukemia, non-Hodgkin's lymphoma; shock, trauma	
Myoglobin	*men*: <92 ng/ml *women*: <76 ng/ml	Myocardial infarction	
Phosphorus (inorganic), serum	3.0–4.5 mg/dL	Chronic glomerular disease, hypoparathyroidism Milk-alkali syndrome Sarcoidosis	Hypoparathyroidism, rickets, osteomalacia, renal tubular necrosis, malabsorption syndrome, vitamin D deficiency
Potassium, serum	3.5–5.0 mEq/L	Diabetic ketosis, renal failure, Addison's disease, excessive intake	Thiazide diuretics, Cushing's syndrome, cirrhosis with ascites, hyperaldosteronism, steroid therapy, malignant hypertension, poor dietary habits, chronic diarrhea, diaphoresis, renal tubular necrosis, malabsorption syndrome, vomiting
Protein, serum (albumin/globulin)	*Total*: 6.4–8.3 g/d *Albumin*: 3.5–5.0 g/dL *Globulin*: 2.3–3.5 g/dL	Dehydration Multiple myeloma	Chronic liver disease Myeloproliferative disease Burns
Serum glutamic oxaloacetic transaminase (SGOT)—see Aspartate aminotransferase	---	---	---
Sodium, serum	138–144 mEq/L	Increased intake, either orally or IV; Cushing's disease; excessive sweating; diabetes insipidus	Addison's disease, sodium-losing nephropathy, vomiting, diarrhea, fistulas, tube drainage, burns, renal insufficiency with acidosis, starvation with acidosis, paracentesis, thoracentesis, ascites, heart failure, syndrome of inappropriate antidiuretic hormone
T_3 uptake	24–34%	Hyperthyroidism, thyroxine-binding globulin (TBG) deficiency	Hypothyroidism Pregnancy Thyroid-binding globulin, excess
Thyroxine	5–12 mcg/dL	Hyperthyroidism Pregnancy	Hypothyroidism Renal failure
Troponin T	<0.1 ng/ml	Myocardial Infarction	
Troponin I	<0.1-3.1 ng/ml	Myocardial Infarction	

Test	Normal Values	Possible Significance	
		Increases	**Decreases**
Urea nitrogen, serum (BUN)	10–20 mg/dL	Acute or chronic renal failure, heart failure, obstructive uropathy, dehydration	Cirrhosis Malnutrition
Uric acid, serum	*Men*: 2.1–8.5 mg/dL *Women*: 2.0–6.6 mg/dL	Gout Chronic renal failure Starvation Diuretic therapy	
BLOOD GASES			
Bicarbonate (HCO_3)	21–28 mEq/L	Metabolic alkalosis	Metabolic acidosis
Carbon dioxide pressure (PCO_2), whole blood, arterial	35–45 mm Hg	Primary respiratory acidosis, loss of H^+ through nasogastric suctioning or vomiting	Primary respiratory alkalosis
Oxygen pressure (PO_2), whole blood, arterial	80–100 mm Hg	Oxygen administration in the absence of severe lung disease	Chronic obstructive lung disease, severe pneumonia, pulmonary embolism, pulmonary edema, respiratory muscle disease, ARDS
pH, serum	7.35–7.45	*Metabolic alkalosis*-alkali ingestion; *respiratory alkalosis*-hyperventilation	*Metabolic acidosis*— ketoacidosis, shock; *respiratory acidosis*— alveolar hypoventilation
IMMUNODIAGNOSTIC STUDIES			
Carcinoembryonic antigen	<3 mg/mL	Cancer of: colon, lung, metastatic breast, pancreas, stomach, prostate, ovary, bladder, limbs; also neuroblastoma, leukemias, osteogenic carcinoma. *Noncancerous* conditions such as: hepatic cirrhosis, uremia, pancreatitis, colorectal polyposis, peptic ulcer disease, ulcerative colitis, regional enteritis	
Prostate specific antigen (PSA)–screening for prostate cancer	0–4 ng/mL	Prostate tumor	
URINALYSIS			
Casts	Negative	Nephrosis Glomerulonephritis Lupus erythematosus Infection	
Catecholamines (VMA) (vanillylmandelic acid)	*Epinephrine*: 0.5–20.0 mcg/24 h *Norepinephrine*: 15–80 mcg/24 h	Pheochromocytoma Severe anxiety Numerous medications	

Test	Normal Values	Possible Significance	
		Increases	Decreases
Chloride	110–250 mEq/L/24 h	Chronic obstructive lung disease Dehydration Salicylate toxicity	Gastric suction HF Emphysema
Color	Normal yellow	*Abnormal: red to reddish brown*—hematuria; *brown to brownish gray*—bilirubinuria or urobilinuria; *tea-colored*–possible obstructive jaundice	*Almost colorless*: chronic kidney disease, diabetes insipidus, diabetes mellitus
Creatinine clearance	90–139 mL/min		Renal failure
Glucose	Negative	Diabetes mellitus	
17-Hydroxycorticosteroids	2–10 mg/24 h	Cushing's disease	Addison's disease
Ketosteroids	*Men*: 7–25 mg/24 h *Women*: 4–15 mg/24 h	Hirsutism Adrenal hyperplasia	Thyrotoxicosis Addison's disease
pH	4.8–8.0	Metabolic alkalosis	Metabolic alkalosis
Potassium	25–120 mEq/L/24 h	Diuretic therapy	Renal failure
Protein	Negative	Nephrosis Glomerulonephritis Lupus erythematosus	
Red blood cells	Negative	Renal calculi Hemorrhagic cystitis Tumors of the kidney	
Sodium	40–220 mEq/L/24 h	Salt-wasting renal disease Syndrome of inappropriate antidiuretic hormone Dehydration	Heart failure Primary aldosteronism
Specific gravity	1.010–1.030	Dehydration Pituitary tumor Hypotension	Distal renal tubular disease Polycystic kidney disease Diabetes insipidus Overhydration
White blood cells	Negative	Inflammation of the kidneys, ureters, bladder	
URINE TESTS			
Schilling test	Excretion of 8%–40% or more of test dose should appear in urine		Gastrointestinal malabsorption Pernicious anemia

Index to 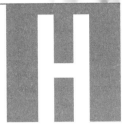 Mnemonics/Memory Aids

Condition	Mnemonic	Page
Acid-base Balance	RAMS	115
Angina: Precipitating Factors	3 E's	50
Asthma: Sx, Cause, Dx, Tx	WHISTLE	90
Atelectasis: Characteristics, Tx	COLLAPSE	90
Blood Glucose: Sx, Implications	(rhyme)	173
Bronchitis: Sx, Tx	COUGH	90
Cancer: Client Care	CANCER	338
Circulation: Assessment	4 P's	141
Compartment Syndrome: Assessment	5 P's	275
C.P.R.	ABC's	50
Cushing's Syndrome: Signs	3 S's	237
Diabetes: Assessment	3 P's	173
Heart failure: Signs/Symptoms	OVERLOAD	51
Histoplasmosis: Characteristics	SOIL	90
Hypertension: Assessment	ELEVATED	22
Hypertension: Complications	4 C's	22
Hypoglycemia: Signs, Sx	DIRE	173
MI: Signs/Symptoms	INTENSE PAIN	50
Pain: Assessment	$P^2QR^2S^2T$	147
Pain: Management	ABC's	148
Pneumonia: Signs, Sx, Tx	FRAPPÉ	90
Postoperative Complications: Tx	4 W's	141
Pulmonary Edema: Signs/Symptoms	FOWLER'S	51
Pulmonary Embolism: Signs, Dx	SUDDEN	90
Traction: Nursing Care Plan	TRACTION	275
Transient Ischemic Attacks: Assessment	3 T's	291
Trauma Care: Complications	TRAUMA	369
Tuberculosis: Cause, Dx, Sx, Tx	SPREAD	90
Varicose Veins: Assessment	TWISTED	22

Index to ☞ Common Tubes

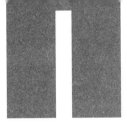

For a quick reference as you study or review, use this index to locate **approximately 25 tubes** that are covered throughout the book as they are used in various conditions.

Tube	Condition	Page
Cantor	Intestinal obstruction	138, 201
Catheterization	Prostatic hyperplasia	222
Chest tubes	Hemothorax	86, 87, 88, 133
	Pneumothorax	81, 86, 87, 88
	Post-op cardiac surgery	31, 86, 87, 88
	Sucking chest wound	80
	Thoracic surgery	82, 86, 87, 88
Endotracheal	Post-cardiac surgery	31
	Sucking chest wound	80
Three-way Foley	Prostatectomy	139, 222, 223
Gastrostomy tube	Hiatal hernia	139, 191
Hemovac	Laryngectomy	84, 85
	Mastectomy	139
	Total hip, knee replacement	139
Jackson-Pratt	Mastectomy	139
	Total hip, knee replacement	139
	Wounds	139
Levin	Gastric surgery	128, 138, 192
Linton	Esophageal varices	181
Miller-Abbott	GI surgery	128, 138
	Intestinal obstruction	201
	Paralytic ileus	136
Nasogastric (NG)	Aneurysm	18
	Gastric distention	135
	Gastric surgery	191, 192
	Intestinal obstruction	136
	Paralytic ileus	136
	Splenectomy	64
	Wound dehiscence, evisceration	135
Oropharyngeal airway	Post-operative	132, 133
Penrose drain	Bowel resection	138
Pulmonary artery catheter	ARD	79
	Burns	348
	MI	47
	Pre & post op cardiac	30, 31
	Shock	122
Salem sump	Gastric surgery	128, 138, 192
Sengstaken-Blakemore	Esophageal varices	181
Shunts	Dialysis	216, 218
Suction	Post-cardiac surgery	31
Suprapubic catheter	Prostatectomy	139, 222, 223
T tube	Cholecystectomy	139, 171
Tracheostomy	Laryngectomy	83, 84, 88
Ureteral catheter	Cystoscopy, pyelotomy	139, 223
Urinary catheter	Shock	122

Index: Nursing Treatments

APPENDIX **J**

☞ **Hands-On Care, Skills, Activities and Procedures**

Use this index as a quick checklist of **over 100** essential **skills and procedures** with page references to selected conditions mentioned in this book that nurses need to know about or be able to perform in giving client care. **Bold face** page number indicate **key** points.

Index to 👉 Positioning the Client

 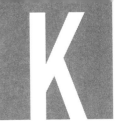

For a quick reference as you study or review, use this index to locate **40 positions of choice** (or contraindications) in various conditions.

AVOID:

Chair, high	Varicose veins	19
High-Fowler's	Uterine cancer	327
Hip flexion/sitting	Aneurysm	18
	Arterial insuffiency	22
	Ileofemoral bypass	140
	Polycythemia vera	62
	Vein ligation, stripping	22
Leg elevation	Arterial insufficiency	22
	Ileofemoral bypass	140
Standing, prolonged sitting	Varicose veins	19
	Vein ligations, stripping	22
Trendelenberg	Lobectomy	140
	Shock	122, 123, 134

🏠 Home Health Care/Health Teaching APPENDIX

For a quick review of essential information related to health care teaching covered in this book, refer to the pages listed to locate what you need to know to provide **basic home care teaching in 40 conditions/situations**.

Most Common Diagnoses for Home Care Clients:
1. Diabetes mellitus.
2. Hypertension.
3. Heart failure.
4. Osteoarthritis.
5. Stroke.
6. Chronic skin ulcers.
7. Chronic obstructive pulmonary disease.
8. Heart disease.

Risk Indicators for Clients Needing Home Care Services
1. Unexpected readmission to acute care facility within 30 days, or frequent readmissions.
2. Significant change in health problem or regimen.
3. Change in client's mental status
4. Noncompliant behavior.
5. Terminal condition.
6. Received physical, occupational, or speech therapy while in the hospital.
7. Post-amputation, hip or knee replacement.
8. New assistive devices, e.g. cane or walker
9. Indwelling urinary catheter, or urinary or bowel diversion.
10. Complex medical equipment required, such as a special bed.
11. Pain management.
12. Intravenous antibiotics or chemotherapy.
13. Draining wounds.
14. Complex health care regimen.
15. Drainage tubes.
16. Enteral feeding tubes.
17. Ventilator dependent.

CONDITIONS SEEN IN HOME HEALTH CARE

System/Condition	General, Selected Home Health Care Goals
PULMONARY SYSTEM	
Asthma	*Teaching*: medication regiment to prevent or control attacks, prevent upper and lower respiratory tract infections, **p. 77.**
COPD	*Teaching*: medication regimen that involves various routes, use of assistive mechanical ventilation, **p. 76.** Infection control.
Pneumonia	*Teaching*: anti-infective medication regimen, **p. 70-71.** Prevention of complications.
Tracheostomy/ laryngectomy	Respiratory care Patency of tube. *Teaching*: tube changes, dressing and tie changes, **p. 83, 84.** Prevention of complications. ↓ Emotional problems associated with artificial airway.
Tuberculosis	*Teaching*: personal hygiene, rest, nutrition, medication regimen, **p. 74.**
CARDIOVASCULAR SYSTEM	
Coronary artery disease	*Teaching*: medication regimen, control of risk factors, compliance with exercise and diet, **p. 46.**
Heart failure	Assessment. *Teaching*: medical regimen to prevent heart failure, **p. 49.**
Coronary artery bypass surgery	*Postoperative teaching:* medical regimen to prevent complications, lifestyle changes (i.e., limitations) made necessary by this surgery and underlying cardiac condition, **p. 32.**
Hypertension	*Teaching*: medication regimen to control condition, preventive measures to control risk factors, **p. 15-16.**

CARDIOVASCULAR SYSTEM (*Continued*)

System/Condition	General, Selected Home Health Care Goals
Myocardial infarction	Assessment. *Teaching*: medication regimen, control of risk factors to prevent recurrence or complications, measures to prevent further damage, **p. 48.**
Pacemaker	Monitor pacemaker function and heart rate to prevent complications, **p. 36.**
Peripheral vascular disease	*Teaching*: medical regimen to enhance circulation in extremities, prevent complications, **p. 17, 19.**
Thrombophlebitis	*Teaching*: control of factors that contribute to thrombus formation, **p. 21.** Prevention of chronic venous insufficiency or pulmonary emboli.

NEUROLOGIC SYSTEM

System/Condition	General, Selected Home Health Care Goals
Alzheimer's disease	*Teaching*: safety. Preservation of cognitive, social, physical, and psychological function.
Amyotrophic lateral sclerosis	*Teaching*: preservation of muscle function and independence, **p. 309.**
Brain attack (stroke)	*Teaching*: medical regimen to treat underlying codition, **p. 288.** Rehabilitation and aftercare to maximize potential.
Parkinson's disease	*Teaching*: administration of medication, self-care to meet own basic needs, **p. 308.**
Seizure disorder	*Teaching*: medication administration to control seizures, **p. 286.** Prevention of physical and psychological trauma resulting from seizures.
Spinal cord injury	Rehabilitation and aftercare to maximize function, **p. 298.**

GASTROINTESTINAL SYSTEM

System/Condition	General, Selected Home Health Care Goals
Cirrhosis	Ongoing assessment. Elimination of underlying causes, if possible. Prevention of further liver damage and complications, **p. 181.**

GASTROINTESTINAL SYSTEM (*Continued*)

System/Condition	General, Selected Home Health Care Goals
Hepatitis	Testing and treatment to prevent spread of disease in the community. *Teaching*: care in acute stage, **p. 179-180.** Prevention of permanent liver damage.
Ulcerative colitis/ Crohn's disease	*Teaching*: measures to prevent exacerbation, **p. 200.**

ENDOCRINE SYSTEM

System/Condition	General, Selected Home Health Care Goals
Diabetes mellitus	*Teaching*: medication regimen, monitoring glucose level, measures to control disease and prevent complications, **p. 168.**

HEMATOLOGIC SYSTEM

System/Condition	General, Selected Home Health Care Goals
AIDS	*Teaching*: prevention of transmission of infection, **p. 152.** Activities of daily living.
Anemias (iron deficiency and pernicious)	*Teaching*: compliance with medical regimen to control condition or prevent recurrence, **p. 60, 61.**

MUSCULOSKELETAL SYSTEM

System/Condition	General, Selected Home Health Care Goals
Amputation	*Teaching*: stump care, prosthesis care, compliance with rehabilitation regimen, **p. 274.**
Osteoarthritis/ rheumatoid arthritis	Care of involved joints. *Teaching*: medical regimen to prevent progression of the disease, **p. 160, 264.** Prevention of injury to the joints.
Fractured hip; knee or hip prosthesis/ replacement	Optimal mobility. *Teaching*: medical and rehabilitative regimen, **p. 271, 273, 274.**
Fractures/cast care	Ensuring immobilization. Prevention of complications of the fracture. *Teaching*: care for the body part, **p. 261-262.**
Laminectomy/spinal fusion (lumbar or cervical)	*Teaching*: postoperative care to promote healing and function, **p. 296.** Prevention of complications.
Osteomyelitis	Symptomatic treatment. Prevention of secondary infection. Prevention of transmission of infection to others.

MUSCULOSKELETAL SYSTEM (*Continued*)

System/Condition	General, Selected Home Health Care Goals
Osteoporosis	*Teaching*: medical regimen to prevent or control progression of bone mass loss and fractures, **p. 269**.

RENAL SYSTEM

System/Condition	General, Selected Home Health Care Goals
Kidney transplant	*Teaching*: immunosuppressive therapy, **p. 218-219**. Monitor for signs and symptoms of rejection.
Prostatic hyperplasia with prostatectomy	Maintenance of urinary output pre- and postoperatively. Wound care postoperatively. *Teaching*: medical regimen, **p. 222**. Prevention of complications.
Chronic renal failure	Providing for activities of daily living. Administration of peritoneal dialysis prn. *Teaching*: fluid and diet restrictions, compliance with hemodialysis, prevention of complications, **p. 215**.
Urinary tract infection	*Teaching*: medication regimen to prevent or control bladder infection and spread to kidneys, **p. 212, 264**.

INTEGUMENTARY SYSTEM

System/Condition	General, Selected Home Health Care Goals
Burns	Rehabilitation phase of burn care. *Teaching*: care of wounds, **p. 346**. Support of compliance with physical therapy regimen.
Decubitus ulcer	Care of existing ulcer. *Teaching*: prevention, **p. 270**

REPRODUCTIVE SYSTEM

System/Condition	General, Selected Home Health Care Goals
Mastectomy	Maintaining function of the operative side (exercise regimen), **p. 325**. Psychological consequences of loss of body part.
CHEMOTHERAPY AND RADIATION THERAPY	Monitoring physical and emotional effects. Assessment of side effects. Care for resulting needs (nausea, diarrhea, oral lesions, skin reaction, fatigue, bleeding tendency, weakness), **p. 316, 318-319**.

System/Condition	General, Selected Home Health Care Goals
POSTOPERATIVE CARE	Reinforcement of hospital discharge plan. Reduction of risk of infection. Wound care and dressing change. *Teaching*: use of incentive spirometer, **p. 132, 214, 266, 272**. Monitoring temperature. Administration of anti-infective therapy. Assessment of respiratory and urinary status.

Adapted from Jaffe, Marie S., *Home Health Nursing Care Plans*, **2nd edition**, St. Louis: Mosby.

NCLEX-RN® Test Plan: ⋈ Nursing Process Definitions and Descriptions/Cognitive Level Definitions and Descriptions

 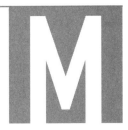

The phases of the nursing process include:

⋈ **I. DATA COLLECTION**

    A. Assessment: Establishing a database.

        1. *Gather objective and subjective information relative to the client.*

            a. Collect information from the client, significant others, and/or health care team members; current and prior health records; and other pertinent resources.

            b. Utilize assessment skills appropriate to client's condition.

            c. Recognize *symptoms* and significant findings.

            d. Determine client's ability to assume care of daily health needs (self-care).

            e. Determine health team member's ability to provide care.

            f. Assess *environment* of client.

            g. Identify own or staff reactions to client, significant others, and/or health care team members.

        2. *Confirm data:*

            a. *Verify* observation or perception by obtaining additional information.

            b. *Question* prescriptions and decisions by other health care team members when indicated.

            c. *Observe* condition of client directly when indicated.

            d. *Validate* that an appropriate client assessment has been made.

        3. *Communicate information gained in assessment:*

            a. Document assessment findings thoroughly and accurately.

            b. Report assessment findings to relevant members of the health care team.

⋈ **II. Analysis: Identifying actual or potential health care needs and/or problems based on assessment.**

    A. *Interpret data:*

        1. Validate data.

        2. Organize related data.

        3. Determine need for *additional* data.

        4. Determine client's unique needs and/or problems.

    B. *Formulate client's nursing diagnoses:*

        1. Determine significant relationship between data and client needs and/or problems.

        2. Utilize *standard taxonomy* for formulating nursing diagnoses.

    C. *Communicate results of analysis:*

        1. Document client's nursing diagnoses.

        2. Report results of analysis to relevant members of the health care team.

⋈ **III. Planning: Setting goals for meeting client's needs and designing strategies to achieve these goals.**

    A. *Prioritize nursing diagnoses:*

        1. Involve client, significant others, and/or health care team members when establishing nursing diagnoses.

        2. Establish *priorities* among nursing diagnoses.

        3. Anticipate needs and/or problems on the basis of established priorities.

    B. *Determine goals of care:*

        1. Involve client, significant others, and/or health care team members in setting goals.

        2. Establish *priorities among* goals.

        3. Anticipate needs and/or problems on the basis of established priorities.

    C. *Formulate outcome criteria for goals of care:*

        1. Involve client, significant others, and/or health care team members in formulating outcome criteria for goals of care.

        2. Establish *priorities* among outcome *criteria* **for goals of care.**

        3. Anticipate needs and/or problems on the basis of established priorities.

    D. *Develop plan of care and modify as necessary:*

        1. Involve the client, significant others, and/or health care team members in designing strategies.

        2. *Individualize* the plan of care based on such information as *age, gender, culture, ethnicity and religion.*

        3. Plan for client's *safety*, comfort, and maintenance of optimal functioning.

        4. Select nursing interventions for delivery of client's care.

        5. Select *appropriate teaching approaches.*

    E. *Collaborate with other health care team members when planning delivery of client's care:*

        1. Identify health or social resources available to the client and/or significant others.

        2. *Select appropriate health care team members*

Source: Adapted from: National Council of State Boards of Nursing, Inc., most current *NCLEX-RN® Test Plan*.

when planning assignments.

3. Coordinate care provided by health care team members.

F. *Communicate plan of care:*

1. Document plan of care thoroughly and accurately.

2. Report plan of care to relevant members of the health care team.

3. Review plan of care with client.

⋈ IV. **Implementation: Initiating and completing actions necessary to accomplish the defined goals.**

A. *Organize and manage client's care:*

1. Implement a plan of care.

2. Arrange for a client care conference.

B. *Counsel and teach client, significant others, and/or health care team members:*

1. Assist client, significant others, and/or health care team members to recognize and manage stress.

2. Facilitate client relationships with significant others and health care team members.

3. *Teach* correct principles, procedures, and techniques for maintenance and promotion of health.

4. Provide client with health status information.

5. Refer client, significant others, and/or health care team members to appropriate *resources.*

C. *Provide care to achieve established goals of care:*

1. *Use safe* and *appropriate techniques* when administering client care.

2. Use precautionary and *preventive* interventions in providing care to client.

3. *Prepare client for surgery, delivery,* or other *procedures.*

4. Institute *interventions* to compensate for adverse responses.

5. Initiate *life-saving interventions* for emergency situations.

6. Provide an *environment* conducive to attainment of goals of care.

7. Adjust care in accord with client's expressed or implied needs, problems, and/or preferences.

8. Stimulate and motivate client to achieve *self-care* and independence.

9. Encourage client to follow a treatment regimen.

10. Assist client to maintain optimal functioning.

D. *Supervise and coordinate the delivery of client's care provided by nursing personnel:*

1. *Delegate* nursing interventions to appropriate nursing personnel.

2. *Monitor* and follow up on delegated interventions.

3. Manage health care team members' *reactions* to factors influencing therapeutic relationships with clients.

E. *Communicate nursing interventions:*

1. Record actual client responses, nursing interventions, and other information relevant to implementation of care.

2. Provide complete, accurate reports on assigned client(s) to relevant members of the health care team.

⋈ V. **Evaluation: Determining the extent to which goals have been achieved and interventions have been successful.**

A. *Compare actual outcomes with expected outcomes of care:*

1. Evaluate responses (*expected and unexpected*) in order to determine the degree of success of nursing interventions.

2. Determine impact of therapeutic interventions on the client and significant others.

3. Determine need for modifying the plan of care.

4. Identify factors that may interfere with the client's ability to implement the plan of care.

B. *Evaluate the client's ability to implement selfcare:*

1. Verify that *tests* or *measurements* are *performed correctly* by the client and/or other caregivers.

2. Ascertain client's and/or others' *understanding* of information given.

C. *Evaluate health care team members' ability to implement client care:*

1. Determine *impact of teaching* on health care team members.

2. Identify factors that might alter health care team members' response to teaching.

D. *Communicate evaluation findings:*

1. Document client's response to therapy, care, and/or teaching.

2. Report client's response to therapy, care, and/or teaching to relevant members of the health care team.

3. Report and document others' responses to teaching.

4. Document other caregivers' responses to teaching.

Notes:
1. Throughout the outline in this book, the stages of the nursing process are referred to as: assessment, analysis/nursing diagnosis, nursing care plan/implementation, evaluation/outcome criteria.
2. The practice questions in this book are coded as to the phase of the nursing process being tested; the codes are found following the answer/rationale for each question. *Key to Nursing Process Codes:*

> AS Assessment
> AN Analysis } Data Collection
> PL Planning
> IMP Implementation
> EV Evaluation

For an **index to questions relating to each phase of the nursing process**, see **Appendix N.**

The phases of the **cognitive level** include:

A. **Recall/Knowledge**: Rote remembering of significant facts or terms; to define, to name and to list.
B. **Comprehension**: To understand; to restate; to reorganize; to translate; to find an illustration or example; to interpret by explanation or summary; to determine implications, consequences and effects.
C. **Application**: The use of abstractions in particular or concrete situations. They may be in the form of general ideas, rules, procedures, or general methods. The abstractions may also be technical principles, ideas, and theories that need to be remembered and applied, using a concept or principle in a new situation.
D. **Analysis**: The breakdown of the whole into constituent parts or elements so that a rank priority of ideas can emerge and relationships between ideas can be made clear.
E. **Synthesis**: Putting ideas together to form a new whole.
F. **Evaluation**: Judging material using specific criteria.

Key to cognitive level codes:

> RE/KN Recall/Knowledge
> COM   Comprehension
> APP   Application
> AN   Analysis
> SYN   Synthesis
> EV   Evaluation

For an **index to questions relating to each phase of the cognitive level**, see **Appendix N.**

Index: Questions Related to Nursing Process/Cognitive Level

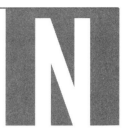

Use this index to locate *practice questions* throughout the book in each of the phases of the nursing process and cognitive level.

Please refer to the following pages for the complete table.

Nursing Process | Cognitive Level

Chapter	Assessment (AS) Question #:	Analysis (AN) Question #:	Planning (PL) Question #:	Implementation (IMP) Question #:	Evaluation (EV) Question #:	Recall/Know. (RE/KN) Question #:	Comprehension (COM) Question #:	Application (APP) Question #:	Analysis (ANL) Question #:	Evaluation (EVL) Question #:	Synthesis (SYN) Question #:
1—Nursing Assessment of the Adult	1, 2, 3, 4					1, 2, 4	3				
2—Peripheral Vascular Disorders	3, 13, 14, 15	1, 6	9	5, 7, 11, 12	2, 4, 8, 10		1, 11, 13, 15	3, 5, 7, 9, 12	2, 8	4, 6, 14	10
3—Cardiac Structure Disorders		2	4	3	1	3			4	1, 2	
4—Cardiac Function Disorders	2, 8, 9, 12			1, 4, 6, 7, 10	3, 5, 11, 13	1	7, 8, 12	4, 6, 9, 10	2	3, 5, 11, 13	
5—Hematologic Disorders	4	1	8, 10	2, 3, 5, 6, 7, 9		2, 3	4, 5, 6	7, 9	1, 8, 10		
6—Respiratory Disorders	1, 2, 7, 16, 18, 22, 23	10, 15, 21, 24, 27	6, 20, 25	3, 4, 5, 8, 9, 12, 14, 19, 26	11, 13, 17	4	2, 6, 9, 15, 16, 19, 20, 22, 24, 26	1, 3, 5, 8, 10, 12, 14, 27	17, 18, 21, 23, 25	7, 11, 13	
7—Fluid and Electrolyte Imbalances	5, 15, 21	3, 10, 12, 14, 22, 23, 25	24	2, 4, 6, 7, 8, 9, 16, 17, 18, 19, 20	1, 11, 13	24	20	7, 8, 9, 16, 17, 18, 19, 22	2, 4, 6, 10, 12, 14, 15, 21, 23, 25	1, 5, 11	3, 13
8—Shock	4	3, 5	1		2				1, 4, 5	2, 3	
9—Perioperative Nursing	3		6	1, 2, 5	4	6	3, 5	1, 2	4		
10—Pain	1, 2			3, 4			1, 2	4	3		
11—Altered Immune System Disorders				1, 2, 3, 4, 5			2, 3	1, 4, 5			
12—Connective Tissue Disorders		2		1, 4	3		3	1, 2, 4			
13—Biliary and Pancreatic Disorders	1	2, 4, 5	6, 11	3, 7, 9, 10, 12	8, 13	1, 2	3, 6, 7, 8, 9	10, 11, 12	4	5, 13	
14—Hepatic Disorders	1, 4, 5, 7	2, 3, 6, 9	8				2, 3, 5	1, 4, 6	7, 8	9	
15—Gastric Disorders	10, 12, 13		2, 5, 7	1, 3, 4, 6, 8, 9, 11			4, 9, 12, 13	2, 3, 7	1, 5, 6, 8, 10, 11		

(continued)

Nursing Process / Cognitive Level

Chapter	Assessment (AS)	Analysis (AN)	Planning (PL)	Implementation (IMP)	Evaluation (EV)	Recall/Know. (RE/KN)	Comprehension (COM)	Application (APP)	Analysis (ANL)	Evaluation (EVL)	Synthesis (SYN)
	Question #:	Question #:	Question #:	Question #:	Question #:	Question #:	Question #:	Question #:	Question #:	Question #:	Question #:
16—Intestinal Disorders	3, 13, 14	8	5, 7, 11	1, 2, 6, 9, 10, 12	4	13	1, 6, 10, 14	5, 7, 12	2, 3, 8, 9, 11	4	
17—Renal Disorders	1, 4, 17, 19	9, 14, 20	10	3, 6, 7, 8, 11, 12, 13, 15, 16	2, 5, 18	12, 14	1, 8, 11, 13, 19	6, 7, 10	2, 3, 4, 5, 9, 15, 16, 17, 18, 20		
18—Endocrine Disorders	2, 4		1, 3			2	4	1, 3			
19—Sensory Disorders	6, 8			2, 4, 5, 7, 9, 10, 11, 12	1, 3	2, 6, 7, 8, 10, 11	4	5	9, 12	1, 3	
20—Musculoskeletal Disorders	3, 6	4, 7	12	1, 2, 5, 8, 9, 10, 11, 13, 14		5, 11, 12, 13	7, 8, 14	1, 2, 6, 9, 10	3, 4		
21—Neurologic Disorders	1, 9	3, 6	5	2, 4, 7, 8		9	1, 3, 8	2, 4, 5	6, 7		
22—Disorders of the Spinal Cord	3	4		1, 2, 5	6		2	1, 3	4, 5	6	
23—Degenerative Neurologic Disorders	1	2, 3		4			1, 2	4	3		
24—Neoplastic Disorders	4, 9			1, 2, 3, 6, 7, 10	5, 8	10	2, 3	1, 4, 6, 7	9	5, 8	
25—Emergency Nursing		1, 2, 3		4				3	1, 2, 4		

Index: Definitions and Questions Related to Categories of Human Functions

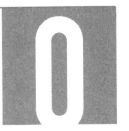

This index lists *practice questions* for you to use in reviewing *categories of human functions* (which are *detailed* examples of what subtopics are covered by the four *broad* client needs categories).

The eight categories of human functions include:

Protective Functions client's ability to maintain defenses and prevent physical and chemical trauma, injury, and threats to health status (e.g., communicable diseases, abuse, safety hazards, poisoning, skin disorders, and pre and postoperative complications).

Sensory-Perceptual Functions client's ability to perceive, interpret, and respond to sensory and cognitive stimuli (e.g., auditory, visual, verbal impairments, brain tumors, aphasia, sensory deprivation or overload, body image, reality orientation, learning disabilities).

Comfort, Rest, Activity, and Mobility Functions client's ability to maintain mobility, desirable level of activity, adequate sleep, rest, and comfort (e.g., pain, sleep disturbances, joint impairment).

Nutrition client's ability to maintain the intake and processing of essential nutrients (e.g., obesity, gastric and metabolic disorders that primarily affect the nutritional status).

Growth and Development client's ability to maintain maturational processes throughout the life span (e.g., child bearing, child rearing, maturational crisis, changes in aging, psychosocial development).

Fluid-Gas Transport Functions client's ability to maintain fluid-gas transport (e.g., fluid volume deficit/overload, acid-base balance, CPR, anemias, cardiopulmonary diseases).

Psychosocial-Cultural Functions client's ability to function (intrapersonal/interpersonal relationships; e.g., grieving, death/dying, psychotic behaviors, self-concept, therapeutic communication, ethical-legal aspects, community resources, situational crises, substance abuse).

Elimination Functions client's ability to maintain functions related to relieving the body of waste products (e.g., conditions of GI and/or GU systems).

Chapter	Protective Functions (1) Question #:	Sensory-Perceptual Functions (2) Question #:	Comfort, Rest, Activity, and Mobility Functions (3) Question #:	Nutrition (4) Question #:	Growth and Development (5) Question #:	Fluid-Gas Transport Functions (6) Question #:	Psychosocial-Cultural Functions (7) Question #:	Elimination Functions (8) Question #:
1—Nursing Assessment of the Adult					1,2,4	3		
2—Peripheral Vascular Disorders				9,12		1,2,3,4,5, 6,7,8,10, 11,13, 14,15,		
3—Cardiac Structure Disorders						1,2,3,4		
4—Cardiac Function Disorders		1		6,10		2,3,4,5,8, 9,11,12, 13	7	
5—Hematologic Disorders	5					1,2,4,6,8, 9,10	3,7	

Chapter	Protective Functions (1) Question #:	Sensory-Perceptual Functions (2) Question #:	Comfort, Rest, Activity, and Mobility Functions (3) Question #:	Nutrition (4) Question #:	Growth and Development (5) Question #:	Fluid-Gas Transport Functions (6) Question #:	Psychosocial-Cultural Functions (7) Question #:	Elimination Functions (8) Question #:
6—Respiratory Disorders	24		8	14		1,2,3,4,5, 6,7,9,10, 11,12,13, 15,16,17, 18,19,20, 21,22,23, 24,25,26, 27		
7—Fluid and Electrolyte Imbalances				1,2,14,15, 16,20,24		3,4,5,6,7, 8,9,10,11, 12,13,17, 18,19,21, 22, 23,25		
8—Shock						1,2,3,4,5		
9—Perioperative Nursing	1,2,3,4,6						5	
10—Pain			1,2,4			3		
11—Altered Immune System Disorders	1,2,4,5							3
12—Connective Tissue Disorders	3		1,2,4					
13—Biliary and Pancreatic Disorders	6			2,3,4,5,7, 8,9,10,11, 12,13				1
14—Hepatic Disorders		9		1,2,3,4		7,8		5,6
15—Gastric Disorders	3,6,8,9		1	2,4,5,7, 10,11,13		12		
16—Intestinal Disorders	11			1,6				2,3,4,5,7, 8,9,10,12, 13,14
17—Renal Disorders	20			10,11		19		1,2,3,4,5, 6,7,8,9, 12,13,14, 15,16,17, 18
18—Endocrine Disorders			2,4	1,3				
19—Sensory Disorders		1,2,3,4,5, 6,7,8,9, 10,11,12						
20—Musculoskeletal Disorders	8		1,2,4,5,7, 9,10,11, 12,13, 14			3,6		
21—Neurologic Disorders		2,3,4,5,6, 7,9		8		1		
22—Disorders of the Spinal Cord	4	3	1,2,5			6		

Chapter	Protective Functions (1) Question #:	Sensory-Perceptual Functions (2) Question #:	Comfort, Rest, Activity, and Mobility Functions (3) Question #:	Nutrition (4) Question #:	Growth and Development (5) Question #:	Fluid-Gas Transport Functions (6) Question #:	Psychosocial-Cultural Functions (7) Question #:	Elimination Functions (8) Question #:
23—Degenerative Neurologic Disorders			1,2,3			4		
24—Neoplastic Disorders	2,3,4,8,10		1,5			9	6,7	
25—Emergency Nursing	4					1,2		3

Index: Definitions and Questions Related to CLIENT NEEDS/ *Client Subneeds*

 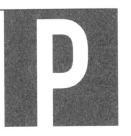

To *practice questions* in each of the 4 categories of **client needs** and *6 client subneeds* that are tested on NCLEX-RN®, refer to the questions listed on the following pages.

CLIENT NEEDS/*Client Subneeds:*

1. SAFE, EFFECTIVE CARE ENVIRONMENT
    Management of Care
    Safety and Infection Control

2. HEALTH PROMOTION AND MAINTENANCE—**has no** *client subneeds.*

3. PSYCHOSOCIAL INTEGRITY— **has no** *client subneeds.*

4. PHYSIOLOGICAL INTEGRITY
    Basic Care and Comfort
    Pharmacological and Parenteral Therapies
    Reduction of Risk Potential
    Physiological Adaptation

The four broad categories of **CLIENT NEEDS** include:

SAFE, EFFECTIVE CARE ENVIRONMENT—coordinated care, environmental safety, safe and effective treatment and procedures (e.g., client rights, confidentiality, principles of teaching/learning, control of infectious agents).

HEALTH PROMOTION AND MAINTENANCE—normal growth and development from birth to death, self-care and support systems, prevention and early treatment of disease (e.g., newborn care, normal perinatal care, family planning, human sexuality, parenting, end-of-life process, lifestyle choices, immunity).

PSYCHOSOCIAL INTEGRITY—psychosocial adaptation, coping (e.g., behavioral norms, chemical dependency, communication skills, family systems, mental health concepts, psychodynamics of behavior, psychopathology, treatment modalities).

PHYSIOLOGICAL INTEGRITY—physiological adaptation, reduction of risk potential, provision of basic care (e.g., drug administration, emergencies, nutritional therapies).

The six categories of *client subneeds* include:

1. *Management of Care*—staff development, collaboration, supervision of multidisciplinary health team; delegation; client rights; prioritization, ethical and legal responsibilities; referrals.

2. *Safety and Infection Control*—protecting clients, family/significant others and health care personnel from health and environmental hazards; e.g., disaster planning, home safety, medical and surgical asepsis, use of restraint/safety devices, safe use of equipment, standard precautions.

3. *Basic Care and Comfort*—performing routine nursing activities of daily living.

4. *Pharmacological and Parenteral Therapies*—expected and unexpected effects, chemotherapy; blood products; pain management; calculations; TPN, IV; central venous access devices.

5. *Reduction of Risk Potential*—monitoring, and reducing likelihood of complications related to existing conditions, treatments or procedures.

6. *Physiological Adaptation*—meeting acute, chronic or life-threatening physical health conditions

Chapter	CLIENT NEED: SAFE, EFFECTIVE CARE ENVIRONMENT (SECE)		CLIENT NEED: HEALTH PROMOTION/ MAINTENANCE (HPM)	CLIENT NEED: PSYCHOSOCIAL INTEGRITY (PsI)	CLIENT NEED: PHYSIOLOGICAL INTEGRITY (PhI)			
	Client Subneed: Management of Care Question #:	Client Subneed: Safety/Infection Control Question #:	Question #:	Question #:	Client Subneed: Basic Care/ Comfort Question #:	Client Subneed: Pharmacological/ Parenteral Therapies Question #:	Client Subneed: Reduction of Risk Potential Question #:	Client Subneed: Physiological Adaptation Question #:
1—Nursing Assessment of the Adult			1,2,4					3
2—Peripheral Vascular Disorders					9	3,5,7,8,11,12	4,6,10,15	1,2,13,14
3—Cardiac Structure Disorders			1			3		2,4
4—Cardiac Function Disorders			12	7		1,2,5,6,10,11,13	3,4,8	9
5—Hematologic Disorders				7		6,8,9	1,5	2,3,4,10
6—Respiratory Disorders	10	3,15	21,24,26		8,14	4,11,12,19,20,22,27	6,7,17,25	1,2,5,9,13, 16,18,23
7—Fluid and Electrolyte Imbalance	23				1,2,20	6,9,14,16,17,18, 19,24	7,8,21	3,4,5,10,11, 12,13,15,22,25
8—Shock				5	1	1,2	4	3,5
9—Perioperative Nursing			6				2,3,4	
10—Pain				2		1,4		3
11—Altered Immune System		1,3,4,5				2		
12—Connective Tissue Disorders					4	3	1	2
13—Biliary and Pancreatic Disorders					3,4,12	6,7,8,9,10,13	2	1,5,11
14—Hepatic Disorders					5	6	1,4	2,3,7,8,9
15—Gastric Disorders	6,9		2			3,5,7	1,4,11	8,10,12,13
16—Intestinal Disorders	7,8		12,13		1,6,14	5,10,11	2,4	3,9
17—Renal Disorders	9,18,20		8		10,11	7,13	2,3,5,6,15	1,4,12,14, 16,17,19

(continued)

Chapter	CLIENT NEED: SAFE, EFFECTIVE CARE ENVIRONMENT (SECE)		CLIENT NEED: HEALTH PROMOTION/ MAINTENANCE (HPM)	CLIENT NEED: PSYCHOSOCIAL INTEGRITY (PsI)	CLIENT NEED: PHYSIOLOGICAL INTEGRITY (PhI)			
	Client Subneed: Management of Care Question #:	Client Subneed: Safety/Infection Control Question #:	Question #:	Question #:	Client Subneed: Basic Care/ Comfort Question #:	Client Subneed: Pharmacological/ Parenteral Therapies Question #:	Client Subneed: Reduction of Risk Potential Question #:	Client Subneed: Physiological Adaptation Question #:
18—Endocrine Disorders					1,3		4	2
19—Sensory Disorders	7,9,10,11		1,8	5	4		2,12	3,6
20—Musculo-skeletal Disorders	1,4,11		5,14			8,13	2,3,7,9,10,12	6
21—Neurologic Disorders	5		4		8		2,7	1,3,6,9
22—Disorders of the Spinal Cord	2			4	1	5	3	6
23—Degenerative Neurologic Disorders	3					4	2	1
24—Neoplastic Disorders	3,7			6	1,2,8	4	5,9,10	
25—Emergency Nursing						4		1,2,3

Resources

 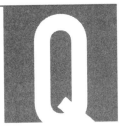

These are **selected sources of information and services.** (Every effort has been made to provide current names and addresses; however, addresses do change frequently.)

Health and Welfare Agencies/Associations

ACTION (programs for older adults)
806 Connecticut Ave. NW
Washington, DC 20525
202-254-7310

Administration on Aging
Department of Health and Human Services
200 Independence Ave. SW
Washington, DC 20201
202-245-0724
www.aoa.dhhs.gov

American Association of Kidney Patients
3505 E. Frontage Rd. Suite 315
Tampa, FL 33607-1756
800-749-2257
www.aakp.org

American Burn Association
Shriner's Burn Institute University of Cincinnati
202 Goodman St.
Cincinnati, OH 45219 513-751-3900
www.ameriburn.org

American Cancer Society
1599 Clifton Rd. NE
Atlanta, GA 30329
404-320-3333
www.cancer.org

American Diabetes Association
National Center
1660 Duke St.
Alexandria, VA 22314
800-232-3472
www.diabetes.org

American Foundation for the Blind
15 W. 16th St.
New York, NY 10016
212-620-2000
www.afb.org/

American Liver Foundation
1425 Pompton Ave.
Cedar Grove, NJ 07009
800-223-0179
www.liverfoundation.org

American Lung Association
1740 Broadway
New York, NY 10019
215-315-8700
www.lungusa.org

American Pain Society
PO Box 186
Skokie, IL 60076
312-475-7300
www.ampainsoc.org

American Parkinson's Disease Association, Inc.
116 John St.
New York, NY 10038
212-732-9550
www.apdaparkinson.org

American Speech-Language-Hearing Association
10801 Rockville Pike
Department AP
Rockville, MD 20852
301-897-5700
www.asha.org

American Spinal Injury Association
2020 Peachtree Rd. NW
Atlanta, GA 30309
www.asia-spinalinjury.org

Arthritis Foundation
1314 Spring St. NW Atlanta, GA 30309
404-872-7100
www.arthritis.org

Asthma and Allergy Foundation of America
1717 Massachusetts Ave. NW
No. 305
Washington, DC 20036
800-7ASTHMA
www.aafawa.org

Centers for Disease Control
Department of Health and Human Services U.S. Public Health Service
Atlanta, GA 30333
404-639-3534
www.cdc.gov

Concern for Dying
250 W. 57th St.
New York, NY 10107
215-246-6962
http://grief.netfirms.com/dying.html

Epilepsy Foundation of America
815 15th St. NW, Suite 528
Washington, DC 20005
202-638-5229
www.epilepsyfoundation.org

Guillain-Barre Foundation
129 North Carolina Ave. SE Washington, DC 20003
202-387-2216
www.guillain-barre.com

Leukemia Society of America
31 St. James Ave.
Boston, MA 02116
617-482-2256
www.mdleukemia.org

Muscular Dystrophy Association
3561 E. Sunrise Ave.
Tucson, AZ 85718
602-529-2000
www.mdausa.org

Myasthenia Gravis Foundation
61 Gramercy Park North
New York, NY 10010
212-533-7005
www.myasthenia.org

National Association to Control Epilepsy
22 E. 67th St.
New York, NY 10012
www.epilepsyfoundation.org/

National Cancer Institute
Office of Cancer Communications
Building 31, Room 10A24
National Institutes of Health
Bethesda, MD 20892
800-4-CANCER
www.cancer.gov

National Center for the American Heart Association
7320 Greenville Ave.
Dallas, TX 75231
214-373-6300
www.americanheart.org

National Foundation for Ileitis and Colitis
444 Park Ave. South
New York, NY 10016
212-685-3440

National Head Injury Foundation
333 Turnpike Rd.
Southborough, MA 01722
508-485-9950
www.biausa.org

National Hemophilia Foundation
110 Greene St., Suite 406
New York, NY 10012
212-219-8180
www.hemophilia.org

National Institute of Allergy and Infectious Diseases
Building 10, National Institutes of Health
Bethesda, MD 20892
301-496-4000
www.niaid.nih.gov

National Institute of Arthritis and Musculoskeletal and Skin Diseases
National Institutes of Health
Bethesda, MD 20892
301-496-4000
www.niams.nih.gov

National Jewish Center for Immunology and Respiratory Medicine
1400 Jackson St.
Denver, CO 80206
800-222-LUNG
www.njc.org

National Kidney Foundation
30 E. 33rd St.
New York, NY 10016
212-889-2210
www.kidney.org

National Multiple Sclerosis Society
205 E. 42nd St.
New York, NY 10017
212-532-3060
www.nmss.org

National Parkinson's Foundation
1501 NW 9th Ave.
Miami, FL 33136
305-547-6666
www.parkinson.org

National Psoriasis Foundation
6443 Southwest Beaverton Hwy., Suite 210
Portland, OR 97221
503-297-1545
www.psoriasis.org

National Safety Council
444 N. Michigan Ave.
Chicago, IL 60611
800-621-7619
www.nsc.org

National Society to Prevent Blindness
500 E. Remington Rd.
Schaumburg, IL 60173
312-843-2020
www.eyeinfo.org/national

National Spinal Cord Injury Association
600 W. Cumming Park, #3200
Woburn, MA 01801
800-962-9629
www.spinalcord.org

Office for Handicapped Individuals
Department of Education
Room 3106, Switzer Building
400 Maryland Ave. SW
Washington, DC 20202
202-245-0080

Osteoporosis Foundation
612 N. Michigan Ave., Suite 510
Chicago, IL 60611
www.nof.org/

Paget's Disease Foundation
PO Box 2772
Brooklyn, NY 11202
718-596-1043
www.paget.org

Phoenix Society (assistance following burn injuries)
11 Rust Hill Rd. Levittown, PA 19056
215-946-BURN 800-888-BURN
www.phoenix-society.org

Self Help for Hard of Hearing People (Shhh)
4848 Battery Ln.
Department E
Bethesda, MD 20814
301-657-2248
www.shhh.org

United Network for Organ Sharing
3001 1100 Boulders Parkway Suite 500
Richmond, VA 23225
(804) 330-8500
www.unos.org
crowmg@unos.org

AIDS Information and Hotlines

American Foundation for AIDS Research	212-682-7440
American Red Cross AIDS Education Office	202-737-8300
Centers for Disease Control—Statistics:	
AIDS cases and deaths	404-330-3020
Distribution-categories	404-330-3021
Demographics	404-330-3022
Hearing Impaired AIDS Hotline	800-243-7889
National AIDS Hotline	800-342-AIDS
National AIDS Information Clearing House	800-458-5231
National AIDS Network	202-293-2437
National Gay/Lesbian Crisis Line	800-767-4297
Project Inform (Drug Information)	800-822-7422
Spanish AIDS Hotline	800-344-7432

Professional Organizations/Associations
American

Academy of Ambulatory Nursing Administration
N. Woodbury Rd., Box 56
Pitman, NJ 08071
www.aaacn.org

American Academy of Nurse Practitioners
45 Foster St., Suite A
Lowell, MA 01851
www.aanp.org

The American Assembly for Men in Nursing
P.O Box 31753
Independence, OH 44131
www.aamn.org

American Association of Critical-Care Nurses
101 Columbia
Aliso Viejo, CA 92656
949-362-2000
www.aacn.org

American Association of Nurse Anesthetists
216 Higgins Rd.
Park Ridge, IL 60068
www.aana.com

American Association of Occupational Health Nurses, Inc.
50 Lenox Pointe
Atlanta, GA 30324
www.aaohn.org

American Association of Office Nurses
109 Kinderhook Rd.
Montvale, NJ 07645
www.aaon.org

American Association of Spinal Cord Injury Nurses
75-20 Astoria Blvd.
Jackson Heights, NY 11370-1178

American Holistic Nurses' Association
4101 Lake Boon Tr., Suite 201
Raleigh, NC 27607
www.ahna.org

American Nephrology Nurses' Association
N. Woodbury Rd., Box 56
Pitman, NJ 08071
888.600.2662
www.annanurse.org

American Radiological Nurses Association
7794 Grow Drive
Pensacola, FL 32514
850-474-7292
www.arna.net

American Society of Ophthalmic Registered Nurses, Inc.
PO Box 193030
San Francisco, CA 94119
http://webeye.ophth.uiowa.edu/asorn/

American Society of Plastic Surgical Nurses
3220 Pointe Parkway Suite 500
Atlanta, GA 30092
678-966-3065
www.aspsn.org

American Society of Post Anesthesia Nurses
11512 Allecingie Pkwy.
Richmond, VA 23235
www.aspan.org

Association of Nurses in AIDS Care
3538 Ridgewood Road
Akron, Ohio 44333
800.260.6780
www.anacnet.org/

Association of Operating Room Nurses (AORN)
2170 S Parker Road. Suite 300
Denver, CO 80231
800-755-2676
www.aorn.org

Association of Rehabilitation Nurses
5700 Old Orchard Rd., 1st floor
Skokie, IL 60077
www.rehabnurse.org/

Dermatology Nurses Association
N. Woodbury Rd., Box 56
Pitman, NJ 08071
www.dnanurse.org

Emergency Nurses Association
230 E. Ohio, 6th floor
Chicago, IL 60611
www.ena.org/

Hospice and Palliative Nurses Association
One Penn Center West, Suite 229
Pittsburg, PA 15276
412-787-9301
www.hpna.org

International Association for Enterostomal Therapy Inc.
2081 Business Center Dr., Suite 290
Irvine, CA 92715

Intravenous Nurses Society, Inc.
Two Brighton St.
Belmont, MA 02178
www.ins1.org

National Association of Hispanic Nurses
6905 Alamo Downs Pkwy.
San Antonio, TX 78238
www.thehispanicnurses.org

National Association of Home Care (NAHC)
519 C St. NE
Washington, DC 20002
www.nahc.org

National Association of Orthopaedic Nurses, Inc.
N. Woodbury Rd., Box 56
Pitman, NJ 08071
www.orthonurse.org

National Black Nurses Association, Inc.
1012 Tenth St. NW
Washington, DC 20001
www.nbna.org

National Gerontological Nursing Association
3100 Homewood Pkwy.
Kensington, MD 20895
www.ngna.org

North American Nursing Diagnosis Association
3525 Caroline St.
St. Louis, MO 63104
www.nanda.org

Nurses Environmental Health Watch
33 Columbus Ave.
Somerville, MA 02143

Oncology Nursing Society
1016 Greentree Rd.
Pittsburgh, PA 15220-3125
www.ons.org

Society of Gastroenterology Nurses and Associates, Inc.
1070 Sibley Tower
Rochester, NY 14604
www.sgna.org

Society of Otorhinolaryngology and Head/Neck Nurses
439 N. Causeway
New Smyrna Beach, FL 32169
www.sohnnurse.com

Society for Vascular Nursing
7794 Grow Drive
Pensacola, FL 32514
888/536-4786
www.svnnet.org

Society of Respiratory Nursing
5700 Old Orchard Rd., 1st floor
Skokie, IL 60077
www.respiratorynursingsociety.org

Texas Society of Infection Control Practitioners
P.O. Box 341357
Austin, TX 78734
www.tsicp.org

Transcultural Nursing Society
Department of Nursing
Madonna College
36600 Schoolcroft Rd.
Livonia, MI 48150
www.tcns.org

World Federation of Neuroscience Nurses
6214 Craigmont Rd.
Baltimore, MD 21228
www.wfnn.nu

Patient Education Materials

Abbott Laboratories
Professional Services—D383
Abbott Park
N. Chicago, IL 60064
www.abbott.com/

American Cancer Society
1599 Clifton Rd. NE
Atlanta, GA 30329
www.cancer.org

American Diabetes Association
National Center
1660 Duke St.
Alexandria, VA 22314
www.diabetes.org

American Liver Foundation
1425 Pompton Ave.
Cedar Grove, NJ 07009
www.liverfoundation.org

American Lung Association
1740 Broadway
New York, NY 10019
www.lungusa.org

Arthritis Foundation
1314 Spring St. NW
Atlanta, GA 30309
www.arthritis.org

Eli Lilly and Company
Educational Resources Program
PO Box 100B
Indianapolis, IN 46206
www.lilly.com

National Head Injury Foundation
333 Turnpike Rd.
Southborough, MA 01772
www.biausa.org

National Kidney Foundation
30 E. 33rd St., Suite 1100
New York, NY 10016
www.kidney.org

National Multiple Sclerosis Society
205 E. 42nd St.
New York, NY 10017
www.nmss.org

National Safety Council
444 N. Michigan Ave.
Chicago, IL 60611
www.nsc.org

Nutrition Education Association
PO Box 20301
Houston, TX 77225

Phoenix Society (assistance following burn injuries)
11 Rust Hill Rd.
Levittown, PA 19056
www.phoenix-society.org

Ross Laboratories
Creative Services and Information Department
625 Cleveland Ave.
Columbus, OH 43216
www.rosslearningcenter.com

Schering Corporation Professional Film Library
Galloping Hill Rd.
Kenilworth, NJ 07033
www.schering-plough.com

Skin Cancer Foundation
245 Fifth Ave., Suite 2402
New York, NY 10016
www.skincancer.org

United Ostomy Association
36 Executive Park, Suite 120
Irvine, CA 92714
www.uoa.org
Note: UOA ceased operation in September 2005, but
educational materials are still available on the website.

Alternative and Complementary Therapies

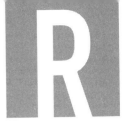

TABLE R.1 SUMMARY OF COMPLEMENTARY AND ALTERNATIVE MEDICINE THERAPIES

ALTERNATIVE MEDICAL SYSTEMS

	Focus/Purpose	Strategies
Art therapy	Goal: promote recovery or healing from past distress or trauma.	Facilitates expression of emotions, memories, and conscious and unconscious concerns through variety of artistic mediums.
Ayurveda	Developed in India. One of world's oldest medical systems Focuses on balance of mind, body, and spirit.	• Diet • Medicial herbs • Detoxification • Breathing exercises • Meditation • Yoga
Environmental medicine	Diagnosis, treatment, and prevention of environmentally triggered illnesses. Emphasis on preventing harmful effects of environmental toxins, chemicals, air and water pollution, radiation, and communicable diseases.	Client teaching: • Customized diets • Detoxification • Immunotherapy • Counseling • Environmental protocols to reduce exposure to toxins
Homeopathy	Developed in 1700s. 2 main principles: "like cures like" and "healing occurs from the inside out". Has been shown to be *effective* for: asthma, rheumatoid arthritis, migraines, diarrhea, fibromyalgia, allergic rhinitis.	Uses very small doses of specially prepared plant and mineral extracts intended to assist body's innate healing processes.
Meditation	Self-directed practice for focusing, centering, and relaxing. Used for stress management and health promotion. Shown to be effective for: ↓ heart rate, respiratory rate, BP; ↓ muscle tension and chronic pain; ↑ immune response; ↑ memory, Enhance a peaceful state of mind.	
Music therapy	Listening to music for therapeutic purposes, e.g. reducing stress or pain	Client preferences about type of music influences the effectiveness of the intervention
Naturopathy	Developed in USA. Emphasizes restoration and maintenance of overall health rather than symptom management. Focuses on enhancing body's natural healing responses. Shown to be *effective* for: ear infections, female reproductive problems, infectious diseases, respiratory conditions.	• Clinical nutrition • Herbology • Hydrotherapy • Homeopathy • Acupuncture • Physical therapies • Counseling and psychotherapy

TABLE R.1   SUMMARY OF COMPLEMENTARY AND ALTERNATIVE MEDICINE THERAPIES (*Continued*)

Prayer and mental healing	Uses a variety of intercessory approaches; often used at distance from the client.	Incorporates compassion, caring, love, or empathy
Qigong	Similar to Tai Chi. Ancient system of exercise that focuses on: breathing, visualization, and movement. Creates balance and enhances self-regulation of the body.	Focuses on developing skills in appreciation and manipulation of internal flow of energy. Many systems exist, from simple calisthenics to complex autoregulatory systems.
Traditional Chinese medicine (TCM)	One of the world's oldest medical systems. Focuses on restoring and maintaining the balanced flow of vital energy (Qi—pronounced "chee").	• Acupressure • Acupuncture • Chinese herbology • Diet • Meditation • Tai chi • Qigong.

BIOLOGIC-BASED THERAPIES

Aromatherapy	Uses plant extracts (essential oils) to promote and maintain overall health.	Essential oils can be applied topically or inhaled; should *not* be taken internally.
Herbal therapies	Have been used extensively in many Eastern cultures:	Includes: • Ginkgo biloba • Echinacea • Milk thistle
	Chinese herbal remedies: most remedies are derived from over 50,000 medicinal plant species; few animal or mineral sources. Ayurvedic herbs; used extensively for 2000 years	• Phytoestrogens • Saw palmetto • Panax ginseng • Fresh ginger • Chinese foxglove root. • Eclipta alba • Commiphora mukul • Picrorrhiza kurroa.
Macrobiotic diet	Part of an overall approach focused on harmonious and healthy interactions between client and diet, lifestyle, and environment.	Diet high in: whole grain cereals, vegetables, beans and sea vegetables, and vegetarian soups Fish and seafood used occasionally *No* meat, animal fat, eggs, poultry, dairy, simple sugars, or artificial foods.
Orthomolecular diet	Based on theory that each client has unique needs for various nutrients. Focus on achieving nutritional balance.	May use vitamins, essential amino acids, essential fats, minerals often in excess of recommended amounts.

MANIPULATIVE AND BODY-BASED METHODS

Acupressure	Improves energy flow. Relieves pain. Stimulates body's innate healing abilities.	Pressure point technique; applied finger and hand pressure on specific areas of body (acupoints). Other techniques include: *shiatsu, reflexology, myotherapy, jin shin do.*
Alexander technique	Movement re-education therapy; develop awareness of unhealthy movement patterns. Emphasis on alignment of head, neck, and spine. Goal: achieve balanced, graceful, coordinated, and relaxed style of moving.	Other techniques include: • *Educational kinesiology* • *Feldenkrais method* • *Trager approach.*

(continued)

TABLE R.1   SUMMARY OF COMPLEMENTARY AND ALTERNATIVE MEDICINE THERAPIES (*Continued*)

Chiropractic therapy	Intended to restore and maintain health by properly aligning spine, using adjustment and manipulation techniques.	Correct spinal alignment facilitates self-healing and reduces interference from the nervous system.
Rolfing	Structural bodywork based on assumption that fascia has become thickened or tight. Goal: improve freedom of movement and alignment of the head, neck, shoulders, thorax, pelvis, and legs.	Therapist manipulates and realigns fascia through systematic process of deep tissue work.
Therapeutic massage	Soft tissue manipulation. Reduces pain and stress; promotes relaxation.	Involves use of stroking, kneading, and friction techniques.

ENERGY THERAPIES

Magnetic therapy	Goal: improve blood flow and reduce pain.	External application of magnets and magnetic energy in a variety of configurations.
Therapeutic touch	Biofield therapy Goal: improved sense of well-being and decreased sense of stress and discomfort.	Involves use of hands to direct or modulate human energy fields. Other types include: *healing touch, quantum touch, Reiki, pranic healing.*

Source: adapted form the National Center for Complementary and Alternative Medicine (NCCAM). See website for more information: www.nccam.nih.gov

BIBLIOGRAPHY

Corbett, J. (2004). *Laboratory tests and diagnostic procedures with nursing diagnoses* (6th ed.). Appleton & Lange: Stamford, CT.
The book covers common laboratory tests and diagnostic procedures, and provides reference values across the lifespan. The nursing process is used as a framework.

Elkin, M., Perry, A., & Potter, P. (2004). *Nursing interventions and clinical skills* (3rd ed., pp. 294-346). St. Louis, MO: Mosby.
Text includes a summary of essential steps of skills, nursing process framework, two-column format with 1,000 color illustrations, communication tips, recording and reporting guidelines.

Gray-Vickery, P. (1999). Taking charge in a geriatric emergency. *Nursing 99*. January 1999. (*classic article*)

Jarvis, C. (2004). *Physical examination and health assessment* (4th ed.). Philadelphia: W.B. Saunders.
Provides the foundation for holistic health assessment across the life span. The physical examination unit is organized by body system, that includes structure and function, subjective and objective data collection, and expected findings as well as variations of normal, and selected abnormal findings. The text also includes sample documentation, clinical case studies, and nursing diagnoses.

Lewis, S.M., Heitkemper, M.M.., & Dirksen, S. R. (2004). *Medical-surgical nursing: Assessment and management of clinical problems* (6th ed.). St. Louis, MO: Mosby.
The book covers nursing assessment and nursing management of medical-surgical problems, grouped by body systems.

Potter, P.A. & Perry; A.G. (2005). *Fundamentals of nursing* (6th ed.). St. Louis, MO: Mosby.
This text uses a nursing process framework with an emphasis on critical thinking, and care in multiple settings. This new edition addresses evidence-based practice, safety concerns, and end-of-life care. Care plans clearly explain assessment findings leading to nursing diagnoses, as well as evaluation of outcomes.

Skidmore-Roth, L. (2004). *Mosby's nursing drug reference*. St. Louis, MO: Mosby.
Covers approximately 1300 generic drugs, 4500 trade-name drugs, and 75 herbal products. The book organizes drugs alphabetically according to generic names, and contains basic information on: uses, dosages, side effects, syringe compatibilities, interactions, precautions, and contraindications, and herbal interactions, as well as client teaching guidelines for treatment.

INDEX

This is an abbreviated general index because this book already includes a unique set of indexes by special topics. Please also look at all the special indexes by separate topics listed under: *Index to: Diets*, p. 385; *Pharmacology*, p. 387-420; *Index to: Mnemonics*, p. 433; *Common Clinical Signs*, p. 421; *Index to: Diagnostic Tests and Procedures*, p. 423-426; *Laboratory Values*, p. 427-432; *Index to: Common Tubes*, p. 435, *Hands–on Care*, p. 437-438, *Positioning*, p. 439-441, and *Home Healthcare/Health Teaching*, p. 443-445.

A

Abdominal injuries, 358
Acid-ash diet, 220, 221, 271
Acid-base imbalances, 101-106, 107, 108-109
Acidosis, 101
    Metabolic, 106, 108 , 111, 115
    Respiratory, 106, 108, 115
Acquired immune deficiency syndrome (AIDS), 151-152, 156
Acronyms and abbreviations, 371
Acute glomerulonephritis, 212-214
Acute lymphocytic leukemia (ALL), 62
Acute myelogenous leukemia (AML), 62
Acute nonlymphocytic leukemia (ANLL), 62
Acute renal failure, 214-215
Acute respiratory distress syndrome (ARDS), 78-79
Addison's disease, 235-236, 237, 238
Adrenal disorders, 233-237
Adrenalectomy, 234-235
Adult respiratory distress syndrome (ARDS), 78-79
    Medications for, 93
AGN (acute glomerulonephritis), 212-214
AIDS (Acquired immune deficiency syndrome), 151-156
Air embolus
    From intravenous therapy, 112
    From total parenteral nutrition, 115
Alkalosis, 101
    Metabolic, 106, 109, 111, 115
    Respiratory, 106, 109, 115
ALL (acute lymphocytic leukemia), 62
ALS; Lou Gehrig's disease (Amyotrophic lateral sclerosis), 308-309
Altered immune system disorders, 151-152, 156
Alternative therapies, App R
Amputation, 273-274, 276
Amyotrophic lateral sclerosis (ALS; Lou Gehrig's Disease), 308-309
Anaphylactic shock, 121
Anemia
    Hemolytic, 60
    Hyperchromic macrocytic, 61

Hypochromic microcytic, 59
Iron deficiency, 59-60
Medications for, 66
Normocytic normochromic, 60
Pernicious, 61
Medications for,66
Anesthesia, 129-130
Aneurysms, 17-18
    Aortic, 348
    Dissecting, 45
    Medications for, 23
Angina pectoris, 45, 46, 50, 51, 52
Angiocardiography, 51
Angiography, 51
    Celiac, 182
    Cerebral, 290
    Pulmonary, 91
    Renal, 224
Angioplasty, percutaneous transluminal coronary, 30, 33
Anthrax, 366
Antrectomy, 192
Aortic insufficiency, 27, 29
Aortic stenosis, 27, 29, 30
Aphasia, 281-282
Appendicitis, 197-198, 206
ARDS (Acute respiratory distress syndrome), 78-79
Arrhythmias, cardiac, 38
    Comparison of, 39-44
    Medications for, 52
    Normal rhythms *vs.*, 37
Arteriosclerosis, 16
Arteriosclerosis obliterans, 16-17, 22, 23
Arterial ulcers, 19
Arteriography, 51
Arteriosclerosis, 16
Arteriovenous fistula, 216, 217, 218
Arteriovenous shunt, 216, 217, 218
Arthritis, 275
    Osteo-, 271
    Rheumatoid, 159-160, 162
Arthroscopy, 275
Artificial skin, 347
Aspiration pneumonia, 69
Assessment, Analysis, and Nursing Diagnosis of the Adult, 1-8
    Cultural and ethnic variations in, 4
    Nursing history, 1

Objective data, 1-8
Of older adult, 4-6
Routine laboratory studies in, 6-7
Subjective data, 1
Asthma, 76-77, 79, 90, 93
Atelectasis, 71, 90, 92
Atrial fibrillation, 41
Atrial tachycardia, 40
Atrioventricular (AV) blocks, 43, 44
Autonomic dysreflexia, 299-300
Autonomic hyperreflexia, 299-300
Avascular necrosis, from fracture, 257
AV (atrioventricular) blocks, 43, 44

B

Bacterial meningitis, 288-289
Bennett ventilator, 89
Biliary and pancreatic disorders, 165-173
Biopsy
    Breast, 323
    Cervical, 326
    Liver, 182
    Renal, 224
    Small bowel, 205
Bioterrorism
    Agents of, 366-368
Bird ventilator, 89
Bladder cancer, 328
Blindness, 247-248
Blood and body fluid precautions, 153-155
Blood gas variations with acid-base imbalance, 106
    Causes of, 107
Blood products, for transfusion, 58-59
Body mass index, 4
Botulism, 367
Bowel sounds, 205
Bradycardia, sinus, 39
Brain attack (Stroke), 287-288
Brain injury, 282-283
    Medications for, 291
Brain scan, 290
Breast biopsy, 323
Breast cancer, 323-325
Breast self-examination (BSE), 324
Bricker's procedure, 220
Bronchitis, 77-78